# MATERIALS FOR BUILDING
## VOLUME 2

# MATERIALS FOR BUILDING
## VOLUME 2

Water and its Effects—1

**LYALL ADDLESON,** B.Arch., A.R.I.B.A., Dip.T.P., A.M.T.P.I.

Head of Design Section
Faculty of Environmental Science and Technology
Polytechnic of the South Bank, London

**London**
**Iliffe Books**

THE BUTTERWORTH GROUP

England
Butterworth & Co (Publishers) Ltd
London: 88 Kingsway, WC2B 6AB

Australia
Butterworth & Co (Australia) Ltd
Sydney: 586 Pacific Highway Chatswood, NSW 2067
Melbourne: 343 Little Collins Street, 3000
Brisbane: 240 Queen Street, 4000

Canada
Butterworth & Co (Canada) Ltd
Toronto: 14 Curity Avenue, 374

New Zealand
Butterworth & Co (New Zealand) Ltd
Wellington: 26–28 Waring Taylor Street, 1
Auckland: 35 High Street, 1

South Africa
Butterworth & Co (South Africa) (Pty) Ltd
Durban: 152–154 Gale Street

First published in 1972 by
Iliffe Books, an imprint of
the Butterworth Group



ISBN 0 592 00236 5

Printed in England by Chapel River Press

# contents

# preface

*Materials for Building* uses a considerable amount of the material that originally appeared in the series of articles of the same name in *The Architect and Building News* between 1964-68. The decision to publish the articles in book form provided an opportunity to correct mistakes, add or delete, and as important, to bring everything up-to-date, including complete metrication. In the light of present practice, some may find the metric values 'too accurate'. Generally speaking the metric equivalents of imperial values rather than sensible metric values are given. In many cases experimental or test results have had to be converted, and here too much rounding off or over-simplification would have been inappropriate.

Materials used in buildings have to meet a number of different functional requirements while they are exposed continuously to a wide variety of destructive agencies. Factors associated with both of these include strength, water, heat, fire, sound and production. In building practice materials have to be selected to meet specific functional requirements and to ensure that harmful deterioration is delayed for as long as is practicable.

In order to obtain the best out of the materials available it is necessary to have an understanding not only of the properties of the materials themselves but also of the factors which influence their performance and durability. This series of books aims to provide a systematic coverage, on a comparative basis, of the relationship between materials for building as a whole and the factors against which materials are expected to perform. Consequently each of the factors in terms of its nature and characteristics are explained separately and then related to a specific range of materials. The properties of all materials relative to each factor are also included.

In this study an attempt has been made to gather together a considerable amount of diversified information from a number of sources and to relate it in a particular way. It is to be hoped that the form of presentation used particularly the graphics and the extensive use of photographic examples will facilitate an understanding of the problems involved and of their possible solution. Perhaps even stimulate further study.

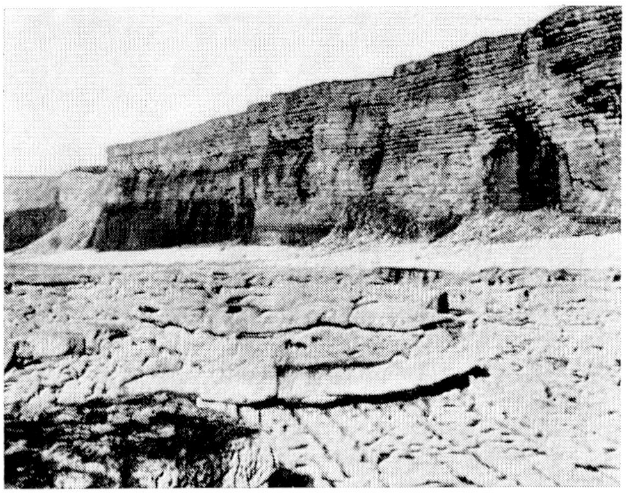

*Undercutting of rocks caused by high water waves (Courtesy: Lake, P. 'Physical Geography', Camb. Univ. Press)*

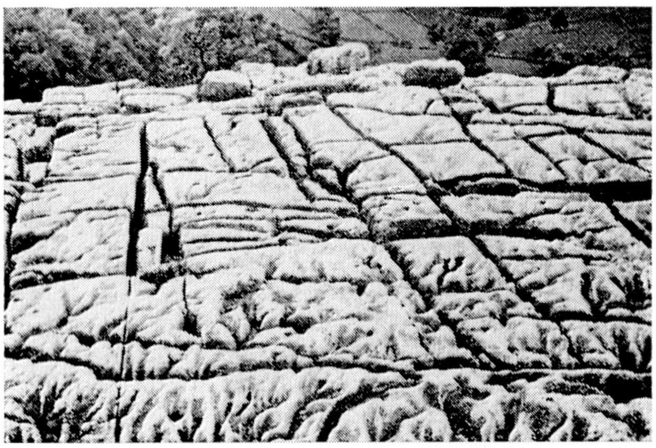

*Limestone weathering and joint formation (Courtesy: Controller of HMSO)*

*In the natural environment the results of the effects of water are usually equated with the 'balance of nature' but in the built environment they are considered to be deleterious. The natural environment provides good examples of the effects of extreme conditions of exposure. Although the materials are different the processes resulting in decay are much the same for both environments. The lesson to be learned is that in time all materials will decay; in the built environment careful selection, proper detailing and execution coupled with proper care can retard the rate of decay*

*The following photographs show some examples of the decay of various building materials*

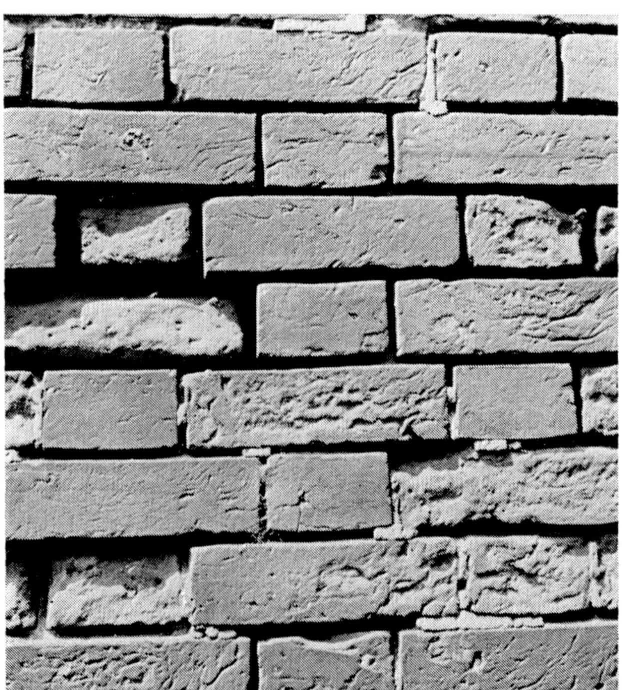

*Erosion of less resistant bricks*

might be obtained of the significance of water insofar as its effects on the use and selection of materials are concerned. This part concentrates on the deleterious effects of water.

At this point it is worthwhile noting that, within the whole context of building, the deleterious effects of water cannot necessarily be confined to what is commonly known as the durability of materials and which is directly related to maintenance. Of equal importance within buildings are the adverse effects which dampness may have on health. Whereas in the past dampness was primarily associated with the manner in which it could influence or aggravate disease or infirmity, nowadays it is not unreasonable, within the wider meaning of the word 'health'* and the demands of higher standards of comfort, to associate dampness with environmental comfort. The reduction in thermal efficiency of many materials (particularly those classified as porous) which does occur as a result of increases in moisture content is, therefore, as important a consideration as keeping out the 'elements' which, among other things, is traditionally associated with the exclusion of rain. As it is the materials which make up the entire fabric of buildings that provide the medium, so to speak, through which water may be transferred or in which it may be held, it follows that the problems associated with dampness are closely inter-related so far as durability of materials and health of occupants are concerned and should, therefore, be envisaged as part of the overall problem.

It is usually convenient to consider water in the widest meaning of the term. When so doing cognisance has to be taken of the fact that this substance seldom 'performs' in its pure chemical form, in any one particular physical state or, for that matter, in isolation. For movement and change of state water depends on other sources such as the atmosphere or solar radiation for the energy necessarily required, while for chemical efficiency it is perhaps better regarded as the vehicle for destructive agencies such as acids, alkalis and salts. In a similar context it also serves as a carrier of solid matter such as rock, grit, dust and constituents of smoke and, when associated with wind, may become an abrasive. It is in the *wider meaning* of the term that water is considered in this part.

If the significance of and the possible methods of dealing with the effects of water on buildings, and particularly the materials of which they are composed, are to be fully understood, it would appear reasonable that all related factors must be considered. Thus in this part some consideration will also be given to those factors which influence the behaviour and

*The definition of health used by the World Health Organisation and which is pertinent to this consideration states, 'Health is a state of complete physical, mental and social well-being, and not merely an absence of disease and infirmity'.

quality of water. (This includes sources of water.) In this way it is then possible to include elementary considerations of meteorology, climatology, hydrology, geology, atmospheric pollution, etc. In addition to being directly related to the 'performance' of water, it is more convenient to include these important aspects here rather than in any other part. However, it should be noted that these factors are only to be considered in sufficient detail to indicate their relevance to the overall problem. (References for further detailed study will be given as necessary.) Furthermore, factors related to condensation will be included in detail in *4.00 Heat and its effects* and, therefore, are only referred to in outline in this part. (It is perhaps axiomatic that the effects of water resulting from this source will be implied in the general considerations of this part.)

In order to deal with all those factors which influence the behaviour and quality of water and the resulting effects on materials, it has been considered convenient to sub-divide the subject matter into the general headings outlined below. It should be noted that, in order to try and make each subject as self-contained as possible, some repetition and/or cross-referencing is inevitable. From this it might be obvious that problems associated with water cannot necessarily, in practice, be clearly thought of in separate compartments, but require to be considered as a whole.

**1. General considerations**

The considerations included here are intended to serve as the nucleus for the whole problem of water and buildings. Accordingly, the basic properties, sources and cycle of water as generally encountered in the natural environment are considered first and then related to the built environment, in which such factors as flow of water, dampness, durability and maintenance are included. Attention is also drawn to the increasing need for and use of quantitative methods of assessing the severity of conditions which are now slowly becoming available.

**2. Exposure**

Exposure of any element in a building is a basic consideration in the assessment of the severity of the conditions under which materials may have to operate. Such exposure is related, firstly, to the various sources of water in and about buildings (including the quantities likely to be involved) and, secondly, the degree of pollution of the water (including the sources of such pollution). Both these interrelated factors are considered.

**3. Moisture content**

Under this general heading the causes and effects of changes in moisture content in those materials in which such changes may take place, that is those generally classified as porous, are con-

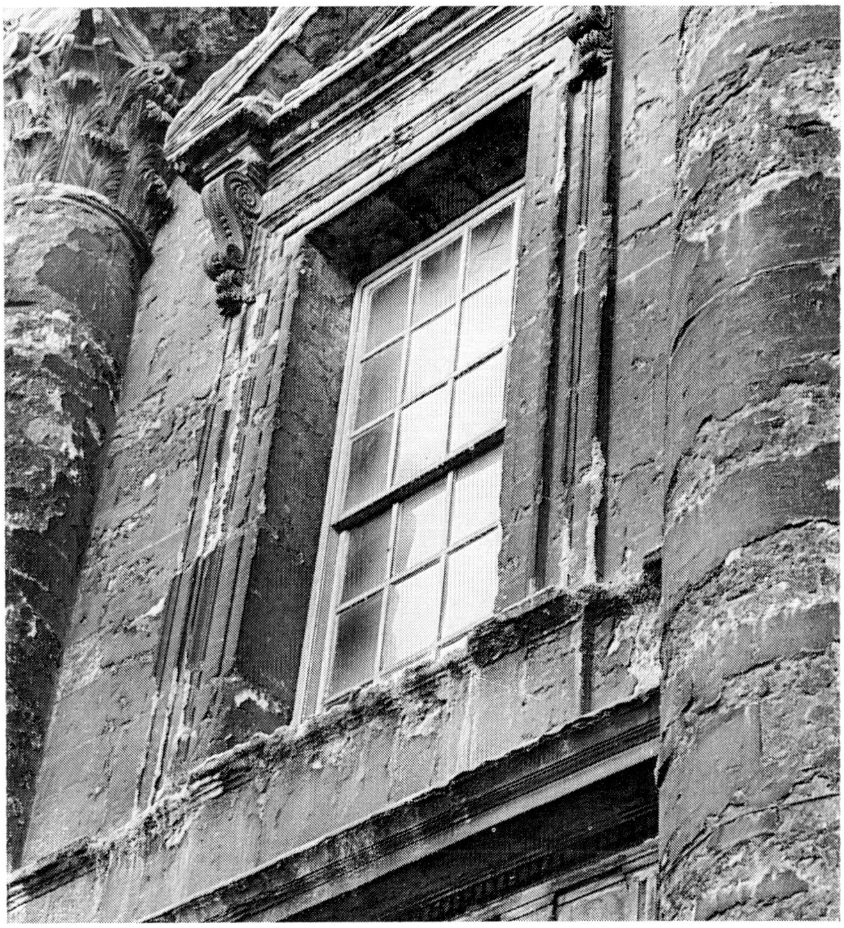

*Decay of stonework at the well-publicised Oxford examples*

*Timber rot*

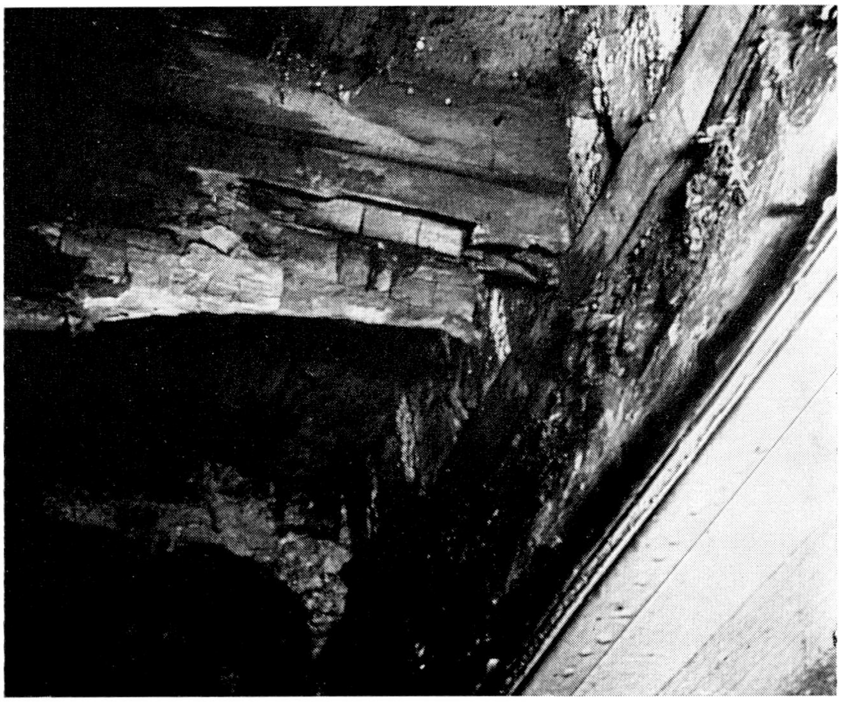

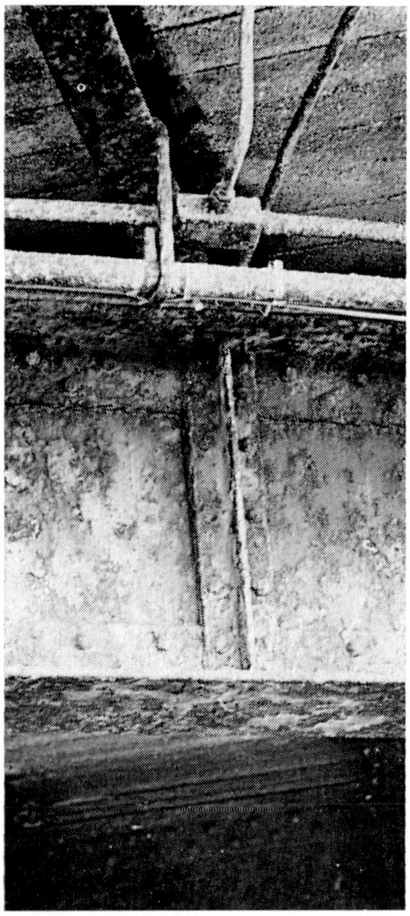

*Corrosion of steel*

*Decay of stonework*

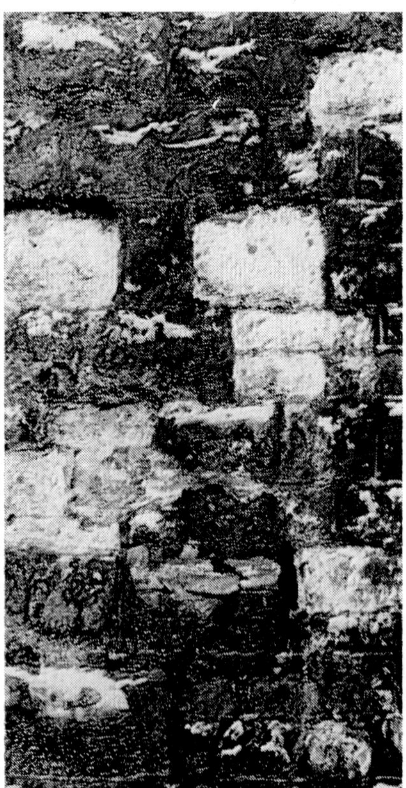

sidered. Included are such factors as absorption, permeability, capillarity and evaporation which influence moisture transfer and the quantities of water actually held. In addition the causes of dimensional fluctuations due to changes in moisture content (the effects have already been considered in *Section 2.03*), together with the extent of movements likely to be encountered and possible methods of allowing for such movements in various materials are tabulated and illustrated.

**4. Exclusion**

In practical terms only that portion of water which is likely to cause dampness of materials and of the internal air and which may have deleterious results must normally be excluded from buildings. In this context the chief sources of water which require consideration are rain, ground water and atmospheric humidity. This section is solely concerned with the methods by which water may be excluded from the main elements of buildings such as walls, ground floors and roofs. The external elements, i.e. walls and roofs (here termed the building envelope), are related mainly to exclusion of rainwater with the differences in behaviour and use of porous and non-porous materials and the effects of shelter discussed. The properties and uses of damp-proof courses and damp-proof membranes are considered in relation to ground water and to those situations in walls and roofs where they are required to meet special problems of rain exclusion such as occur at junctions, openings, etc. Water vapour barriers are considered in outline in relation to problems associated with condensation. A detailed examination of joint design relative to walling units is included together with a consideration of the general properties of mastics. The problems associated with entrapped water in flat roofs are covered in detail.

**5. Efflorescence**

Efflorescence is another problem primarily associated with porous materials (albeit, in practice, only some of them) and at the same time influenced partly by moisture transfer. Although efflorescence may, under some circumstances, result in subsequent chemical actions taking place, the main considerations here include the mechanics of this phenomenon; the basic effects on materials; the sources of salts; the positions in which and the circumstances under which it is likely to occur; and, finally, the precautions which may be taken to avoid its occurrence.

**6. Chemical attack**

Almost all materials for building may be subjected to chemical attack. Under this heading chemical attack usually associated with porous materials only are considered, and include unsound materials; acid action; alkali action; sulphate attack (confined essentially to cement-based products) and fungal attack in timber. In addition to covering the causes and effects of the reactions which take place, an indication of the precautions which can be taken to avoid the deleterious results are noted.

**7. Corrosion of metals**

Corrosion of all metals is considered, with particular emphasis placed on electro-chemical theory, but also including the effects of polluted water, i.e. acids, alkalis, etc. The conditions under which corrosion is likely to occur and the effects of corrosion, both on the metals concerned and other related materials, together with protective methods and procedures available, are also discussed.

**8. Frost action**

Although changes in temperature play an important part in frost action, the deleterious results would not occur if water was not present. Thus, despite the close relationship, insofar as the mechanics of frost action is concerned, with factors which are to be considered in *4.00 Heat and its effects* (particularly temperature gradients), it is more convenient to include this problem here, which is associated with porous materials. As in the other problems the effects on materials, the positions in which it is likely to occur and the precautions which can be taken are discussed. The problems associated with winter building and the precautions that should be taken to minimise the effects of low temperatures and frost on building materials together with the provision of better working conditions for the operatives are included.

**9. Weathering**

Weathering is normally associated, in geological terms, with the disintegration and decay of solid rock. In building the term is associated with the disintegration and decay of the external surfaces of buildings, and particularly of brick, stone and concrete. For the purposes required here the term is used to include all changes in appearance of the external surfaces of buildings, whatever the material. Thus it is possible to include the combined effects of sun, rain and wind, i.e. 'the elements', and also the sometimes annoying problem of staining. This heading then serves to act usefully as a general summary of all the problems in which water plays a major part, plus others in which water may not necessarily be important.

Sections 3.05–3.09 are to be found in Volume 3 but brief details of them are included in this introduction to show how the subject matter is subdivided and to give a clearer picture of the total influence water exerts on materials.

# 3.01 general considerations

The basic properties of water together with its occurrence and behaviour in the natural environment provides, so to speak, the necessary background for any consideration of the effects of water on the materials of those elements and components which collectively make up the built environment. In addition to the relationship between the occurrence and behaviour of water in the natural environment and the built environment there are general factors which must be considered relative to the materials used for buildings. This section includes both considerations under the following general headings: (1) Basic Properties of Water; (2) The Water Cycle; (3) Weathering; (4) Dampness; (5) The Flow of Water; and (6) Assessment of Severity of Conditions. The first three of these are primarily concerned with the natural environment,* the last three with the built environment.

## Basic properties of water

The term 'basic' has been purposely used to imply that all the properties of water are not considered in detail as this is far beyond the scope of this study. In addition to the Table of Properties (Table 3.01/1 on p. 6) in which an attempt has been made to compare water with other substances, some notes are included on those aspects which can usefully be amplified or on which emphasis is important in relation to those problems discussed later. Consequently the notes do not necessarily follow the Table in chronological order, and also include a comparison of the chemical composition of fresh water and sea water.

It is worthwhile noting that in both the Imperial and MKS Systems water was used, in some circumstances, as the standard against which other substances might be compared as, for example, specific gravity, specific heat and viscosity. On the other hand, definitions of quantities of heat, such as the British Thermal Unit or the calorie, used water as one of the governing elements in the standard quantity. However, in all these the precise state of water, either physically or chemically (or both), was always clearly noted. This is important because of the 'ease' with which water can change state and which is later on referred to as the 'instability of water'.

*References: (1) Kuenen, P. H., *The Realms of Water* (Cleaver-Hume Press Ltd., 1955). An extremely lucid coverage of the properties behaviour and occurrence of water. Essentially non-technical language is used. (2) Fox, Sir Cyril S., *Water* (The Technical Press Ltd., 1951). (3) Monkhouse, F. J., *Principals of Physical Geography* (University of London Press Ltd.), 5th Ed., 1963. (4) Lake, Philip, *Physical Geography* (Cambridge University Press), 4th Ed., 1958. (5) *A Course in Elementary Meteorology* by the Meteorological Office, HMSO, 1962. (6) Holmes, Arthur, Nelson, *Principles of Physical Geology*, New and Fully Revised Edition, 1965. Profusely illustrated with diagrams and photographs.

### 1. Chemical formula

Chemically one molecule of water has the formula $H_2O$, that is two atoms of hydrogen to one atom of oxygen. There are variations in the manner in which these molecules may be arranged or in the kinds of hydrogen and oxygen atoms making up the molecules, which give rise to 'special' types, such as 'heavy water'. Because of the minute quantities in which these occur they are generally considered of little importance in the natural environment.

### 2. Instability of water

Water, as generally found in the natural environment, can be distinguished from nearly all other substances and especially fluids in two important ways. Firstly, it is the only substance which occurs *in all three states of aggregation*. that is solid, liquid and gas. As important, it can occur in these states under normal conditions of temperature and pressure and in this it departs from the normal when compared with other substances, Secondly, *the solvent power* of water is more than that of any other fluid. Consequently it is seldom found in its pure state, when it would be odourless and have an insipid taste. (In this state it is said to be colourless, transparent, tasteless and scentless.)

Both of these factors are highly significant. They do in some measure account for the difficulty of defining water in concise terms.* Thus it is suitably descriptive to refer to the instability of water. In fact, this instability underlines the importance of always considering water in all three states of aggregation and as being 'polluted'. For almost obvious reasons, water in its visual perceptible states, that is as liquid or solid, is readily appreciated. However, in the invisible state, that is as a gas, this may not be as apparent. Nevertheless, even in this state it can be active, chemically and physically, while in addition its occurrence, especially in this country, is extensive and ubiquitous. And finally, in many situations water in the gas state may readily and profusely be converted into the liquid state, without changes of either temperature or pressure in the general atmosphere but by contact with colder surfaces, as commonly occurs, for example, in the formation of dew.

### 3. Transportation by water

The ability of water to transport not only small particles of matter but also vast land masses must again, in addition to its greater specific gravity and internal friction, be associated with its three states of aggregation, although more usually with the solid and the liquid states.

Although water may carry the smaller fragments of matter, such as mud, or roll small grains and pebbles, it also has a *lubricating effect* which allows broken particles to slide over one another more easily. The breakdown of large masses of rocks, for instance, into smaller particles is facilitated by the solvent action of water. In this it acts as the vehicle for the actual corrosive agents, such as acids, which may themselves be transported relatively great distances. In this context the corrosive agents are in their dissolved form, although this does not necessarily reduce their

*The Concise Oxford Dictionary* defines water as 'Colourless transparent tasteless scentless compound of oxygen and hydrogen in liquid state convertible by heat into steam and by cold into ice, kinds of liquid consisting chiefly of this seen in sea, lake, stream, spring, rain, tears, sweat, saliva, urine, serum, etc.' This helps to illustrate the difficulties involved.

**Table 3.01/1 Properties of water**

| *Property* | *Ref.* | *Value* | *Comparison with other substances/Notes* |
|---|---|---|---|
| 1. Quantity in the outermost 5km of the earth | a | — | 3 times that of all other substances together<br>6 times that of felspar, the next in abundance |
| 2. State of aggregation | a | — | Almost the only inorganic liquid present in nature and the only substance occurring in all three states of aggregation |
| 3. Solvent power | a | | More general than any other fluid |
| 4. Density: @ 3·98°C<br>@ 0°C | b | 1·000 g/mm³<br>999·87 g/mm³ | Specific gravity of sea water (salinity of 35) @ 0°C = 1·025 |
| 5. Viscosity @ 20°C<br>0°C<br>10°C<br>25°C<br>50°C<br>100°C | b | 1·000 × 10⁻³Ns/m³<br>1·7910 ,, (approx.)<br>1·3077 ,,<br>0·8950 ,,<br>0·5490 ,,<br>0·2338 ,, | Used as standard of viscosity<br>@ 25°C: benzene = 0·649 × 10⁻³Ns/m³<br>kerosene = 2·375 ,,<br>spindle oil = 92·000 ,,<br>castor oil = 620·000 ,,<br>Affected by temperature and pressure: values given for normal atmospheric pressure |
| 6. Specific latent heat | b | 4·187kJ/kg°C | (*Note:* For comparative purposes, the specific latent heat of the materials listed below have been compared to that of water (i.e. water = 1·0) and are therefore *ratios*. To find the actual value of any material in kJ/kg°C multiply by 4·187)<br>Most rocks vary from 0·21 to 0·19<br>Sea water 0·940<br>Ice 0·502<br>Steam (av.) 0·488<br>Common metals vary from 0·22 to 0·0395<br>Alcohol 0·60<br>Benzene 0·41<br>Helium 1·25<br>Hydrogen 3·402<br>Oxygen 0·242<br>Nitrogen 0·235 |
| 7. Boiling point | b | 100°C | Sea water (normal) 104°C<br>Mercury 356·7°C<br>Olive oil (about) 300°C<br>Turpentine 159°C<br>Alcohol 78·3°C<br>Ether 34·6°C<br>Sulphur melts 115°C<br>Tin ,, 232°C<br>Lead ,, 327°C |
| 8. Freezing point | b | 0°C | Expansion on freezing is very exceptional (about 10 per cent by volume)<br>Sea water (normal) −9°C<br>Benzene 5·4°C<br>Turpentine −10°C<br>Mercury −38·8°C<br>Alcohol −115°C |
| 9. Latent heat of vaporisation | a<br>b | 2 253kJ/kg°C (under normal atmospheric pressure) | Greatest of all substances |
| 10. Latent heat of fusion of ice | b | 334kJ/kg°C (under normal atmospheric pressure) | To convert one kilogramme of ice into steam requires:<br>latent heat of fusion 334kJ/kg°C<br>heating from 0° to 100°C 419 ,,<br>latent heat of vaporisation 2 253 ,,<br>3 006 ,, |
| 11. Thermal capacity | a | — | After ammonia, thermal capacity and heat of fusion, the greatest of all fluids and solids |
| 12. Thermal conductivity | a | — | Greatest of all fluids except mercury |
| 13. Surface tension @ 20°C | a | 73·5 × 10⁻³N/m | Highest of all fluids except mercury (see comparative chart C.1.11/1) |
| 14. Transparency | a | | Very considerable and almost equal for all visible rays |
| 15. Electrolytic dissociation | a | — | Very small |
| 16 Dielectric constant | a<br>b | 80 | Highest of all fluids |

*References:* a: Kuenen, P. H., *The Realms of Water,* Cleaver-Hume Press Ltd., 1955
b: Fox, Sir Cyril S., *Water,* The Technical Press Ltd., 1951

potential destructive powers. Breakdown may also occur when water, in the liquid state, trapped or otherwise held in cracks and fissures, subsequently freezes. The 'abnormal' property of water to expand on freezing results in extremely great pressure being exerted. Thus, in addition to actually assisting the physical and chemical breakdown of particles, water also has the ability of subsequently transporting these. Kuenen has aptly described that 'water takes the lion's share of all transport on earth'.

### 4. Derivation of energy

The power of movement apparently inherent in water is dependent on kinetic energy (except that due to tides) derived from the action and movements of the atmosphere. The primary source of these displacements is energy derived from solar radiation.

### 5. Surface tension and capillarity

The surface tension of water is also greater than any other liquid. (A comparative graph of surface tension, C.1.11/1 is included in *Section 1.11.*) This has a marked effect on drop formation (important in precipitation), wave formation, flow and capillarity. The latter, while also associated with the 'wetting' power of water, plays an important part in the transfer of water, mainly in the liquid state, in and about the earth (rocks and soils). Capillarity is also of significance in the transfer of water in and about building materials, wherever capillary paths may be formed. These may be *either* within materials, as in porous materials, *or* at the junction (overlapping or abutting joints) of two or more materials. The latter could be either a combination of porous or non-porous materials. Both methods of the formation of capillary paths have been outlined in *Sections 1.11* and *1.12*

### 6. Thermal properties

The thermal properties of water, namely its great capacity for absorbing, transmitting and storing heat, together with heat of vaporisation, heat of fusion of ice and specific heat, all of which are significantly different from other substances, play an important part in regulating thermal conditions everywhere. The effects of all these properties are closely interrelated. Nevertheless, in general terms water does act as a moderator of temperature fluctuations. The amount of water vapour in the atmosphere is important for the part it plays in what has been described as the 'hothouse effect' of the atmosphere. Control of the amount of vapour evaporated from the earth, which affects the amount of vapour present in the atmosphere, is partially influenced by the great heat of vaporisation of water.

### 7. Density and freezing

The expansion which takes place when water freezes is another significant departure from the normal. Because of this expansion, which is roughly 10 per cent by volume, ice has a lower density than liquid water. (This accounts for floating ice and also for the preservation of much underwater life during winter conditions.) The maximum density of water is reached at 4°C at which contraction ceases. Thereafter further reductions in temperature result in expansion taking place. As already mentioned, water which freezes in entrapped situations induces great pressures on the 'walls of the container' in which it is held, and this accounts for some considerable breaking up of rocks, etc., in the natural environment. As will be seen later under *3.08 Frost action,* this process is equally important in the built environment.

It is relevant to note that the properties of sea water are completely different from fresh water. Contraction on cooling, as with other substances, proceeds steadily until freezing takes place. In addition, the actual temperature of freezing, namely −9°C, is lower than that of fresh water.

### 8. Electrolytic dissociation and dielectric constant

The extremely small degree of electrolytic dissociation of water together with the large dielectric constant, when compared to other liquids, are important factors which affect all solutions in water.

### 9. Compressibility

The compressibility of water is extremely small.

### 10. Chemical composition of fresh water and sea water

Under '2. Instability of water' reference is made to the fact that for most general purposes it is desirable to consider water as being 'polluted'. This has been done in order to emphasise that water usually contains other substances (often referred to as solids) and is therefore seldom found in its pure form.

River water is a useful representative of fresh water. On average, sea water contains nearly 200 times as much dissolved solids as river water* A comparison of the salt content of river water and sea water is given in Table 3.01/2. The analyses given in the table are average values.

The degree of salinity, on the total salt content of water is usually expressed in parts per thousand. Although the saltiness of sea water is due mainly to the presence of the chloride of sodium, other salts are also present. On average, the salinity of sea water is said to be 35, that is 35 parts of dissolved solids per thousand grammes of sea water, and these solids are constituted as shown in Table 3.01/3.

**Table 3.01/2**
**Comparison of salts in river water and sea water**

| River water | | Sea water | |
|---|---|---|---|
| *Salt* | *Per cent* | *Per cent* | *Salt* |
| Calcium carbonate | 42·90 | 0·30 | Calcium carbonate / Magnesium carbonate |
| Magnesium carbonate | 14·80 | | |
| Sodium chloride | 2·20 | 77·70 | Sodium chloride |
| | — | 10·80 | Magnesium chloride |
| Calcium sulphate | 4·50 | 3·60 | Calcium sulphate |
| | — | 4·70 | Magnesium sulphate |
| Sodium sulphate | 4·20 | — | |
| Potassium sulphate | 2·70 | 2·50 | Potassium sulphate |
| Sodium nitrate | 3·50 | — | |
| Aluminium and iron oxide | 3·60 | — | |
| | — | 0·20 | Magnesium bromide |
| Silica | 9·90 | — | |
| Other salts | 1·30 | 0·20 | Other salts |
| Organic substances | 10·40 | — | |
| | 100·00 | 100·00 | |

*Reference:* Values taken from *Water* by Sir Cyril Fox, p. 12.
*Note:* Percentages are of total anhydrous solids.

**Table 3.01/3 Analysis of dissolved solids per 1 000 grammes of sea water**

| | | *per cent* |
|---|---|---|
| Sodium chloride ($NaCl$) | 27·213 | (2·7213) |
| Magnesium chloride ($MgCl_2$) | 3·807 | (0·3807) |
| Magnesium sulphate ($MgSO_4$) | 1·658 | (0·1658) |
| Calcium sulphate ($CaSO_4$) | 1·260 | (0·1260) |
| Potassium sulphate ($K_2SO_4$) | 0·863 | (0·0863) |
| Calcium carbonate ($CaCO_3$) | 0·123 | (0·0123) |
| Magnesium bromide ($MgBr_2$) | 0·076 | (0·0076) |
| | 35·000 | (3·5000) |

*Reference:* Values from *Physical Geography* by P. Lake, Table 2, p. 143.
*Note:* Percentage values have been added as they illustrate the relative concentration of salts.

It should be emphasised that the degree of salinity is not the same everywhere, although the proportion of the constituents does not change.

Density at a standard temperature (0° or 15°C) is a guide to the degree of salinity.

Thus at a temperature of 15°C.

| *Density* ($g/mm^3$) | *Salinity* |
|---|---|
| 1000·0 | 0·0 |
| 1013·8 | 20·0 |
| 1026·0 | 35·0 |

(Reference: *Water* by Sir Cyril S. Fox.)

## The water cycle

The association of water in the three states of aggregation in which it may be found in the natural environment can be extended to include a related, albeit broad, classification of its distribution. Thus, in its liquid state it occurs in the oceans, lakes, rivers, springs and generally underground, that is, groundwater; in its vapour state it is more easily recognised as cloud or mist, although it is present in invisible form in which case humidity terms are relevant; and finally in its solid state the most common form of occurrence is as ice (particularly the polar regions where it is to be found in abundance, or glaciers). Although useful for the general picture, such a classification does not convey any idea of the constant transfer of water which takes place and during which, among other things, water is changing from one state to another. The emphasis is usually on the change of state from vapour to liquid and vice versa, but the significance of the solid state should not be overlooked.

This continual transfer of water, known as *the 'Hydrolic' or water cycle,* results from the interaction of extremely complex factors in which the thermal and other properties of water play a part in addition to solar radiation, wind and pressure. All these are the primary factors which may, in turn, be affected by local topographical and climatic conditions. The actual method by which the transportation of water takes place is in itself fairly complex. However, in essence the basic process consists of evaporation of the liquid water, subsequently to be condensed and then, finally, to be precipitated more commonly as liquid in the form of rain, although snow as a means of precipitation should be included.* The actual amounts of evaporation, condensation and precipitation vary in general not only from one part of the globe to another, but from one season to another (daily, monthly or local variations may also be significant), depending on the interrelated factors already mentioned.

### 1. Types of cycle

As it is the oceans which act as the main and largest reservoir of all water on earth, they serve as the primary source from which evaporation can take place. However, the amount lost by evaporation is, by and large, eventually returned (it may not necessarily be exactly the same water returned to exactly the same place of origin, but this is immaterial). The 'route' by which it is returned is, on the whole, devious and tortuous. Thus, in general terms, the oceans are at once the points of departure and the points of return of water. Again in general terms, the length of time that it takes for the evaporated water to return depends on whether a short or long cycle is involved. Diagram D.3.01/1 illustrates the principal aspects of the water cycle, including the short and long cycle.

(a) *Short cycle:* During the short cycle water evaporated from the ocean follows the basic pattern of condensation and subsequent precipitation in the form of rain. There is no transfer of the water vapour away from the environs of the ocean, that is over land, and thus there is evaporation from and the immediate return of water to the ocean. (A shorter cycle occurs when condensation in the atmosphere evaporates without reaching the earth's surface.)

(b) *Long cycle:* The long cycle includes evaporation from the sea except that precipitation takes place on 'dry' land. The main route for the return of water to the sea is via rivers. These in turn may be fed by springs, which assist in removing ground water (this, in turn, is partly replenished by precipitation, melting ice and by lakes, etc.) or, as occurs in the longest cycle of all, by glaciers which involves a change of state. The complexity of the long cycle may be appreciated if it is realised that within it shorter cycles also occur.

### 2. Equilibrium and distribution

The interchange and transfer of water is virtually a continuous process, during which there are likely to be both losses and gains of water. The effect of these is to establish, more or less, a

*Reference: Mill, Hugh Robert, *The Realm of Nature* and quoted by Fox, Sir Cyril S., in *Water*.

*Detailed studies of these meteorological factors, together with changes due to local conditions, are not included. The emphasis is being placed on the transfer of water, but this should not undermine the importance of the agencies which cause the transfer to take place.

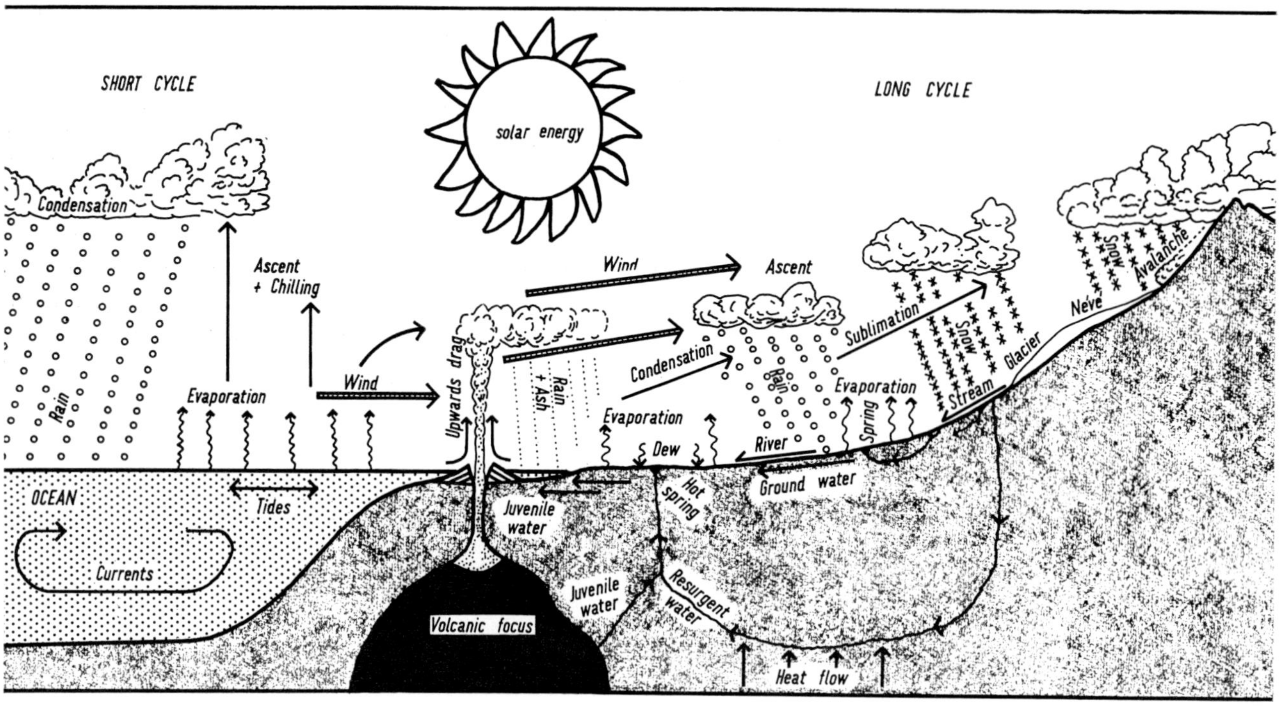


*D.3.01/1*
*Principal aspects of the water cycle.*
*(Based on a drawing in Kuenen, P. H. 'Realms of Water' Cleaver-Hume, 1955)*

balance of the quantities of water distributed over the earth as a whole. Thus, it is estimated that 97 per cent of all the water on earth is in the oceans; of the remaining 3 per cent about one-third occurs as snow and glaciers, while about two-thirds is to be found in rivers, lakes and ground water in soils, etc.; finally, approximately 1/2 000 per cent occurs in the atmosphere.

### 3. Microcosm—land areas

The overall distribution does not take into account the extremely wide variations in the relative distribution which occurs in the microcosm, whatever area this is deemed to include and which is here intended to refer to land areas. In some ways, therefore, the almost disproportionate quantity of water in the oceans may tend to reduce the significance of the relative quantities of water which exist on 'dry' land. As far as the latter is concerned, another point which is important is the fact that wide variations occur in the precise quantities of water present, not only between one area and another but also between one season and another (daily variations may also be important). Thus there may be dry times and wet times in which the general condition of the ground in terms of dryness and wetness can be associated. These variations are of particular significance when considered in relation to the short cycle which occurs within the long cycle. This short cycle, here termed the local cycle in order to avoid confusion with that which occurs over the oceans, is important in the natural environment and virtually fundamental to the problems of the built environment. In both the effect of local variations must always be taken into account. However, an examination, in general terms, of this local cycle is useful.

### 4. 'Local cycle' on land

The sources of water which may be evaporated on dry land include the relatively large and obvious masses, as in lakes, reservoirs, etc., and the surface of the ground itself. Lakes are likely to produce variations not only in the micro-climate, but also in the amount of water in the surrounding atmosphere and ground. They also help to feed underground water courses which may eventually discharge far from the feed point. The possible increases of water in the atmosphere are also likely to modify some aspects of the cycle as, for example, by the formation of local condensation, mist and so on.

Subject to the amount of water present in the surface layers of the ground, the latter can provide an important source for evaporation. Static water in the ground is largely, though not entirely, held in capillaries formed between the grains and particles of the soil. Such capillaries are not necessarily all inter-connected at all levels below the surface. Thus, zones or patches of water may occur at various levels. These zones may, when dry, be filled from above during rain, for example, or from below if they occur immediately above the water table. The latter is almost an underground reservoir, although its top surface may not be level. However, it is the water which occurs at or near the surface which is mainly evaporated and which leads to dry conditions. The quantities of water at lower levels may be reduced as a result of this evaporation, although, in general, this is not considered the primary agency. Water from lower levels may be brought to the surface by thermal and other conditions. This water would discharge into water courses, but inevitably some would return to the ground.

However, after dry periods, it is the surface layers which first absorb water during any subsequent falls, while any excess percolates to lower levels. This excess would either replenish water previously lost or flow to some other place via underground water courses. The latter have more or less the same flow patterns as those which occur on the surface. In all this the precise quantities of water and rate of absorption or percolation are dependent, detailed weather conditions apart, on the nature of the ground which, among other things, may be extremely heterogeneous in its constitution and thus variable. Damp surface layers may also, under certain conditions, encourage local condensation in the form of dew, thus maintaining damp conditions without precipitation. The dew may, of course, change to frost with resulting expansion problems.

Plant life, and especially trees, may also make their own contributions, which in certain situations may be highly significant, to the transfer process. In the ground some transfer of water takes place by 'root action'.

Roots may, in fact, encourage transfer from depths lower than that at which ordinary surface evaporation is effective. During dry periods this may be extremely important. However, through 'respiration' the water is returned, if sometimes only in part, to the atmosphere in the form of vapour, subsequently to take its place in the condensation and precipitation processes. The local concentrations of vapour in the atmosphere may result in almost permanent wet conditions prevailing at ground level, as often occurs, for example, in forests.

**5. Prevailing wet and dry conditions**

Mention has already been made of the wide variations that may occur from one place to another and from one time of the year to another. These variations cannot be attributed to one cause only, but are the net result of the action and interplay of a number of factors among which 'weather' conditions are important. Knowledge, in quantitative terms, of the variations which are likely, between wet and dry extremes, of an area is apparently useful in agricultural undertakings. On the other hand, this knowledge also assists in gauging the probable length of time during which objects are likely to be wet or dry. If this is then related to such other factors as the degree of pollution of water, *a guide*, albeit extremely crude, may be obtained of the likely amount of deterioration which may result. The dampness of the air and the ground may be attributed, in loose terms that is, to high humidity, low temperatures, lack of intensive solar radiation, occurrence and speed of winds and high rainfall.

In this country it is normal to refer to damp conditions in the winter period and to associate this with little drying out, while drier conditions are normally expected in the summer period.

An indication of the effect of micro-climatic conditions in terms of the state of dryness of the soil for instance, can be obtained by comparing average monthly rainfall and evaporation figures. The comparative chart C.3.01/1 compares these figures for six stations in various parts of Britain. Before highlighting some of the relevant facts to be derived from the charts, it is necessary to make a few remarks on the figures presented and which were supplied by the Meteorological Office, on request.*

*Units of measurement*. The amount of both rainfall and evaporation is gauged in terms of millimetres. A millimetre of rain, for example, is that layer of water that would cover a level surface. Quantitatively it would be equal, over an area of $1km^2$ to approximately 1 000 Mg or

*The figures used are 'as supplied' while some of the comments are based on those intimated by the Meteorological Office. In the absence of any authoritative basis for establishing standards of dryness or wetness and drying out times, etc., the charts are intended to assist in a general understanding of the problems being outlined.

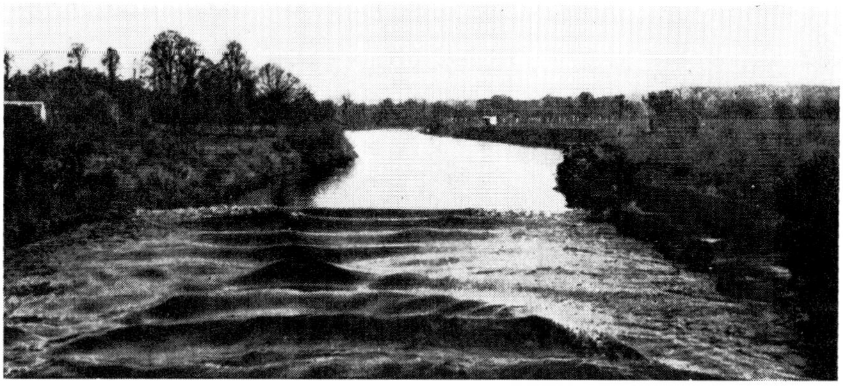

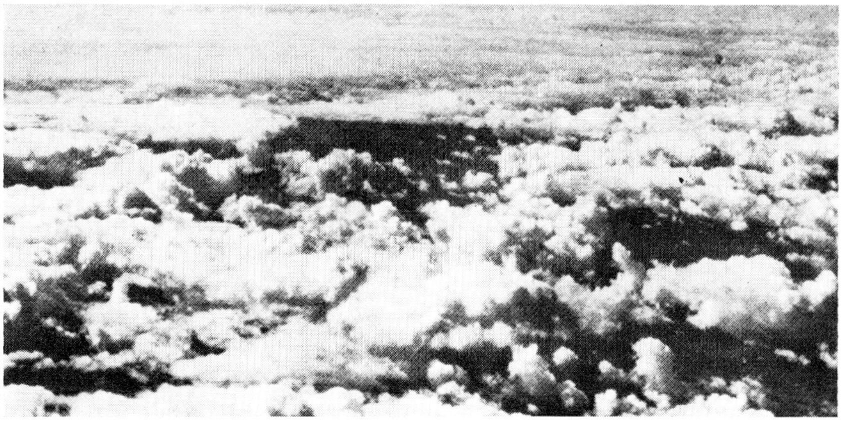

*Some examples of the three states of aggregation of water as found in the natural environment, all of which play a significant part in the water cycle*

*Top picture, liquid state—the 'bore' ascending the river Severn (Courtesy: Keystone Press Agency Ltd.). Above, vapour state—cloud photographed at 7 124m (Courtesy: Ministry of Defence (Air Force Department). Copyright: Ministry of Defence). Below, solid state—glacier (Courtesy: G. P. Abraham Ltd., Keswick)*

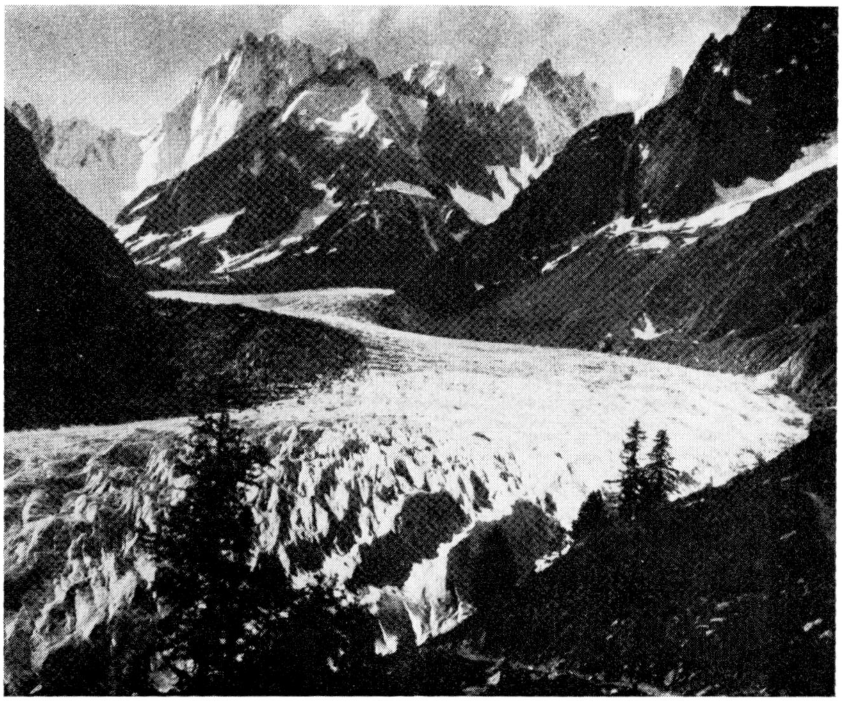

$10^6$ litres of water and exe.'ing a force 9·807MN. On a smaller scale it would be equivalent to approximately 1 litre per $m^2$.

*Evaporation measurements.* These are obtained with a standard Meteorological Office type of evaporation tank, and are therefore not taken from the ground as such. The number of stations for evaporation measurements throughout the country are much sparser than those for rainfall, while the averages are based on comparatively few years (the Cawood figures, for instance, refer to the five years 1960–64 only); those for rainfall are the average for the years 1916–50.

The figures for the winter tend to be less reliable than those for the summer. This is not considered to be of much importance as the figures are, in any case, extremely small.

Returning to the charts and accepting the limitations referred to above, the following points are of note:—

(1) Despite detailed variations, the disparity, during the winter period, between rainfall and evaporation substantiates the generally wet conditions that prevail and offers some support of the slow drying-out concept. The situation is reversed almost completely during the summer period. Subsequent comparison with other meteorological data such as temperature, sunshine, wind, pressure and humidity for the two periods would generally show that these, too, are, for the purposes required here, reversed, although variable.

(2) Most of the annual total of evaporation is accounted for in the half-year from April to September, with the peak rate occurring at about mid-summer at every station.

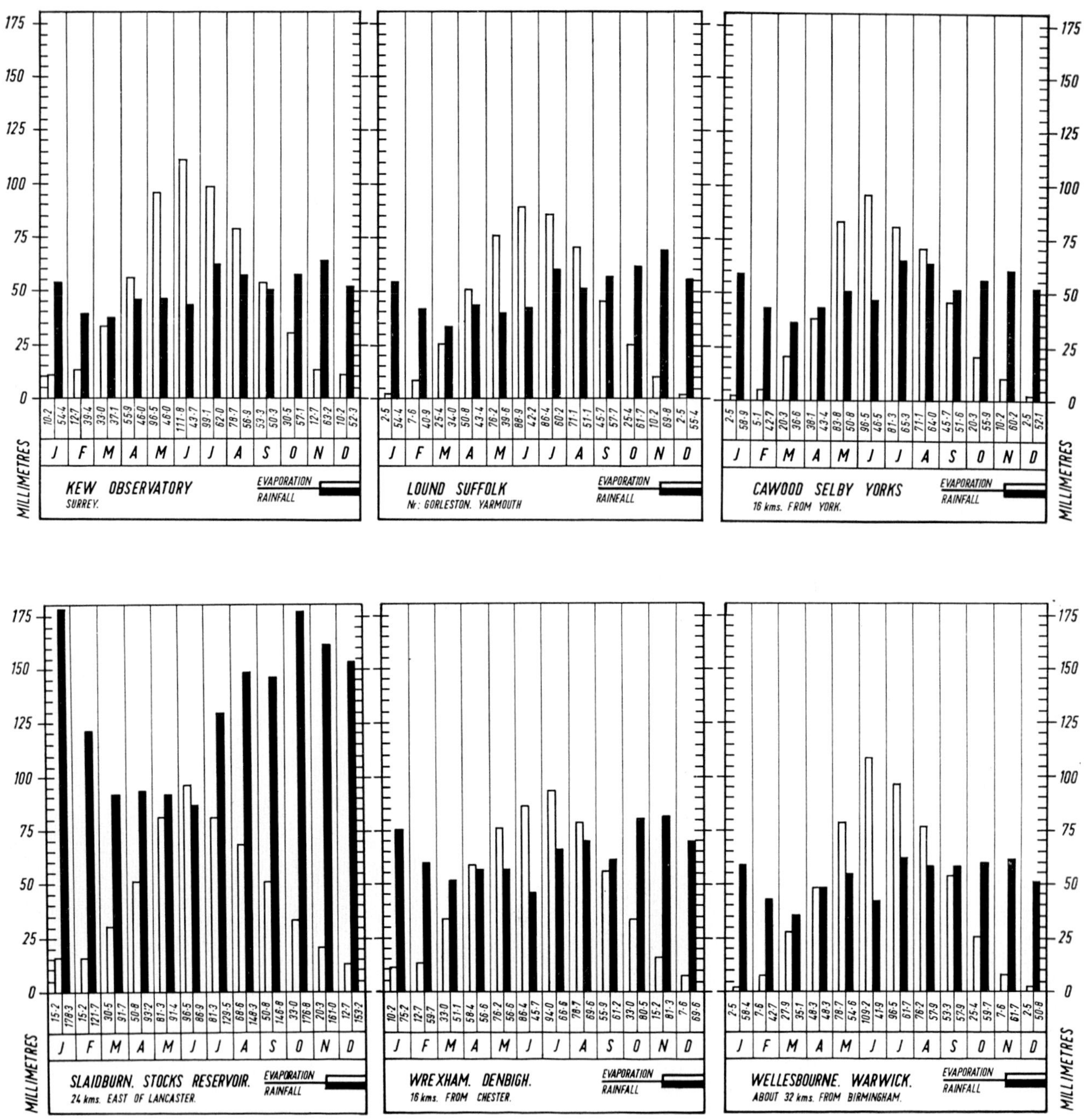


*C.3.01/1*
*Comparative chart of average monthly rainfall and evaporation in millimetres for six stations in Great Britain. Note: Evaporation averages are based on data collected over a few years and are only guides. Rainfall averages based on data for the period 1916–50. (Courtesy: Meteorological Office)*

(3) The average annual evaporation 'rhythm' is generally considered to be roughly the same throughout the country. It is noteworthy that there is a tendency for the windier northern and western districts to evaporate a little more than the southern districts in wintertime. Thus the wind plays as important a role as the sun.

(4) Despite general similarities in the annual pattern, there are notable differences in both rainfall and evaporation figures for each month when the stations are compared. At the Slaidburn Stocks Reservoir there is almost a dramatic increase in the average annual rainfall, where it is 1 580mm compared to, say, Kew Observatory at 608mm (the lowest of the six stations quoted). The comparable evaporation figures (Slaidburn 554mm and Kew 607mm) do not, however, follow the pattern of the rainfall figures.

#### 6. Significance of the cycle

The purpose of presenting, in outline at any rate, the whole of the water cycle has been to draw attention primarily to the fact that water should not be regarded as a static substance. The significance of this lies chiefly in the fact that, because of the constant transfer which is taking place and including the changes of state involved, the aggressive 'nature' of water is in a sense greatly enhanced. This particularly when it is considered that during the transfer processes water has ample 'opportunities', due to its great powers of solvency, to 'pick up' corrosive agencies.

By continual action and interaction, the actual composition of the water along any 'given course' is likely to change as well.

The extent to which the action of water, with or without corrosive agencies, will cause materials to deteriorate is also dependent on the transfer processes, in that these influence the moisture content, that is wetness or dryness, on or within the materials. The moisture transfer in and content of the ground is also significant, especially when it is considered that the most important elements of buildings, that is the foundations, are permanently embedded in it and in some instances at considerable depths. Furthermore, there are a number of other building elements which may be in close contact with or otherwise associated with the ground. Even in the natural environment conditions in the ground are significant.

The inclusion of the whole problem should also serve to emphasise the importance of the interrelation of a great many complex factors, many of which are subject to wide variation. In general, it is of fundamental importance to be able to assess, for any given situation, the severity of conditions which are likely to prevail. In this context the immediate presence of obvious masses of water (oceans, lakes, etc.), for instance, are likely to present severe conditons. As a generalisation, this is sufficient. But at the same time it is as well to be aware of the fact that, subject to other factors, the micro-climatic conditions may, among other things, be such as to lead to conditions as severe as those used in the generalisation. The effect of such variations as may occur may not necessarily be as significant in the natural environment as they generally are in the built environment, where conditions above and below ground are always relevant. In this, the analysis and subsequent synthesis of local conditions cannot be over-emphasised. Intuitive assumptions based on the basic average pattern can very often be misleading.

## Weathering

The agencies which are involved in what is known as the sculpturing of the earth's surface are often covered by the single term *denudation*. Amongst the agencies are included *weathering* (the disintegration and decay of solid rock by the elements *in situ*); *erosion* (the attack and subsequent removal, i.e. transportation, of the 'debris' by the same agent, as for example running water, ice, wind, waves, tides and current); *corrosion or abrasion* (the combined work of the transporting agent and the load which acts as the abrasive in the wearing away process); and, finally, *attrition* (the wearing away of the abrasive medium or load). Although not as conspicuous, these agencies also act in sculpturing the underground world.

In the geological meaning of sculpturing both wearing away and the depositing together with reforming elsewhere of the 'waste' material are normally implied. In the practical terms associated with sculpturing this could be taken as being analogous to shaping processes involving cutting, chiselling, etching, etc., on the one hand, and moulding or casting on the other. (In the natural environment the casting may not necessarily involve a 'mould'.) In building terms the natural wearing away processes are more often taken to be deleterious.

In order to draw attention to the part played by water and particularly the chemical and physical changes involved, the main emphasis is placed here on weathering aspects. However, it is necessary to include the other agencies while some references to those aspects of weathering, in which water plays no part at all, are also made so as to complete the picture. (The use of the term 'solid rock' is not as restrictive as it may appear at first, especially when it is considered that size is not usually stipulated. On the other hand, solid rock does form an overwhelming proportion of the earth's crust, occurring as it does in all shapes and sizes and in an almost inexhaustible range of chemical combinations. However, some reference is also made later on to the part played by decayed organic matter, which can also be said to have disintegrated.)

Under the influence of 'the elements' weathering may take place basically by either *chemical* or *physical means*. Although the manner by which disintegration and decay take place is quite different (in chemical weathering new substances are formed, but no new substances are formed during physical weathering), the effect of either means is essentially to produce a loose layer of material which can be easily removed by the various transportation agents. If the complementary action of the two means are taken into account (a chemical change may facilitate a physical change subsequently to take place and vice versa), then it is true to say that any substance, whatever its constituents, may, in time, be deteriorated. Fortunately, such deterioration requires for each substance, particular circumstances which may not always be 'conveniently' available. Thus in the geological time-scale deterioration is an extremely slow process. The rate of disintegration including decomposition of materials used in buildings may not necessarily be slow when related to the time-scale of buildings.

#### 1. Chemical weathering

All substances may be defined with a definite chemical composition (*Section 1·09*). In the case of rocks, which are aggregates of mineral particles, the latter may also be chemically defined. Under dry conditions the constituent minerals remain unchanged.* However, under damp conditions chemical decomposition may take place, although some minerals, such as quartz, are virtually unaffected, while others, such as rock salt, are removed in solution, These are the extremes. In chemical weathering water is the most influential agent, whether directly or indirectly. As mentioned before, the potency of water is primarily influenced by the corrosive agents which it may carry at any given time. The degree of concentration of these agents is also important. However, another interrelated factor is the actual length of time during which water may be present and hence able to 'act'. The greater part of weathering is often attributed to the effects of standing water, with horizontal surfaces usually suffering far greater than vertical surfaces. (This consideration is particularly pertinent in buildings.) For this reason, any factor which is likely to maintain damp conditions will, in general, increase the amount of weathering which will take place. Nevertheless, this should not detract from the part played by the corrosive agents, the derivation of which is of some importance.

In the natural environment the chief corrosive agents commonly in existence are humic acid, carbon dioxide (only active in the dissolved state—carbonic acid) and oxygen. The action particularly on rocks is important. *Humic acid*, a highly active chemical agent,

*Chemical weathering in desert areas is almost non-existent.

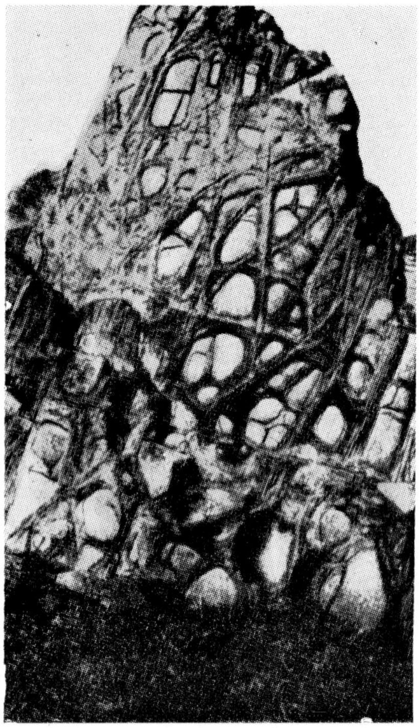

*Spheroidal weathering of dolerite sill. (Courtesy: Controller HMSO)*

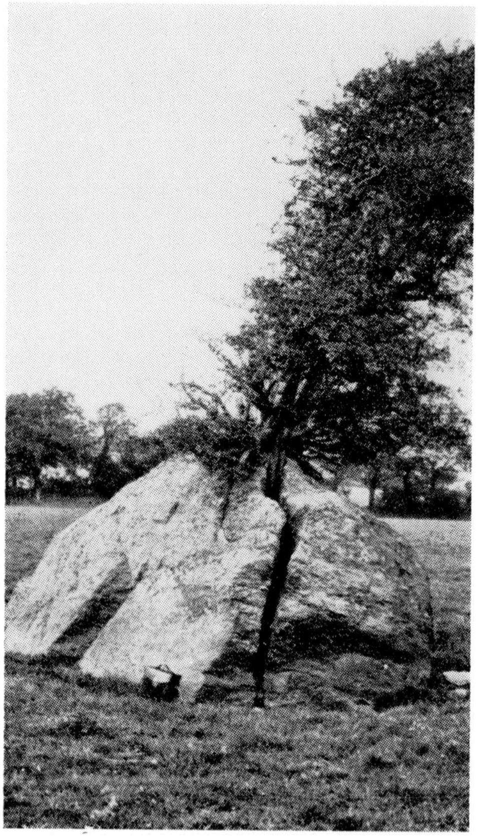

*Crack in ice-transported boulder enlarged by tree root. (Courtesy: Controller HMSO)*

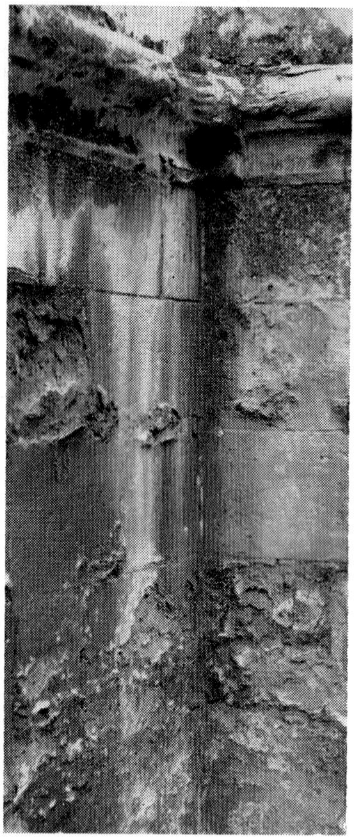

*'Exfoliation' or 'peeling off' of the surface layer of stonework to a building as a result of chemical weathering. Similar results are caused by temperature fluctuations, i.e. physical weathering*

*Frost shattering of igneous rock. (Courtesy: G. P. Abraham Ltd., Keswick)*

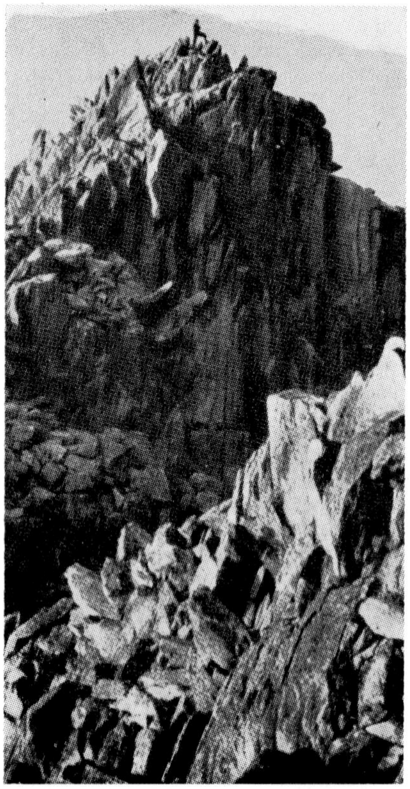

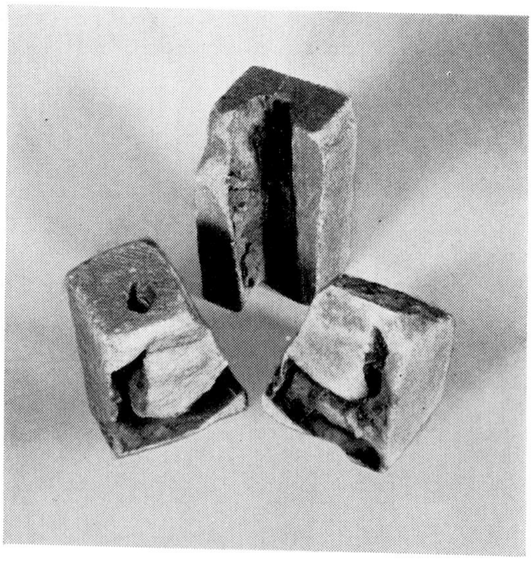

*Action of groundwater 'flowing through' limestone. These quarry samples are unfit for use as stonework in buildings*

is derived mainly from decayed vegetable matter and occurs in groundwater flowing through such matter.* (The decay of the vegetable matter in itself also requires the presence of water, although other agencies may also be at work.) *Carbon dioxide* and *oxygen* are 'freely' available in the atmosphere and are found in both rainwater and groundwater. Often humic acid and carbon dioxide may be present in the same water, thus increasing the corrosive potential of the water.

The decomposition of some of the more common minerals in rocks is given below:

*Felspar.* More than half the volume of the earth's crust is comprised of felspar, which is a common constituent of granite. Decomposition by rainwater (carbon dioxide plays a part) results in the felspar being converted into clay, with calcium and sodium compounds particularly going into solution. Colloidal silica is also removed. The chemical equation is complex. The process is known as hydrolysis.

*Limestone.* Calcite, the crystal constituent of limestone (the rock consists in any case mainly of lime—$CaCO_3$) is the only rock forming mineral which dissolves readily in water. The solvent action of water is considerably increased when carbon dioxide and humic acid are present. The process is known as carbonation. The results of the reaction is to form, among other things, calcium bicarbonate which, when associated with water supply, is a cause of temporary hardness. During the transfer processes the lime solution may, after evaporation, fill in cracks in rocks to form calcium carbonate, or more impressively to form stalactites (downward growth) and stalagmites (upward growth), i.e. columns of 'limestone' in underground caves. The two may join to form one continuous column. The whole process is a long one.

Lime also forms the cementing agent in some sandstones, the decomposition of which can often be attributed to the weakening of the 'cement'. Where the grains are of quartz, as is often the case, these remain unaffected chemically, although physically they will be dislodged from the main body of material. Thus the rock crumbles and in this sense disintegrates. The removal of the cementing agents in any rock has a similar effect, i.e. tendency for the rock to crumble. This may occur at an increasing rate.

*Iron.* Iron is a very common element occurring in many rocks. (Next to aluminium, iron is the most widely distributed metal—each Mg of earth contains about 50kg.) The action of

*The influence of sulphur dioxide (eventually formed into either sulphurous or sulphuric acid) may also be quite considerable in weathering. However, this corrosive agent, essentially although not entirely the result of fuel burning, i.e. a man-made condition, is, in relation to the natural environment, generally not as significant as the naturally occurring agents. However, sulphur dioxide is covered later in *3.02 Exposure* as it is of importance in the built environment.

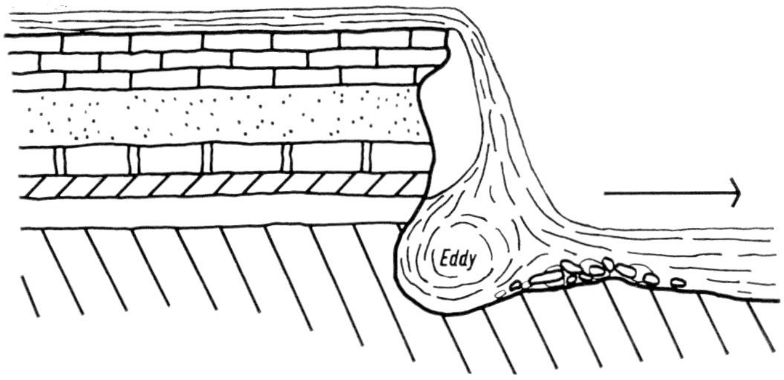


*D.3.01/2*
*The formation of waterfalls. The effect of horizontal beds of resistant rock: undercutting produces a steep overhanging face while less resistant rocks are cut back, thus causing a rapid upstream recession of the fall.* (*Courtesy: Monkhouse, F. J., 'Principles of Physical Geography', 5th Ed., Univ. of London Press, 1963*)

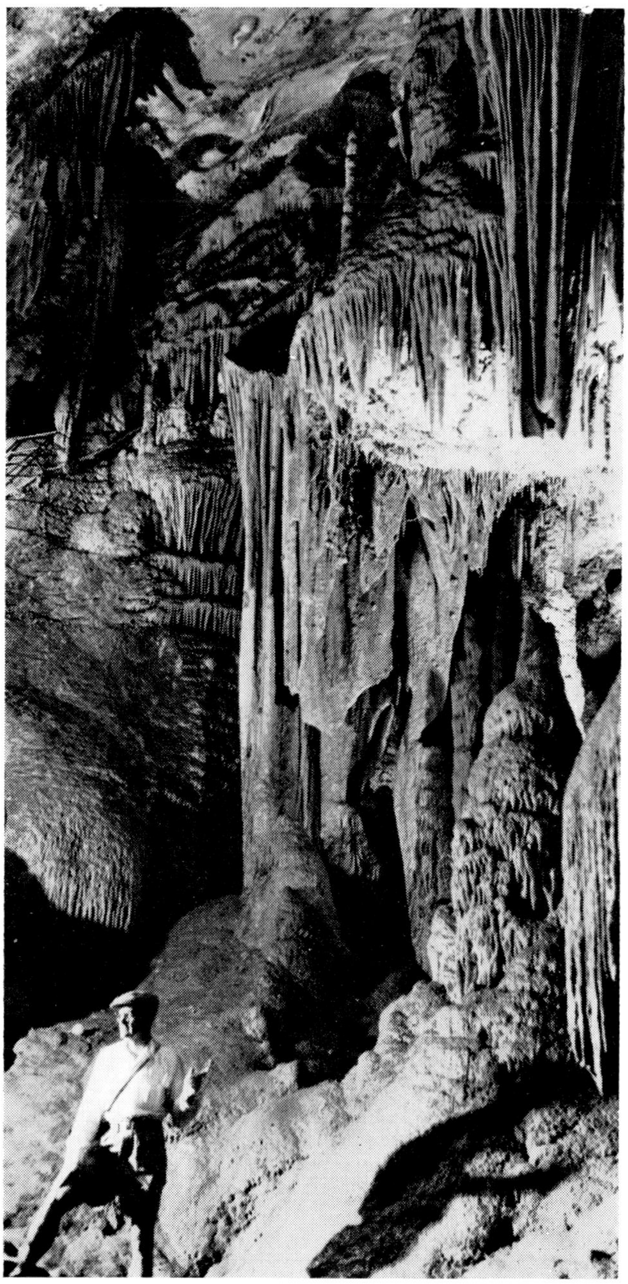

*Stalactites and stalagmites forming columns of limestone in underground caves as a result of water evaporation from lime transferred in solution* (*Courtesy: South African Tourist Corporation*)

oxygen on the iron, during oxidation, is to produce a crust of ferric oxide which readily crumbles.

*Miscellaneous.* Certain minerals which have the property of being able to take up water expand, during a process known as hydration, and thus initiate the break up of the rock containing them. Another effect of rocks such as basalt which are capable of expanding on taking up water is similar to exfoliation, i.e. peeling of the surface layer. The process is known as spheroidal weathering and occurs when the outer surface is affected by penetrating water. The process may continue as fresh layers are exposed. This usually results in the rocks being rounded.

*Effects of other processes.* Although the greatest amount of chemical weathering takes place as a result of standing water, in which could be included contact with moist air, considerable weathering also takes place due to the action of running water, as occurs in the erosive processes. The combined effect of waves, currents and tides on the sculpturing of the sea wall and floor are often extremely impressive. In these processes the abrasive action of the 'debris' removed elsewhere and carried by the water account for some accelerated weathering. In many cases the combined action of erosion and abrasion are extremely significant, particularly as they are, in part at any rate, responsible for the carving of the earth's crust to form watercourses such as rivers, streams, etc. The precise route of these may not always be readily predictable but, once commenced, the weathering processes contribute to their gradual widening and deepening. (The relative resistances of the materials of which the surface is comprised are important. Thus, loosely adhering particles as would be commonly found in soils are more readily removed than the constituents of rock.) This, then, virtually establishes the watercourse along which most subsequent water fed into it will flow. Some dramatic results may occur when less resistant rocks are worn away and undercutting takes place as in waterfalls (Diagram 3.01/2). The continual flow of water down certain parts, particularly of the exposed faces of buildings, may, in miniature, initiate similar watercourses. 'Waterfall effects' may, under some conditions, also occur on the external faces of buildings, particularly those with suitable projections.

In this consideration attention has been drawn to the chief elements affected by weathering. However, it is to be noted that many other elements are involved, all of which contribute, not only to the weathering processes, but also to the pollution of the water. An indication of some of the other substances, many of them corrosive, has been given in the analyses of river and sea water (Tables 3.01/2 and 3). Among these the sulphates (including others which do not occur in the tables) are of particular relevance in building practice, in connection with the problem known as sulphate attack. As mentioned under *The Water Cycle,* any of the corrosive agents may be present during the various water transfer processes, not least those which occur underground in groundwater. Some of the corrosive agents require special consideration in water supply practice, not only for their effects on materials, but also for their effects on health. Others such as the carbonates (a general term usually implied to include bicarbonates) of calcium and magnesium are associated with temporary hardness problems, while the sulphates and chlorides of calcium and magnesium with permanent hardness. (See *3.02 Exposure.*)

### 2. Physical weathering

*Frost action* is the one physical weathering process which requires the presence of water. As mentioned before, water expands roughly 10 per cent by volume on freezing, with the result that rocks may be broken up quite considerably when water in cracks and crevices subsequently freezes.

*Temperature fluctuations,* especially where there is a marked diurnal range, are responsible for the development of cracks (known usually as joints) in rocks as a result of the expansion and contraction which takes place. Ultimately large blocks will break away into smaller units. In those cases where the shell or surface layers of rocks become excessively heated, i.e. in relation to the interior, *exfoliation* or 'peeling off' of the shell takes place.

*Wind,* like water, is more commonly considered as an agent which transports abrasive materials and, in this way, is regarded as being capable of assisting in physical weathering. The effect of wind action can be quite pronounced on loosely adhering or relatively soft materials.

*Rain,* one of the most important of the 'elements', is also one of the more obvious sources of water, and in this way can be said to assist in physical weathering such as frost action, erosion, or where it acts as a lubricant (whole slopes may become unstable after heavy rain). In some processes changes in moisture content may also result in a physical breakdown. As in the case of wind, the action of rainwater on loosely adhering and soft materials (soils are again obvious examples) can be considerable.

Finally, a process of physical disintegration can take place during what is known as 'unloading' or '*pressure release*'. If the weight-caused pressure of overlying rocks is removed as a result of denudation, the newly exposed rocks may then be able to expand, thus causing joints to form. This facilitates 'frost shattering'.

### 3. Effects of biological agencies

The chief way in which plants particularly may assist in chemical weathering is to maintain damp conditions on the surface of rocks, although they may also 'exude' acids. On the other hand, plants may assist in preventing rapid deterioration by binding the surface layers together and thus increasing the difficulty of removal of the debris. Soil erosion is more often than not accelerated by the removal of trees and other vegetation. Other things being equal, the rate of deterioration can be increased by exposure of fresh surfaces.

Mechanical weathering can be influenced to some degree by the root system of plants. Roots do have extraordinary penetrating and expanding powers, thus being able to break open or widen existing cracks and crevices. Such opening up then allows access for water and air, and subsequent chemical weathering.

### 4. Significance

As there may, at first sight, seem to be such a marked difference between the materials of the natural environment when compared with those used in the built environment, it may not be readily apparent what the significance of the weathering, already outlined in general terms, has for the built environment. However, despite recognisable differences in materials, both environments have one thing in common. Subject to variations which, in the present context, are not really significant, both environments are, in general, exposed to the same aggressive agencies, which would also include 'the elements'. In the built environment, moreover, some of these agencies may occur internally, i.e. within buildings, while the effects of other corrosive agents, such as sulphuric acid, 'by-products' from fuel burning and manufacturing processes, have to be considered. In some cases, albeit local, these may be pertinent to weathering.

Similarity between the materials is, therefore, more important than any apparent dissimilarity, especially as chemical weathering must be related to chemical composition and the 'laws' implied by this, rather than to what can best be termed colloquial description whether this is technical or not. As an example consider iron. This substance occurs in abundance in the natural environment but in forms not easily recognisable. It is converted into iron oxide during oxidation and may, among other things, stain other materials. The fact that iron, as commonly used in buildings, is not recognisable as the same substance* which occurs naturally does not detract from the fact that, given the right conditions, the 'man-made' material will also be changed into iron oxide, more commonly known as rust. And so similar analogies could be drawn of many other substances which occur in the

*It is appreciated that this is an over-simplification. In both the natural and built environments iron is associated with other substances. However, this does not materially alter the fact that in both cases iron can be oxidised, nor the principle being outlined.

natural environment and subsequently in materials used for buildings, albeit differently arranged and composed during manufacture. Physical weathering of materials is not restricted to those of a specific composition, although the latter will influence the likelihood of disintegration. Thus, even here there is a parallel with the problems of the built environment.

Weathering in the natural environment also illustrates, sometimes extremely dramatically, the effects and interaction of variations in both the agencies which cause disintegration and the resistance of materials to these agencies. The results of the, so-to-speak, 'free for all' are usually quite marked. The fundamental and perhaps most obvious difference when dealing with the built environment is that choice of materials to resist specific conditions is possible. Such *choice* may very often be limited, but nevertheless to this can be added the vital element of direct *control* which is possible. Thus, for example, the life of materials may be prolonged by protection, i.e. by the use of additional materials ('coatings') or by shelter from the aggressive agents on the one hand, and by maintenance, particularly cleaning, on the other. Choice and control are themselves dependent on the potential of aggressive agents likely to be present in any given situation. Accurate assessment of these is often extremely difficult. Resort has, therefore, to be made to the most accurate guide available. And, if necessary, a suitable factor of safety, so far as the materials are concerned, has to be incorporated.

## Dampness

There are a number of good reasons, some of which may appear all too obvious in the present context, why it is necessary in building work to define the meaning and use of the term 'dampness'.* By implication, the meaning and use of the term 'dryness' is also relevant. Both terms are usually, though not always, restricted to porous materials—restriction to porous materials is being made here. These aspects, together with a brief outline of the sources of dampness and some methods by which it may be measured, are considered. Other aspects, such as the manner in which porous materials may absorb and give off moisture, are included in more detail under *3.03 Moisture content.*

### 1. Meaning and use

The term 'dampness' (or 'dryness' for that matter) is difficult to define with precision. In general terms it can most conveniently be associated with those quantities of moisture which are likely to lead to deterioration of materials, either during or after construction. (Effects of moisture on health may in another, although strongly related, context be relevant. These aspects are not being considered.) Another factor which accounts for difficulty of precise definition is the fact that the measure of dampness will vary for each material. The quantities of moisture implied when considering dampness may be applicable to surfaces, the interior or the body of the material. Within limits, these are interrelated. Usually damp surfaces imply damp interiors (the whole body of the interior is therefore damp); on the other hand, dry surfaces do not necessarily imply dry interiors. It is normal to expect the surfaces of materials to dry out before the interior; visual and even physical assessments of the surface alone cannot be relied upon to substantiate the condition of the interior.

During the working life of a porous material and after any residual moisture, i.e. from water introduced during construction, has evaporated, the moisture content of the material will mainly be influenced, in addition to its nature, by the prevailing humidity of its environment. However, even under 'dry' conditions in buildings, materials may contain certain quantities of moisture which would not be sufficient to lead to deterioration. An indication of the large range (numerically) of moisture contents that can be tolerated, i.e. they are insufficient to cause harm, not only in individual materials but also in a variety of materials, can be given by examining the following three materials:

Plaster—0·2 to 0·1 per cent moisture content.

Lightweight concrete—up to 5·0 per cent moisture content.

Timber—10·0 to 20·0 per cent moisture content.

From the foregoing it will be seen that the terms 'dampness' and 'dryness' are in reality relative ones. Thus materials may contain moisture but may not necessarily be regarded as damp or, looked at in another way, may be said to be dry. In addition to the deterioration aspects of dampness, which are more commonly associated with the life of materials, another aspect important during building practice must be considered. This is primarily concerned with problems connected with adhesion on surfaces of wet construction,* mainly during initial building. The problems may, of course, also occur during maintenance and repair. Speed of building and other factors have led to the development of physical methods (more reliable than perception by sight or touch) of measuring dampness so that a better guide can be obtained as to whether a surface is dry enough for plastering, painting, receiving a floor finish, etc. (See '3. Measurement' later.)

### 2. Causes of dampness

Dampness, whether on the surface or within the interior of porous materials, may result from any one of the causes set out below. The order in which these are arranged is of no significance. At the same time, dampness may result from one or more of the causes. Looked at in another way, these causes could be regarded as sources of water and are, in fact, considered in this way later under *3.02 Exposure.*

(a) Residual moisture from water introduced during the construction of the building. (Concerns both internal and external elements.)

(b) Moisture rising by capillarity in those elements such as walls and floors in close contact with the ground.

(c) Moisture in the atmosphere and by formation of condensation or absorption by hygroscopic materials, as, for example, deliquescent salts. (Almost universally applicable.)

(d) Rain penetration of building units. (Primarily concerned with external elements.)

(e) Leakage of water from faulty plumbing (including rainwater), drainage, heating and other water-borne services. (Universally applicable.)

(f) Spilling of water during cleaning, etc., (indeterminate) or during actual usage (determinate in most cases) as, for example, in kitchens, laboratories, industrial processes, etc.

### 3. Measurement

In some instances, particularly in existing buildings, it may be sufficient to rely on sight or touch (feelings of undue coldness may be indicative too) for dampness measurements and thus the possibilities of impending deterioration. Often, of course, actual deterioration of materials draws attention to dampness. However, as mentioned earlier, during building practice a need has arisen for more accurate methods of determining dampness where adhesive processes, particularly to surfaces, are involved. Such a need is obviously met by quantitative rather than subjective measurements and this has, therefore, led to the development of a variety of physical methods. The unit most suited for making such quantitative measurements is moisture content, although most meters, for simplicity, are gauged in coloured zones, such as green (dry enough), amber (drying, i.e. not dry enough) and red (still wet) and related to specific materials or a range of materials.*

The basic requirements for 'measuring devices' appears quite simple at first glance. However, difficulties have been encountered relative to normal building, rather than laboratory, conditions.

Some of the difficulties are concerned with the necessity for checking, albeit occasionally; length of time

*Main Reference: *Causes of Dampness in Buildings*, BRS Digest (1st Series) No. 33., HMSO, August 1951.

*It should be remembered that many adhesive processes may involve non-porous materials. Dryness of the surfaces of these materials is in this context also of fundamental importance.

*A recent example of the use of a quantitative method of assessment is illustrated in BRS Digest (2nd Series) No. 55, February, 1965, 'Painting walls', in Table 1, *Dampness of walls and choice of decoration.*

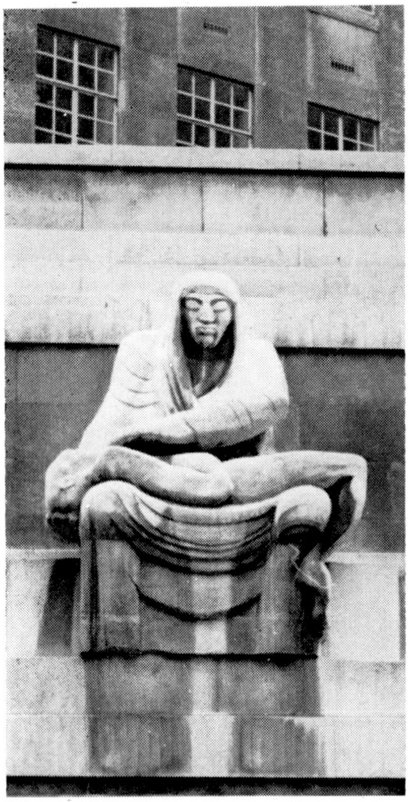

*The weathering of stone sculpture, particularly that of Portland stone, is a useful point of departure for the study of the effects of modelling on the flow of water*

often required before useful readings can be taken; sensitivity to damage and perhaps also cost relative to accuracy obtained, i.e. greater accuracy usually implies greater capital cost.

Some of the meters available rely on the measurement of relative humidity of the air, i.e. types of hygrometers.* With these meters overnight readings are advisable. Coloured indicator papers are probably the simplest, being fixed to a surface and changing colour according to the moisture present. However, there has been a further development of meters, based on electrical resistance, originally intended for use with timber† but which may now be used, in modified form, with other materials. These meters, by and large, have prongs and are more accurate for measuring surface dampness or the depth of penetration possible by the prongs. The latter may be restricted by the hardness of many materials, such as brick and concrete. For greater reliability when using coloured indicator papers or electrical moisture meters, methods have sometimes to be devised (when measuring the condition of a new wall to take paint for example) for encouraging any moisture in the interior to come to the surface. This would be done by covering at least $0{\cdot}1m^2$ of the surface with a piece of glass, metal or polythene sheet for several hours (preferably overnight) before taking a reading in the centre of the area covered.

More recently a moisture meter using micro-wave techniques, and commercially available, has been devised by the Building Research Station primarily to facilitate the measurement of the total moisture content of constructions. The meter has a transmitter and receiver and, when compared to other meters available, is costly and less versatile although more accurate, giving direct and instantaneous readings.

The difficulties involved, and especially doubt which many still have of the accuracy of those meters economically available, together with lack of enough practical experience, have probably accounted for the comparatively limited use of physical measurement. It is also conceivable that the necessity of making some kind of quantitative assessment has not been fully realised.

**Methods of determining the dryness of a sub-floor*, BRS Digest (2nd Series) No. 18, p. 4, January 1962.

†*Causes of dampness in buildings*, BRS Digest (1st Series) No. 33, p. 1, August 1951.

## Flow

The term 'flow' is here restricted to the transfer of water, in its liquid state, over exposed faces of buildings and with particular emphasis on vertical faces. The main objective is to outline, in general terms, the manner in which the flow of water is influenced by modelling of the exposed faces which may be due either to the surface characteristics of materials or to projections and recessions in the profile of vertical surfaces.* Both factors may be operative at the same time. The effect that these have on the *basic* flow of water does in turn determine, in principle at any rate, the extent to which areas or zones of a vertical face are likely to be exposed to or sheltered from water. Both are important in any consideration of the effects of water. No detailed consideration is given here of the actual effects of water as it flows over any surface, or of the manner in which any of the water may be absorbed into materials or the joints between materials in any element. As the main consideration is concerned with the paths taken by water over surfaces, rather than effects, subsequent transfer and precise quantities involved, the flow of water is clearly defined and self-contained routes, that is in pipes, channels, gutters, etc., are omitted as these aspects are more closely related to problems associated with the servicing of buildings. The transfer of water vapour, on the other hand, is covered in *4.00 Heat and its effects*.

It is axiomatic that the severest problems associated with the flow of water are generally encountered on the external faces of buildings with water falling during rain. Accordingly, this condition is taken as the basis for the principles outlined. However, the principles may be equally applicable to surfaces within buildings where the source of water may result from spraying, spilling, etc. Although some of these sources may be regarded as fortuitous, it is worthwhile noting that usage itself may involve the spraying or spilling of water more or less continuously within certain spaces. An extreme case would be a car washing bay, for example. On the other hand, the likelihood of 'streaming' as a result of condensation may also have to be taken into account.

*The extent to which wind action and other factors are likely to influence the flow of water are noted where relevant, but detailed consideration is generally omitted in order to emphasise the basic pattern of water flow. The significance of these other factors is outlined in *3.02 Exposure*.

Before attempting to outline the mechanics, so to speak, of the flow of water down vertical faces of buildings resulting from rainfall, it is necessary, for a number of different reasons, to first set out some of the difficulties involved. Many find it extremely difficult to appreciate why the flow of water down vertical surfaces should be of any importance at all. They would argue that resistance to water penetration and weathering are of primary importance and, provided it is assumed that all exposed surfaces will receive or be subjected to water, that the associated problems are concerned essentially with selection and use of materials. Accurate assessment of the likely flow of water, it is felt, is also bedevilled by other complex factors which must inevitably become involved. At the same time, they appreciate the necessity for determining the rate of flow along horizontal or sloping surfaces in order to be able to assess sizes of gutters and rainwater pipes.

However, in recent years, mainly because of the development and increased use of impervious claddings, some consideration has been given, among other things, to the rate of flow and quantities of water on vertical surfaces. Investigations into the problems associated with impervious claddings have indirectly drawn attention to the effects on weathering and/or water penetration resulting from the omission of the shelter provided by traditional modelling in the form of mouldings and other projections on a great number of present-day buildings. It has often been suggested that 'traditional' designers of buildings were more fully aware of the effects of the flow of water and related weathering on appearance particularly, and 'manipulated' their mouldings and projections accordingly. The significance of this is that water does appear to play some part in changes of appearance, whatever the profile of buildings may be. Much of the doubt expressed on the necessity of understanding flow patterns can, in many cases, be dismissed. The results due, in part at any rate, to uncontrolled flow are to be found on innumerable present-day buildings (many older buildings can also be included) as can be seen in

*These four photographs illustrate effects of 'uncontrolled' flow of water. The lowermost picture was taken during rainfall*

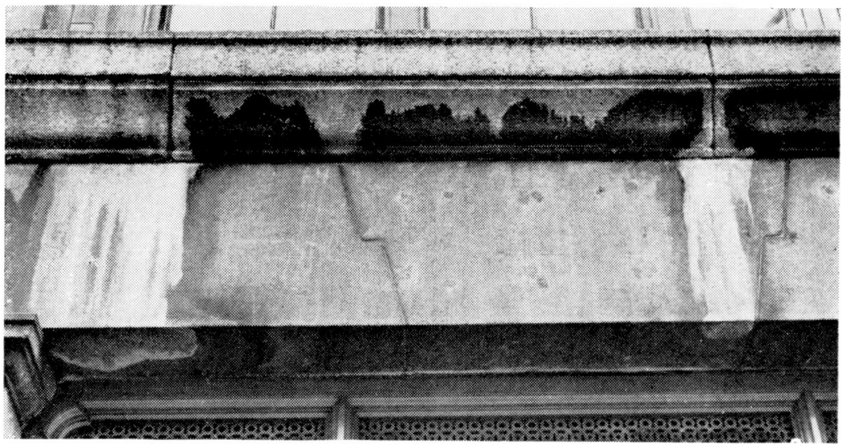

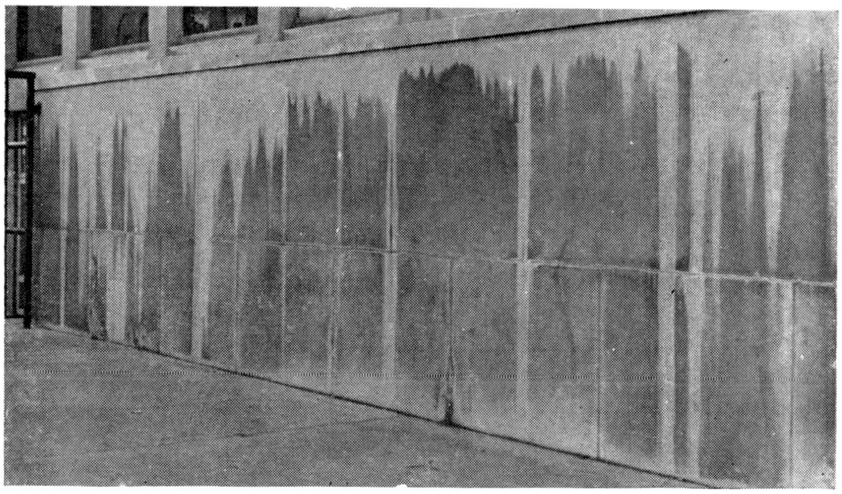

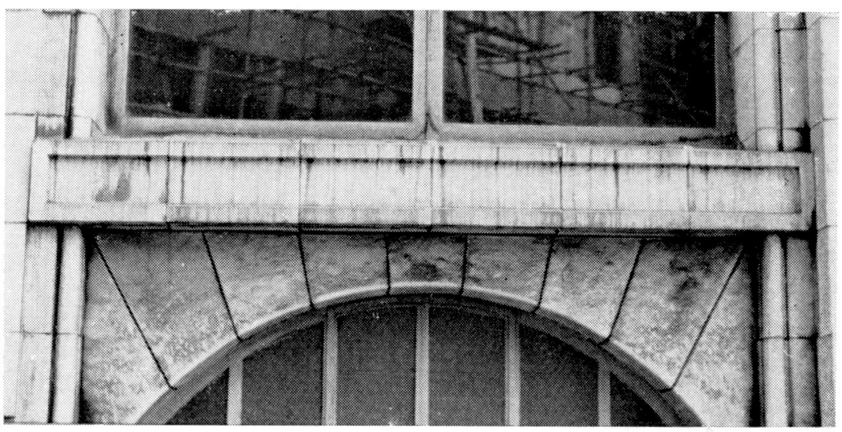

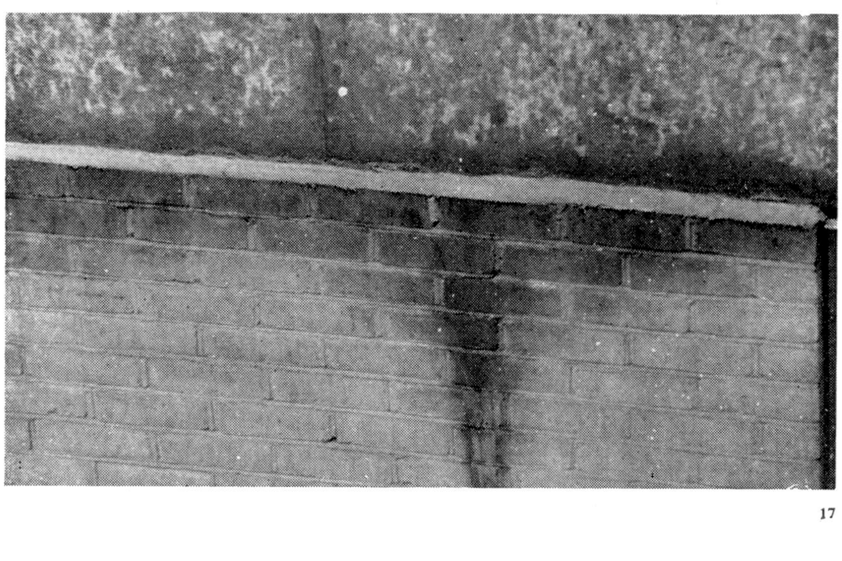

the accompanying photographs.* Thus there would appear to be every reason why some understanding should be gained of at least the basic flow patterns that take place down vertical faces of buildings. Furthermore, there does appear to be good reason to believe that uncontrolled flow of water does place a heavy burden on materials, the selection and use of which require serious reassessment.

In the absence of the results of studies specifically directed at the problems of flow which now seem to be required, it is only possible to outline the basic flow patterns on what can be best termed a subjective basis. In the context of deterioration or changes of appearance it is difficult to isolate the flow of water from all the other factors which must inevitably be involved. For convenience, therefore, the mechanics of flow are considered under the following closely interrelated headings, namely: (1) Exposure conditions; (2) Soffits; (3) Surface characteristics of materials; and (4) Projections and recessions.

**1. Exposure conditions**

It is generally accepted that apart from the comparatively isolated occasions, rainwater falls at an inclined plane. This is due mainly to the effects of wind. The angular measurement of 10 degrees from the vertical, sometimes accepted as a guide of the extent of the inclination, may not always prevail, but is nevertheless sufficient to underline the basic concept and also serves to illustrate the fact that exposed vertical surfaces, i.e. those 'facing' the rain, are capable of receiving water and this may be considerable. Unexposed vertical surfaces may also be subjected to water from horizontal surfaces. Subject to the amount of water which may be absorbed or otherwise retained by the materials constituting the exposed face, the quantities received flow downwards. (Under severe conditions of wind exposure, water has been known to 'flow' upwards.) During this flow, when it is convenient to imagine the water as a film of variable thickness and area, there is a progressive increase in the actual quantities of water with the greatest amounts passing the lowest level.

*It is extremely difficult to illustrate photographically the flow of water down the vertical face of actual buildings without resorting to those examples in which the effects of water (mainly weathering and changes of appearance) are already manifest. Many examples also illustrate the results of localised concentrations. Nevertheless, it is felt that the selected examples should assist in an appreciation of flow and also help to reinforce the fact that, in the final analysis, other factors have always to be taken into account.

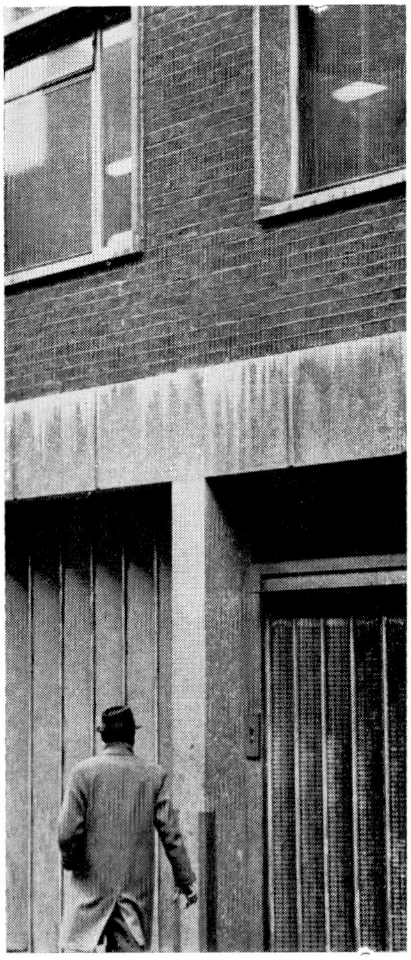

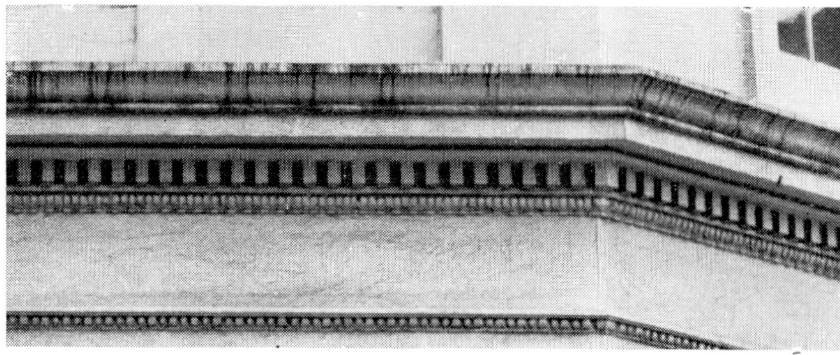

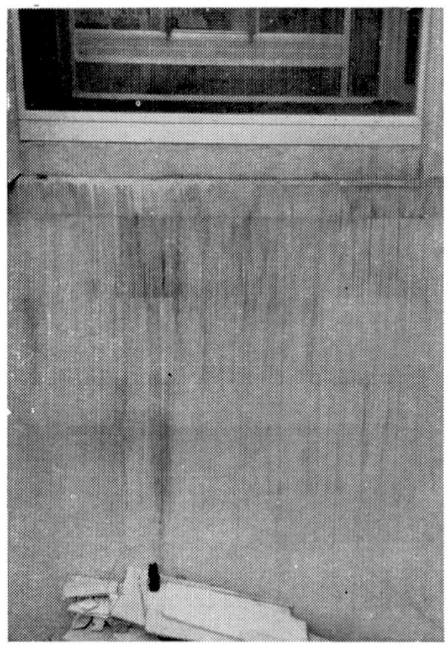

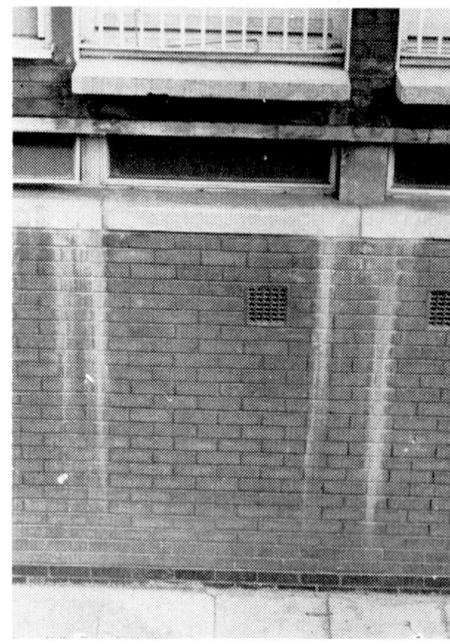

*The photographs above show examples of 'uncontrolled' flow of water*

*Below left, effects of discontinuity of drip, and lack of drip to underside of balcony upstand and lintel to window. Below, omission of drips resulting in some increased exposure of vertical surfaces which would otherwise have been protected*

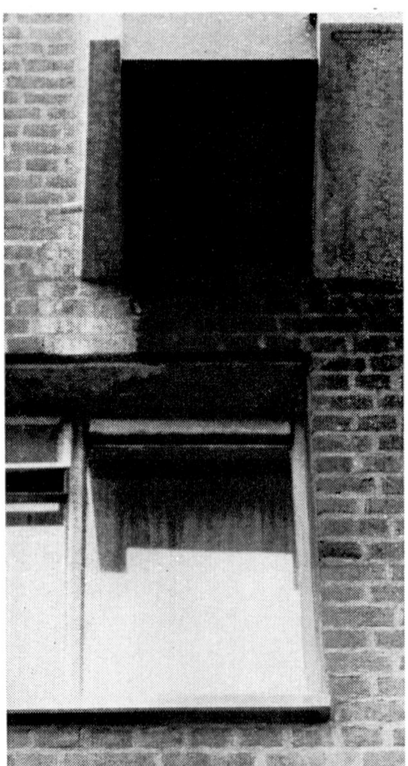

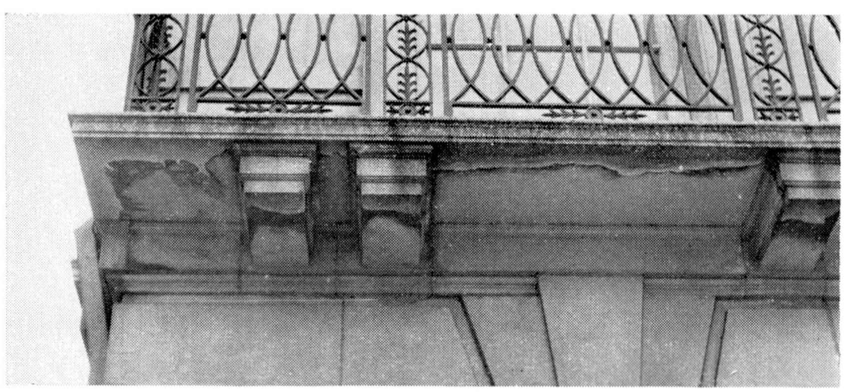

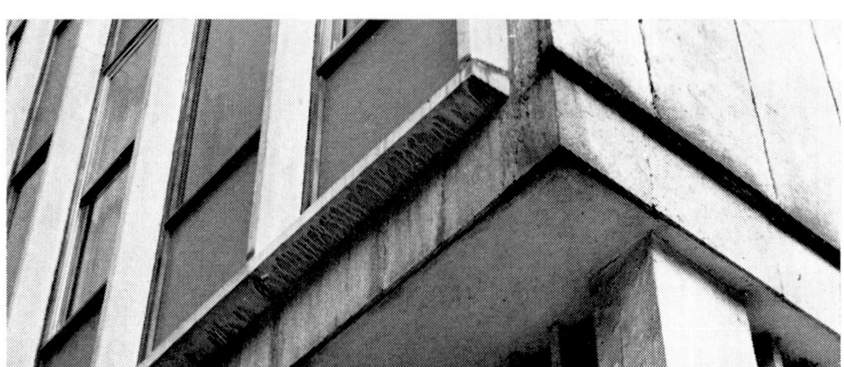

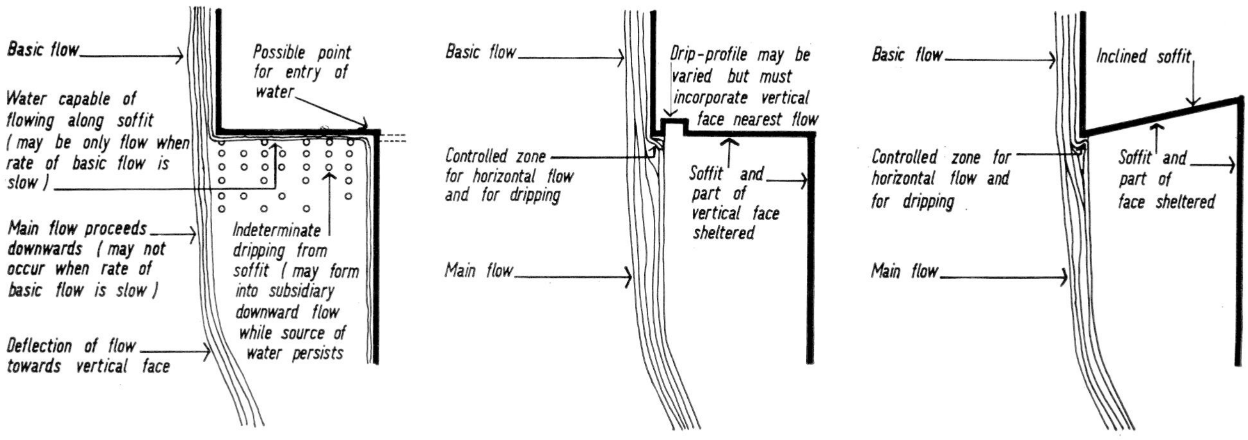


Uncontrolled horizontal flow
(a) BASIC CONDITION

Controlled horizontal flow
(b) USE OF DRIP

Controlled horizontal flow
(c) INCLINED SOFFIT

*D.*3.01/3

*Illustration of uncontrolled horizontal flow of water along soffits (a) with two possible methods of control (b) and (c). Note: in the basic condition no account has been taken of the effects of the surface characteristics of the soffit: the worst condition is shown*

The areas over which water actually passes, that is the pattern of flow, will be influenced partly by the obstructions encountered and partly by the rate of flow. Both are closely interrelated. The effects of the actual obstructions are better considered separately, as it is important first to draw a distinction, in general terms, between two extreme rates of flow, both of which involve different quantities of water.

It is perhaps all too obvious that the rate of flow of water in any given situation will be less during a short shower than during a heavy downpour or even a continuous drizzle. However, for any given intensity of rainfall, the rate of flow at the commencement and end of the fall (water will continue to flow at a progressively slower rate for some time after the fall has ceased) will be less than that which occurs for the duration of the fall. Thus, whatever the intensity of rainfall, there will always be, at some time or another, comparatively slow rates of flow down a vertical surface. To a large extent it is these extremely slow rates which appear, in the final analysis, to manifest themselves (in terms of differential weathering, staining, etc.) and also indicate that obstacles of some kind or another, resulting from various causes (including weathering itself), exist. The water circumvents these obstacles. In general, the slower the rate the greater the influence of obstacles which tend to cause the flow to become 'fragmented' (by analogy broken up into rivers, streams and lakes), and the surfaces, dependent on other factors, such as the properties of materials themselves and pollution of the water, undergo differential weathering, etc. It should be noted that the 'drying out pattern', particularly immediately below projections or recessions, often influences the pattern of 'streaking' which manifests itself and can be seen in many of the photographs. Drying out naturally enough occurs in the opposite direction to that of the flow, i.e. from the bottom upwards. In addition the slower rates of flow may also be responsible for unsuspected rain penetration, particularly at joints where capillary paths may be formed. The main emphasis given to the slower rates of flow should not detract from the fact that accelerated erosion, for example, is possible with the faster rates of flow.

## 2. Soffits

It is not uncommon to find (even in some traditional work) that the ability of water to flow along the soffits of horizontal surfaces, which occur on all projections and recessions to the vertical faces of buildings, has been overlooked. The flow of water along such soffits may result in: (1) the soffit itself being subjected to increased weathering; (2) the vertical surface under the soffit being less sheltered; (3) a possible point of entry for water at the junction of the soffit and the vertical surface being allowed; and (4) a relatively large area for potential dripping being created, either when the rate of flow has been considerably reduced or the source of water causing the flow has ceased—persistent dripping may initiate or accelerate erosion of exposed surfaces lower down.

These points are illustrated in diagram D.3.01/3 (a). Here again account must be taken of the more or less continuous flow that will occur along the soffit when the flow on the vertical surface is slow—some water will also flow during high velocity flow on the vertical surface. Two methods of preventing the horizontal flow of water are shown in diagram D.3.01/3 (b) and (c). In both these cases dripping will occur at the forward edge of the projection, but in this case the zone of potential dripping can be controlled. It is not possible to show clearly that the water proceeding downwards past the soffit will, on the whole, join the general rainfall and thus eventually flow down the lower surfaces. The exceptions to this general statement would have to be related to the distance of fall (for the water), the velocity of flow and wind conditions.

## 3. Surface characteristics of materials

Although it is conceivable that some materials may be manufactured with absolutely smooth and level surfaces, it is not always practicable or economically possible, in building terms, to demand or expect such accuracy. Even if such accuracy was feasible, the physical processes of building, however good the workmanship may be, make absolute smoothness, evenness, levelness or plumbness impossible.* Thus when materials are used to form uninterrupted vertical surfaces, it is unrealistic to anticipate that there will be an even or regular flow pattern of water and particularly during slow rates of flow. Similarly the edges of projections cannot be regarded as capable of producing even flow patterns for water flowing over them. This means that the selection and use of materials have to be related to the *degree* of smoothness, evenness, levelness and plumbness that can be expected. For any given situation flow patterns must then be related to other properties of materials.

Roughness of surfaces has the effect of breaking up the pattern of flow. The more even the distribution of roughness, often coupled with the degree of roughness, the more even

*Drafting practice employing as it does lines drawn with the aid of a straight edge can, within the present context, be quite misleading.

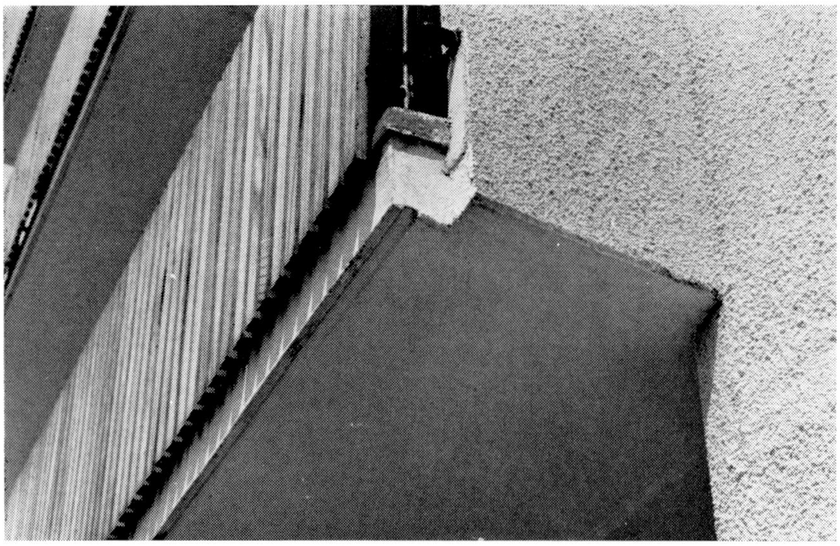

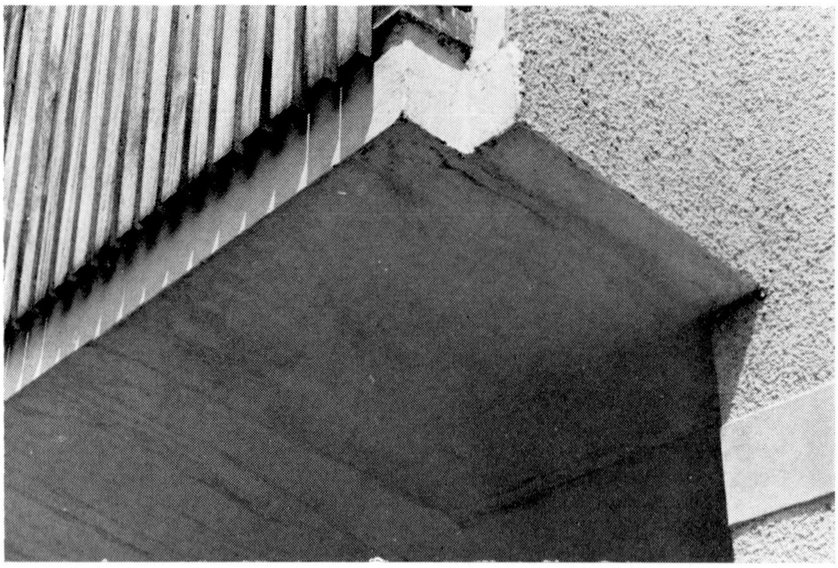

*Examples illustrating the importance of drips in controlling the flow of water along soffits, including in some cases the significance of consideration of returns to projections. — Compare with diagram D.3.01/3. The photographs above show the soffits of two balconies from the same building, one (top picture) with a drip to the forward edge and the other without. The roughness of the vertical face to the return appears to have acted as a drip in both cases. Below, omission of drip to return with increased exposure of vertical face as a result*

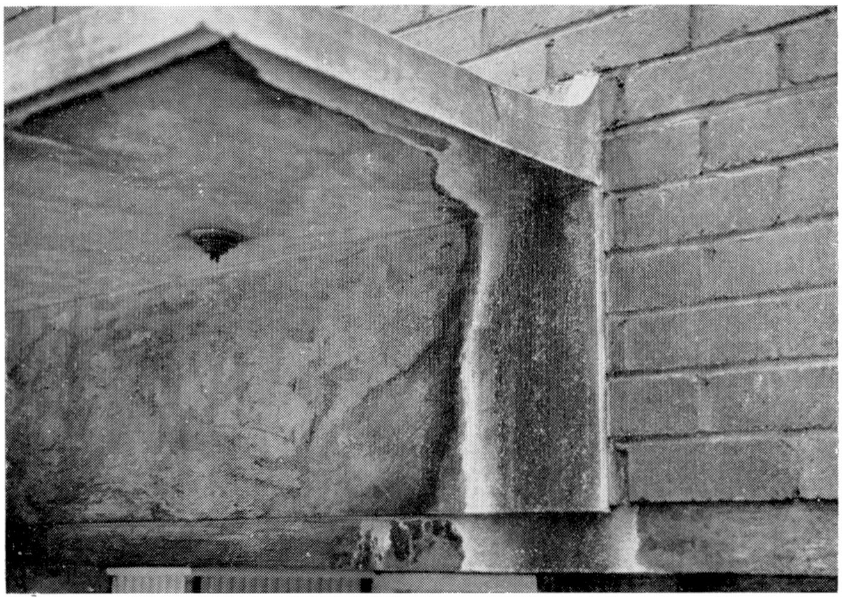

the flow tends to be. Thus, on an essentially smooth surface, but which may have some isolated obstacles of relative weakness or unevenness, the flow pattern may *eventually* become recognisable (usually due to the relative weakness of material in relation to the amount of water it receives and resulting in weathering) whereas on an extremely rough surface this is, under normal conditions, unlikely to occur. The fact that an uneven pattern does not manifest itself in any given situation cannot be taken, by itself that is, to imply that the pattern, which does in fact take place, is even. Thus the surface texture of a vertical face, excluding in this instance horizontal projections, does influence the pattern of flow. Whether or not any of the patterns formed are likely to result in differential weathering or other forms of disintegration and disfigurement is dependent on the quantities of water involved (local concentrations, many of which can be seen in the photographs, play an extremely important part) relative to the properties of the materials concerned. Despite the complexities which are inevitably involved, the basic differences between the two extreme conditions which may occur serve as useful *guides* in any assessment of the severity of conditions which can then be related to the selection and use of suitable materials for the particular exposure.

**4. Projections and recessions**

The vertical faces of buildings are seldom without projections and recessions of one kind or another. The provision of openings for windows, for example, immediately implies the formation of a recession, and the accompanying sill, a projection. The extent of either the recession or projection is dependent on detailed design and liable to innumerable variations. It is interesting to note that, even in those present-day examples where a flush face, that is as between window and wall, is sought, some recessions are formed, with, in many cases, the omission of the traditional sill. The recessions so formed, and which are not necessarily restricted to window/wall details, are sometimes termed 'flashgaps'. As important, flashgaps may run either in a horizontal or in a vertical direction. Other elements such as balconies, canopies, string courses, etc., also create projections.

Any interruption in the vertical plane, whether this is a projection or a recession, has the effect of altering the pattern of the flow of water down the face. The primary effect of projections is to throw water away from the main face and by so doing to afford some shelter to the faces underneath the projection. However, at the same time the water thrown off will, subject to conditions, join the general fall and thus increase, albeit locally, the rate of flow at the zone of meeting. The extent of local concentrations of water is important. Although the extent of the projection will basically influence, in the vertical plane that is, the amount of shelter, account has also to be taken of the amount of shelter in the horizontal direction. The latter will be influenced primarily by the length of the projection. Recessions, and particularly those which run vertically, also contribute to local concentrations of water; on the other hand the tops of horizontal surfaces of recessions (the same would also apply to horizontal surfaces of projections) present vulnerable zones.

Concentrations of water flow imply, naturally enough, that materials must be selected to resist these flows which represent the worst or most severe condition. On the other hand, it is conceivable that advantage may be taken of concentrations of water flow to actually allow or encourage differential weathering, that is between sheltered and unsheltered areas of the same material, to take place. The pattern of flow resulting from the occurrence of projections and recessions can be considered under various headings.

(a) *Profile of front edge*

The extent to which water will be thrown off the face of a building and thus the degree of shelter provided, is dependent on a number of interrelated factors, chief of which are:

(1) Quantity of water reaching the projection, that is either before the run-off commences or subsequent to the initial flow; (2) slope of the projection (the steeper the slope the faster the rate of run-off for any given quantity of water); and (3) the extent of the projection. However, in addition to these factors, the profile of the front edge of the projection is important. It is convenient to consider the basic effects of the two extremes which are illustrated in diagram D.3.01/4. In example (a) the front edge of the projection is rounded (which would always occur in pressed metal work and this is worthwhile remembering). Generally, the water will follow the rounded profile. In example (b) where the front edge has a sharp arris, the water is thrown clear of the projection itself. Thus the projection results in a greater throw off than in the previous example. Although water may be thrown clear of the projection with the rounded front edge when the intensity of flow is great enough, this will, in general, be less than would occur with a similar intensity on the projection with a sharp arris. Thus the profile of the front edge of a projection will influence, in principle at any rate, the degree of shelter provided by a projection.

(b) *Eddies*

As mentioned before, the water thrown off by any projection will, subject to circumstances, be 'deflected' towards the vertical surface. Projections or

*Bridging of a drip causing localised flow*

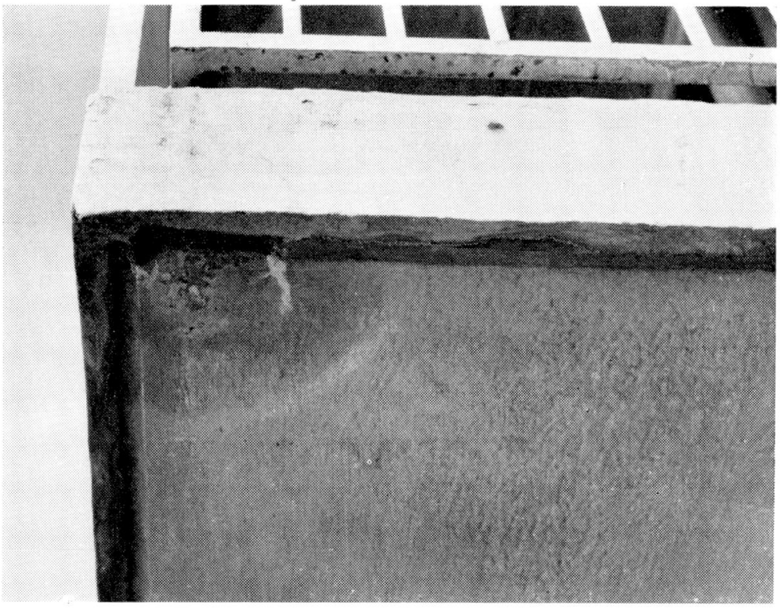

*Omission of drip to return; bottom right, general view and below, detail of another balcony on the same building*

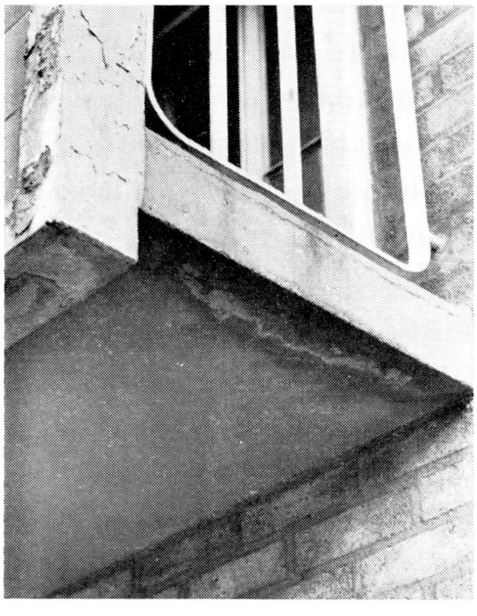

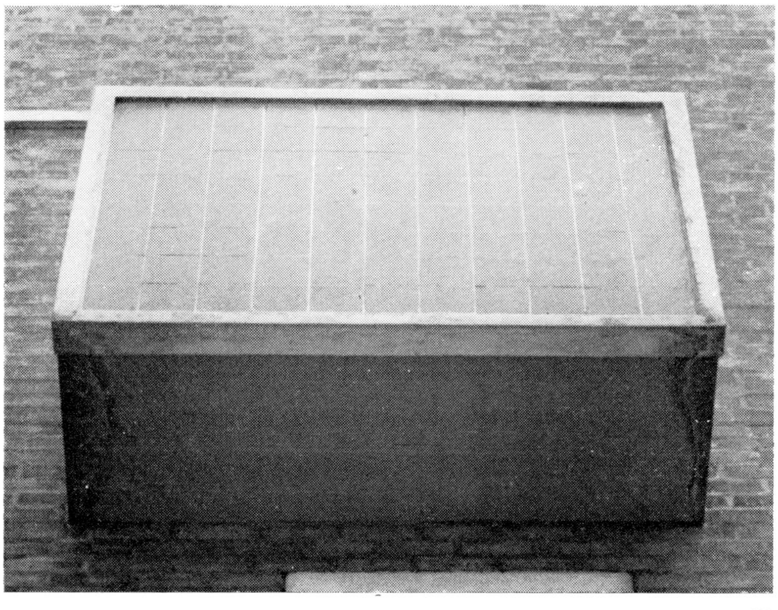

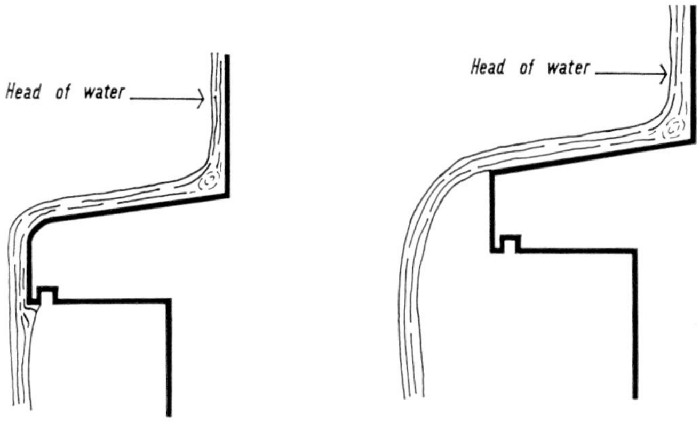


D.3.01/4

*The effect of the profile of the top front edge of a projection on the flow of water. Note: the illustrations are intended to compare extreme cases and do not take the effects of intensity of flow into account*

*The photographs below show that failure of detail (triangular raised block at corner of front edge) to direct water over the front edge has been partially due to the failure of the mastic jointing. The sills of both examples are identical. Due to differences in surface characteristics and properties leakage is not visible on the brickwork (below) but is on the stonework (bottom picture). The horizontal surface of the stone under the sill has commenced to erode*

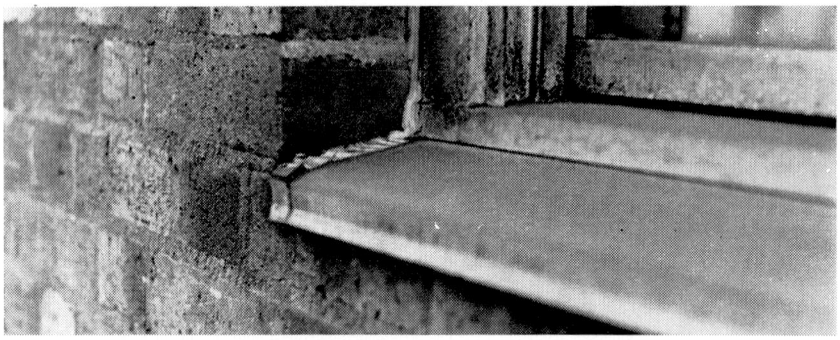

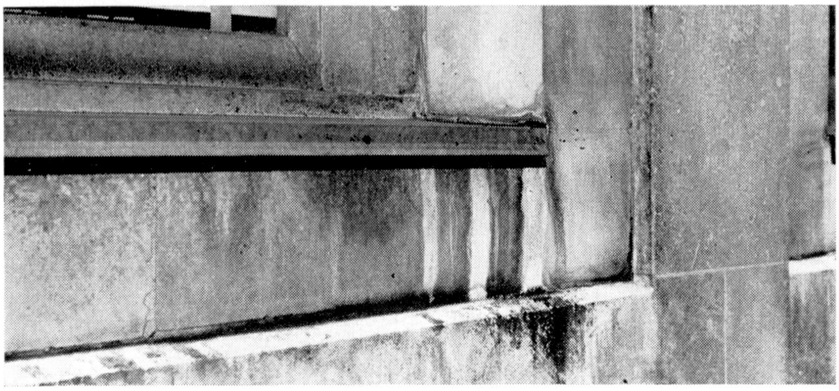

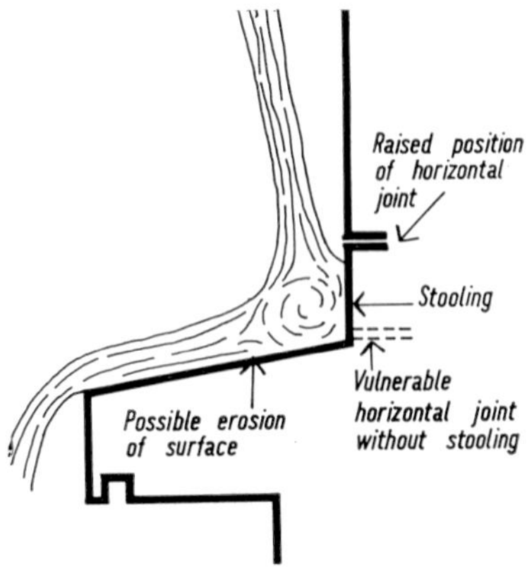


D.3.01/5

*Possible effect of angular downward flow of water at the junction of the top of a projection and the vertical face. (Similar effects may be obtained even when downward flow is perpendicular). Stooling, i.e. 'turning up' of the horizontal surface, is also illustrated*

recessions which occur below may, therefore, receive water at an angle, almost in the form of a 'sheet'. The possible effect of this is the creation of an eddy as shown in diagram D.3.01/5, with the resultant increase in erosion, plus the possibility of an upwards flow, albeit only for a comparatively short distance. The latter would imply an inherent weak point at the junction of the vertical and the horizontal; this junction requires special consideration to prevent any lateral transfer of water due to capillarity. Traditionally this problem was more usually overcome by *stooling* of sills and other projections, that is by ensuring that no joint occurred at the junction of the vertical and horizontal. To do this requires the material of which the projection is composed to be 'turned up' at the junction. This is also shown in the diagram. It should be noted that the advisability of employing the principles used in stooling may be necessary for reasons other than those suggested. For example, when there is any possibility of water remaining at the junction of the horizontal and the vertical for any period of time.

(c) *Returns*

The return of any projection, and particularly the junction of the return and the general vertical face, requires special consideration. Water will, subject to detail, usually flow over the edges of these returns and result in local concentrations, although the major flow will still occur over the forward edge. Thus the assumption that all water will flow over the forward edge may be wrong. The principles to be employed in preventing water flow over edges of returns, based essentially on the formation of a 'tray', are concerned more with details than with generalities. The application of the principle of the tray is illustrated in diagram D.3.01/6, where a window sill has been used as an example, and in which (a) shows the basic condition and problem involved, and (b) a possible solution. The importance of detail cannot be over-stressed. In many cases the use of upstands to the returns to form a tray have not been effective due to 'leakage' which has occurred at the junction of the upstand and the reveal of an opening. The importance of stooling can be seen in those examples which have allowed leakage of water at the junction of a sill and the reveal to the opening, and where the junction has been sealed with a mastic. (See photographs.)

(d) *Exposure of horizontal surfaces and joints*

Although the nature of the top surface of a projection or horizontal recession does influence the pattern of the flow of water, other factors are worthwhile noting. All horizontal surfaces are likely to suffer a greater exposure than vertical surfaces; the materials

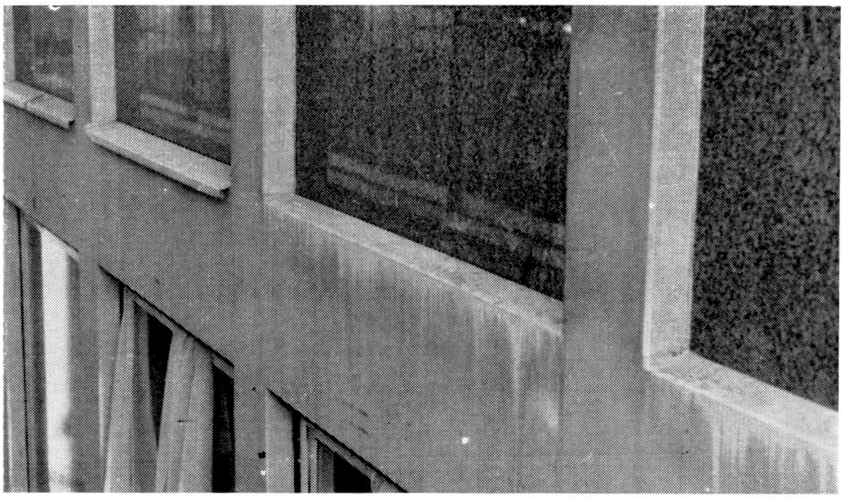

*In the photograph above right the sills incorporated in some of the bays have prevented undue staining and washing; they have also assisted in protecting the inherently weak stone horizontal surface. The picture below shows limewashing of brickwork where water has been allowed to run continuously over the stone projections without any throw off*

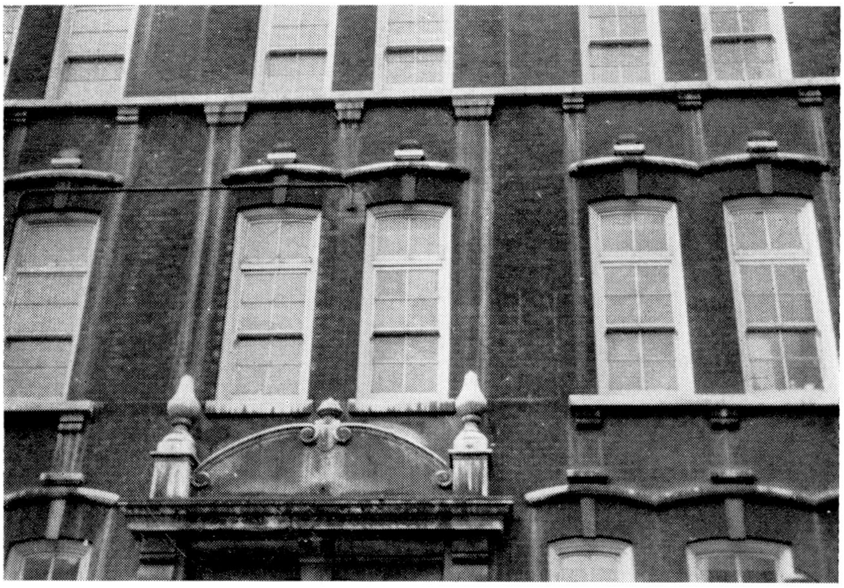

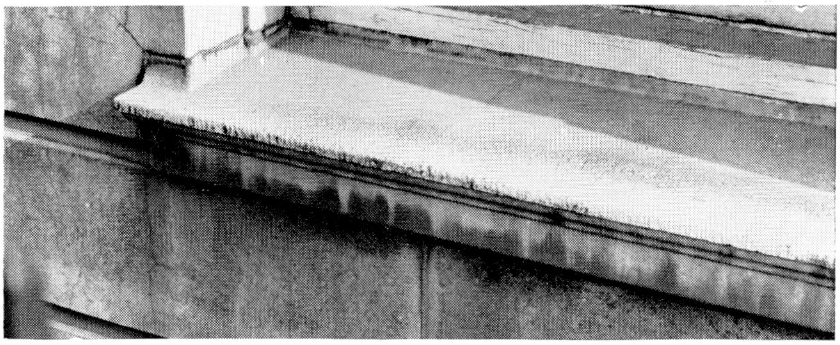

*Right, two examples of stooling of stone sills; the upper is in London atmosphere and is much older than the lower sill which is in a rural atmosphere*

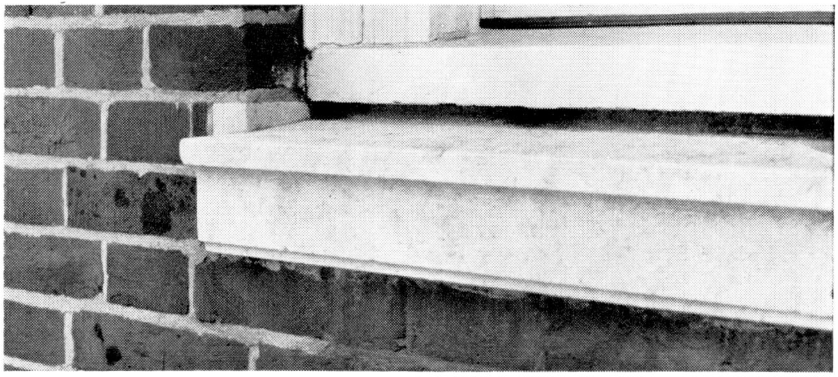

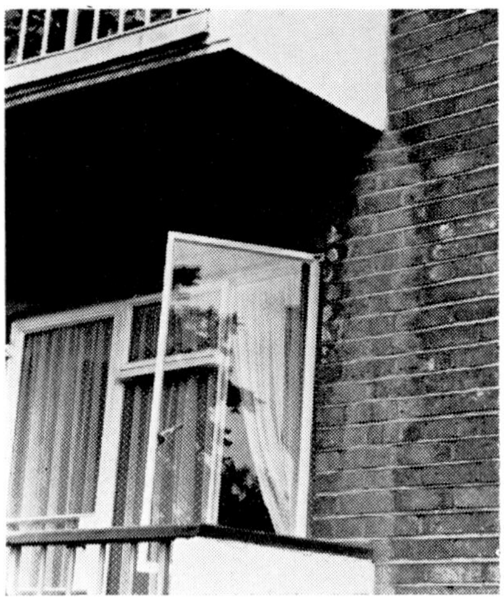

*Limewashing on brickwork as a result of water flowing over balcony upstand*

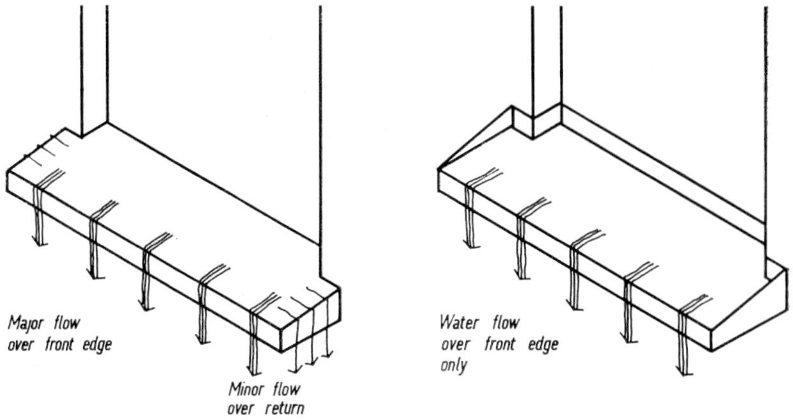


(a) BASIC CONDITION & PROBLEM (b) POSSIBLE SOLUTION - TRAY PRINCIPLE

D.3.01/6 *Application of the 'tray' principle to a window sill to reduce the likelihood of water flowing over the return. (The principle is equally applicable to other forms of projections which have returns)*

*Below, attempts at producing a tray. In the first example no leakage or local concentration of water is visible but similar details elsewhere in the same building show local concentrations very much like those to be seen in the bottom picture which is an example from another building*

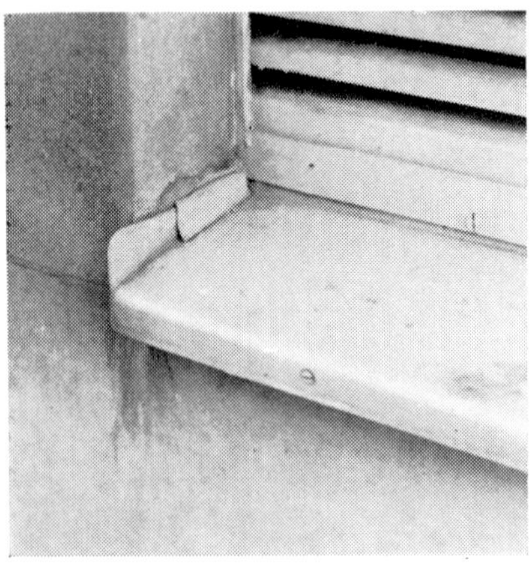

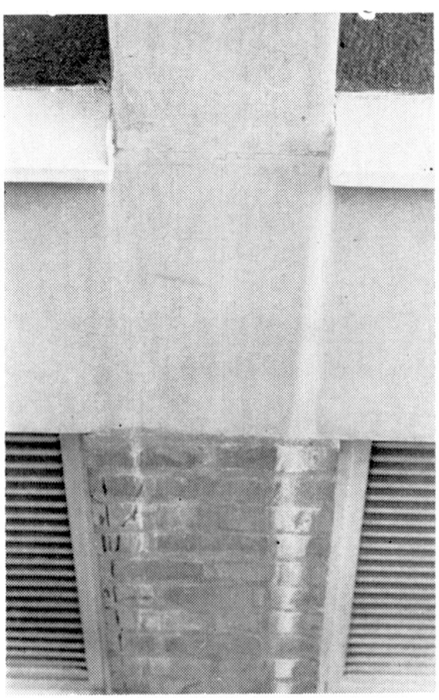

*Below, local concentration at lower junction of box projection and vertical face. No drip to return which in this instance is of little consequence. Solutions require either the use of different materials or changes in elevational treatment—an uncontrolled change of the elevation has in any case occurred as a result of the lines made by lime washing*

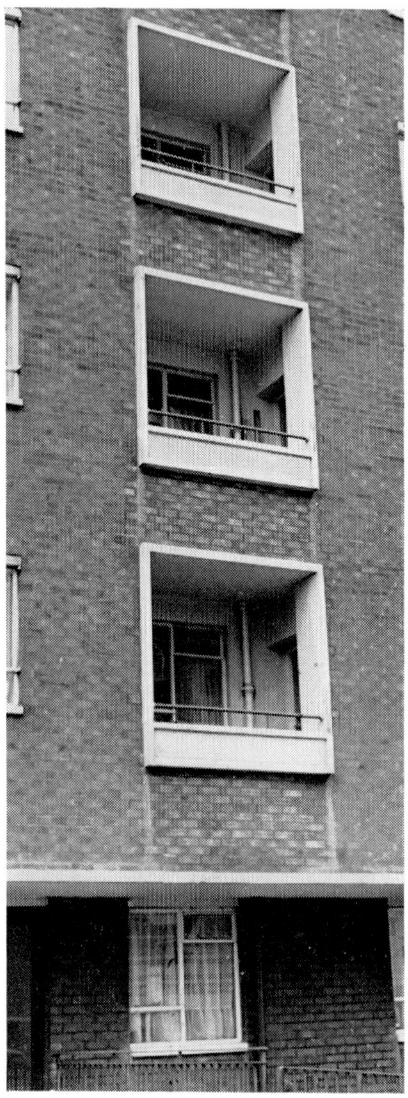

*Below, horizontal surfaces are ideal collectors of dust, dirt, grit and sooty deposits, which may be washed over other surfaces and subsequently deposited to stain as can be seen in the bottom picture where normal weathering has not yet commenced*

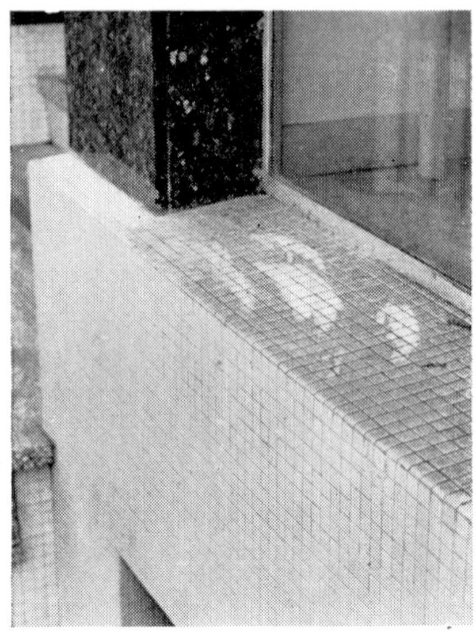

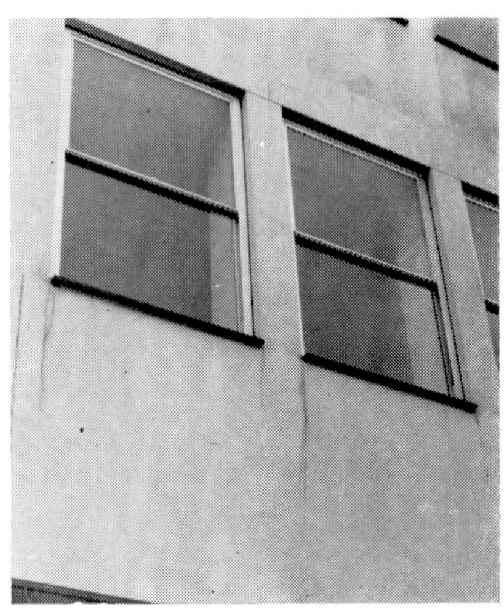

of which they are composed require, accordingly, special consideration. The effects of standing water cannot be overlooked and thus slope is important. Slope is also relevant to rate of flow; shallow slopes encouraging, in general, slower rates of flow.

Joints between units also require special consideration. Localised concentrations of water do occur where joints allow leakage, as can be seen in the photographs, and thus reduce considerably the degree of protection which a projection may otherwise afford.

Finally, horizontal surfaces provide ideal areas for the settlement of dirt, grit, soot, etc. Water flowing uncontrolled over such surfaces, and particularly when this water is not suitably thrown away from the general face of the building, as often occurs with many horizontal recessions, is likely to lead to uncontrolled staining of vertical surfaces. It would appear that if water is thrown clear of a vertical face sufficiently, the staining particles are dispersed adequately enough during the subsequent 'bombardment' of vertical surfaces below any projection so as to reduce considerably the possibilities of staining. It is also possible to regard the 'debris' resulting from erosion in the same way. Wind action may also assist in the dispersal process and thus mitigate the effects of an otherwise shallow projection. Factors such as these often account for the variations of weathering to be found on various faces of the same building with standard projections on each face. The effects of uncontrolled flow due to the omission of suitable projections are illustrated in the photographs.

## Assessment of severity of conditions

### 1. Scope

If materials are to be used to their fullest possible advantage, that is with as little waste as possible—this would appear to be an implied aim in most building work—then it follows that the *known* properties of any one material must be closely related to the conditions to which it is *expected* to be exposed during its working life. The extent to which such advantages may be taken at any given time in the development of building is primarily dependent on the *degree* of accuracy which can be practically achieved in the determination of the variables which are involved. The need for any degree of accuracy in connection with problems associated with water and its effects (as in other fields) will be dependent on a number of factors chief among which are social/economic relationships. Greater advantage in the use of any material also implies the use in some senses of smaller factors of safety. However, as in the case of the mechanical properties of materials (outlined in *Section 2.02* under 'Factor of safety'),

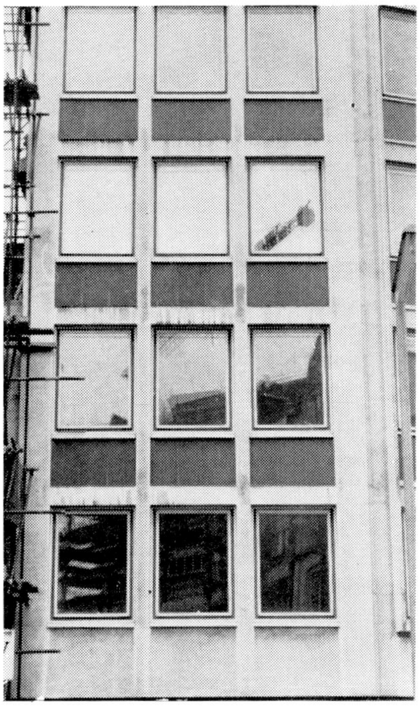

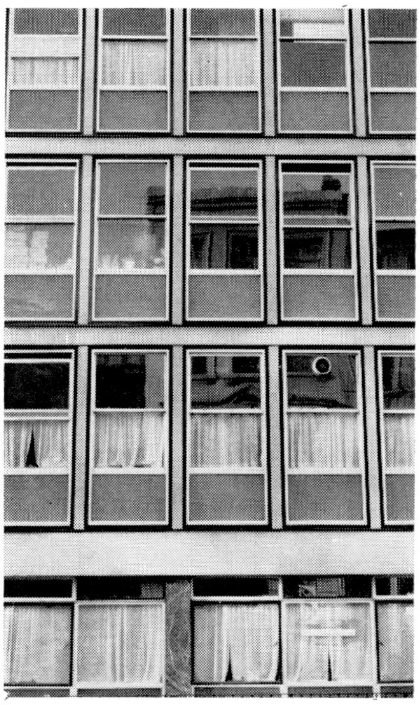

*Uneven 'washing' of the thin horizontal stone bands above the windows may have been averted by the inclusion of a sill as is illustrated by the protection afforded to the stonework under the lower low row of windows and by the example, top right (basically similar but differently 'modelled') where the additional staining of the junction of the horizontal and vertical members has been avoided by recessing the latter. Right, sheltered and unsheltered vertical faces. Note stains appearing under the sill are from humic acid action often found with new Portland stone. Below, failure of sill to allow even throw-off due to insufficient projection relative to levelness of front edge, which is rounded. Photograph was taken during light rainfall. Bottom right, 'flashgap' type detailing which results in no throw-off of water and so 'staining' the stonework (Portland)*

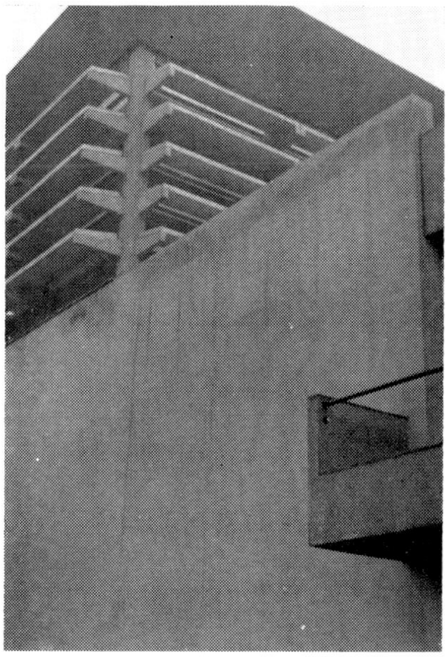

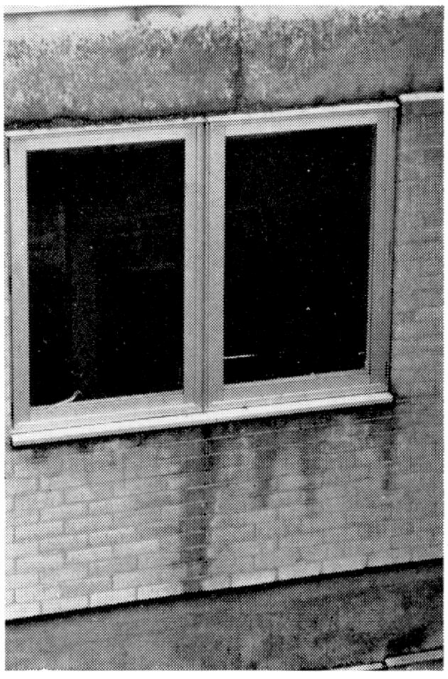

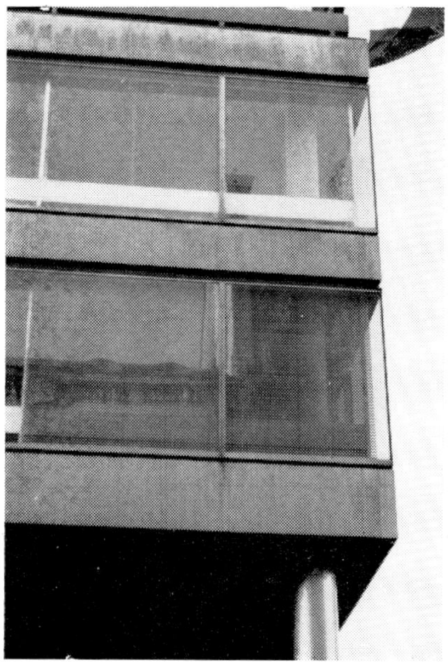

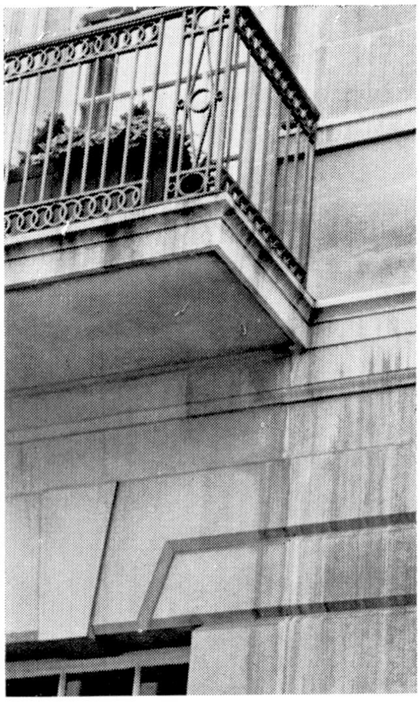

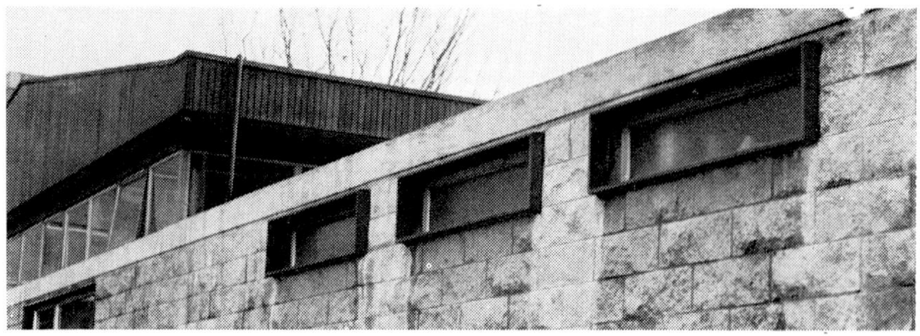

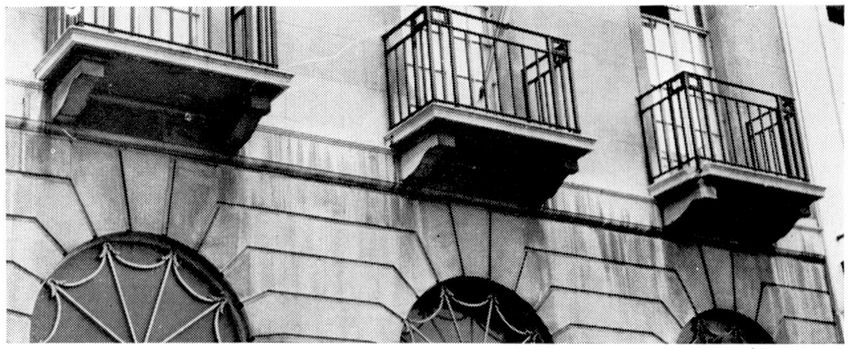

*Shelter provided by projections*

*Below, some examples of local concentrations of water*

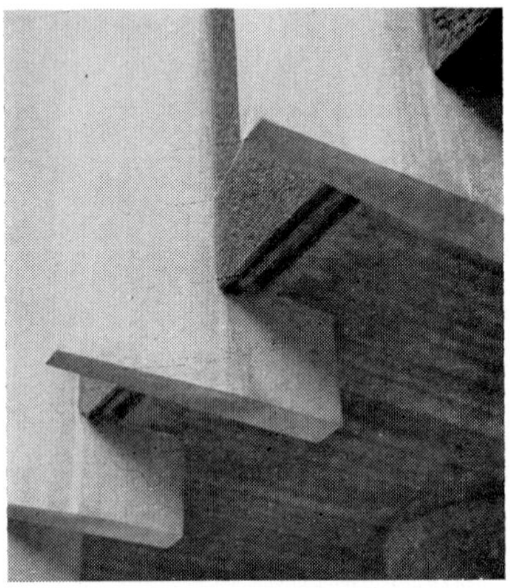

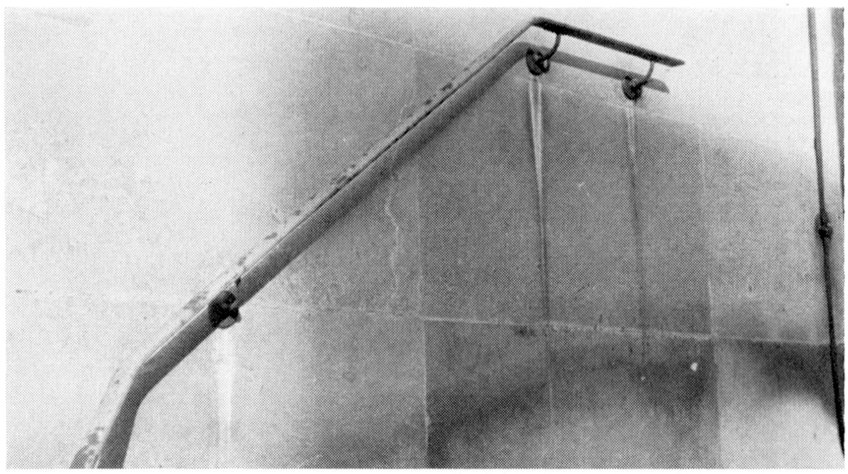

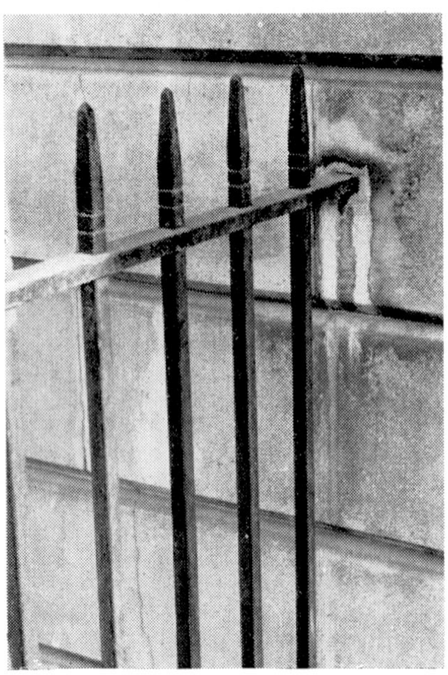

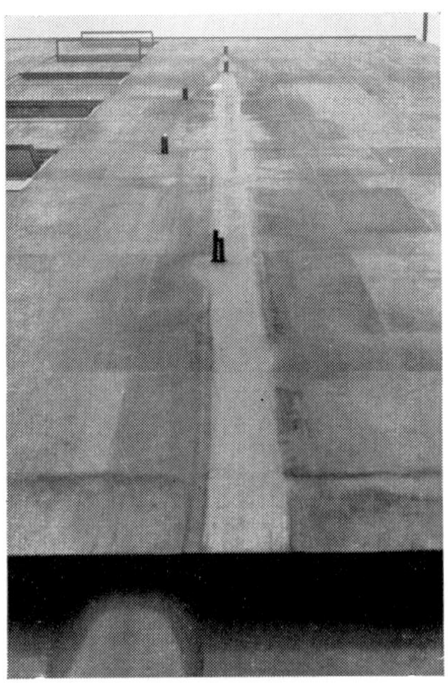

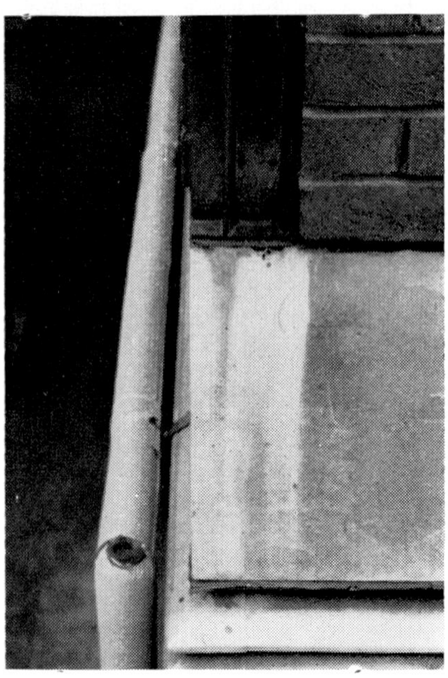

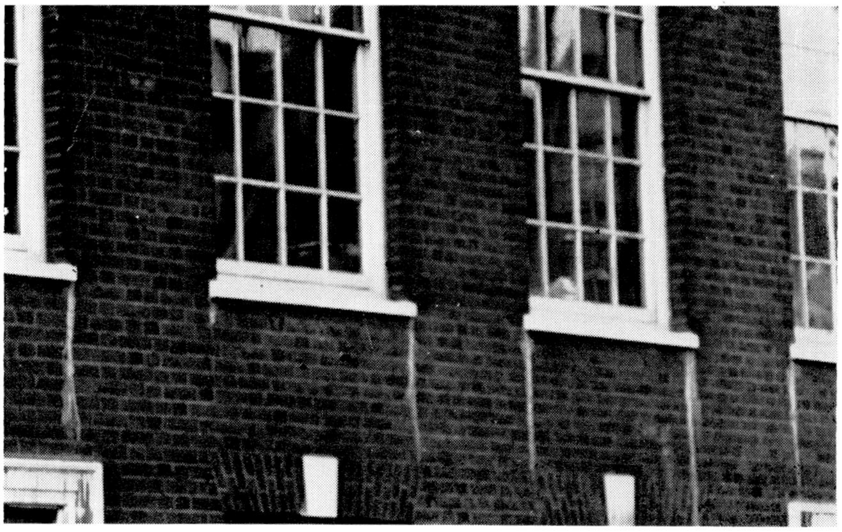

*Local concentration at return to sill*

three criteria, namely knowledge, quality and variations, will be operative in the determination of the actual factor of safety applicable in any given circumstance.

In recent years a need does appear to have arisen for more accurate methods of assessing the severity of conditions than have been generally available. In general terms these have tended to rely far more on practical 'empiricism' resulting essentially in rule-of-thumb methods. Assessment based on 'scientific' empiricism and resulting in quantitative methods of assessing the severity of conditions provide, despite their own limitations, far more reliable guides. Consequently, attempts have been, and continue to be, made to increase the number already available. Compared to the structural mechanical field the development of these methods is more difficult. The purpose of this section is chiefly aimed at drawing attention to some of the problems involved and to some of those methods which are now available. By so doing it is hoped that some understanding might be gained of the reasons for many of the 'gaps' in knowledge, which perforce leads, in many instances, to the use of somewhat generalised statements often strictly qualified. Detailed values are not generally given here, as these are included in those sections to which they essentially belong.

**2. Precedent**

Many of the classifications which have been used in the past included such comparative and descriptive terms as *'severe'*, *'moderate'* or *'sheltered'*. In general terms these are of little practical value, particularly for comparative purposes, unless accompanied by wide experience of the use of a particular material or of a particular location, when it is then possible to take into account variations such as might exist between, for example, macro- and micro-conditions. The number of qualifications necessary, whether by way of general comparison or other means, in order to allow for the widest use of a particular classification, often become misleading. In many cases, however, the key to the difficulty would appear to rest with the non-measurable basis used which generally leads to hazardous guesswork. All classifications are, within limits, only useful as guides, should always be regarded as such and accordingly require intelligent interpretation in all applications. However, in providing guidance they should aim to reduce the amount of guesswork needed to the absolute minimum. Thus classifications become of far greater practical value and far more reliable as guides when they can be related to some quantitative method of measurement. This then allows measurements to be made for a specific building problem on a similar basis to that used for the classification. On the other hand, some of the information necessary to enable a suitable assessment to be made may very well be obtainable from other published sources.

The use of quantitative methods of assessment, particularly those based on calculation, are more common (and have been for a considerable time) in structural mechanical work in which the shape and size of members are determined, in general terms that is, by relating stress analysis to the mechanical properties of materials. In the newer sciences associated, for instance, with the use of thermal and acoustic properties of materials, great reliance is also placed on the use of methods of calculation. Although the methods used in these fields may prove on the whole to be fairly reliable, in addition to overcoming many of the hazards of guesswork, they are not necessarily practical or feasible when considering problems associated with water and its effects. Revaluation leading to certain modifications of known methods and, in a sense, innovations are usually necessary.

**3. Difficulties**

There are a variety of reasons why a different approach is necessary when dealing with water and its effects, but chief among these would appear to be the difficulty of resolving the many factors involved in terms of methods of calculation. On the other hand, to be of any significant value a method of assessment based on quantitative methods of measurement must also be capable of being related to methods of measuring the related properties of materials and other factors. Among other things, the units of measurement used are usually required to be the same in all cases or, if not the same, at least capable of being related to each other simply.* In many cases methods of assessment are, or could be, easily made available but these may not have been adequately related to the properties of materials or, for that matter, to buildings as a whole. Finally, the requisite properties of all types of materials may not be available—in the past there may not have been the need to have available values of such properties.

**4. Examples**

Among the examples included, the one on 'Rain penetration', developed by the Meteorological Office and the BRS, is described in detail in order to illustrate the difficulties which are normally encountered in devising quantitative methods of assessment and the manner in which these are being overcome. The remainder are dealt with in general terms and, where necessary, 'gaps' in knowledge are highlighted.

*Simplicity would appear to be an essential requirement of any methods used if such methods are to find wide acceptance amongst designers and many others associated with practical building problems.

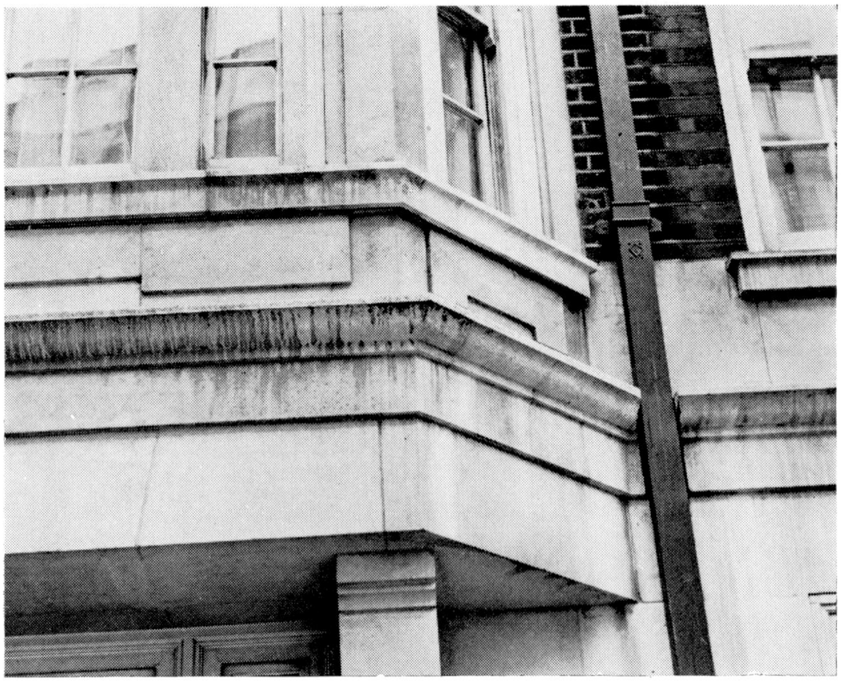

*Change in exposure does influence weathering patterns as can be seen in this example where the modelling is identical to the front and oblique return*

*Horizontal surfaces usually suffer greater exposure than vertical surfaces, and should not hold water for longer than necessary. The picture, below right, illustrates standing water, while the left-hand picture shows the erosion to stonework due to 'waterfall' effects and 'bombardment' by rainwater drops*

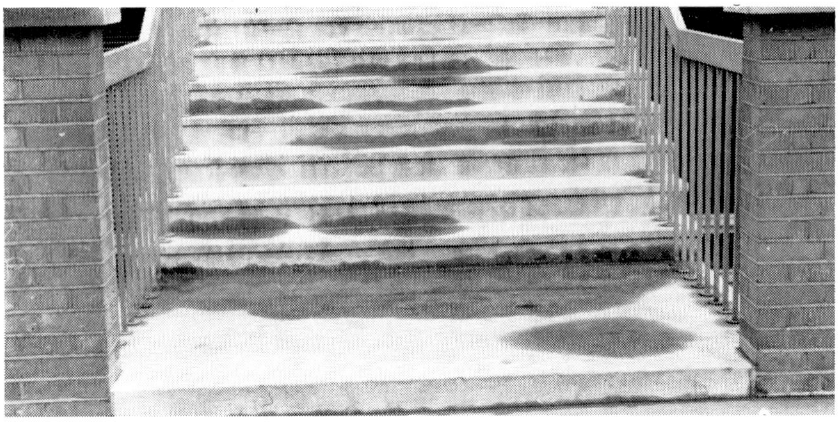

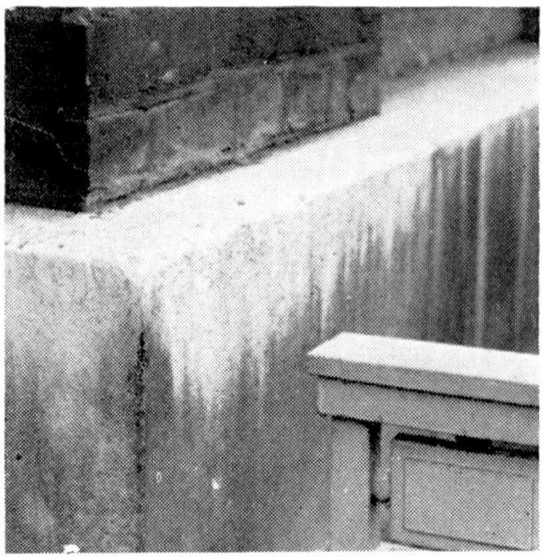

*Below, two examples of the failure of joints in the horizontal surface resulting in local concentrations of water under the joint*

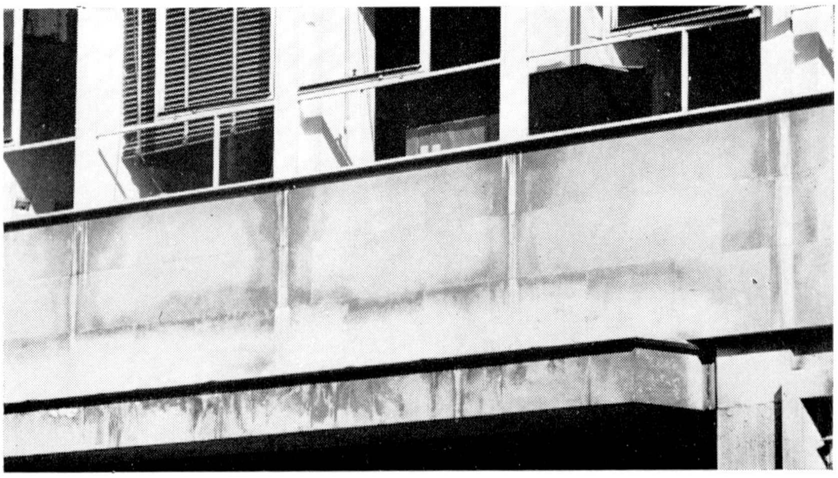

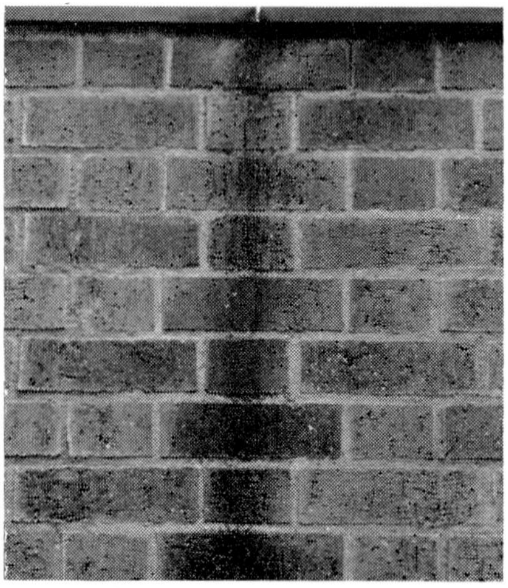

(a) *Rain penetration*

There is a great deal of climatic data available on the elements involved such as rainfall, wind, sunshine, etc., covering many stations throughout the country and in some cases measured over a long period of time. (The time element is important if more accurate forecasts of probable future conditions are to be made.) All these elements are significant when considering, for example, the exclusion of rainwater from a building. However, the methods of measurement, made separately for each element, are seldom if ever undertaken by meteorological authorities so that they may be directly related to the way in which they influence the properties of materials or, as important, the way in which they 'act' on buildings. As an example consider driving rain, that is wind-driven rain, usually carried at an angle so that it impinges on vertical surfaces. This is of far greater importance in making an assessment of the severity of exposure conditions than the amount of rain falling on level ground, as obtained from normal rainfall measurements. In order to make such an assessment of the measure of the severity of exposure it is necessary to know the direction and speed of the wind during any given intensity of rain together with the amounts 'collected' from the vertical faces of buildings. Other factors such as raindrop size and the angle of incidence which vary from rainstorm to rainstorm are also significant. Following investigations into the amount of rain collected from the vertical faces of buildings and other related data, it has been shown that the amount of rain driven on to a wall is directly proportional to the product of the rainfall recorded on level ground and the wind speed during the rain. Thus, once the values of the two elements are known, it is then possible to determine the severity of conditions of exposure which might obtain on a quantitative basis, by the use of a suitable index.

In view of the fact that wind speeds are not normally recorded simultaneously with rainfall, it was proposed to utilise existing available information, and to formulate an index of driving rain, on an annual basis, using annual average rainfall and annual average wind speed data. The resultant index is measured in $m^2/s$, this being the product of the annual rainfall in millimetres and average wind-speed in m/s divided by 1 000. From available information it is assumed that this expedient does not distort the overall picture, and is therefore as reliable as can be currently expected. The index for any particular location indicates the amount of rain which would be driven on to the vertical face of a building in an average year. Although it is appreciated that the worst rain penetration occurs during the most severe storms, the index applicable in such circumstances is unlikely to exceed one quarter of the mean annual index. From the contoured map produced of the British Isles indicating the variations in the index which occur over the whole country, an exposure grading has been determined.* Thus *'sheltered'* areas are now those with an index of $3m^2/s$ or less; *'moderately exposed'* areas have an index of between 3 and $7m^2/s$, while *'severely exposed'* areas have an index of $7m^2/s$ and above. The chief limitation of this map is that it deals with the macro-climatic condition while reasonable interpolation between the contours of indices varying from 2·5 to 20 may not be possible. In order to assess the changes in the micro-climatic condition account must be taken of the effect of variations in topography, proximity to the coast, adjoining buildings, height, etc. Some rules have, therefore, been laid down where, in the absence of the requisite measurements for actual sites, suitable modification of the classification of sheltered, moderate and severe exposure conditions may be made.

The annual driving-rain index succeeds in general to overcome some of the problems associated with the assessment of the severity of conditions to rain penetration. Among other things it does at least offer a useful and more direct method of comparison in that one site with which a designer, for example, may be familiar can be compared with another with which he is unfamiliar. However, the stage has not yet been reached when the properties of materials, particularly in terms of construction, have been related to the various driving rain indices. In this must be included the difficulties associated with the large amounts of water which may be shed from impervious surfaces of materials. Answers to these and other similar problems are for the future.

It should be pointed out that in addition to the map of annual driving-rain index contours, a map has also been prepared showing for 23 stations the annual *relative* driving-rain index for each of eight wind directions. This map contains what are termed 'driving rain roses'. Each 'rose' indicates the proportion of the total index attributable to winds from different directions, and enables an assessment to be made of the faces of buildings liable to be more heavily exposed than others. Both maps are included in *3·02 Exposure*, under 'Rain', diagrams D.3.02/2 and 3.

(b) *Dampness and adhesion*

The measurement of moisture content of materials and the significance of such measurements in the adhesive processes in buildings have already been outlined in this section under the heading of 'Dampness', p. 14. At this point it may be noted that even such general methods of assessment which are available would not be of very much practical value unless the degree of dampness which any of the adhesive processes can 'tolerate' without failure was established. The practicality of the available methods is still to a certain extent limited by the fact that not all the adhesive processes have been fully investigated.

(c) *Sulphate attack*

Among the chemical attacks on materials which have received particular attention is that related to sulphate attack of cement products used below ground level. In this a classification of soil conditions* has been developed in which there are five classes, each based on a stipulated concentration of sulphur trioxide. Precautionary measures which are advisable relative to each of the five basic concentrations and to the type of product concerned have been put forward. It is therefore important that an analysis of the sulphate content of any soil is undertaken so that the necessary measures may be taken to avoid attack. The classification is a useful and simply presented guide. (Sulphate attack is discussed in detail in *Section 3.06*.)

(d) *Atmospheric pollution*

On the whole, atmospheric pollution plays an important part in chemical attack on a variety of materials. Classifications intended to act as guides for the severity of conditions are still general in character and in descending order of pollution are usual given as:† (1) industrial and heavily polluted urban areas; (2) normal urban areas; (3) coastal areas; and (4) rural areas. None of these classes takes into account the increase in the severity of conditions often caused by micro-climatic conditions or of the proximity of the source of pollution. In part this is due to the lack of sufficient quantitative measurements of the degree of atmospheric pollution throughout the country‡ which could then possibly be related to the resistance to deterioration by chemical means which may be expected from various materials. Some guidance is available on the rate of corrosion of mild steel and zinc coatings on steel relative to the four classes of atmospheres quoted above. The rates of corrosion used in conjunction with tables of thickness of steel plate or of zinc coatings enable *an estimation* to be made of the thickness required for

*A detailed description of the method of the preparation of this map and the one illustrating 'rain-roses' together with the problems associated with the formulation and use of the index by Lacy, R. E. (BRS) and Shellard, H. C. (Met. Office), *An Index of Driving Rain*, Meteorological Magazine, July 1962, Vol. 91, No. 1080, pp. 177–184. BRS Digest (2nd Series) No. 23, 'An Index of Exposure to Driving Rain', describes the development of the index, formulates three exposure gradings, indicates the factors which are likely to influence the basic exposure gradings and notes the limitations of the application of the index to practical building.

*Reference: Table 1 in Concrete in *Sulphate-bearing Soils and Groundwaters*, BRS Digest (2nd series) No. 90, HMSO, Feb. 1968.

†Reference: Appendix VI, *Durability*, BS Code of Practice, CP3—Chapter IX (1950).

‡Measurement of atmospheric pollution has in the past been generally confined to the essentially severely polluted areas. Measurements are now being taken throughout the country since the introduction of the national survey on air pollution. Results now available have yet to be correlated.

a given life. The rates of corrosion may also be used to estimate the life of a given thickness of metal, with or without a coating.

(e) *Dimensional fluctuations*

An assessment of the extent of dimensional fluctuations in porous materials due to changes in their moisture content is necessary if the basic shape and size of any member or element, usually determined by other factors, is to be suitably modified so as to limit distortion or prevent the likelihood of cracking taking place. In the main modifications, in addition to changes in the basic dimensions, including area, usually involve the use of movement joints. In this the detailed relationship of two or more elements of different materials may be important.

Among the factors relative to the properties of individual materials which may influence the extent of change likely in any given situation are relative humidity, thermal conditions and air movement of the environment. Most of the information—and there is quite a considerable amount available—on the dimensional changes to be expected in various materials is generally related to relative humidity. It is, therefore, necessary for some estimation to be made of the effect of the other factors involved. Because of these and other difficulties in making the necessary calculations, rule-of-thumb methods, particularly for the 'traditional' materials, are more often used and usually found to be fairly reliable as guides. However, this may not necessarily be true of the newer materials, in which case results based on calculations, despite their own limitations, generally provide sufficient guidance to enable an assessment to be made of the necessity or otherwise of taking precautions. Where it is desired to limit the actual dimensions of any movement joint it is important to take into account the limitations of the calculations. Accordingly, it is always advisable to incorporate a suitable factor of safety. In most cases this means adding a suitable amount to the calculated size.

# 3.02 exposure

All materials are liable, in varying degrees, to exposure to water, from commencement through to completion and during the life of a building. The degree of exposure, that is the severity of conditions under which materials will have to perform, is a primary factor to be considered prior to the selection, use and maintenance of suitable materials and related forms of construction which would include assembly in its broadest sense. An assessment of the severity of conditions requires, among other things, a clear understanding of the source of water relative to a particular element or part of a building together with an indication of the nature, that is the degree of pollution, of the water relative to the source involved.

The purpose of this section is mainly concerned with an examination of those factors which affect the *basic exposure* of materials to water. It therefore excludes the detailed consideration of those factors which may alter this basic exposure, particularly within a material or construction. These together with the principles of the methods which may be adopted to exclude water are covered in *3·04 Exclusion*. Similarly there is no detailed consideration of the resistances which various materials may offer to water, as these are more conveniently included under the specialised headings of the other sections which follow later.

Although a particular source of water and the degree to which it may be polluted are closely interrelated insofar as the performance of materials is concerned, it does not always follow that the pollution of the given source of water will always be the same either in composition or in concentration. It is, therefore, considered more appropriate to deal with (1) the sources of water under one general heading and (2) the pollution of water under another. An indication is given of the significance, mechanics and where relevant the concentration of both the source of the water and the source of the pollution. The manner in which these are related in terms of building practice is also noted.

## Sources of water

Building materials may, subject to the position in which they are included in a building, be effected by water derived from a variety of sources. In many cases the source of water is indicative of those parts of a building likely to be primarily effected. Thus one particular source may not affect all parts of a building at all times during its life, while some may only be relevant during the period of construction of a building, or, in relation to the life of buildings, for a comparatively short period after completion.

For convenience, the various sources of water have been subdivided into the following headings: (1) Rain; (2) Ground; (3) During construction; (4) Atmosphere; (5) Water supply; (6) Faulty services; and (7) Maintenance and general usage. Each of these is dealt with separately. It may be noted here that all these with the exception of 'Water supply' are sources of dampness and were, therefore, included previously in *Section 3.01* 'Dampness' but without any of the elaboration given in this section.

### 1. Rain

The elements of a building which are usually associated with exposure to rainwater are those which make up the external fabric of the envelope of the building above ground and consisting of walls and roofs. One of the functional requirements of these elements, amongst others which are also important, is to prevent the penetration of rain. Another, in which rainwater is concerned, is related to changes in appearance of the exposed surfaces of the materials of which the external elements are composed. Of these two, it is perhaps understandable that prevention of rain penetration is usually regarded as the most important. However, in the long term, it is as well to note that some changes of appearance, implying as they do changes in either the physical or chemical nature of the materials concerned, that is decay and deterioration, may take place.

When considering the exposure of

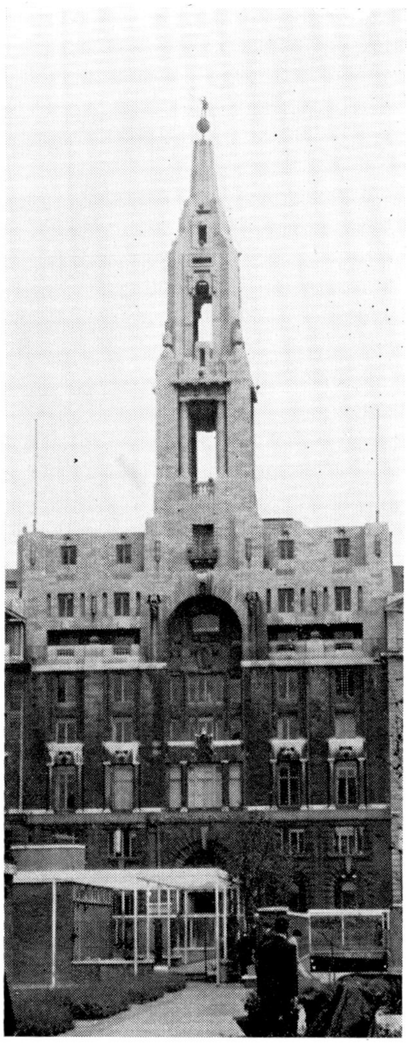

*Changes in the degree of exposure of any element or part of a building to water, whatever the source, are important in all assessments of the severity of conditions. This example illustrates, in general terms, changes in exposure conditions of an external element relative to one particular source of water, namely rain. The more severely exposed surfaces of the Portland stone are 'washed' clean while those which are relatively sheltered retain the dirt and grime encountered in a polluted urban atmosphere*

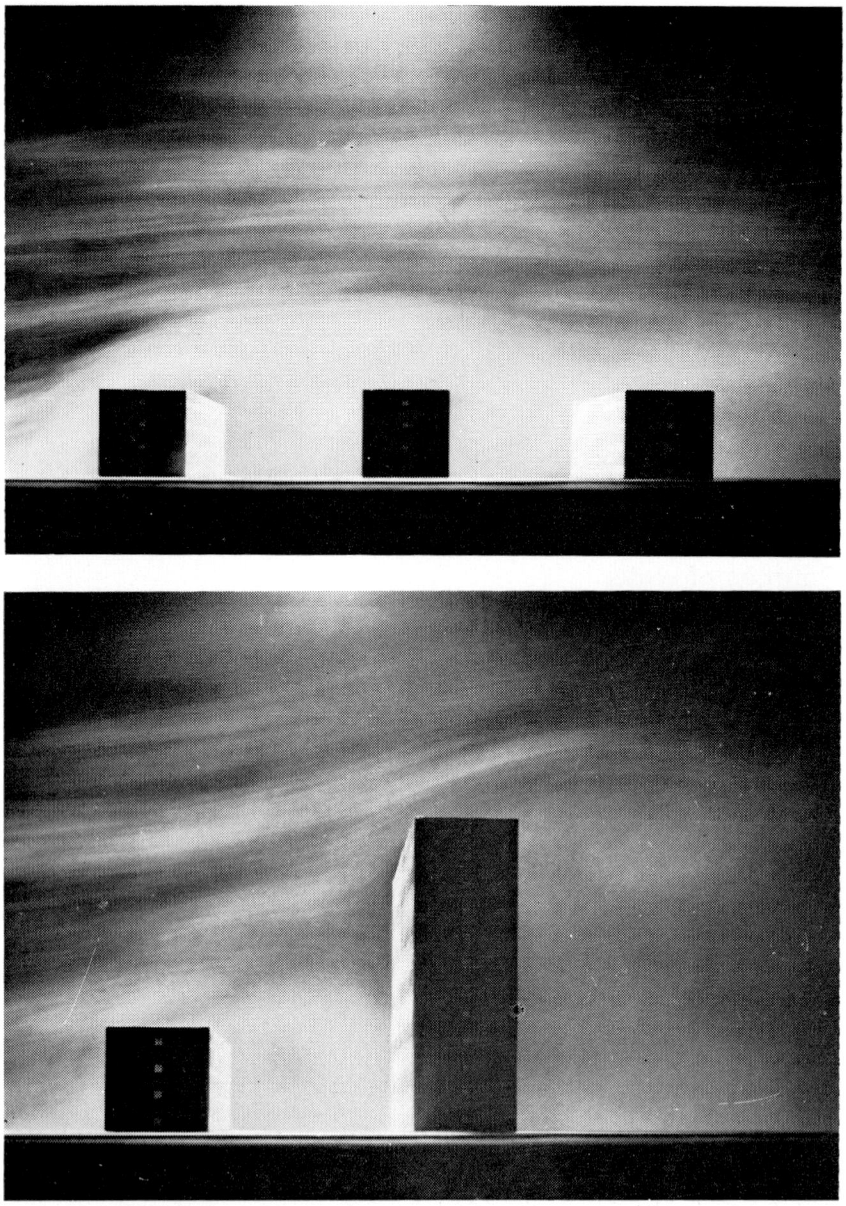

*Photographs of smoke visualisation tests carried out in the BRS wind tunnel showing the effects of low building and, bottom picture, high building on the wind flow pattern (Courtesy: BRS)*

the external elements of a building to rainwater a number of variable factors must be taken into account. These are all interrelated to some extent and may be broken down into the following general headings: (a) The meaning of 'rain penetration'; (b) The significance of wind; (c) Basic exposure of a site; (d) Effects of building design; and (e) Portrait of a building.

(a) *The meaning of 'rain penetration'*

Mention has been made of the fact that one of the functional requirements of the external fabric of a building is to prevent rain penetration. It is normal to consider the problems associated with rainwater in this general way. However, in practice, and taking into account the variability of the properties of the various materials which are available to make up the respective elements of which the external fabric is composed, it is better and more realistic to consider the extent to which the penetration of rainwater should be *controlled*. The exposed surfaces, that is those facing on to the rain, provide the lines of demarcation, so to speak, beyond which the penetration of water should be controlled. This does not in any way conflict with the reasons behind the necessity for the prevention of rain penetration, which are essentially aimed to maintain dry conditions, (i) for human health and (ii) to control the deterioration, physical or chemical, of materials, surface and/or interior, used to make up the external fabric, or others which may be closely associated with it. (With reference to the last reason, it may also be noted here that dampness in certain materials often results in the undesirable reduction in their thermal properties.) None of these reasons requires that the whole thickness of the external fabric should necessarily remain dry at all times.

The extent to which water may be allowed to penetrate past the exposed surface of materials will be dependent on a number of factors, but one of the most important of these is concerned with the 'absorption/evaporation' performance of the materials. (The time element, that is the period during which dampness may persist, is of primary importance.) This immediately allows a distinction to be drawn between (1) *the porous materials* which allow absorption and evaporation, although the quantities involved in each type of material are subject to wide variations, and (2) *the impervious materials* which, in the present context, do not absorb water. Thus control of the penetration of rainwater into porous materials is necessary.

The necessity of the *use of joints* in virtually all materials, whether porous or impervious, requires that special attention should be given to this aspect of an element as a whole. It is extremely common to find that control of penetration of rainwater has been defeated by 'leakage' through the joints.

In the case of *porous materials*, leakage may occur literally through the joints of cladding units using no jointing medium, that is a dry jointing system, as in traditional tiled roofs or tiled wall hanging or as more recently in large-scale claddings; on the other hand, where a jointing medium is used, such as in brick- or blockwork or other large-scale unit systems, structural or otherwise, leakage may occur through the material of which the joint is composed, although it is more common for the weakness to occur at the interface of the jointing material and the unit being joined, due to a loss of adhesion.

In the case of the *impervious materials*, watertightness of the joint between units is of fundamental importance if there is to be no penetration of rainwater. Where joints are designed to allow leakage, then suitable drainage is implied. With impervious materials and especially the metals it is always important to avoid the possibility of water being held in joints or other crevices, unless suitable protective measures have been taken. In roofs the use of interlocking and other methods for effecting a watertight joint do, on the whole, appear to have been more effective than composite joints relying, in many cases, on the efficiency of mastics, used for vertical surfaces of walls. (Here it is appreciated that the methods of jointing used for roofing are not necessarily applicable to vertical surfaces. It must also be noted that in many cases the failure of the 'mastic' joint can very often be related to incorrect choice or detailed use or, as important, to lack of maintenance.)

(b) *The significance of wind*

In *Section 3.01* ('Assessment of severity of conditions', 4. Example (a) 'Rain penetration') the significance of wind in connection with the formulation of the 'Index to driving-rain' has been outlined. For completeness it is desirable to include in this section, in greater detail, some of the aspects previously covered.

One of the fundamental effects of wind during rain is to change the direction of the fall of water. In building terms this implies the deflection of water so that it impinges on vertical surfaces. In the absence of any wind, something which may occur in isolated cases, rain would fall completely perpendicularly. Thus water would only impinge on horizontal or sloping surfaces, while vertical surfaces would be sheltered. A diagrammatic representation of this relative to a section through a hypothetical building is shown in (1) of diagram D.3.02/1. It should be noted that the vertical surfaces only remain sheltered if the water collected by the horizontal or sloping surfaces is adequately drained and therefore prevented from flowing over the vertical surfaces. The effect of wind blowing during rain is shown in the comparative diagram (2) from which it will be seen that, in addition to the horizontal and sloping surfaces, the vertical surfaces facing the wind now receive rainwater. The diagram also serves to illustrate the fact that the run-off from vertical surfaces will increase the load, that is the exposure, of any abutting horizontal or sloping surfaces, unless of course the run-off load is drained away separately.

The diagrams used, it should be appreciated, are an over-simplification but they do illustrate the principle involved. No account has been taken of wind-speed and precise direction, nor the effect of the profile of the building on the 'shape' of the wind flow around the building. Wind-speed is important in determining the basic exposure, as is discussed later. The direction of the wind influences the faces of the building which will be exposed. In diagram (2) and assuming a rectangular building, two faces are likely to be exposed. Both wind-speed and direction are likely to change either during a particular fall of rain or, more important, during rainfalls occurring at different times. In this seasonal variations are important. Another factor which is likely to cause those surfaces which may be potentially sheltered (as shown in (2) for instance) to become exposed, are the effects of the shape of the building on wind flow. Such flow patterns may also be important when the rain has ceased (water may still be flowing down surfaces) but the wind is still blowing. An indication of some of the effects of the profile of a building on wind flow patterns is shown in the accompanying photographs. The examples which the photographs illustrate were not intended specifically for driving-rain studies but nevertheless they do appear to substantiate the basic principles being outlined. In addition they also give some indication of the possibilities of upward flow of water

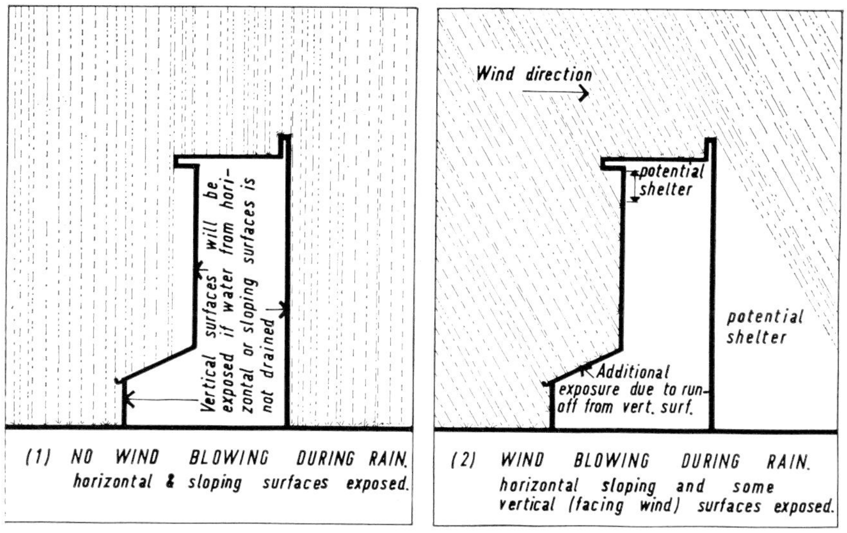


*D.3.02/1 Diagrammatic representation of the basic effect of wind during rain relative to the exposure of horizontal sloping and vertical surfaces using the section through a hypothetical building*

*The angular direction of rain, due to the action of wind, can be seen in the photograph below as white streaks against the roof guardrail and the facing windows. Bottom picture, an example illustrating the manner in which rainwater splashing on vertical surfaces manifests itself when horizontal and vertical surfaces abut one another*

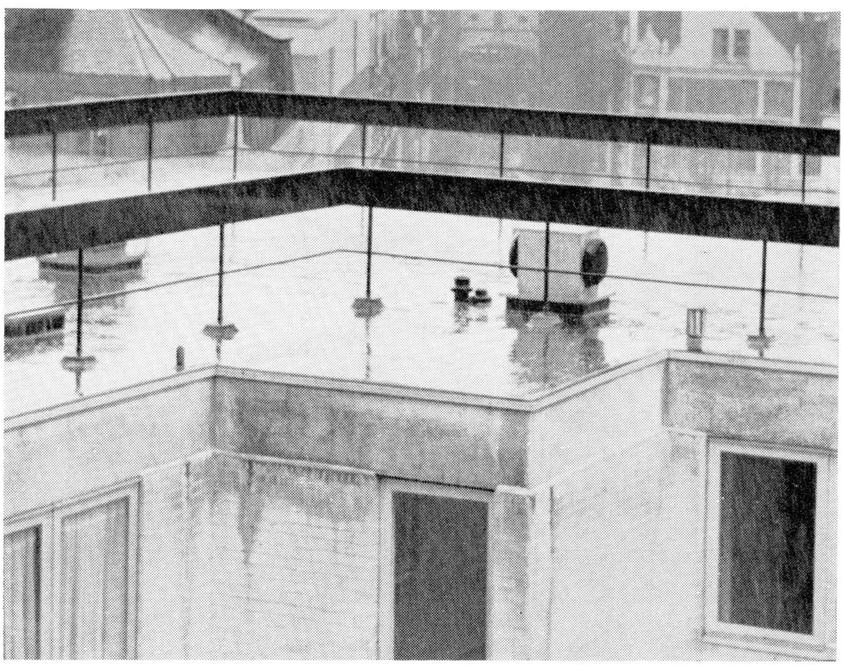

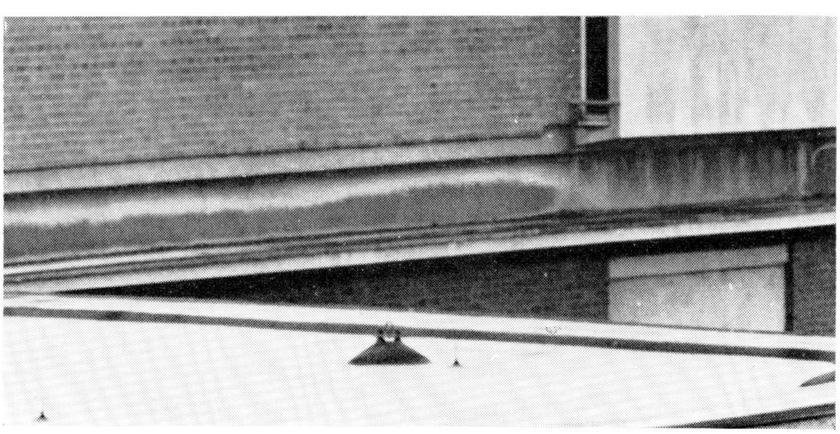



c

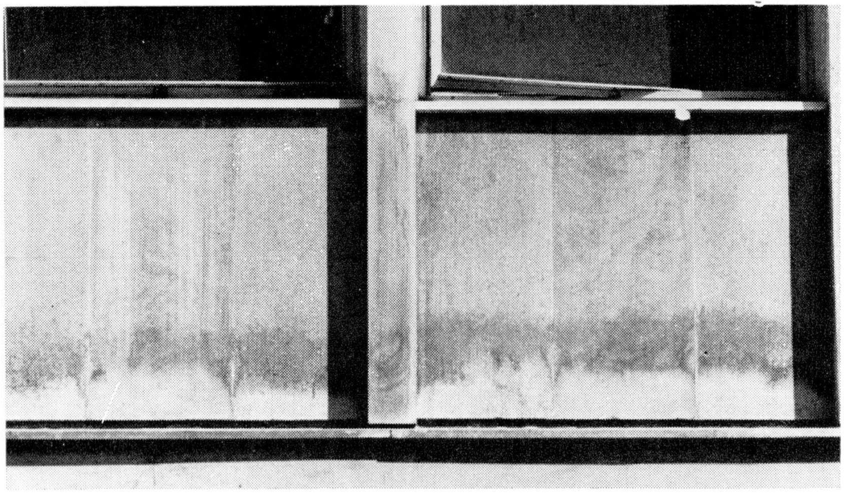

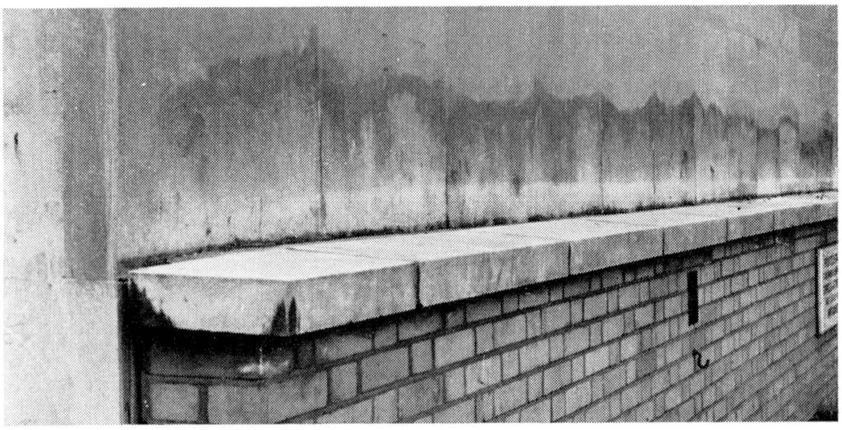

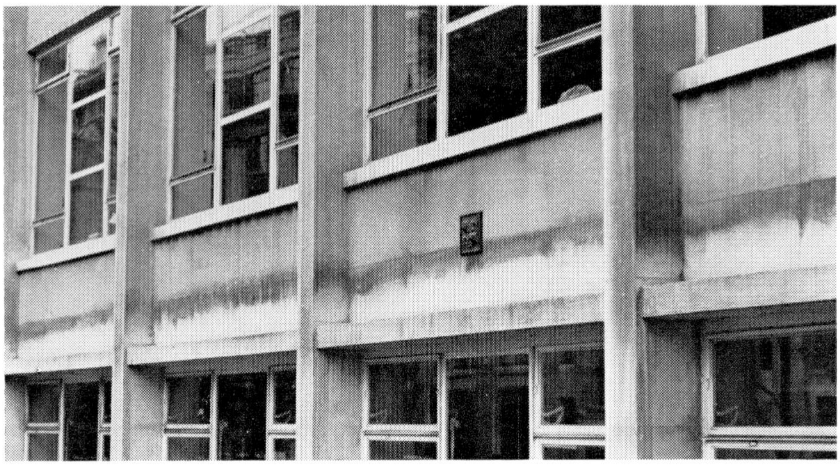

*Three more examples illustrating the manner in which rainwater splashing on vertical surfaces manifests itself when horizontal and vertical surfaces abut one another. With porous materials there is also a vertical rise of water as shown by the 'tide' marks generally above the clean zone in these stonework examples*

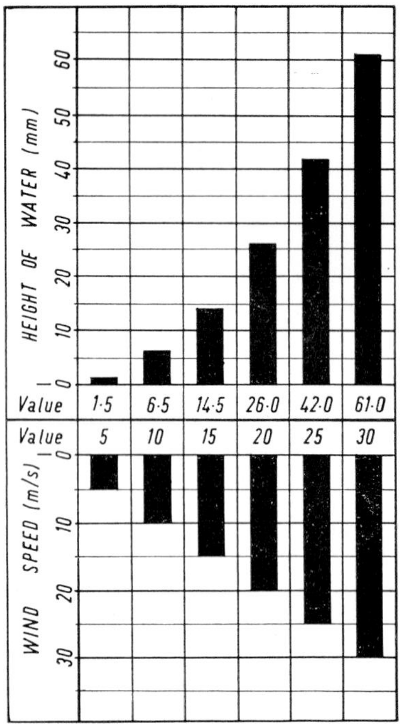


*C.3.02/1*
*Relation between wind-speed and height of a water column which can be supported. (Reference: 'Principles of Modern Building', Vol. II, p. 103, HMSO, 1961)*

on vertical faces, in which case joints and junctions require special consideration. It is also possible to see how wind may result in the *scouring* of the surfaces of materials used in vertical planes of buildings. Such scouring effects are greatly increased when rainwater contains abrasive material, usually derived from polluted atmospheres.

There is another aspect of wind occurring during rain particularly applicable to *roofs* (sloping or flat) and related to the fact that water may be driven uphill by wind into joints and over upstands, and the fact that wind exerts pressure. The pressure exerted by wind is capable of supporting a column of water, the height of which is dependent on the wind speed. The relationship between wind speeds of from 5 to 30m/s and the height of a water column which can be supported at various speeds in the range is given in the comparative chart C.3.02/1. From the values given in this chart it is possible to calculate the size of lap or upstand necessary during rain accompanied by a particular wind speed. If, for example, the design condition is taken to be 20m/s, then the laps in the pitched roof or the upstand joints in a flat roof would have to be of sufficient size to avoid a head of water of 26mm to cause leakage. In other words, a head of water of more than 26mm would have to be capable of moving upwards before leakage occurred. It is perhaps unnecessary to emphasise that the worst condition to be expected (including sudden variations which may take place over a short period of time) must be used as the design condition. For convenience, it may be noted here that the dimensions of laps and upstands are governed by tradition. However, there is some evidence to suggest that these may be excessive and therefore changed, in which case the future use of the values given in the chart, together with other available information, may be fully exploited.

The run-off from vertical surfaces will add to the load of water on any abutting horizontal or sloping surfaces, as indicated in diagram D.3.02/1 (2). However, wind may assist in causing the water flowing over the sloping or horizontal surfaces to be 'whipped up' and in this way cause splashing of the vertical surface at or near the junction with the horizontal or sloping surfaces. Pavings abutting vertical surfaces at ground level must also be included in this consideration. Splashing does, therefore, tend to increase the exposure

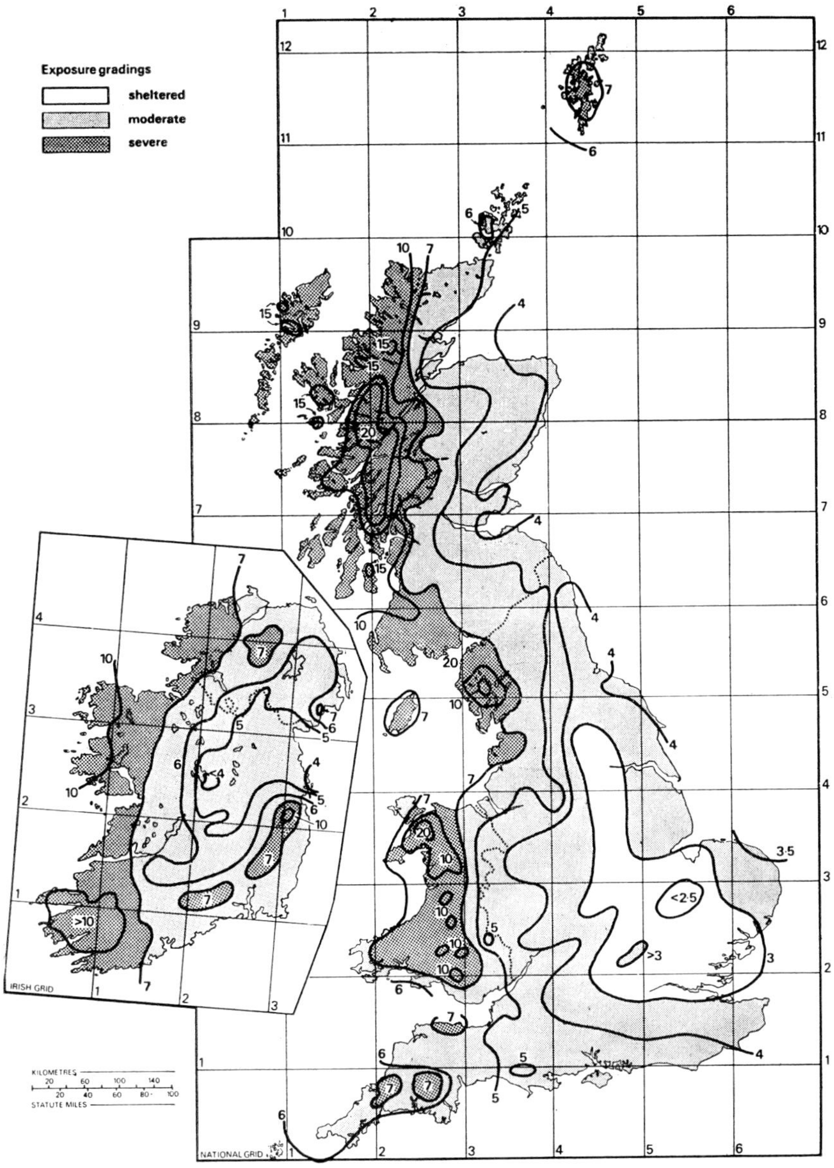


*D.3.02/2*
*Annual driving-rain index for the British Isles (units: m²s). Read with Table 3.02/1 (From: 'An Index of Exposure to Driving Rain', BRS Digest 127, Fig. 1, p. 3, March 1971 (Crown Copyright))*

of parts of vertical surfaces.The accompanying photographs indicate the manner in which splashing may manifest itself, and have been included to illustrate that splashing increases exposure.

(c) *Basic exposure of a site*

The annual driving-rain indices for the British Isles (diagram D.3.02/2) and the driving-rain 'roses' attributable to wind from different directions at 23 places* (diagram D.3.02/3) are, as already outlined in *Section 3.01* ('Assessment of severity of conditions', 4. Example (a) 'Rain penetration') only indicative of the values applicable in general to an area, that is the macro-condition. In the case of the driving-rain indices, these have been graded into *sheltered, moderate* and *severe* conditions, as noted in diagram D.3.02/2. However, some allowance must be made in order that account may be taken of the manner in which the grading applicable to an area may modify the exposure applicable to a building site in that area, due to local circumstances. Of these, proximity to the coast and the elevation of the site or building above their surroundings are of particular importance. Rules which may be applied to the basic exposure grading of an area in order to determine the exposure of a given site in that area have been tabulated in Table 3.02/1.

Further modifications may be necessary to take into account the effects of building design on exposure (see (d)). However, the basic exposure grading of a site provides, at the

*Originally driving-rain 'roses' for each of eight wind directions at 20 stations were published. These 'roses' were expressed as a percentage, i.e. the length of each vector represented the percentage for that direction, of the total index for the station.

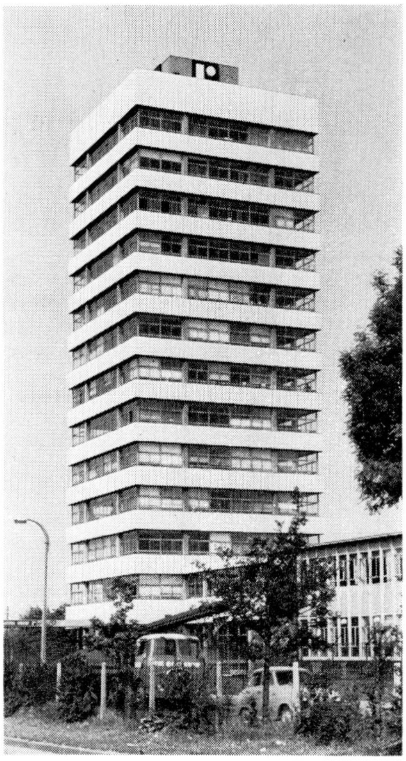

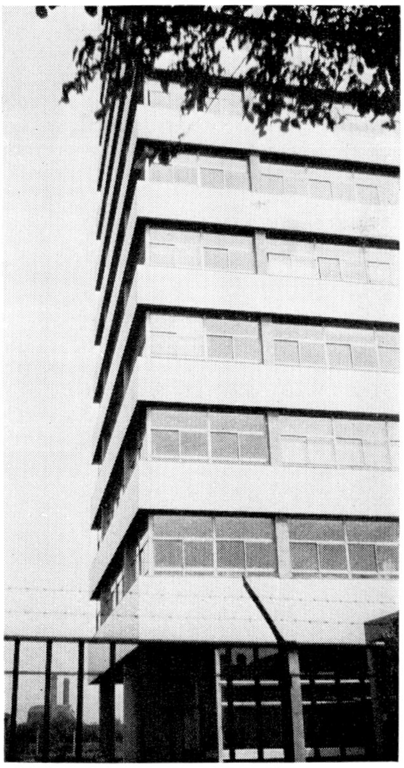

*In some buildings horizontal gutters have been incorporated on the vertical faces in order to reduce the cumulative run-off load of rainwater. In the building above (the lower picture is a detail) the gutters replace the sill at all levels on all four faces (architect: D. Pugh)*

D.3.02/3

*Driving-rain 'roses' attributable to wind from different directions at 23 places in the British Isles. The length of each of the twelve 'petals' is proportional to the annual mean driving-rain index from that direction (From: 'An Index of Exposure to Driving Rain', BRS Digest 127, Fig. 2, p. 4, March 1971 (Crown Copyright))*

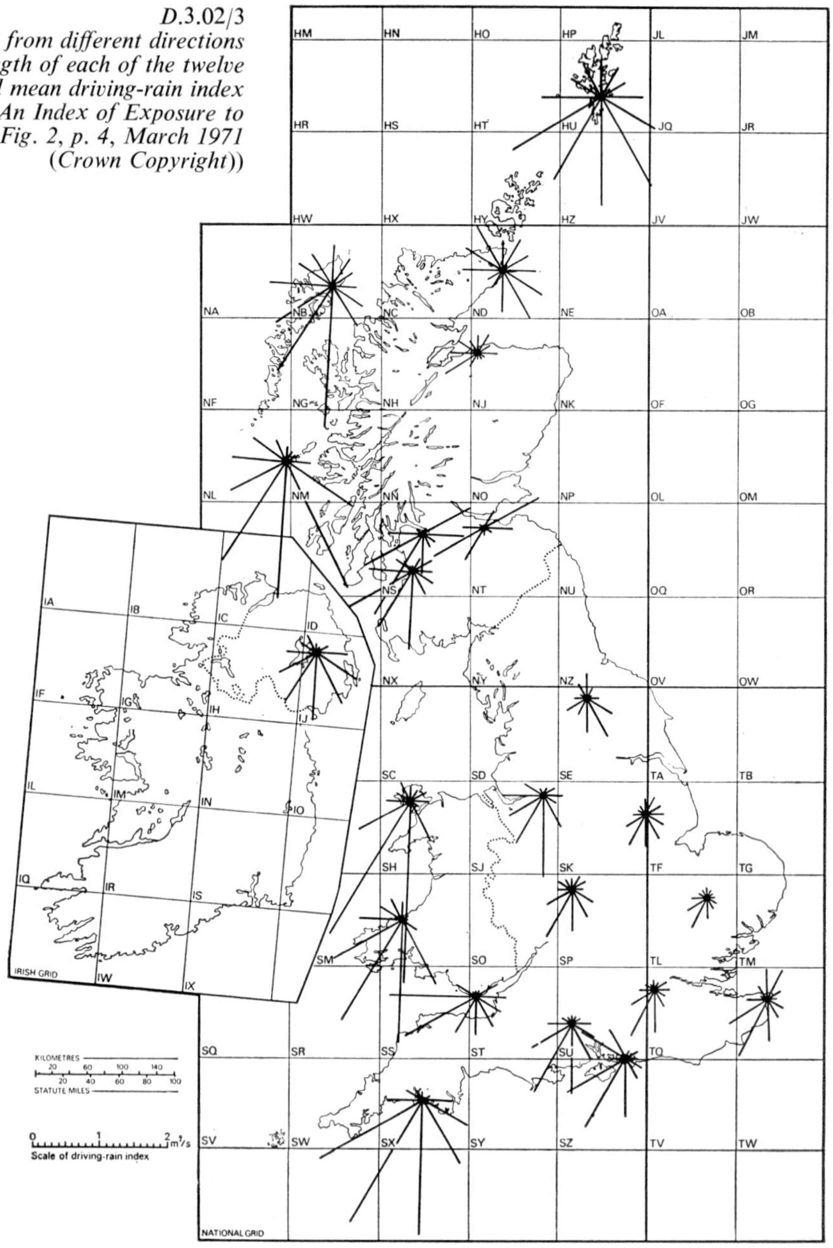


moment, a means of comparison with other sites with which a designer may be familiar. Such comparison as might be made then allows for some revaluation to be undertaken in order to assist significantly in the selection and use of materials for a given condition. In addition, the exposure grading for a given site might serve as a warning signal of the necessity for special precautions to be taken. Subject to the results of further research it may be possible in the future to relate the basic exposure grading of a site more specifically to selected materials and constructions. At present there is some correlation between the driving-rain index and masonry constructions, particularly brickwork. In the main the annual driving-rain index is applicable essentially to vertical surfaces, that is walls. In the case of roofs the problems involved are somewhat different and, as a result, information of a different kind is normally required. As already noted, the problems of rain driven into joints or over upstands can be related to wind-speed. However, the major problem associated with roofs is concerned with drainage, via gutters and downpipes, of the water collected by flat or sloping surfaces. The principle involved here is, in addition to ensuring that no leakage occurs, to prevent water collected by roofs from flowing on to vertical surfaces and thus increasing the exposure of the latter. This principle, although not always practised, is in many cases also applicable, if not essential, to many projecting surfaces (sloping or horizontal). The hydraulics connected with the design of gutters and downpipes with associated design flow

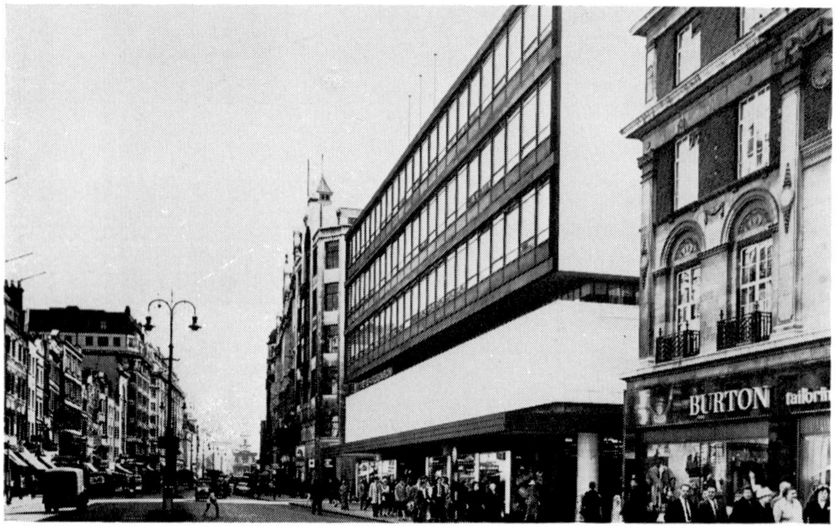


*Another example of horizontal gutters. In the building on the left the gutters have been incorporated in a special projecting member in the lower part of the spandrels to the upper three floors. The gutters in this example also prevent the run-off of rainwater from the bronze cladding staining the stone-work underneath (architects: Denys Lasdun and Partners)*

| PLACE | | | DRIVING RAIN INDEX $m^2/s$ | | MAX. HOURLY DRI | |
|---|---|---|---|---|---|---|
| Name | Alt. (m) | Map Ref. | Annual Mean | Max.✱ Hourly | Dir. of wind | Month of occurence |
| LERWICK | 82 | HU | 10·60 | 0·117 | 180° | Dec. |
| WICK | 36 | ND | 6·37 | 0·169 | 030° | Aug. |
| STORNOWAY | 3 | NB | 9·34 | 0·104 | 240° | Aug. |
| KINLOSS | 5 | NJ | 2·99 | 0·099 | 030° | Jun. |
| EDINBURGH Turnhouse | 35 | NT | 3·68 | 0·096 | 060° | Sep. |
| TIREE | 9 | NL | 10·25 | 0·181 | 150° | Sep. |
| GLASGOW Renfrew | 5 | NS | 5·51 | 0·205 | 060° | Jun. |
| PRESTWICK | 16 | NS | 5·69 | 0·125 | 030° | Aug. |
| DISHFORTH-LEEMING | 32 | SE | 3·39 | 0·211 | 240° | Jun. |
| WADDINGTON | 68 | SK | 3·46 | 0·107 | 120° | Aug. |
| MILDENHALL | 5 | TL | 2·33 | 0·104 | 270° | Aug. |
| BIRMINGHAM Elmdon | 97 | SP | 3·88 | 0·094 | 360° | Nov. |
| LONDON Heathrow | 25 | TQ | 3·37 | 0·140 | 090° | Jul. |
| KEW | 5 | TQ | 2·75 | 0·078 | 030° | Jul. |
| MANSTON | 44 | TR | 4·45 | 0·086 | 240° | Jan. |
| THORNEY ISLAND | 3 | SU | 4·42 | 0·110 | 210° | Sep. |
| BOSCOMBE DOWN | 126 | SU | 4·82 | 0·147 | 300° | Aug. |
| MANCHESTER Ringway | 76 | SJ | 4·87 | 0·167 | 090° | Sep. |
| HOLYHEAD Valley | 10 | SH | 8·18 | 0·178 | 210° | Sep. |
| ABERPORTH | 133 | SN | 7·67 | 0·146 | 240° | Dec. |
| CARDIFF Rhoose | 62 | ST | 5·82 | 0·199 | 360° | Aug. |
| PLYMOUTH Mt Batten | 27 | SX | 9·08 | 0·404 | 090° | Jul. |
| ALDERGROVE | 69 | IJ | 5·74 | 0·112 | 090° | Dec. |

✱ Shown solid within bar for annual mean DRI.

*C.3.02/2*
*Annual mean driving-rain index at 23 places, with greatest hourly driving-rain index (mostly in ten years 1957-66) and corresponding wind direction.*
*(Reference: BRS Digest No. 127, Table 1, p. 6, March 1971)*

**Table 3.02/1 Basic exposure gradings and rules for decision**

| *Basic exposure grading* | | *Modifications to be applied to basic exposure grading** | |
|---|---|---|---|
| *Classification of conditions* | *Related annual driving-rain index* ($m^2/s$) | *Districts or special conditions to be excluded* | *Districts or special conditions to be included* |
| Sheltered | 3 or less | (1) Areas that lie within 8km of the sea or large estuaries—exposure to be regarded as 'moderate' (2) High buildings standing above their surroundings, or buildings of any height on hill tops—exposure to be regarded as 'moderate' | None |
| Moderate | between 3 and 7 | (1) Areas that have an index of 5 or more and lie within 8km of the sea or large estuaries—exposure to be regarded as 'severe' (2) High buildings standing above their surroundings, or buildings of any height on hill tops—exposure to be regarded as 'severe' | (1) Areas that lie within 8km of the sea or large estuaries situated in districts generally classified as 'sheltered' (2) High buildings standing above their surroundings, or buildings of any height on hill tops situated in districts generally classified as 'sheltered' |
| Severe | above 7 | None | (1) Areas that have an index of 5 or more and lie within 8km of the sea or large estuaries situated in districts generally classified as 'moderate' (2) High buildings standing above their surroundings, or buildings of any height on hill tops situated in districts generally classified as 'moderate' |

*Note:* *Any of the gradings may in addition be altered by local circumstances. For example:
(1) Exposure of a site may be *less* than that of its surroundings when high ground is on the windward side or if there is a belt of trees;
(2) Exposure of a site may be *more* than the average for the area if it lies on the windward slope of even a slight hill, or in a valley facing into the strongest rain-bearing winds.
All local circumstances, details of which can be studied on large-scale maps, must, therefore, be taken into account. In cases of doubt consult the Advisory Offices of the Meteorological Office.

Reference: *An index of exposure to driving rain*, BRS Digest No. 127, March 1971.

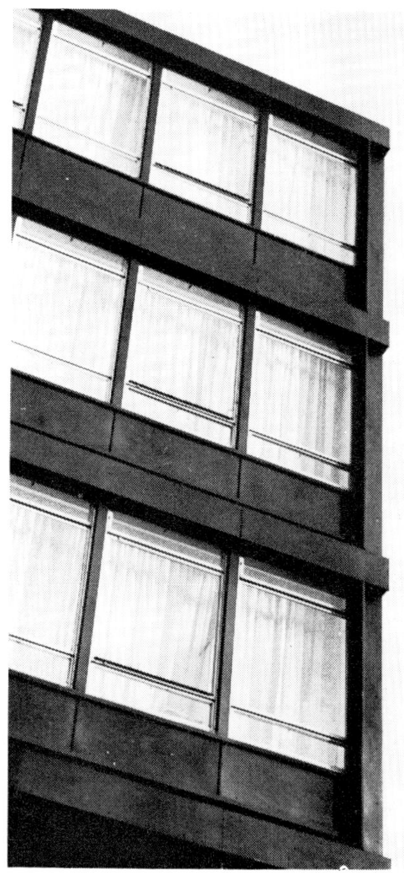

*Above, detail from the building shown on the opposite page. Note, the projecting lower section of the spandrels which house the gutter*

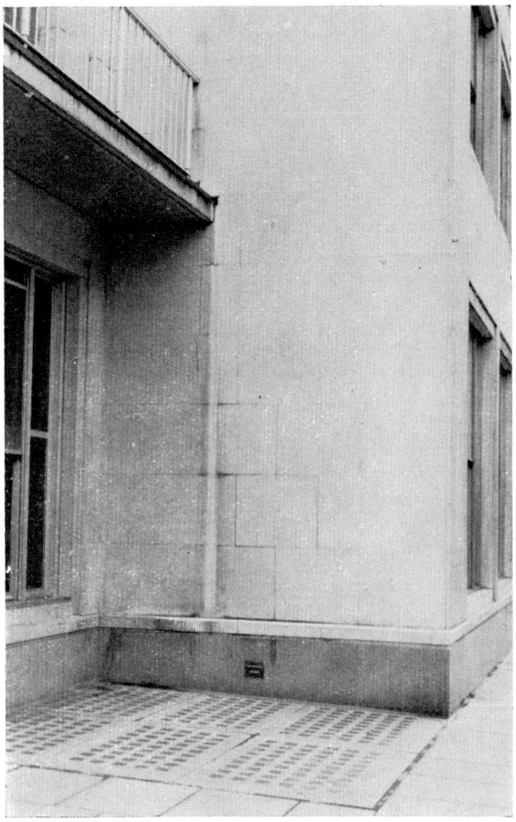

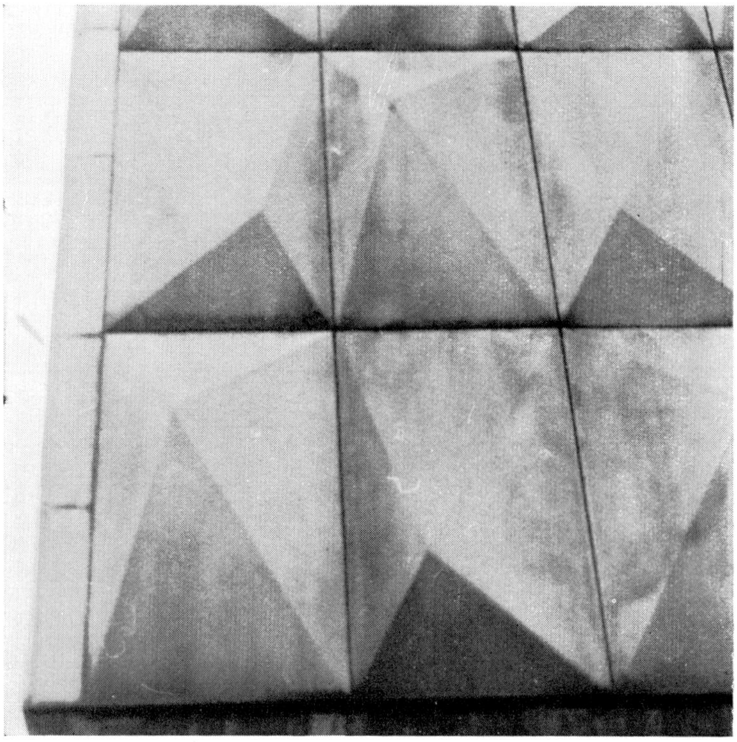

*Projections and recessions to the vertical face of a building may act both as a means for reducing or increasing exposure*

loads* from all types of roofs is outside the scope of this study and is therefore excluded.

Recently an analysis of hourly values of driving-rain index at 23 places has been made by the Meteorological Office giving the values shown in chart C.3.02/2. These are indicative of intense driving rain that can occur in heavy showers lasting for a few minutes, or on occasion up to an hour or so. (Most driving rain is caused by more or less prolonged storms.) The maximum hourly driving-rain index has been experienced at each place during 10 years. With one exception the maximum hourly index lies within the range of 0·09 to 0·21m²/s.

The use of the annual driving-rain index relative to materials and construction is still in its formative stage. However, it may be noted that greater attention is now being given to the run-off of water from exposed impervious materials. This is due mainly to the fact that 'traditional' walling, with its essentially porous materials in which absorption is possible, does not present the problems which have been encountered with impervious claddings for example. Solution of the problems involved may in part be found, it is thought, by ensuring that the run-off water is suitably drained. This should reduce the quantity of water which may be 'whipped up' by the wind and thus driven into joints and junctions. (Some buildings incorporating gutters on vertical surfaces have, in fact, already been erected.) Recent measurements taken show that in a place with a driving-rain index of 7m²/s a run-off of 100 litres/m²h can take place in a period of a few minutes, and may occur once in five or ten years. An hourly maximum driving-rain index of about 0·1 to 0·2m²/s (to be expected once in ten years) corresponds to an actual volume of rain of about 20 to 40 litres/m² in the hour on the vertical. By using measurements such as this as a guide, a useful indication of the total run-off to be accommodated can be obtained.

*Guidance on flow loads of roofs and the hydraulics of gutters and downpipes is given in two BRS Digests—
(1) *Roof drainage*, BRS Digest (1st Series), No. 116, November, 1958.
(2) *Design of gutters and rainwater pipes*, BRS Digest (2nd Series), No. 34, May, 1963.

### (d) *Effects of building design*

Whereas it may be possible to obtain a measure of the basic exposure of a building site, the extent to which this exposure may be *further* modified from place to place on a building by details of building design itself is subject to wide variations. Some details, which here includes the disposition of elements relative to one another, may assist in reducing exposure; others in increasing it. Accordingly, it is only possible to refer in general terms to the effect of some common details, most of which are related to vertical surfaces.

Increases in exposure may be anticipated on freely exposed surfaces of a building, when the speed of the wind is increased due to deflection from its normal course as it passes the building. Such deflection may occur at corners or cornices, in which case the wind speed may be twice that when undisturbed. This increase naturally enough also increases the driving-rain index.

Projections and recessions to the vertical face of a building may act both as a means of reducing or increasing exposure. With details of this kind flow patterns and particularly local concentrations become important as illustrated in *Section 3.01* under 'Flow'.

Obstructions also provide another means whereby exposure conditions may be materially affected. Surrounding buildings, whether on the same site or not, may appear as potential sources of shelter. However, cognizance must be taken of wind flow patterns which may result from the surroundings. In present-day circumstances it is now becoming more common for wind-tunnel tests to be undertaken in order to establish design criteria for structures and other purposes. The results of such tests may also provide useful information on exposure conditions. In the case of roofs, projections, such as chimneys, above the general roof level, are indicative of obstruction to the flow of water. Associated details involving flashings, soakers and similar devices to ensure watertightness require special consideration.

*All the photographs on this page are examples of increases in exposure due to leakage of water at joints*

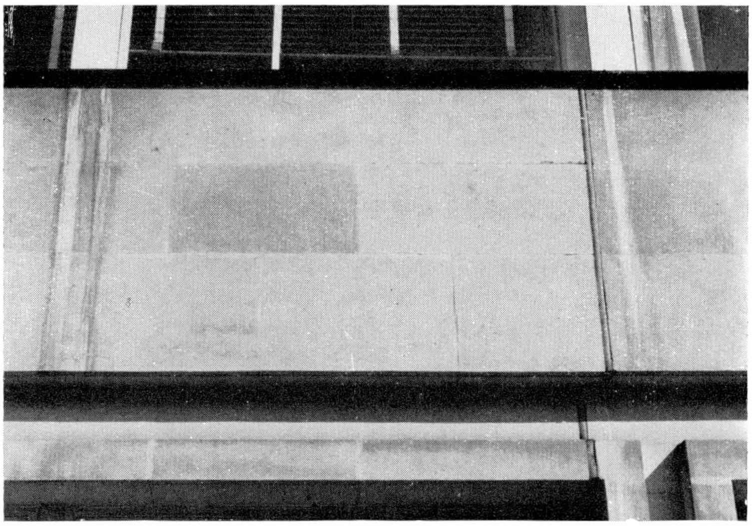

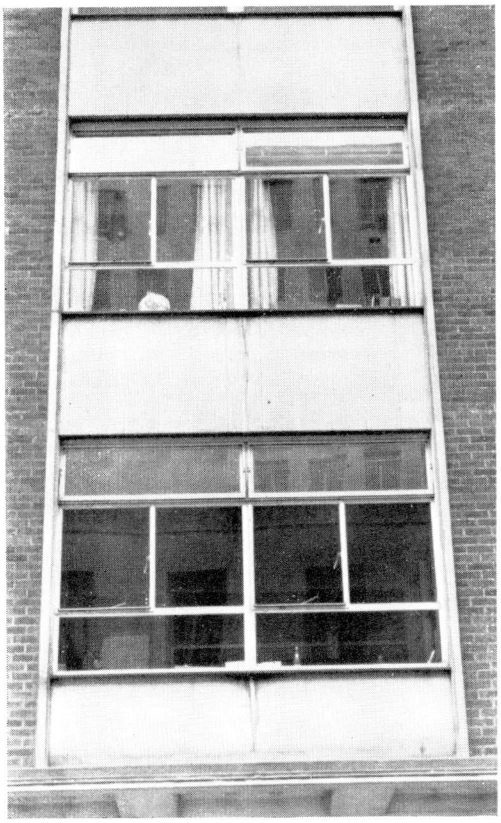

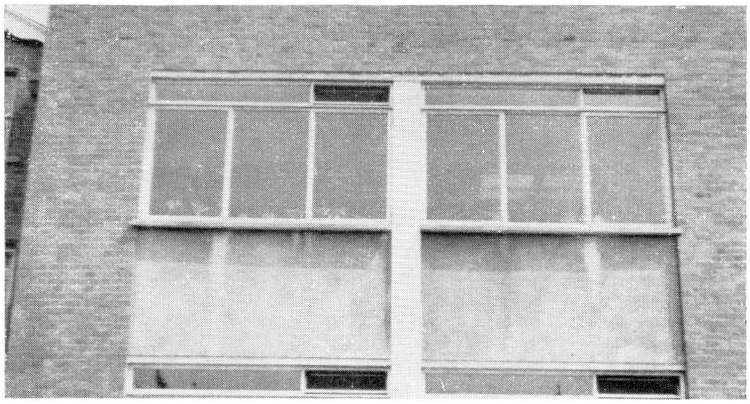

*Sills. Materials used in the top right-hand picture and the picture above are impervious, those in the lower right-hand picture are porous*

*Lack of maintenance*

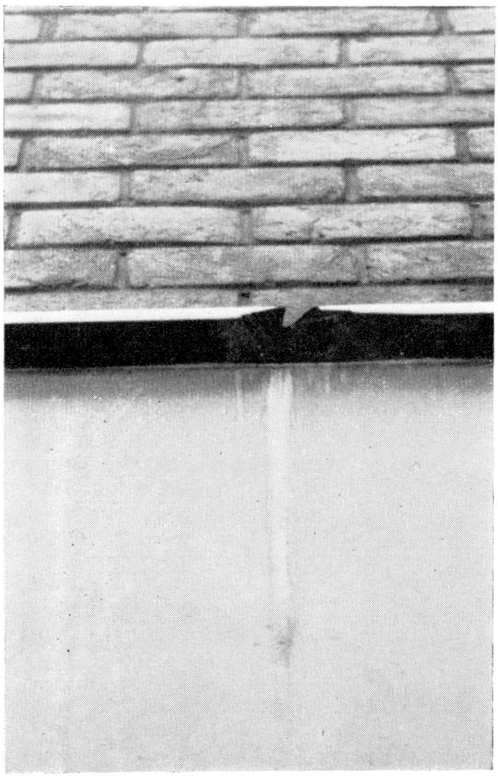

*The pictures below, reading from top to bottom, illustrate :*
1. *Cornice. Lead dressing does not protect the joint.* 2. *Coping. Lime washings correspond exactly with joints.* 3. *Failure of construction joints in concrete due to lack of impervious protection to top surface of projection*

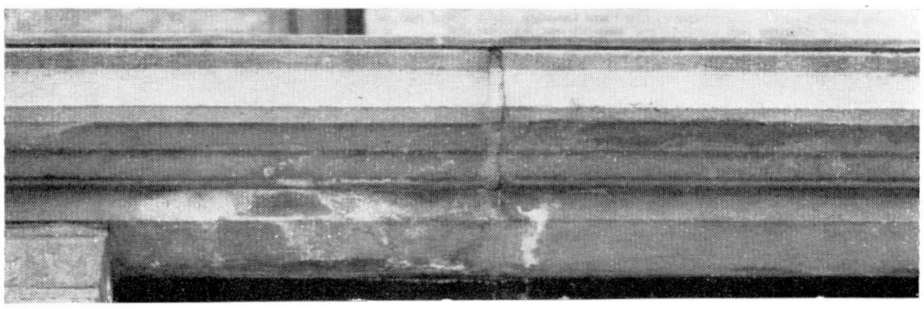

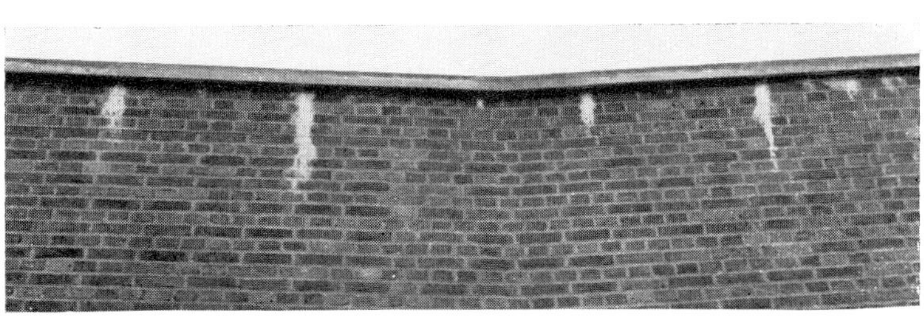

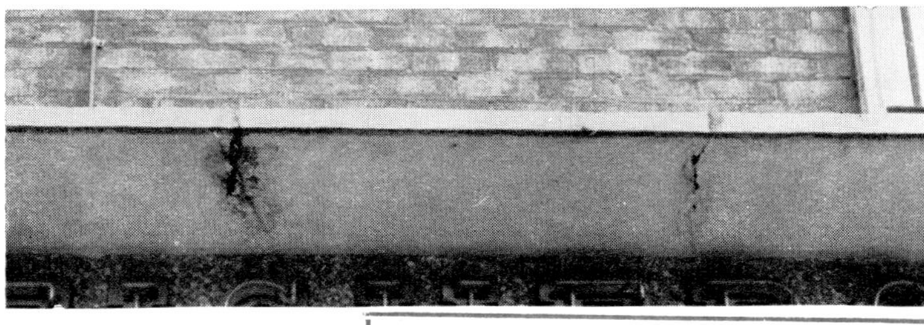

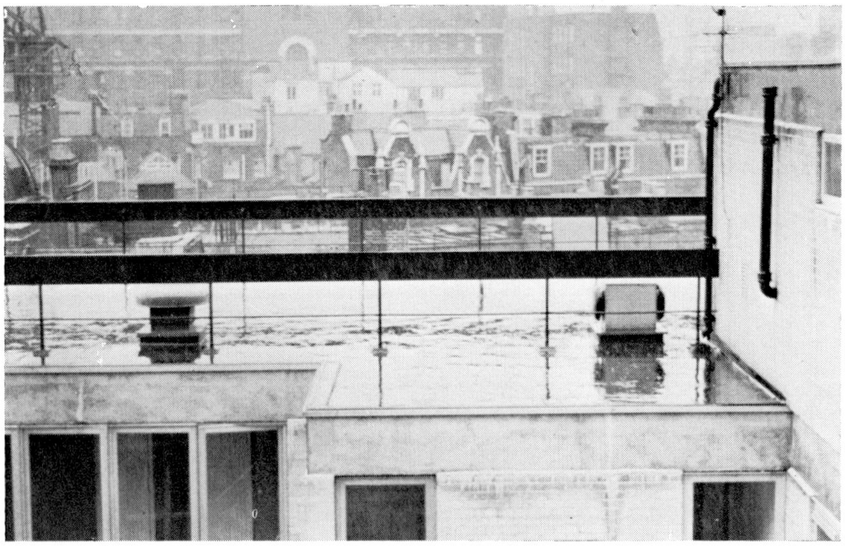

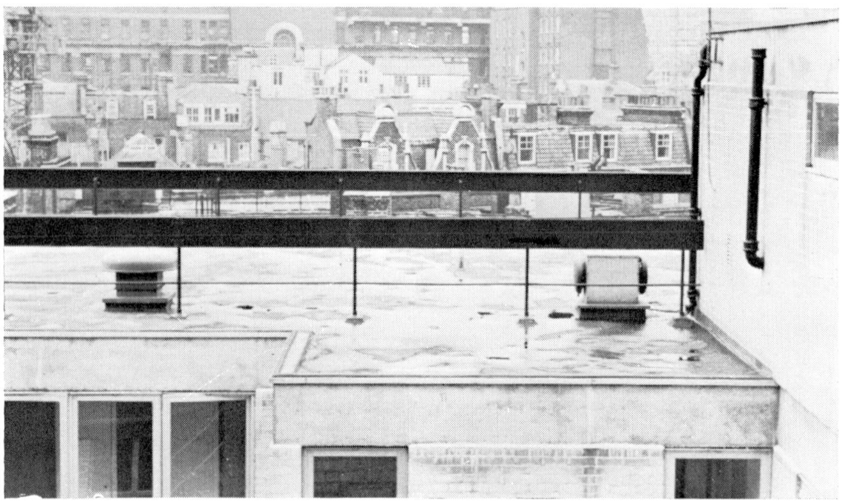

*Illustration of 'ponding' on a flat roof. The top picture was taken during rain and the one beneath it shortly after the rain had ceased. The photographs also illustrate local concentrations of water due to faulty joints and the increase in exposure to exposed horizontal surfaces, particularly that to the brickwork which in this case has an ineffective sloping fillet of mortar at the top*

*The example below shows a general increase in exposure of a parapet wall. Concentrations of leakage generally occur at the zone of joints in the coping, although in this case there does appear to have been rain penetration through the porous coping. Note how the top of the wall to the penthouse has remained unaffected despite its theoretical greater exposure due to increased height. In this case the projection of the flat roof has provided sufficient shelter*

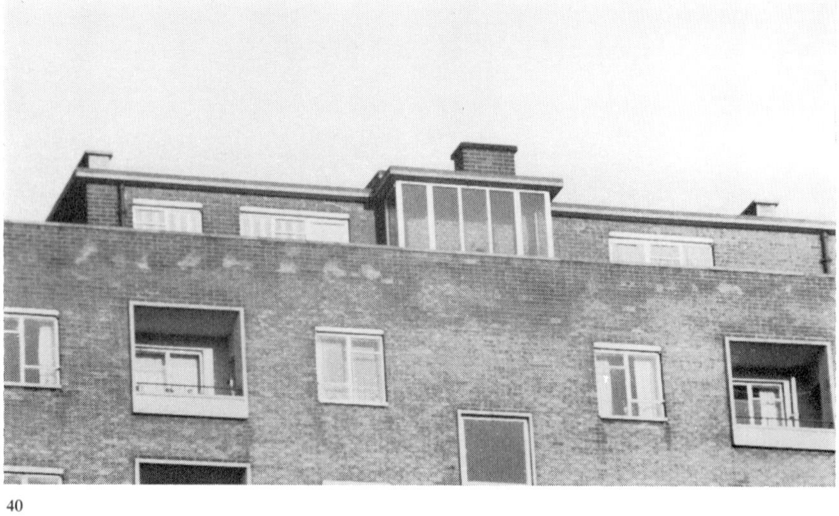

Finally, a special point on horizontal or near horizontal surfaces. These, when compared with vertical surfaces are, in general, always exposed to rain irrespective of wind. Whereas the run-off on vertical or sloping surfaces is fairly rapid, the run-off from horizontal surfaces is dependent essentially on the falls provided and, as in the case of roofs, the efficiency of the drainage system. Falls are important if 'ponding', which creates a head of water, is to be prevented. The effect of standing water even for fairly short periods on horizontal surfaces composed of porous materials, such as copings for example, is to increase exposure significantly. During rainfall the effect of water impinging continuously on horizontal surfaces with poor throw-off may, within limits, be considered as analogous to the effects of standing water. Joints between the units making up the coping of a parapet wall, for example, often provide 'leakage' points with subsequent increases in exposure in the zone of the joint. Window sills and other similar elements must also be included.

### (e) *Portrait of a building: exposure to driving-rain*

As previously explained the present usefulness of the BRS annual driving-rain indices (diagrams D.3.02/2 and 3) is that they provide the designer with a means of comparing known and unknown situations. Their full potential relative to the performance of materials and constructions has yet to be developed.

All the examples shown so far in this study have been concerned with certain specific aspects of exposure to rain and consequently have not been related to the indices as such. However, by way of summarising most of the factors which influence exposure to rain relative to the indices, it would seem that the *annual relative index*, which uses the 'rain rose', offers a convenient point of departure. Accordingly in this 'Portrait of a Building' an attempt has been made to relate the performance of the various faces to the rain rose for the macro-condition of the locality. There is no intention, it should be emphasised, of dealing with the performance of the external faces in terms of decay, deterioration or rain penetration as such—for the building chosen, see below, there has already been an examination of these aspects*—but rather to illustrate the basic relationship between the rain rose and the various faces of a building in terms of their comparative exposure. Among other things this should help to reinforce the fact that exposure is likely to be altered, in some cases significantly, by a number of different factors which

***A qualitative study of some buildings in the London area*, National Building Studies, Special Report No. 33, Chapter 11, pp. 109–125, HMSO, 1964.

must be taken into account in the selection and use of materials.

For the present purposes a building complex which has been considered most suitable for illustrating the manner in which exposure varies is 'The London University: The Senate House'. There are two main reasons why this is a particularly good example to examine. These are:

(1) The complex consists of buildings of varying heights, including a tower rising well above its surroundings, presenting four orientations and accommodated on an island site. The complex is shown on the location plan, while the aerial photograph*, taken from the SW, indicates the general nature of the environment and the building.

(2) The external faces are generally of Portland Stone†, which, because of its solubility, is washed 'clean' when sufficiently exposed to rainwater and accordingly eventually shows, sufficient for comparative purposes, which faces or parts are more heavily exposed than others.

As this examination is not intended to be exhaustive in detail but mainly aimed at concentrating on the principles involved, presentation is essentially by way of a number of photographic views of the building complex (the positions from which the views were taken are indicated on the plan—diagram D.3.02/4). These together with the text and captions, it is hoped, will to a large extent 'speak for themselves'. The purpose of the text is to briefly outline those aspects illustrated by the photographs; in some cases it is necessary to refer to groups of photographs which have been arranged accordingly; in others a particular aspect may be seen on all or some of the photographs, but in the text reference is made specifically to some. In general the text is intended to act as a guide.

The rain rose for London‡ is included with the location plan and has been orientated for the plan (diagram D.3.02/4). It should be noted that the rain rose is that for London in general and not for the site in particular. This is an advantage in this study as it facilitates illustration of the occurrence of changes in the basic exposure conditions.

From the rose it will be seen that the greatest exposure should occur with those faces orientated to the south and south-west. Each of these faces should receive about 30 per cent, making a total together of 60 per cent, of the total for rain from all directions. The orientations of the various faces of the buildings are SW, SE, NE and NW.

*D.3.02/4*
*The location plan shows the Senate House building complex and its environments*

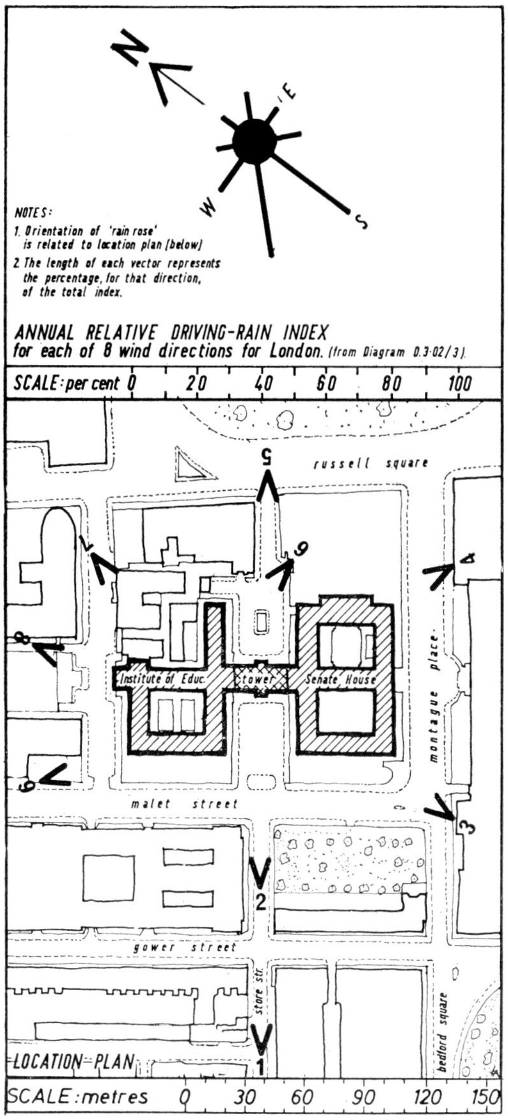


*Photograph taken from the SW with Gower St. in the foreground, the British Museum in the SE corner and Russell Square in the NE corner (Courtesy: Aero Pictorial Ltd.)*

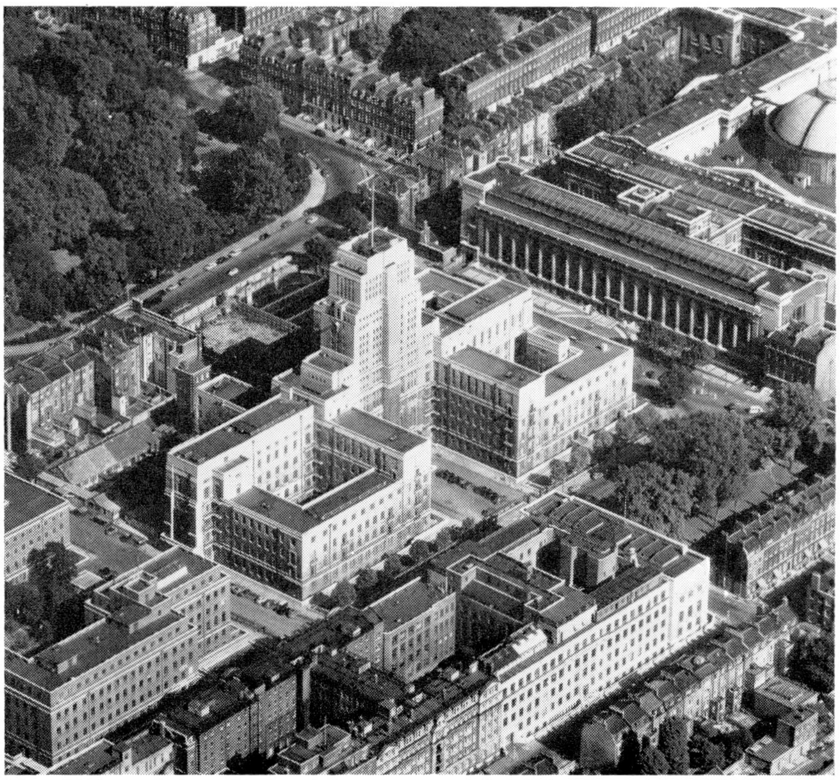

*The aerial photograph was taken in August, 1955, two years before the stonework was cleaned. All the other photographs were taken in June, 1965. There are therefore slight, although insignificant, differences to be seen.

†Granite was used on the lower floors of some of the building, but this does not affect the present consideration.

‡The rain rose used here is the one originally issued. It has 8 petals instead of 12 and is relative instead of proportional. However, the principles of application remain essentially the same.

The upper parts of the tower being relatively free from the effects of their environs illustrate the changes in exposure of the various faces (views 3, 4, 7 and 9), the severity of which coincides with the information given by the rain rose. For a comparison of two extremes, representing opposite faces so to speak, namely SW and NE, views 1 and 5 are particularly useful.

An examination of the aerial photograph illustrates that even those parts of the lower buildings relatively unaffected by their environs 'respond' to the rose. Note the differences between the SW and NW faces. A detail of one of the latter can be seen in view 8.

Changes in the basic exposure condition outlined above due to the nature of the environs, i.e., obstructions, can best be seen in view 2, where the lower part of the tower is generally 'sheltered' by the projecting lower wings. The lower buildings are also 'sheltered' by the tower (views 2 and 6).

The effects of projections is noticeable in all views but particularly on the less exposed faces (views 5 and 8).

Increased run-off of rainwater from impervious faces manifests itself in the window sills which are generally clean (views 2, 6 and 8).

*Least exposed face according to rain rose; increases in exposure to the 'parapet zone' are probably due to the deflection of wind with resultant increases in wind speed*

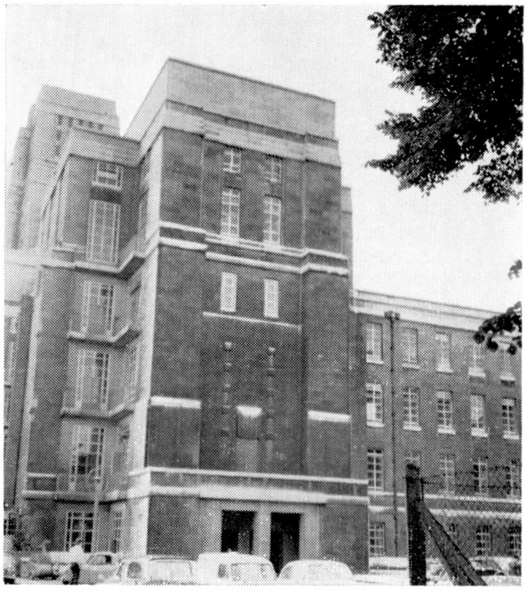

V8 NW

### 2. Ground

The elements or parts of a building which are exposed to groundwater* are essentially those which are either (1) *placed in,* that is buried, in the ground and consisting of foundations (all types), lower parts of walls and columns (generally from foundation level to d.p.c. level), retaining walls (in basements, on sloping sites, in manholes, etc.), or service components such as pipes, conduits, cables, etc., or (2) those in *close contact* with the ground, such as floor slabs. In all cases any form of direct connection between any of the elements with other parts of the building must be taken into account. Although suspended timber floors occurring immediately above ground level should not be connected directly or indirectly with the ground itself, they may nevertheless be exposed to groundwater in the vapour state. Such exposure occurs if there is inadequate ventilation to the outside air of the plenum space between the ground and the under-side of the floor and may, in the long term, be sufficient to cause serious rotting of the timber.

Although the elements which are exposed to groundwater are limited, a number of conflicting reasons make quantitative assessments of exposure extremely difficult. Accordingly, it is only possible to indicate, in general terms, the relationship between the factors involved and upon which assessments have to be made. For convenience these have been divided into

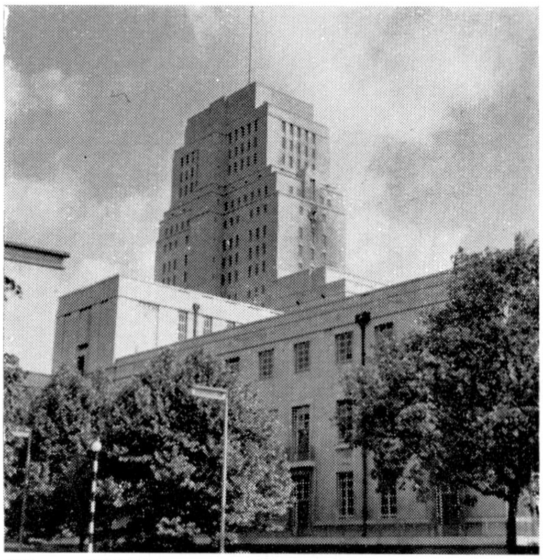

V3 SW/SE

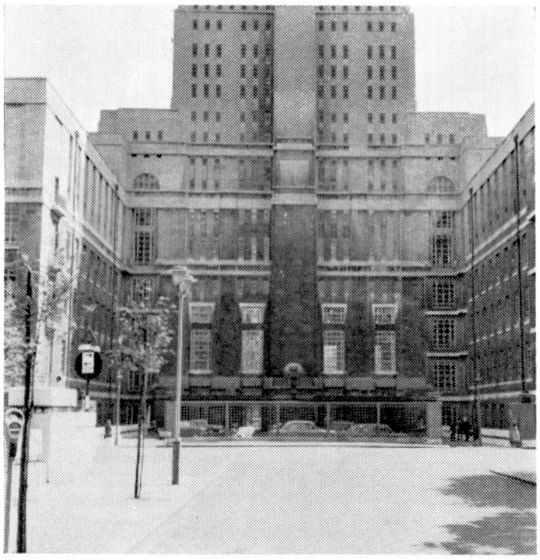

V2 SW

*The term 'groundwater' must, in the present context, include not only 'free flowing' water but also water contained in or held between the particles of any substance making up the ground as a whole. The latter is perhaps more general, but at the same time the former cannot be excluded. In this section both are implied unless the term is specifically qualified.

*The first row of photographs including the one on the opposite page, give a comparison of the change in exposure of the four upper faces of the tower which, being relatively free from the effects of their environs, respond to the severity of exposure indicated in the rain rose. Clean faces represent severe exposure; dirty faces sheltered exposure. Note : allowance should be made when comparing the photographs for the differences in lighting—all photographs were taken during one morning. In the bottom row V1 and V5 give a comparison of two extremes of exposure, SW severe, NE sheltered. V2 and V6 show modification of basic exposure as given by rain rose caused by obstruction*

the following general headings: (a) Significance of exposure to groundwater ; (b) Variable factors involved ; (c) Pressure build-up ; (d) Capillarity and vapour ; and (e) Pollutants.

(a) *Significance*

Unlike most other conditions of exposure, exposure to groundwater is not only perennial but also lasts throughout the whole life of the building. Exposure to groundwater is, therefore, the most severe encountered in building when compared to other exposure conditions, and particularly when the importance of most of the elements involved in exposure to groundwater are taken into account.

The severity of conditions is not dependent only on the fact that water is, in general, always present, but is also dependent on the fact that the water is usually polluted to some extent. In many cases the fact that the water, or the ground for that matter which in this context can usually be regarded as damp, is polluted, will dictate the precautions which must be taken in the selection and use of materials.

(b) *Variable factors*

Although the precise quantities of water together with the degree of pollution which may constitute the worst condition in any given situation would assist in determining the materials to be associated with groundwater, there are a number of variable factors involved which make this extremely difficult. Of these factors the following are the most important:

(1) Variations in the composition of the substances making up the ground, in which the differing water transfer or water holding capacities of different types of soil and rocks are significent ;

(2) Variations in the actual source of the groundwater, that is whether entirely from local rain or whether derived from other source or sources which could be near or far from a given site (see *3.01 Water cycle*);

(3) Climatic conditions affecting rainfall and evaporation.

Experience of local conditions and the results of site surveys (the latter always being advisable) may help in determining the effect of most of these factors on the actual exposure condition which may be anticipated. In

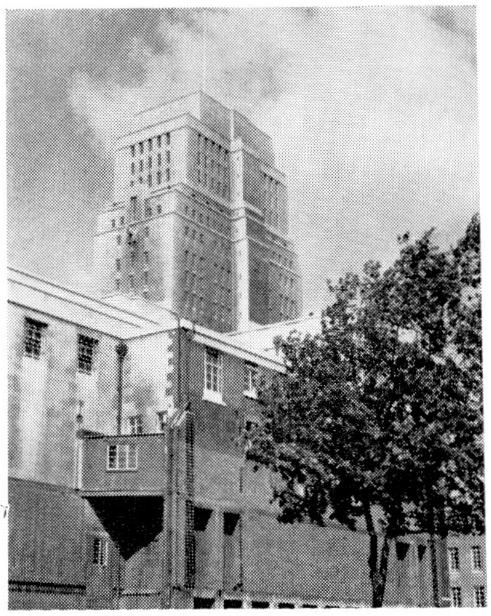
V4 SE/NE

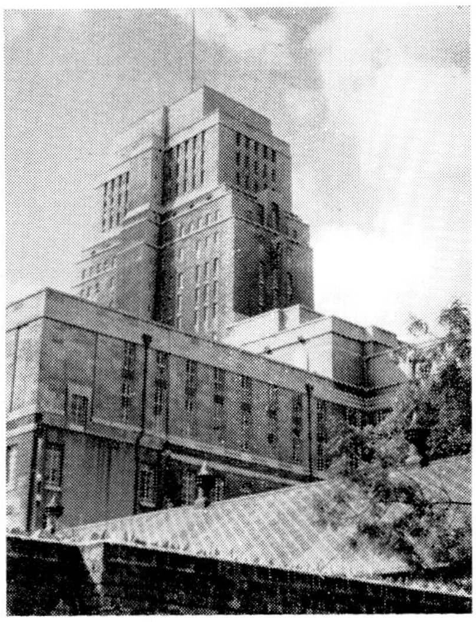
V7 NE/NW

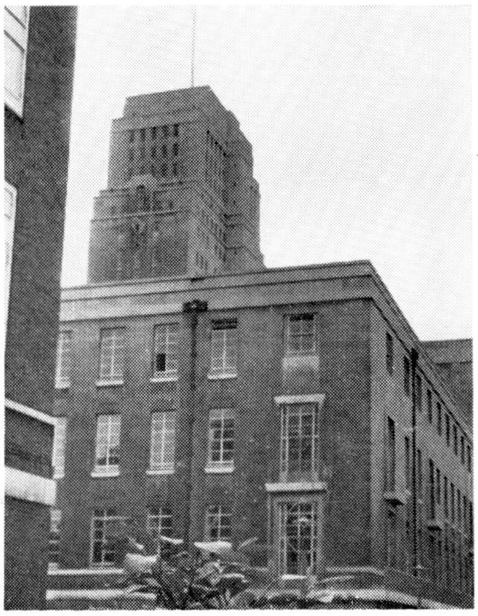
V9 NW/SW

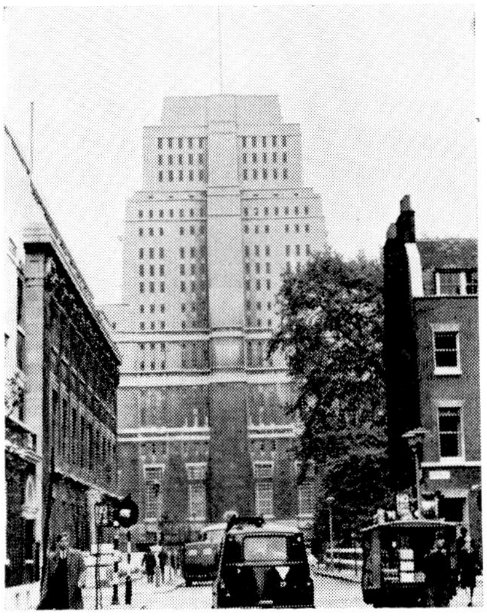
V1 SW

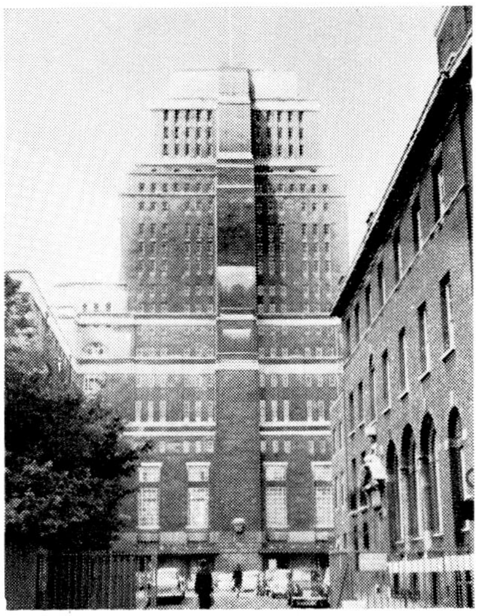
V5 NE

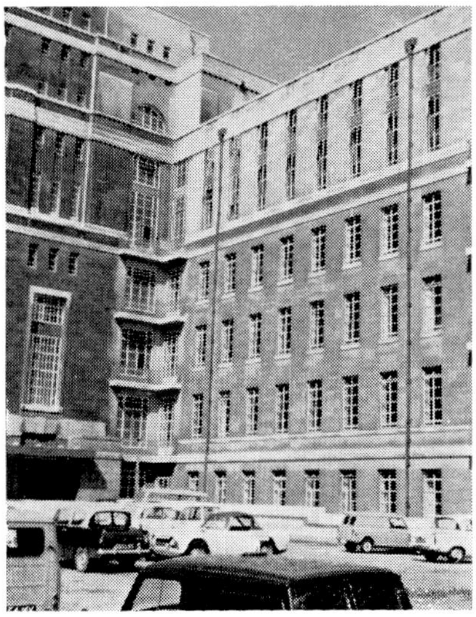
V6 NE/SE

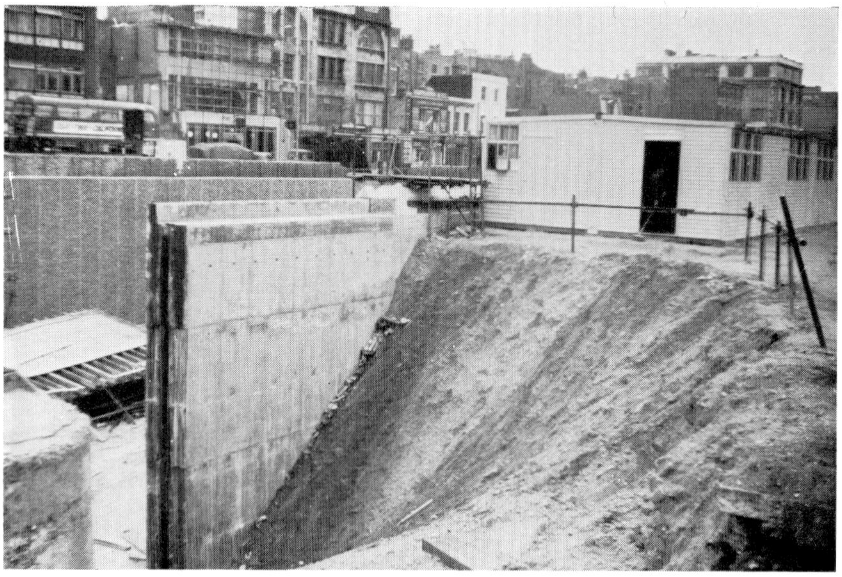

*Some examples of elements or parts of buildings placed in close contact with the ground. Above, retaining walls*
*Below, pipes*

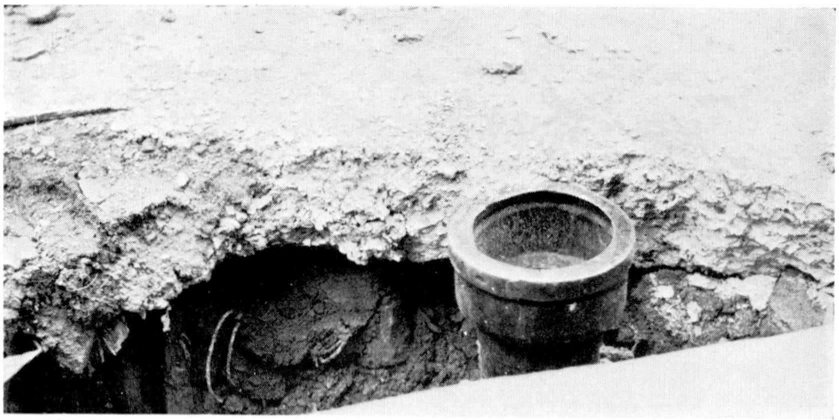

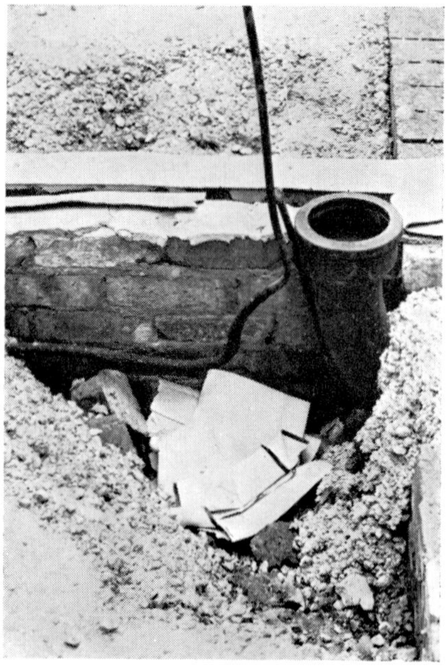

*The photograph above shows pipes and conduits and the bottom picture illustrates walls below d.p.c., manholes and drains*

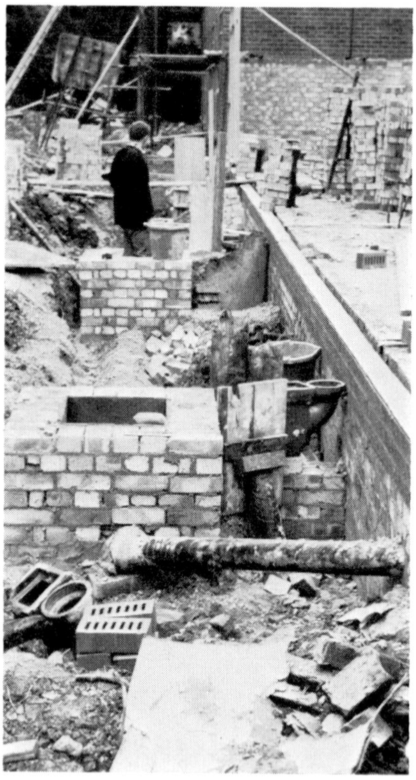

*Foundations*

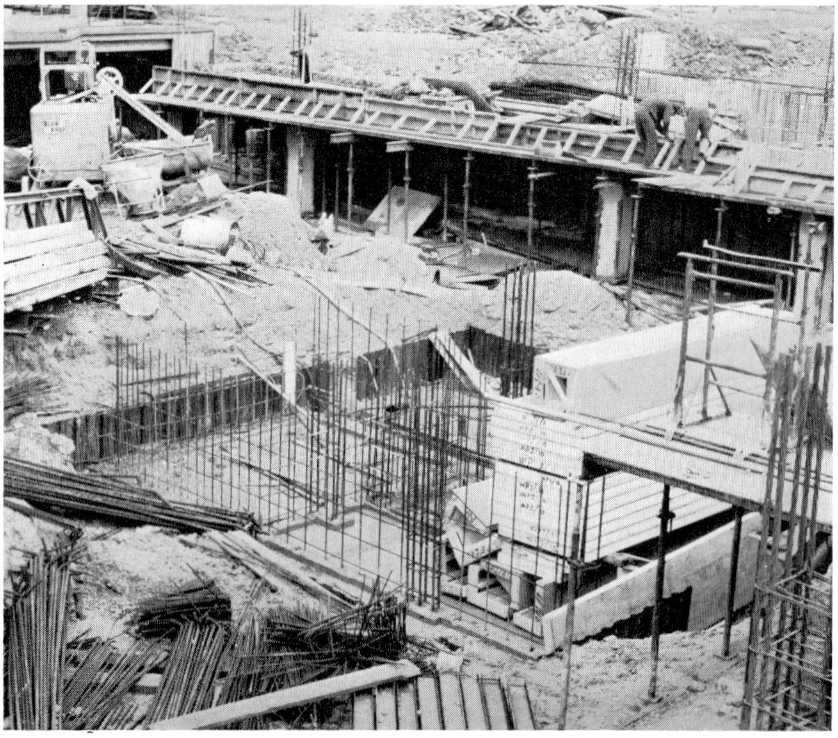

general it may be noted in connection with soil types that the cohesive soils, such as clays, are always likely to transfer and/or hold considerably more water than the non-cohesive soils, such as the gravels, sands, etc. The latter generally permit fairly rapid drainage to lower depths of, for example, rainwater, although they are capable of holding water in the interstices between the particles. (A description of the main classes of soil types is included in *2.03 Cracking due to soil movements.*)

(c) *Pressure*

Special mention should be made of 'free flowing' groundwater which may be encountered on a site during a survey or the dig for foundations. Groundwater such as this usually implies that the source is at some distance from the site, in either a horizontal or downwards direction. In this the water table is significant. If the 'flow' is 'dammed up' by the construction of the building there is the possibility of pressure being exerted on those elements causing the obstruction. In most cases pressure build-up, which may be overcome by diverting the water course or by adequate pumping, are significant because of their structural implications. However, they do also accelerate the rate at which groundwater may be transferred through porous materials associated with the ground.

(d) *Capillarity and vapour*

The manner in which the groundwater in close contact with the relevant elements of a building is depleted and subsequently replenished (a continual process) is, as already noted, complex. However, transfer of water into and through materials by means of capillarity plays an extremely important part. In this cognisance has to be taken of the fact that most of the structural elements referred to earlier are composed of porous materials, all of which, in varying degrees, are capable of 'encouraging' water transfer, either horizontally or vertically, by capillarity. Some of the materials used, and concrete is a notable example, may be highly resistant to water transfer in the liquid state even under pressure, but they may not be sufficiently resistant to the transfer of water in its vapour state. In all cases the control of the transfer of water, in any of its states, is effected at a predetermined level (or levels) by the incorporation of an impervious layer of some kind or another (damp-proof courses and membranes). Subject to conditions, the 'route' of such a layer may be quite complex. One of its main requirements is that it should be continuous in order to avoid local leakages.

It may be useful here to quote an example which should illustrate the importance of transfer of groundwater in the liquid state, particularly in floor slabs. Where concrete ground-floor slabs have been laid on hardcore, without the incorporation of a damp-proof membrane, on what were considered to be dry soils, dampness has often occurred underneath essentially vapour resistant floor finishes such as linoleum. In these cases vapour has permeated through the concrete only to condense when it has come into contact with the vapour resistant material, which has acted as a damp-proof membrane. This unfortunately has been 'incorporated' in the wrong position.

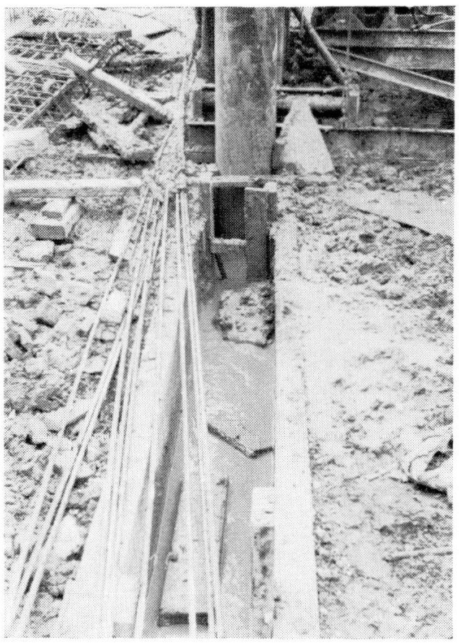

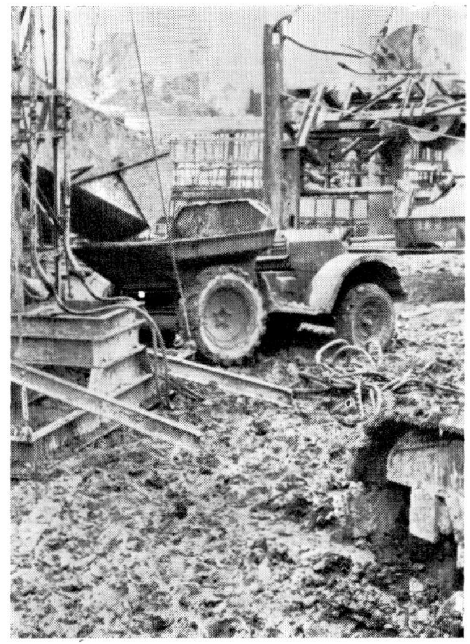

*Removing 'free flowing' groundwater on a site. Note general wetness and mud Below, an attempt to avoid increases in exposure to rainwater during construction of walls to a house. In this case the spirit was willing but . . .*

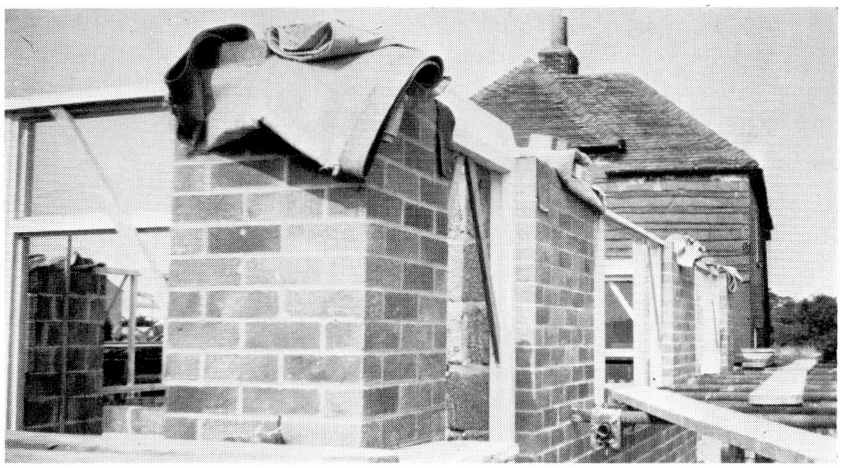

(e) *Pollutants*

In view of the fact that pollutants, many of which may be comparatively easily transferred in solution with water, play such an important part in any consideration of the effects of groundwater on materials, it follows that both source and pollution are closely interrelated. The wide variations as regards the degree of pollution which may exist necessitates each case to be considered separately. An analysis of soil conditions for both source and pollution of groundwater is always advisable.

**3. During construction**

It is perhaps all too obvious that water must be introduced during construction involving all the wet trade processes in brick and block laying, concreting, plastering, screeding, some painting, etc. However, the quantities of water necessary to make any of these processes chemically and physically possible in the first instance are, in a sense, a nuisance after any of the operations concerned have been completed. If the water remains behind too long it can also cause inconvenience by way of delay for the following trades. Under winter conditions, too much water in the elements may, under certain conditions, lead to frost action and related deterioration. For a number of different reasons, therefore, drying out commensurate with other requirements, such as avoidance of cracking (see *2.03 Cracking due to moisture movement*), should be accomplished as soon as possible. Where the drying out time cannot be speeded up sufficiently it is sometimes possible to use forms of construction which will allow drying out to proceed after a particular operation has been completed, and thus reduce delay. In winter special precautions are necessary.

Part of the problem of controlled drying out is seen to be best effected under controlled factory conditions, usually off the site, such as takes place with many large panel systems. However, wherever the drying out is to take place it should be properly controlled. In many cases units or elements which may have been properly dried out, are then left unprotected, either during storage prior to use or while actually in position in a building under construction, only to be rewetted during rain or by careless spilling during cleaning and other operations. These all aggravate an already difficult and time-consuming task. Materials such as timber, timber products or other fibrous products, not normally associated with the water-bound problems of the wet-trade processes are, however, also highly susceptible to moisture content changes. They, too, should not be left exposed to rain or other sources of water both on or off the site.

It is not always appreciated that fairly vast quantities of water are, in fact, used during the construction of most buildings. Despite the increased use of 'dry' forms of construction, it has been considered advisable in this study to give some indication of the probable quantities of water which may be used with the wet-trade processes. Table 3.02/2 sets out the quantities of water introduced during construction. From this it will be seen that in a traditional three-bedroom house, for example, it is estimated that between 6 364 and 8 183 litres are actually used in the construction. This is equivalent to about 6 364 to 8 183kg of water or a weight of between 62·4 and 80·2 kN. These figures, it should be noted, do not include the quantities of water spilt, used for cleaning (cement mixers, etc.) or a variety of other site uses. The total quantity including these contingencies is estimated in the example quoted to be about 8 092–22 730 litres. There is, therefore, a considerable amount of 'waste' water, the destination of which cannot be realistically accounted for.

An indication of the significance of some of the quantities of water introduced during construction relative to drying out times might be given by taking an extreme example of a screed or concrete slab laid on an impervious membrane as would occur in a ground-floor slab. It is estimated that, under normal conditions, the rate of drying out would be at least 1 month per 25·4mm.* Thus, a 50·8mm screed would take two months to dry out; a 152·4mm combined screed and concrete slab six months. On the other hand, the importance of protection from rainfall in order not to delay drying out can be obtained by considering the fact that 13mm rain is equivalent to 13 litres/m². In the case of a lightweight concrete screed (aggregate or aerated cement) to a flat roof it is estimated that only a small proportion of this quantity would be shed, except in heavy showers. In an experiment carried out at the BRS* it was shown that an unprotected dry aerated concrete screed, 76·2mm thick, laid to a fall of 1 : 60 picked up 9·24 litres/m² of rainwater in four wet days. Of the 9·24 litres/m², only 1·08 litres/m² could be drained off. In eight days of excellent summer weather half of the remaining water, that is 4·08 litres/m², dried out while the screed was protected from rain and the surface freely ventilated. (The eight summer days are equivalent to about 48 normal winter days.) For complete drying out 36 good summer or 180 winter days were needed.†

The rate of drying out is dependent on a number of factors, but the guides now available are useful in that they are indicative of the period that should reasonably be left before it is worthwhile actually measuring the degree of dampness with measuring devices (see *Section 3.01* 'Dampness'). On the other hand they may indicate when an alternative form of construction or special precautions are necessary. It may also be noted here that greater attention is now being paid to moisture contents than hitherto, and consequently more quantitative information may be expected.

Pollutants derived from the materials used in many of the wet-trade processes must always be taken into account especially when considering following trades. Cement is notable, for instance, for producing alkaline solutions which may have deleterious effects on paints and adhesives. In brickwork efflorescence may occur during drying out which may cause plaster or paint to deteriorate.

**Table 3.02/2 Quantities of Water Introduced during Construction**

| *Material/Construction* | | | *Quantity of water* |
|---|---|---|---|
| *Ref.* | *Description* | *Unit* | |
| a | Brickwork, average | m³ | up to 178·38 litres |
| a1 | Brickwork, average, 229mm thick | m² | up to 40·8 litres |
| a1 | Brickwork, average, 114mm thick | m² | up to 20·4 litres |
| a1 | Brickwork, average | per brick | up to 0·38 litre |
| a | Concrete, average | m³ | up to 178·38 litres |
| b | Concrete, 1 : 2 : 4 mix, water/cement ratio 0·45 | m³ | 140·63 litres |
| b | Concrete, 1 : 2 : 4 mix, water/cement ratio 0·65 | m³ | 200·00 litres |
| a | Plaster undercoat, 6·4mm thick | m² | about 2·72–4·08 litres |
| a | Plaster scim coat | m² | about 1·36 litres |
| c | Screed, lightweight aggregate or aerated cement, 76·2mm thick | m² | about 5·44–10·87 litres |
| d | Traditional 3-bedroom house | complete | about 6364–8183 litres |
| e | 2 tower blocks of flats, each 13 storeys high—see photograph. (combined floor area = 969m² combined cube = 716 761m³) | complete | about 3·705 × 10⁶ litres |

References:
(a) National Building Studies, Bulletin No. 2, *Painting New Plaster and Cement*, HMSO, 1948. *Important note:* Quantities are only rough estimates.
(a1) Calculated from 'a'.
(b) Calculated from values given in *Report on concrete practice*, part one, table 12, p. 56 (Cement & Concrete Association), 1963.
(c) *Developments in roofing*, BRS Digest (2nd Series), No. 51, p. 1, October 1964.
(d) From the BRS. *Note:* Total quantity used, i.e. including cleaning, spilling etc. estimated to be between 8 092–22 730 litres.
(e) From Widnell and Trollope, Surveyors, S.W.1. *Note:* The total quantity of water used on the job, i.e. including waste, was metered as 7·410 × 10⁶ litres. The figure of 3·705 × 10⁶ litres quoted in the table assumes 100% waste (see (d) above).

## 4. Atmosphere

Water vapour is always present in the atmosphere. The comparative ease with which gases are transferred from place to place or even through materials means that virtually all parts of a building, whether these occur internally, externally or within the thickness of a construction, are perpetually exposed to water.

Although water in the vapour state cannot necessarily be entirely discounted from the point of view of exposure, it is perhaps more realistic to consider the actual degree of severity of exposure when the vapour has been 'converted' into the liquid state. In this context it is more common for liquid water to be derived from the atmosphere during condensation which results from thermal differentials. On the other hand, deliquescent salts, particularly on surfaces of materials, are capable of absorbing moisture from the atmosphere, and in so doing convert this

*Reference: *Damp-proofing solid floors*, BRS Digest (2nd series) No. 54, p. 4, January, 1965, 'Drying out time'.

*Reference: *Developments in roofing*, BRS Digest (2nd series) No. 51, p. 1, October, 1964, 'Drying wet screeds'.

†Note: Methods of providing ventilation so as to reduce the time before the impervious roofing is laid and to avoid 'entrapped' water problems are now being used. These are described in the digest referred to above and are also included in *3.04 Exclusion*.

moisture into what may be termed a kind of condensation.

The whole problem of condensation, covering all aspects, is discussed fully in *4.00, Heat and its effects*. Accordingly, only general points related to exposure are included here.

Condensation as a source of dampness in building does appear to be far more significant nowadays than rain penetration. As the results of years of research and experience, particularly in the more traditional forms of construction, have shown how the problems associated with the exclusion of rainwater may be effectively solved, so the increased use of more efficient and rapid forms of heating during winter has resulted in increases of condensed water vapour forming not only on surfaces of an enclosure but also within the thickness of the enclosing fabric.

Both forms of condensation, either surface or interstitial, are attributable to a number of factors among which higher internal air temperatures and better thermal insulation are, paradoxically, important. Local concentrations of surface condensation are usually due to the lack of continuity in the thermal insulation of the enclosure, resulting in 'cold bridges' being formed, on which moisture contained in the warm air may condense. (The term 'cold' is used relative to the temperature and the thermodynamic properties of air in which 'dew point' is significant.) Uninsulated cold water pipes also provide 'suitable' cold surfaces for the formation of condensation—such condensation is very often mistaken for 'a leaky' pipe.

Interstitial condensation, resulting mainly from differential vapour pressures (temperature differentials are also involved), must be carefully considered whenever 'sandwiched' forms of constructions, including within their thickness materials of high thermal insulation, are proposed. The actual position of the insulation is critical. The use of vapour barriers also requires careful consideration. When such barriers are to be incorporated account must be taken of the probable necessity for the adequate drainage of water which may condense on the barrier itself. An example of the 'unwitting' use of a vapour barrier may be noted here. Impervious claddings used on the exterior of buildings do automatically form vapour barriers and water vapour permeating from the inside air can condense behind such claddings. Drainage of the condensed vapour is important.

The probable quantities of water which may result from condensation can be calculated for a design condition. However, the purpose of calculations is generally to act as a guide of the probability of condensation occurring under given environmental conditions relative to particular forms of construction so that suitable precautions may be taken to ensure either its avoidance or its harmless collection and drainage. This may involve a

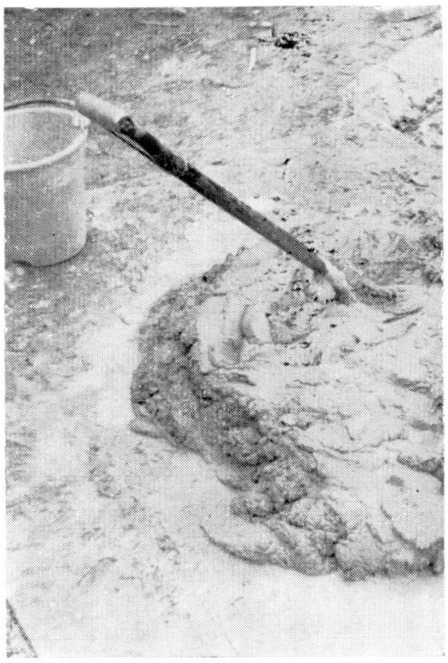

1

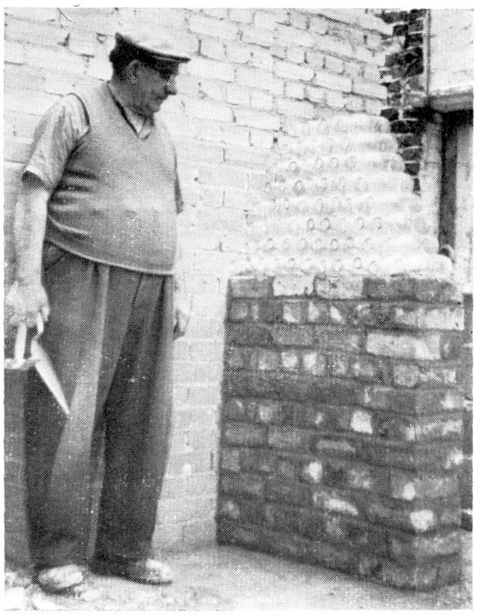

2

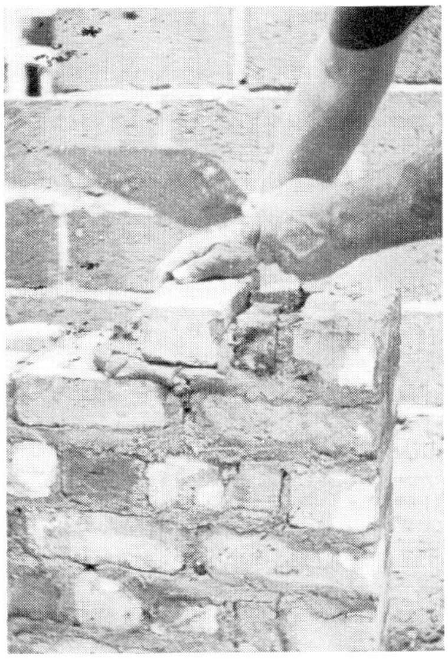

3

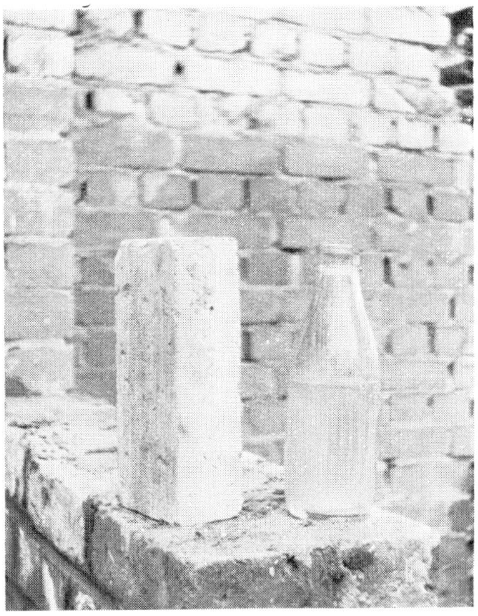

4

*Vast quantities of water are used in the construction of most buildings (see Table 3.02/2). The examples below are in British Units, but the SI equivalents are given in brackets.*

1. *Mortar requires water.* 2. *It is estimated that up to 7½gal of water is contained in 1 sq yd of 9in brickwork when freshly laid. (Equivalent to 40·8 litres in 1m² of 229mm brickwork.) In this photograph the water is represented by the 60 pint milk bottles, while Mr. J. Francis, who specially built the wall from old Belgian bricks, looks on.* 3. *Building the wall.* 4. *Each brick plus its surrounding mortar accounts for up to ¾pt of water. (Equivalent to 0·38 litre.) (Courtesy: G. W. Wooldridge Esq. (contractor) and the South Coast Dairies Ltd.)*

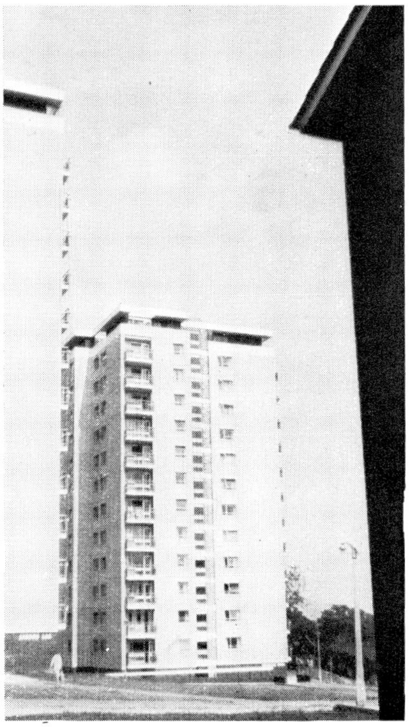

*The two point blocks of flats, each 13 storeys high, referred to in Table 3.02/2. During the contract 7·410 × 10⁶ litres of water was metered; if account is taken of wastage an estimated 3·705 × 10⁶ litres of water was introduced during construction*

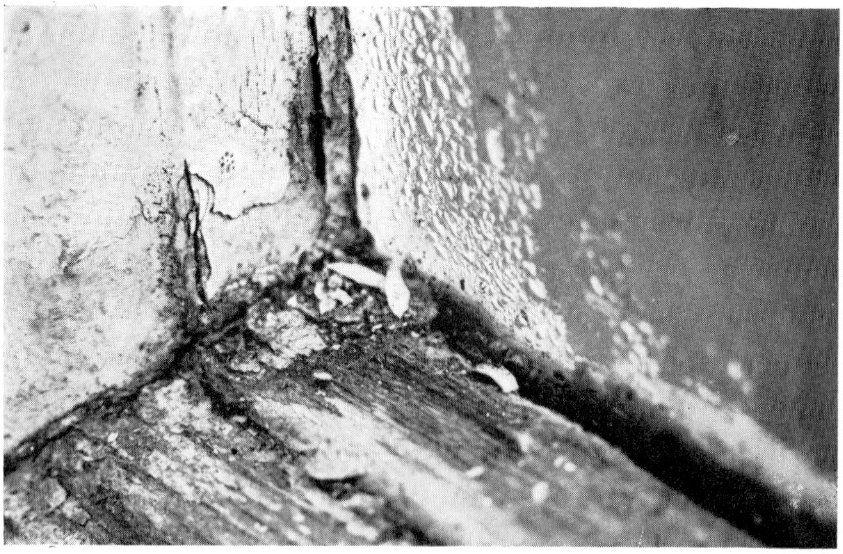

*'Condensation as a source of dampness in buildings does appear to be far more significant nowadays than rain penetration.' Both surface and interstitial condensation must be taken into account.*

*Above, surface condensation on a window pane and the deterioration of the timber frame due to continuous wetting and insufficient protection.*

*Below, discoloration of glass cladding due to the formation of interstitial condensation. An example of the 'unwitting' use of a vapour barrier*

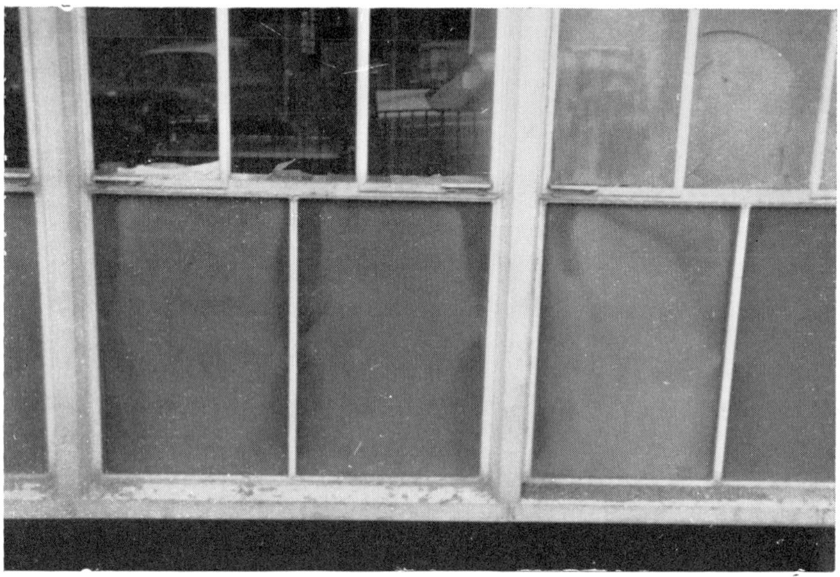

change in the conditions or a change in the form of construction, including materials. It is perhaps all too obvious that certain user requirements (kitchens, bathrooms, swimming baths and many industrial processes) imply, without the need for calculation, severe conditions of exposure.

Although greater emphasis has been given to condensation occurring internally, it should be noted that condensation, often referred to as dew, does occur frequently externally. Thus, external elements are not entirely exempted from due consideration. In general, it is the metals which require special care in that suitable precautions should be taken to ensure that condensed vapour is not allowed to remain in cracks, crevices, etc.

Finally, condensed flue gases provide an important source of water in chimneys. Furthermore, such condensed vapour may be highly polluted. Special precautions are, therefore, necessary in the selection and use of materials making up the flue.

**5. Water supply**

Water as supplied by a water authority or as obtained from other 'private' sources such as wells, rain collecting tanks, etc., is required in buildings for a number of different reasons, among which are included human consumption (cooking, drinking, etc.); human cleanliness (ablutions, etc.); human comfort (heating, cooling, etc.); and industrial and other processes. All the water required is contained, distributed and eventually carried away by means of some form of piped system. In addition to pipes, many other component parts are also used. Despite the number and diversity of pipes and components which may be involved in the piped system as a whole, the problems of exposure are at least confined. On the other hand, the surfaces of the materials used, consisting mainly of the metals although plastics are now being increasingly used, are *always* exposed and, in this sense, present the severest conditions of exposure of all elements in a building. In view of the permanency of exposure implied with water supply, the severity of exposure is determined, in the final analysis, by the degree of pollution of the water. As will be seen later, there are likely to be considerable variations in the degree of pollution which may be expected in water as supplied to the piped system. Further pollution may take place during distribution, while the nature of pollutants to be found in 'wastes' which are eventually drained away must also be taken into account.

**6. Faulty services**

Water, which may leak from any of the component parts of the piped system of the water supply *or* from pipes, gutters and other component parts used to drain rainwater from horizontal or sloping surfaces, constitutes conditions of exposure which may seem, at first glance, to be completely fortuitous.

However, this does not detract from the fact that a condition of exposure exists when a leak has occurred. The severity of the exposure will be dependent on the position in which the leak takes place, the rate of leakage and the speed with which the requisite repair is carried out. Subject to the relationship between these factors, faulty services may be a major cause of dampness. This means then that some serious consideration must be given at the design stage of the manner in which such a contingency is to be dealt with during the life of a building. This involves basically the relationship between materials selected and maintenance. It may be noted here that pipes, for instance, which may be buried within the fabric or under the structure of a building, present special cases, particularly so far as effects of leaks and replacement of parts are concerned.

Faulty services may also imply bad design. In this context the detailed positioning, size and projection of overflow pipes, which are in any case specifically incorporated in a piped system to deal with faults in some of the water containing components, are important. A number of examples are to be found in buildings where this aspect has not received due attention. The result is invariably a change in appearance of materials underneath the overflows caused by local concentrations of water. One example is

*Conditions of exposure due to faulty services may seem, at first glance, to be completely fortuitous. However, a condition of exposure does exist when a leak occurs. In the example, far right, continuous dripping from the taps has enabled water, initiated by splashing, to be transferred up the vertical face of the porous wall. At the time of taking the photograph water had commenced to 'bridge' the line of the d.p.c. Due consideration should be given to the effects of leaks or replacements of parts for pipes which may be wholly or partially buried within the fabric or under the structure of the building*

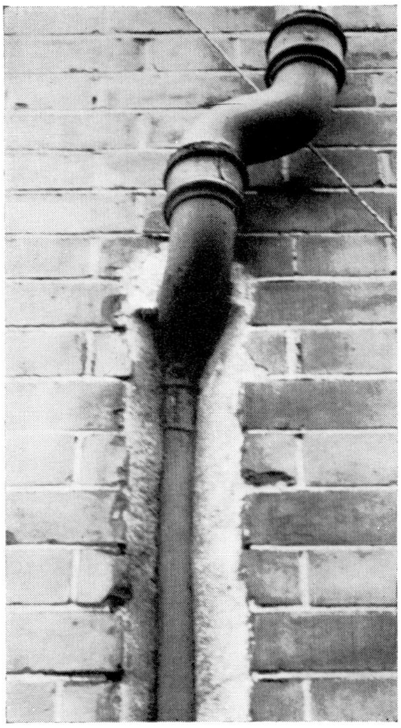

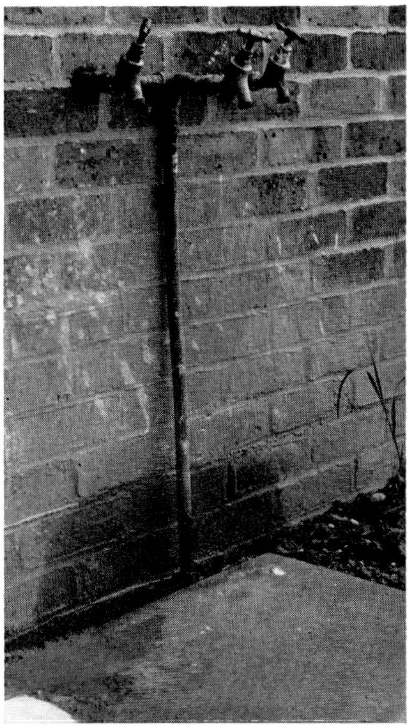

*The examples below illustrate some of the effects, mainly changes in appearance, resulting from increases in exposure to water in overflow pipes due mainly to incorrect positioning or slope*

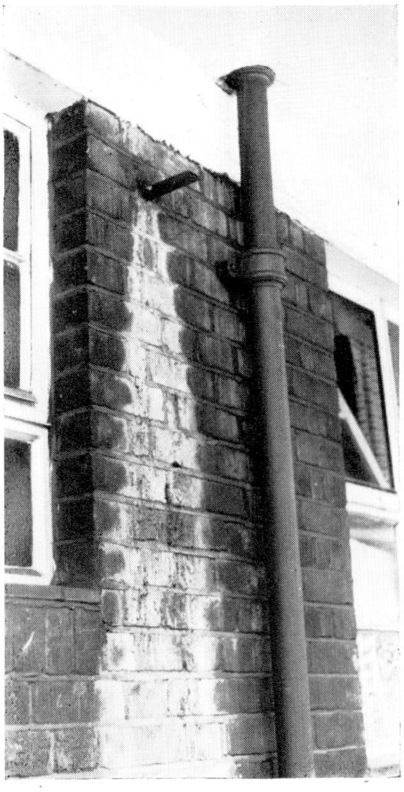

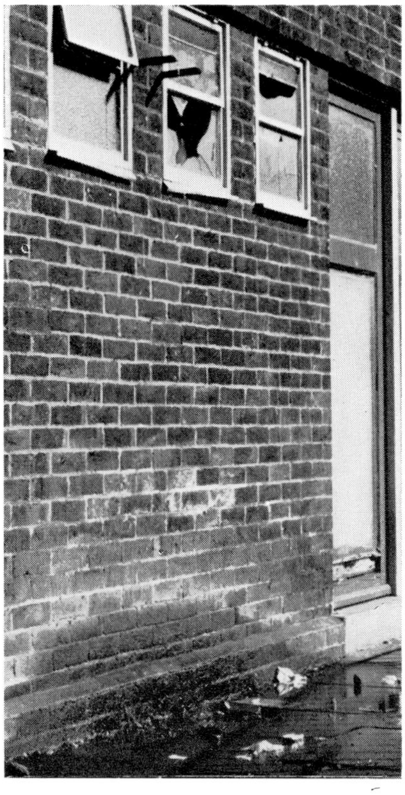

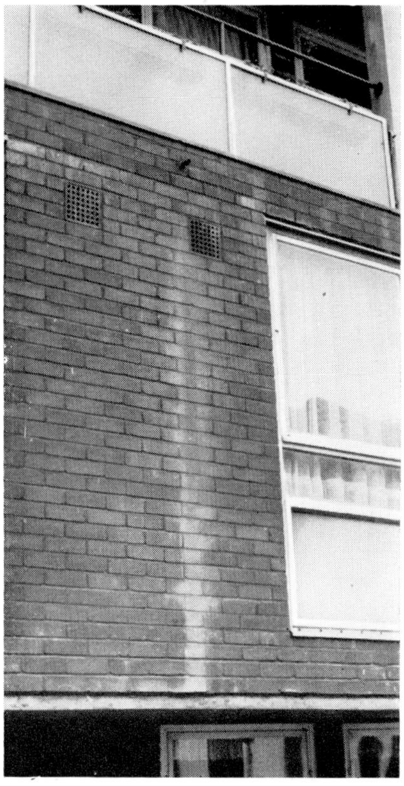



D

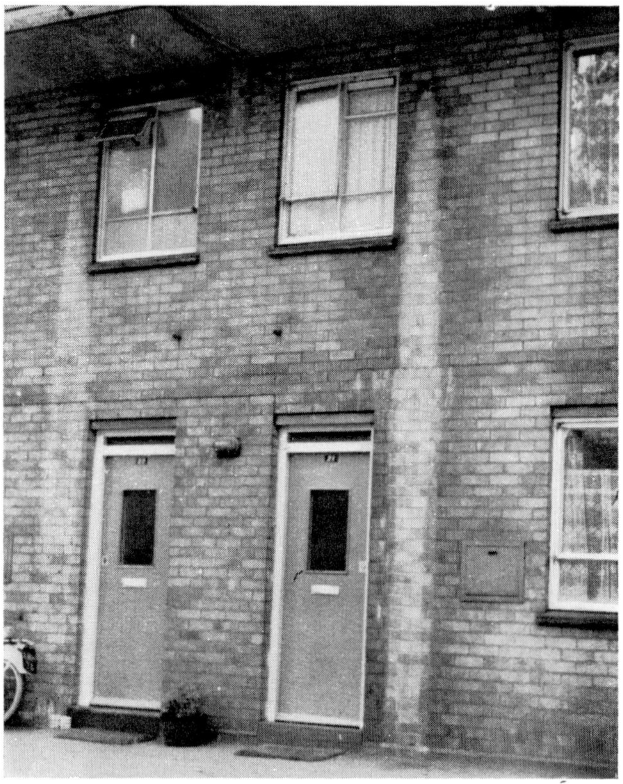

*Overflows from appliances such as water cisterns normally considered essential for use when appliance is faulty, i.e. occasionally. Most by-laws require these to be in noticeable positions*

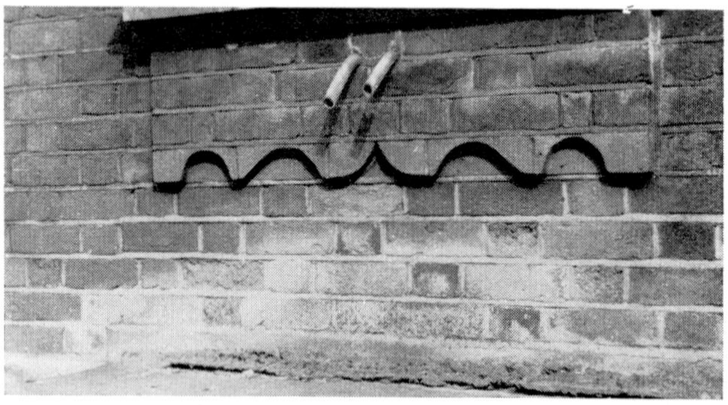

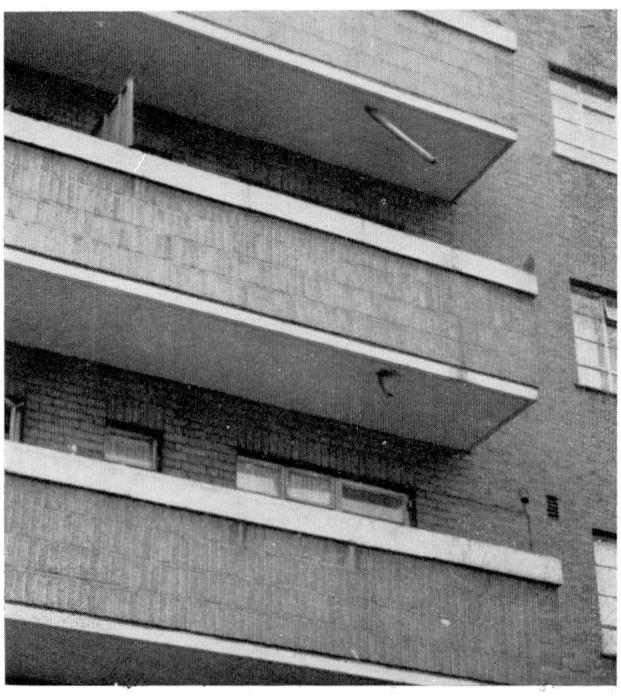

*Pipes designed for continuous flow during rainfall for drainage of water from horizontal surfaces. In these cases balconies*

included in *Section 3.01* 'Flow', others are shown in the accompanying photographs.

The severity of exposure conditions resulting from faulty services may be significantly increased by pollutants. Services as such are, of course, liable to contain a variety of these.

**7. Maintenance and user requirements**

Maintenance and especially regular cleaning of surfaces of materials used in buildings may involve the use of water. Similarly, there are a number of user requirements, such as occur in kitchens, bathrooms, swimming baths, and many industrial and other processes, which necessitate the use of water. In all cases the quantities of water and the relationship between these and the materials concerned are subject to wide variation. However, what is significant is the fact that the continual or occasional presence of water is, or should be, known in advance. This is important and of some considerable advantage in the final selection and use of materials to meet particular conditions. However, it should be noted that a careful analysis is required of the conditions which are likely to prevail, with particular attention paid to the possibility of pollutants being involved in any of the processes concerned.

## Pollution of water

Water may 'pick up' pollutants throughout the whole of the water cycle. In the context of buildings this cycle is indeed extremely complex plus the fact that the wide range of materials available for building also 'offer' many pollutants. It is, therefore, extremely difficult, in this study, to take into account fully the effects of any 'chain reactions' that do occur as water follows its cycle, whether in the liquid or vapour state (in building the solid state is usually of little significance as regards pollution). Accordingly, and also to avoid unnecessary repetition, it has been considered convenient to deal with the causes of pollution separately under the following general headings: (1) Atmosphere; (2) Ground; (3) Water supply; (4) Solution of building materials; and (5) Processes and cleansing agents. In each case an indication is given of the sources of water which are likely to be affected. As already mentioned, account must be taken of the whole of the water cycle in a building when making an analysis of the severity of conditions for a particular case.

**1. Atmosphere**

Atmospheric or air pollution plays an important part in causing water to contain corrosive agencies more potent than would be the case in the absence of the pollution. Additional abrasive particles may also be present in the water as well as the chemical substances. In general it is perhaps more usual to consider the contamination of rainwater, either in the chemical or physical sense, caused by impurities present in a polluted atmosphere.* However, in the context of building materials, and taking into account the comparative ease with which gases can be transferred, it is far more realistic to include the effects of air pollution on water formed during condensation, both surface and interstitial. In this the action of flue gases in chimneys requires special consideration. The fact that polluted water vapour may often be in contact with building materials, if not transferred through them, makes it necessary to pay some attention to this aspect too. In short, the destructive effects of atmospheric pollution when associated with water can be widespread and are, therefore, applicable to all parts of a building whether these are inside or outside. This is extremely important when considering exposure.

Although quite a substantial quantity of water becomes corrosive as the impurities present in a polluted atmosphere are 'picked up' and dissolved during rainfall, the corrosive agencies may also be formed as a result of water wetting the surfaces of buildings and subsequently absorbing impurities which are then oxidised. The importance of this method of formation lies chiefly in the fact that on evaporation the corrosive agencies are liable to become highly concentrated. The destructive effects of such concentrations are accentuated if they are held by materials for any length of time. A further related point may also be noted here. The corrosive agencies of polluted rainwater may be changed when there is a reaction between the contaminated water and certain other substances. As an example consider any building material containing carbonates. In addition to the fact that the material itself will suffer damage, soluble sulphates and chlorides are formed as a result of the action of polluted rainwater on the insoluble carbonates. The 'new' substances may, of course, be transferred to other materials which, in turn, may suffer damage.

(a) *Basic constituents*

The air normally contains many basic constituents, the major of which, expressed as a percentage by weight, are: nitrogen (75 per cent), oxygen (23 per cent), argon (1·26 per cent), water vapour (0·70 per cent) and carbon dioxide (0·04 per cent). Neon,

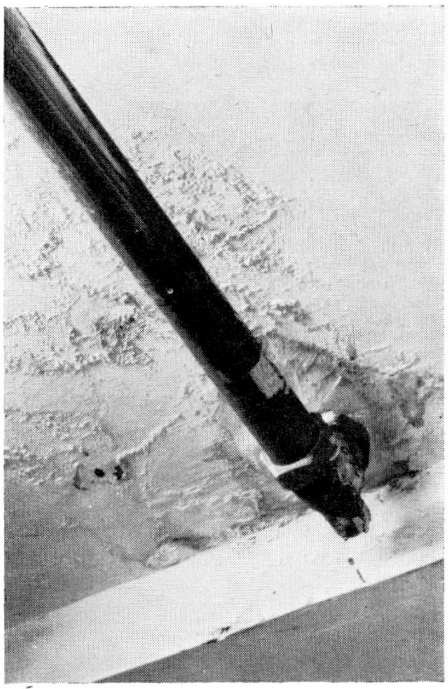

*The example above shows a fault in a kitchen waste running across an office*

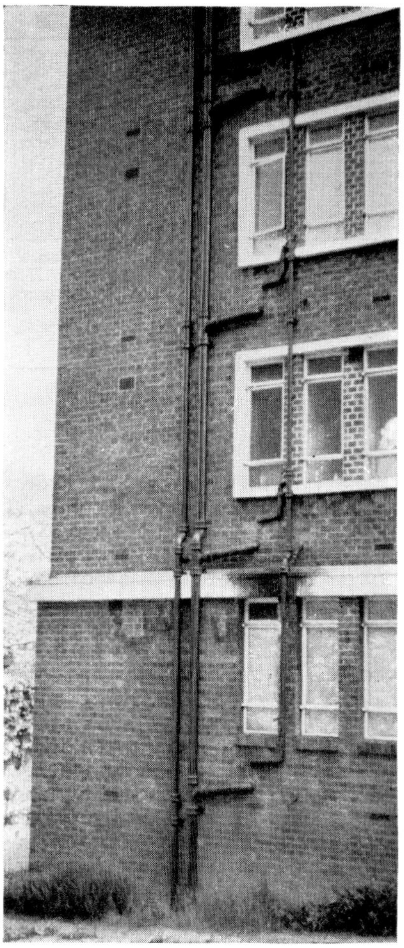

*The severity of exposure conditions resulting from faulty services may be significantly increased by pollutants. Services as such are, of course, liable to contain a variety of these*

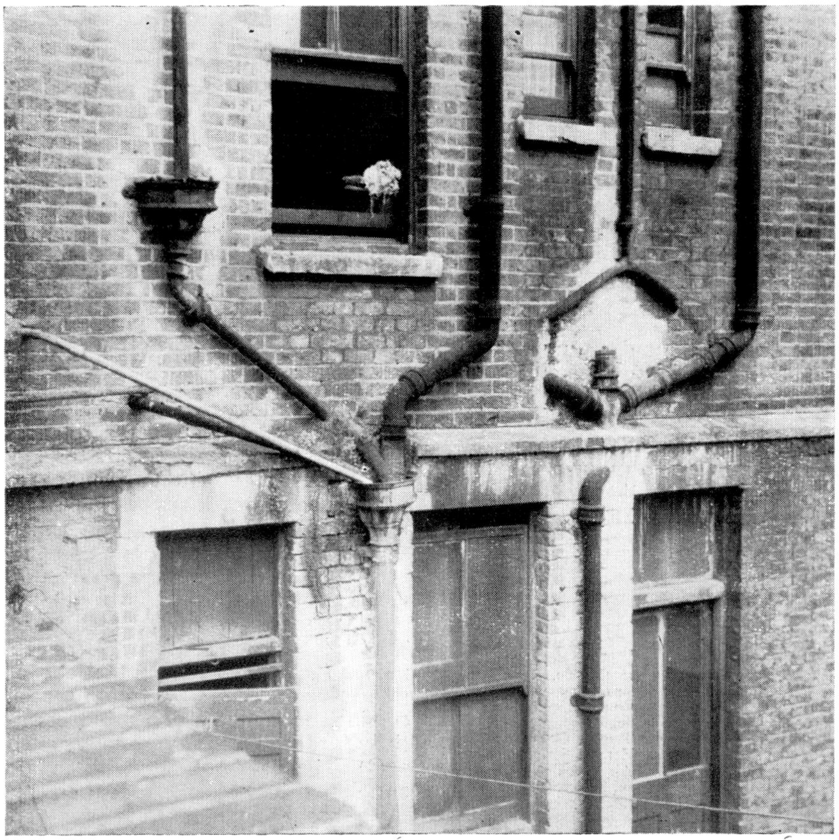

* References and Notes:

(1) Meetham, A.R., *Atmospheric Pollution, Its Origins and Prevention*, rev. 3rd Ed. Pergamon, 1964. This has been used as the main reference. (2) Report of the committee on air pollution, The Beaver Report, Cmd 9322, November, 1954. (3) *The destructive effects of air pollution on materials*, the 6th Des Voeux Memorial Lecture by Parker, A., September 28, 1955 (National Smoke Abatement Society)—now National Society for Clean Air (NSCA). (4) *Meteorology and Air pollution*, the 8th Des Voeux Memorial Lecture by Sutton, Sir Graham, October 4, 1957 (National Smoke Abatement Society)—now National Society for Clean Air (NSCA). (5) Notes on Air Pollution issued by the Warren Spring Laboratory (DSIR), Gunnels Wood Road, Stevenage, Herts. (6) *Durability*, BS Code of Practice, CP3—Chapter IX (1950). (7) *The Investigation of Atmospheric Pollution* 1958-1966, 32nd Report, Warren Spring Laboratory, Ministry of Technology, HMSO, 1967.

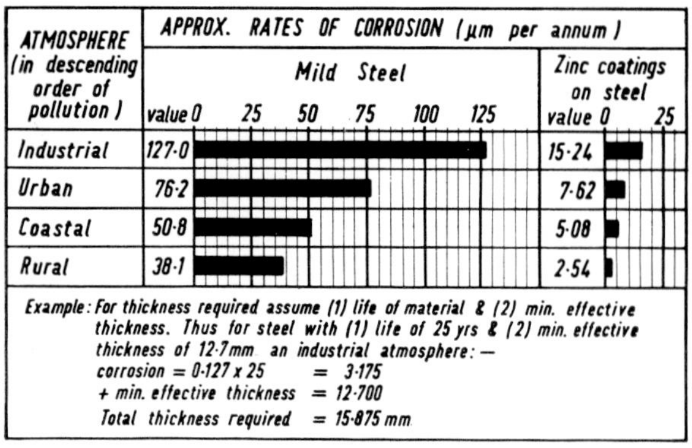


C.3.02/3
*Approximate rates of corrosion of mild steel and zinc coatings on steel in atmospheres of differing pollutions. (Values from: Durability, B5 CP3, Chapter IX, Table 2, p' 18, 1950)*

krypton, helium, xenon and hydrogen are also present but in a comparatively minor way. Some of these when combined with water (free carbon dioxide forming a weak acid—carbonic acid—is a notable example) may be corrosive. However, within the present context, none of the major or minor constituents of air is usually considered to be a cause of atmospheric pollution.* Other substances, such as the oxides of sulphur, the chlorides, chlorine and fluorine compounds, resulting essentially from fuel burning, fuel handling and chemical processes (in order of importance) or, on the other hand, the salts from a natural source such as the sea and found in areas at or near the coast, form the main constituents of a polluted atmosphere. All of these are capable of causing water to be corrosive and occur in a wide range of concentrations. When compared to the major constituents of air, the quantities of the pollutants which may be present even in a highly polluted atmosphere are small. In some cases they are also small when compared with the quantities of the minor constituents of air. An indication of the scale of the difference may be obtained by considering the fact that the major constituents of air may be measured in $g/m^3$, whereas the minor constituents and the atmospheric impurities in $mg/m^3$. However, despite the comparatively small quantities involved, the potential (and, in fact, actual) aggressiveness of the impurities, particularly when associated with water, cannot be under-estimated.

The Beaver Report contained some illuminating estimates of the additional or direct *annual* costs of maintenance of buildings in polluted atmospheres.† For painting and decorating the sum was estimated to be approximately £30m (one-fifth of the total expenditure in the country as a whole); for cleaning and depreciation of buildings other than houses approximately £20m (the cost being two and a half times as much in a dirty area as compared with a clean area); finally the corrosion of metals due to atmospheric pollution was estimated as approximately £25m.

(b) *Problems of assessment*

In the past the greatest attention has naturally enough been given to those materials which were commonly found in practice to be most affected by atmospheric pollution in the presence of water. Accordingly, stone and metals (particularly the ferrous metals) have received considerable study. However, others such as sacrifice coatings (paint, galvanizing, etc.), bricks and mortar may also be included. From the point of view of exposure, classifications were made according to the type of atmosphere. In descending order of severity these are given as Industrial, Urban, Coastal and Rural. On the basis of these classifications an indication of the probable performance of a material could be given. Few attempts have been made to classify atmospheres relative to building performance, that is, in terms of the precise degree of pollution which may be expected in any area. (A guide of the approximate rates of corrosion for both mild steel and zinc coatings on steel in atmospheres graded in terms of severity of pollution is given in the comparative chart C.3.02/3). There are a number of reasons for this, some of which are:

(1) The wide variation in the degree of pollution, including the substances present, which may occur in any locality. These variations are due to the interaction of many variable factors including the effects of human activity and weather.

(2) The lack of systematic measurements over the whole country, that is polluted as well as non-polluted areas. The great number of measurements made since 1933 with a variety of measuring devices have mostly been confined to polluted areas and essentially for local needs.

(3) The lack of any systematic correlation between the measurements of airborne pollution and the performance of materials, particularly when water is present.

(4) There has been no apparent need on a large scale for any greater degree of accuracy.

Some of the 'gaps' are now in the process of being filled. Since the publication of the Beaver Report on Air Pollution, 1954,—the committee was set up following the disastrous effects particularly on human health of the 1952 London smog—and the subsequent passing of the Clean Air Act, 1956, there has been a greater interest in all aspects of air pollution. In 1961 'The National Survey of Air Pollution' was inaugurated. The Warren Spring Laboratory (DOE), has encouraged the use of standard methods of measurement by local authorities. The laboratory also publishes annually the results from stations now covering all parts of the country. Thus polluted and non-polluted areas are being covered. Information more detailed than that published can often be obtained, very often from the local authority concerned. In the main, measurements are made of the main pollutants *at ground level*; they are not concerned particularly with the pollution of rainwater as such, although measurements of the pollution of rainwater are made by many authorities. Investigations into other aspects of atmospheric pollution are also carried out by the Warren Spring Laboratory, such as the effects of chimney heights, the weather and obstructions.

It will probably be some time before the results of the national survey—the first period is to extend over five years—and other research currently taking place will be related to the performance of building materials. The existing classifications will therefore have to suffice. A better understanding of these and of the precautions which should be exercised in applying them in practice should be obtained if some of the more important aspects of air pollution are known. It is, therefore, the main aim of this part to outline these aspects and, where possible, to indicate the manner in which any of the pollutants influence the basic corrosive nature of water.

Despite the inherent difficulties involved in any assessment of the severity of atmospheric pollution relative to buildings as a whole, it is convenient to note here that local authorities and other interested bodies, such as the Warren Spring Laboratory, should be consulted where special problems appear to exist. The Scientific Adviser to the LCC (now the GLC) mentions in his Annual Report, 1963 (page 51) that advice on air pollution aspects relative to the problems of high buildings in the vicinity of existing power stations and factory chimneys were increasingly being sought at the planning stage. Some of the work carried out by the council in this connection had been found to the helpful, although it was recognised that further study of the problem was still required.

*The pollution of water by the 'natural' constituents of air is extremely important relative to decay and deterioration of materials. However, this aspect has been purposely omitted from this section in order that detailed consideration may be given to those pollutants which are essentially 'man-made' and therefore potentially controllable. The effects of the natural constituents of air on materials are noted as relevant in the other sections dealing mainly with decay and deterioration in detail.

†Members of the Beaver Report Committee have since stated that they consider the figures to be too conservative. 'The Cost of Air Pollution', Clean Air Year Book 1964–65 (National Society for Clean Air), p. 29. Note: No revised figures are included in this ref.

| | CLASS OF CONSUMER | FUEL USED Value (Tg) | SMOKE Value (Tg) | SULPHUR DIOXIDE Value (Tg) | GRIT & DUST Value (Tg) |
|---|---|---|---|---|---|
| COAL | Domestic | 37·39 | 0·91 | 0·91 | 0·10 |
| COAL | Electricity works | 37·28 | small | 1·02 | 0·30 |
| COAL | Railways | 14·05 | 0·30 | 0·41 | 0·10 |
| COAL | Industrial & misc. | 65·63 | 0·81 | 1·83 | 0·30 |
| COAL | Coke ovens | 26·31 | small | 0·10 | small |
| COAL | Gas works | 27·63 | small | 0·20 | small |
| COKE (excl. gas wks. & blast furnaces) | | 14·94 | nil | 0·41 | small |
| OIL | Diesel & gas oil | 3·05 | — | 0·10 | nil |
| OIL | Fuel oil | 5·38 | — | 0·30 | nil |
| OIL | Creosote-pitch mixt. | 0·71 | — | small | nil |

NOTES: (a) Includes general industry, collieries, patent fuel works, non-industrial establishments, waterworks and the service departments.
(b) Certain types of plant used and particularly the older coke oven plants may discharge smoke and grit in sufficient quantities to cause serious local concentrations.
(c) To this column must be added approx. 0·51 Tg. from industrial processes other than steam raising.

C.3.02/4

*Main supplies and uses of fuels and estimates of pollutants discharged in Great Britain during 1953. (Values from: 'Committee on Air Pollution Report', Nov. 1964, Cmd. 9322, p. 7)*

| | FUEL & CLASS OF CONSUMER | FUEL USED value (All values in Tg) | SMOKE value (All values in Tg) | SULPHUR DIOXIDE value (All values in Tg) | GRIT & DUST value (All vs. in Tg) |
|---|---|---|---|---|---|
| COAL | Domestic (a) | 33·6<br>25·6 | 1·20<br>0·80 | 0·86<br>0·66 | 0·10<br>0·30 |
| COAL | Electricity Works | 61·4<br>69·0 | small | 1·77<br>2·05 | 0·30<br>0·10 |
| COAL | Railways | 6·2<br>1·7 | 0·10<br>0·03 | 0·18<br>0·05 | 0·10<br>small |
| COAL | Industrial & Misc. | 43·9<br>36·6 | 0·20<br>0·11 | 1·26<br>1·06 | 0·30(h)<br>0·20(h) |
| COAL | Coke ovens | 23·9<br>24·7 | small | 0·08<br>0·09 | small |
| COAL | Gas works | 22·5<br>17·0 | small | 0·16<br>0·12 | small |
| COKE (excl. gas wrks. & blast furnaces)(b) | | 15·8<br>13·0 | nil | 0·36<br>0·29 | small |
| OIL | Domestic (c) | 1·8<br>2·2 | v.small | 0·01<br>0·01 | nil |
| OIL | Industrial (d) | 28·9(g)<br>40·0(g) | small | 1·40<br>1·92 | nil |
| OIL | Road & Rail transp.(e) | 12·4<br>16·6 | small | 0·06<br>0·08 | nil |
| OIL | Marine craft (f) | 1·2<br>1·1 | small | 0·04<br>0·04 | nil |

KEY: ■ values for 1962; □ values for 1966; ( ) values in brackets in the notes are for 1966; unbracketed values for 1962.

NOTES: (a) Includes miner's coal.
(b) Includes domestic coke + other solid smokeless fuels and industrial + misc.
(c) Includes kerosene and domestic oils.
(d) Includes kerosene gas/diesel fuel oils and creosote pitch.
(e) Includes motor spirit gas/diesel and fuel oils.
(f) Includes gas/diesel and fuel oils.
(g) The amount of 28·9 Tg (40·0 Tg) of oil equivalent to about 48·8 Tg (68·1 Tg) of coal which if used for the same purpose would have produced about 0·2 Tg (0·2 Tg) of smoke; 1·3 Tg (1·9 Tg) of sulphur dioxide and 0·3 Tg (0·2 Tg) of grit.
(h) Excluding grit and dust emissions, estimated at about 0·5 Tg (0·4 Tg) from industrial processes other than steam raising.

C.3.02/5

*Comparison of main supplies and uses of fuels and estimates of pollutants discharged in Great Britain during 1962 and 1966. (Values from: 'Clean Air Year Books,' 1964/65 and 1968/69, tables on pp. 38 and 28 respectively, prepared by Dr. A. Parker)*

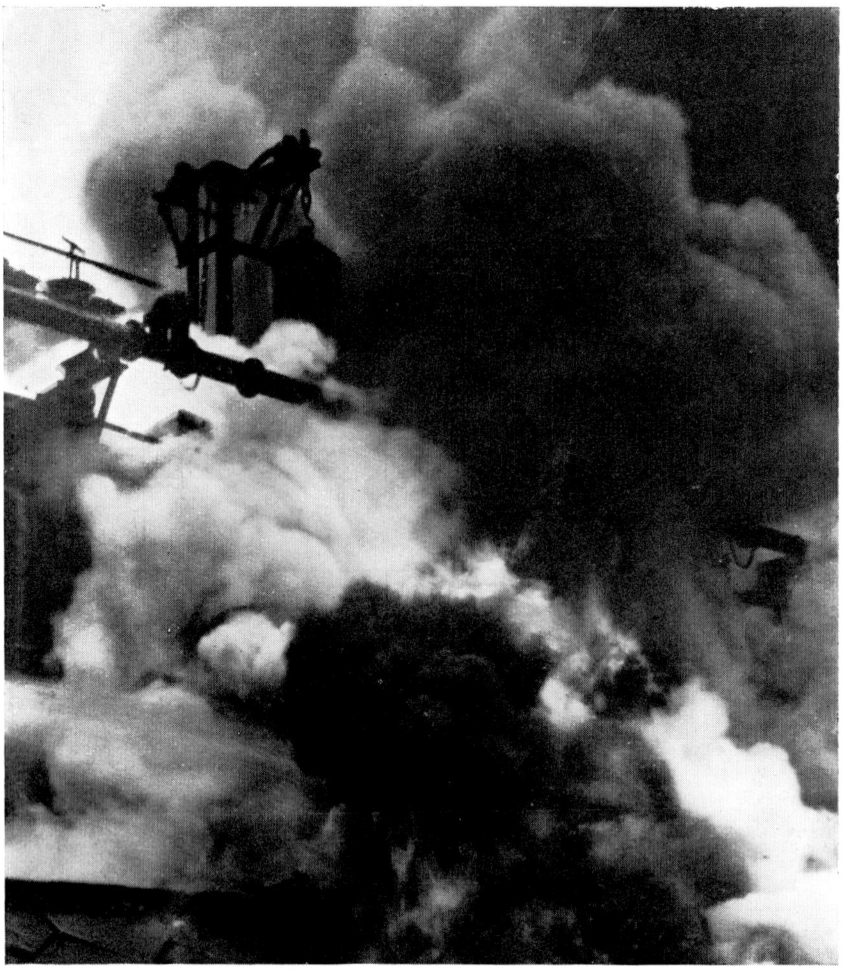

*'The greatest amount of air pollution in Great Britain is made from the burning of fuel of various kinds.'* *Pollutants being discharged from a coke oven (Courtesy: National Society for Clean Air)*

(c) *Impurities from fuel burning*

In general the greatest amount of air pollution in Great Britain is made from the burning of fuel of various kinds. The resultant impurities or pollutants which include solids, liquids and gases are chiefly smoke, grit and dust, sulphur dioxide, carbon monoxide, chlorine and fluorine. These are dealt with separately below, but before doing so it is convenient to note the amounts of the pollutants which are discharged annually over the whole country. Smoke and sulphur dioxide are in the first instance the most important—the amounts of these are usually much higher than the others, while they are the major destructive agencies—and are accordingly the ones most commonly measured. They also form the basis of assessment of the degree of pollution in an area. The comparative chart C.3.02/4 gives the amounts of these pollutants, plus the amounts of grit and dust discharged in Great Britain during 1953 from the main fuels used. Some of the changes in the amounts since 1953 can be seen in the comparative chart C.3.02/5 (discharges in 1962 and 1966) which excludes grit and dust from industrial and miscellaneous users. It is important to note that the amounts quoted in both of these charts are only indicative of the *potential* of air pollution. The quantities are those *discharged* rather than those which are deposited at or near ground level. The concentrations of deposited matter are, in general, far more significant. In the context of the contamination of water, and taking into account tall buildings, this may not necessarily be the case. Conclusive evidence on this point is, however, not generally available.

*Smoke*

The term 'smoke' is applied to the visible products of imperfect combustion, and commonly seen in smoke trails from chimneys which may be short or long. The particles in smoke are extremely small (not to be confused with grit and dust which consist of much larger particles) and behave like a gas. Thus smoke ultimately becomes so well mixed with air that it is invisible except as a bluish haze which obscures distant objects. Despite the mixing which takes place, smoke in this 'diluted' form still remains a potential cause of dirt and damage.

Coal contains a high proportion of carbon. Thus the finely divided particles resulting from its incomplete combustion consist of carbon or carboniferous matter, which when viewed in bulk are nearly black. In addition, coal also contains tarry hydrocarbons which add to the sticking power of the particles and a tendency for the formation of *sooty deposits*. In this connection domestic smoke is far more tarry than industrial smoke. An important aspect of the finely divided nature of the particles is that they are supported by air and unlike the heavier particles do not fall readily to the ground. (The average time for the suspension of smoke particles in air is estimated to be two days. In Great Britain a considerable proportion is blown to sea.) Thus they may be carried in currents of air, sometimes great distances from the source of emission, and eventually enter buildings via windows, cracks, vents, etc., with the incoming air. Whereas ordinary gas molecules will 'bounce off' the enclosing surfaces of an interior which they are continually bombarding, the smoke particles will, because of their adhesive qualities, remain behind. This then accounts for the progressive accumulation of dirt.

A similar procedure takes place on the external surfaces of buildings where, per force, greater quantities of smoke are available. The resultant sooty deposits are not, unfortunately, readily removed by rainwater unless the material on which they have been deposited is soluble, as in the case of limestones. In addition to spoiling appearance, the sooty deposits are generally *hygroscopic* and are thus capable of holding fairly large amounts of water which, because of the chemical nature of the deposits, becomes corrosive. An analysis of soot, C.3.02/6, shows that, in addition to the tarry matter and carbon which causes the blackening effect, soot also carries with it free acids and soluble salts. (The action of acids and the effects of solubility of stones on decay and appearance are discussed in detail in *3.06 Chemical attack,* under 'Acid action'.)

*Grit and dust*

Grit and dust are emitted from furnaces whether or not there is visible smoke. Generally the particles are large enough to fall under the influence of gravity. Ash, which is the unburnable solid material that is set free when fuel is burnt, mainly escapes with the flue gases, although some does remain behind. Some of the ash particles, it should be noted, may be so finely divided as to remain suspended in air. Unlike smoke particles, grit and dust tend to be deposited near the source of emission.

*Sulphur dioxide*

Sulphur dioxide ($SO_2$) is formed in considerable quantities as a result of the burning of fuels such as coal, coke and certain fuel oils. Other sulphur compounds are also formed but in far smaller quantities. The percentage of sulphur, from which the sulphur dioxide is formed when combined with oxygen during combustion, in various types of fuels in common use is given in the comparative chart C.3.02/7. Only 80 to 90 per cent of the sulphur in coal and coke is emitted from a chimney as sulphur dioxide, the remainder being retained in the ashes; in the case of oil, all the sulphur is emitted as sulphur dioxide.

The corrosive action of sulphur dioxide, itself soluble in water, is due to the formation of sulphurous or sulphuric acid. Some of the sulphur dioxide is removed from the air by solution in cloud droplets falling as rain and in surface water. It is estimated that only one-fifth of the sulphur dioxide emitted into the atmosphere is brought down with rain; a further one-fifth is blown into the sea, while the remainder (three-fifths) is mostly dissolved in water on buildings, soil and vegetation, after rain and at other times. (It is estimated that the average time for sulphur dioxide to remain in air is less than 12 hours.)

The formation of sulphuric acid as a result of rainwater wetting surfaces of buildings is of particular interest. (The process involved is, of course, also applicable to surfaces other than those of buildings.) Rainwater wetting the surfaces of buildings when combined with the sulphur dioxide present in the atmosphere forms a weak solution of sulphur dioxide. On evaporation a concentrated solution of sulphur dioxide is formed and when this is oxidised sulphuric acid results.

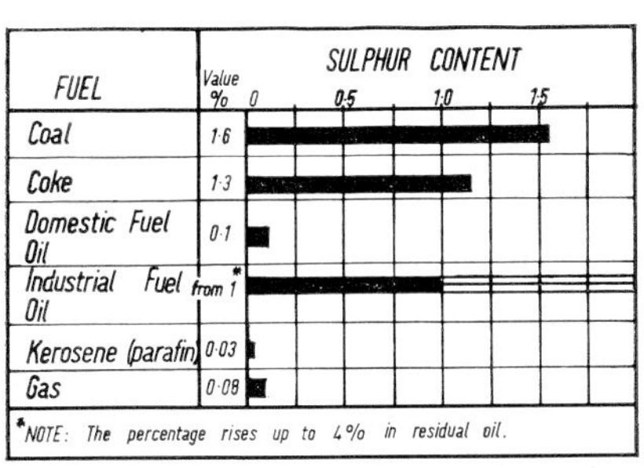


C.3.02/7
*Percentages (by weight) of sulphur in fuels in common use (average values for the U.K.) (From: Notes on Air Pollution, No. 4, 'Pollution by Sulphur Dioxide': Revised April, 1963. Warren Spring Laboratory (DOE) )*

C.3.02/6
*An analysis of soot (values are percentages). (Analysis carried out by Voelcker in 1864 and quoted in 'Weathering of Natural Building Stones' by Schaffer, R., DSIR, BRS Special Report No. 18, Appendix 1, p. 109, 1932)*

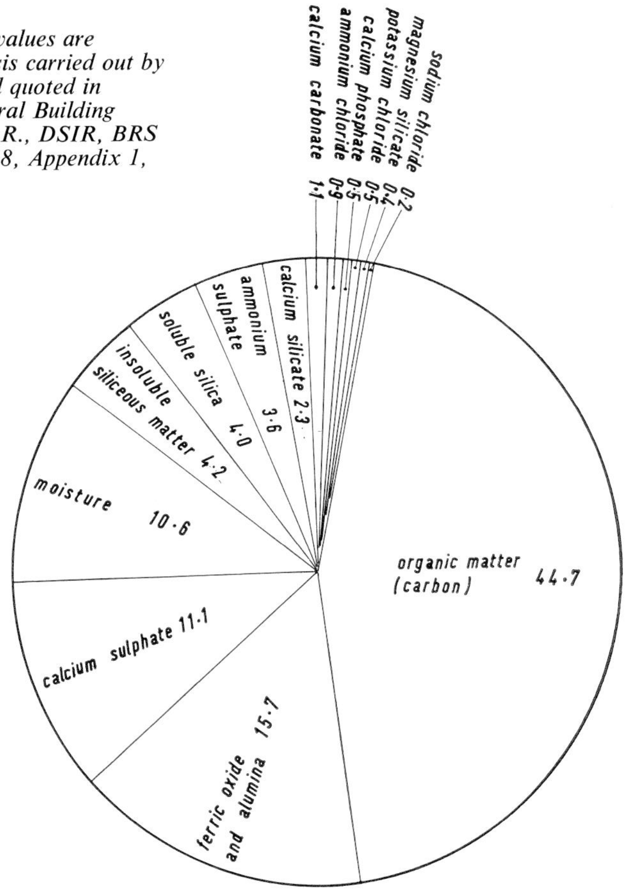


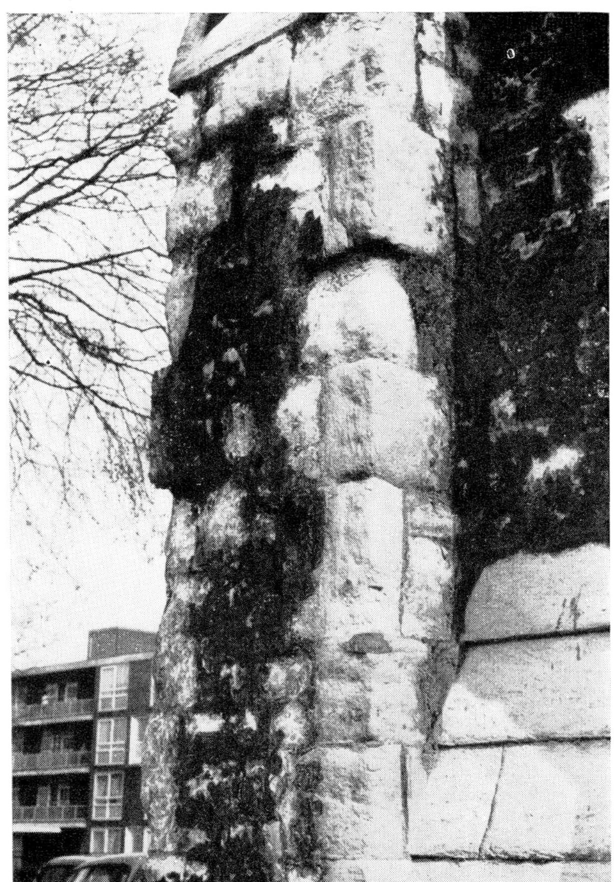

*In addition to spoiling appearance, sooty deposits are hygroscopic and may become corrosive. The photograph shows one possible result, namely exfoliation of the soot and stone*

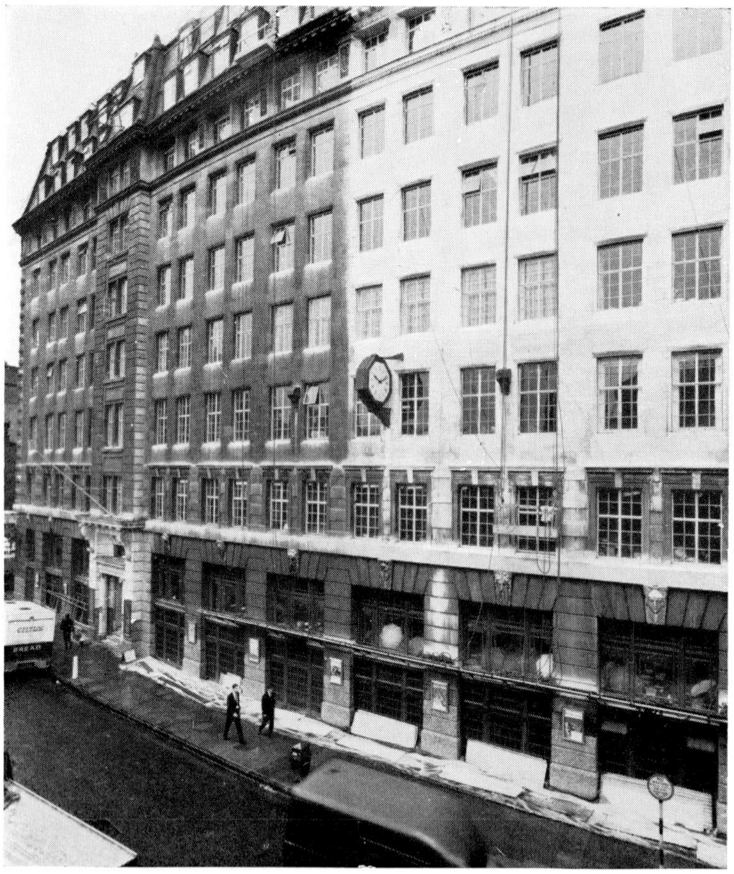

As already mentioned, the sooty deposits on surfaces are hygroscopic. Accordingly, when they are moist or wet they absorb sulphur dioxide from the polluted atmosphere. The absorbed sulphur dioxide is converted into sulphurous acid and then to sulphuric acid, which slowly becomes more concentrated on drying. The interaction of the sulphuric acid which will eventually flow down surfaces or be absorbed into materials may result in the formation of sulphates, chlorides and other substances which may cause destruction of many materials; these compounds also form powerful electrolytes which accelerate the corrosion of metals in general and the ferrous metals in particular.

*Sources of emission*. In addition to the type of pollutants involved during emission and the velocity of the emission, the height above ground level from which the pollutants are emitted is of some importance when considering dispersion. In general, the higher the chimney (a source of emission) the greater the dispersion. However, other influences should be noted. Domestic chimneys being low do not disperse sulphur dioxide as effectively as the taller industrial chimneys. On the other hand, the quantities of fuel burnt industrially are so large that their contribution to

*The clean and dirty faces of Dorset House photographed during stone cleaning of the building. This is the first time this building has been cleaned (apart from washing down during painting operations) since it was built in 1933*

*Even with some of the soluble sedimentary stones, such as limestone, the degree of exposure to rainwater will determine the amount of soot, etc., which will be washed away. The accumulation of sooty deposits may over the years eventually cover up details as has been discovered during the cleaning of St. Paul's Cathedral recently. Reports of the thickness of deposits collected over nearly 300 years have varied—the greatest thickness reported being 8in. The photograph on the left shows part of the cathedral before cleaning and that on the right after cleaning (Courtesy: Szerelmey Ltd.)*

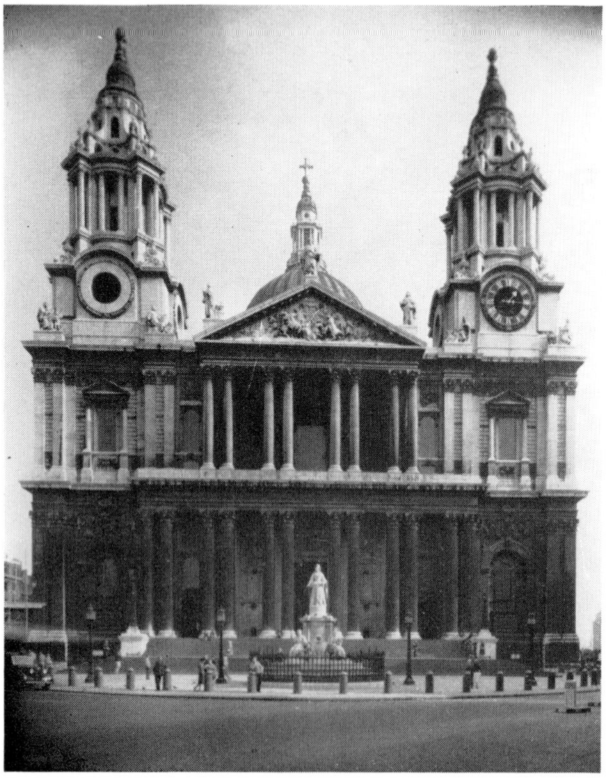

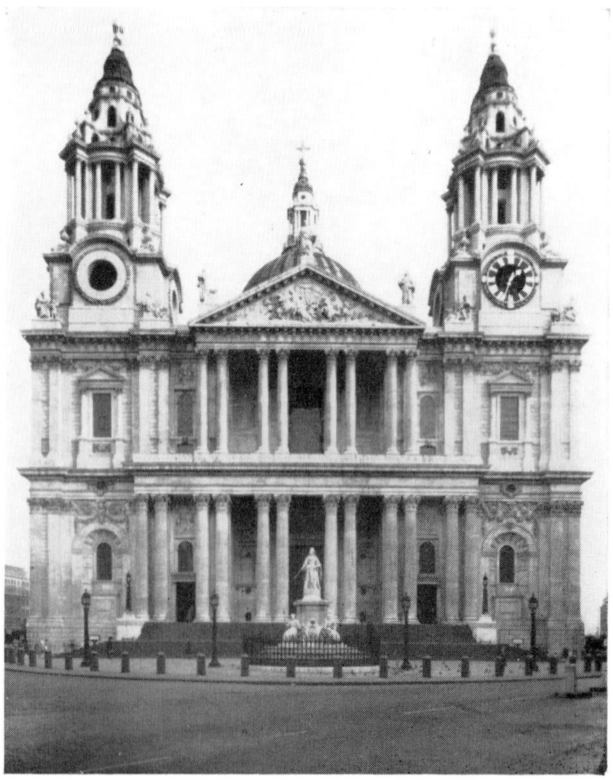

ground level concentrations of sulphur dioxide becomes extremely significant. As regards smoke, domestic chimneys generally account for a far greater proportion of the pollution at ground level than industrial chimneys. Industrial combustion processes being far more efficient, the amount of smoke emitted in relation to fuel burnt is very low. Together with the use of taller chimneys, the industrial contribution to ground level smoke pollution is very small. For this reason, among others, the local density of population is usually indicative of the degree of smoke pollution which can be anticipated.

*Thermal and wind conditions.* Of the meteorological conditions which influence the dispersion of pollution by the atmosphere, thermal and wind conditions are probably the most important. The action of rain, for example, generally causes the pollutants and especially sulphur dioxide to be brought down to ground level in solution. Thermal and wind conditions are inevitably interrelated.

Although wind under normal conditions acts as an efficient mixer with consequential increases in pollution, the worst pollution of all arises when the air temperature increases in height and there is no wind. Under conditions such as these an *inversion* occurs in which case the pollution remains near the level of emission. (When the air temperature of the surroundings decreases with height, dispersal is usually rapid as there is no tendency for the pollution to accumulate.) Although inversions accumulated overnight may be destroyed the following day as a result of solar heat gain, the resultant mixing which takes place due to compensating up and down currents may cause the pollutions to be brought down to ground level in high concentrations. This is known as *fumigation*. Valleys, it may be noted, are usually particularly susceptible to inversions. In these areas fumigation is also a serious problem.

In general, wind is usually regarded as the agency by which pollution may be dispersed away from the source of emission. Although this may well decrease the concentrations of pollution near the source of emission. there is still the possibility of the pollution being carried distances up to 80km away. This aspect is of particular importance when considering areas which may otherwise be regarded as comparatively free from pollution because they do not have immediate major sources of pollution. Topography or buildings around a chimney may influence significantly the degree of localised pollution during a wind. The relationship of the chimney to its surroundings may be such as to cause the pollution to be brought to the ground rapidly. The complex nature of the performance of a plume of smoke from a chimney and particularly relative to tall buildings requires that each case should be considered on its own merits. The help

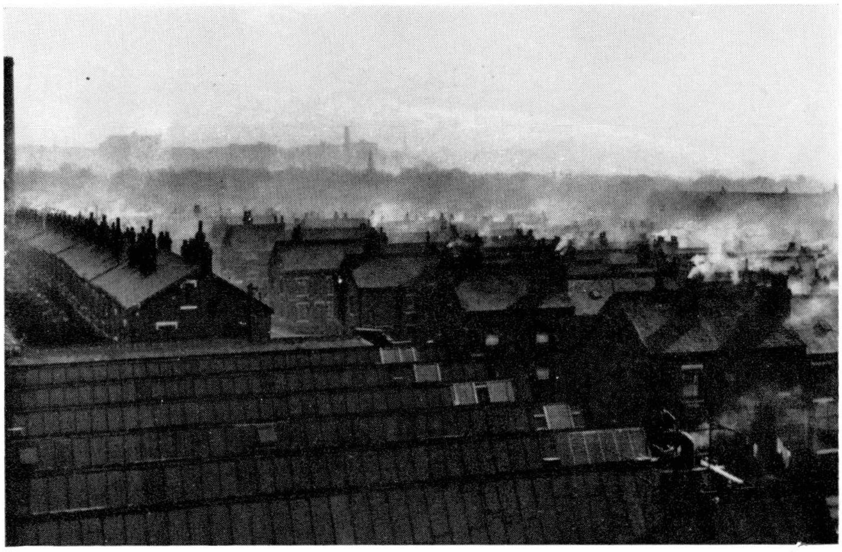

*Chimneys provide the chief sources of emission of pollutants. Many factors affect the degree of pollution at ground level from the two main types of chimney, namely domestic (above) (Courtesy: National Society for Clean Air) and industrial (below) (Courtesy: Mrs W. A. Clark, Chesterfield). See text 'Sources of emission'*

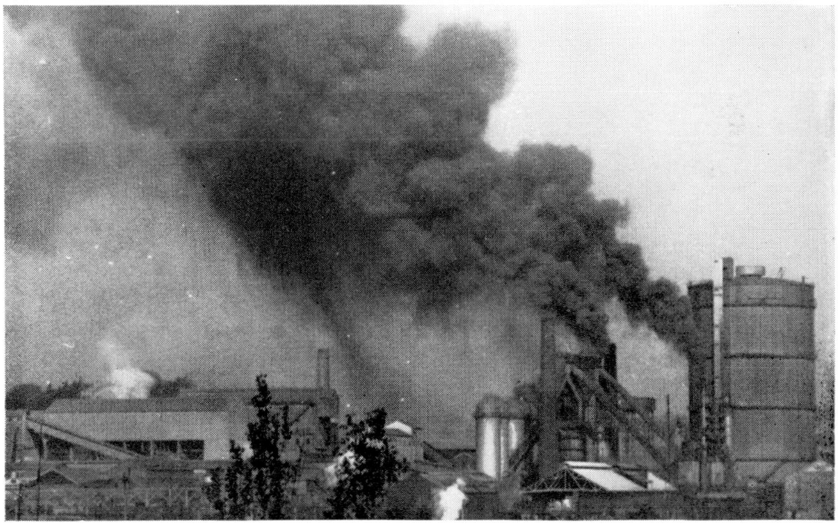

*Below, an example of an 'inversion' to which valleys are usually susceptible (Courtesy: National Society for Clean Air)*

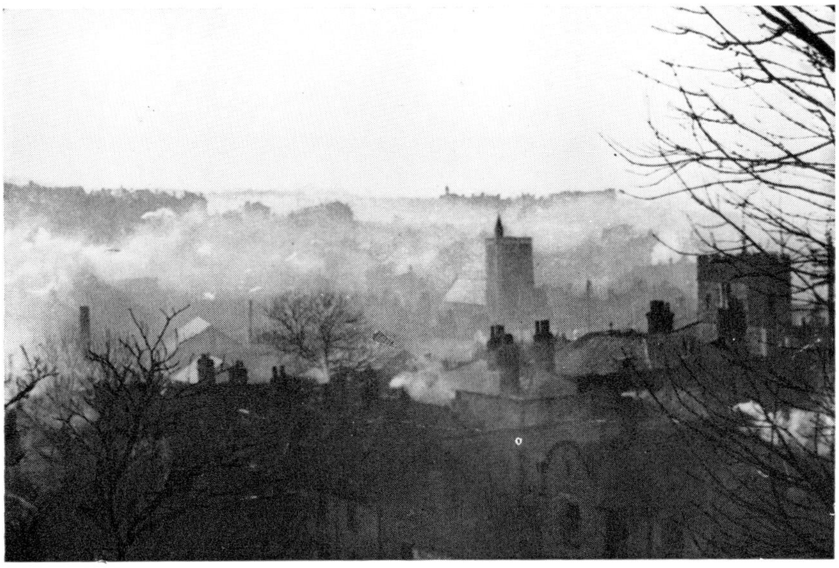

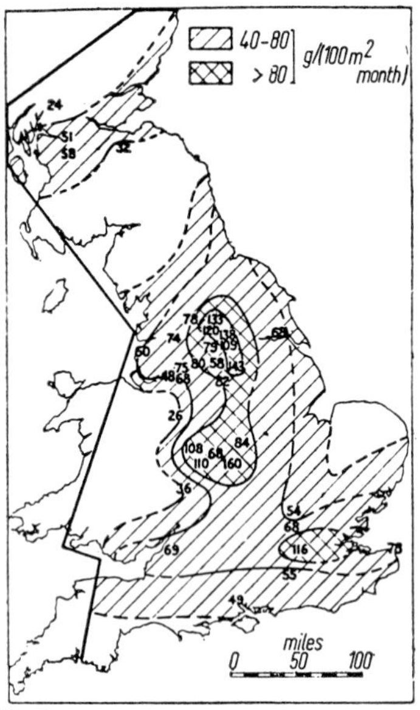


(1) ASH

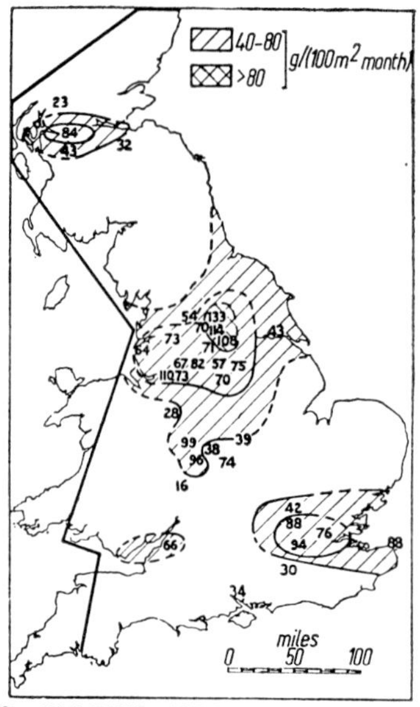


(2) COMBUSTIBLE MATTER

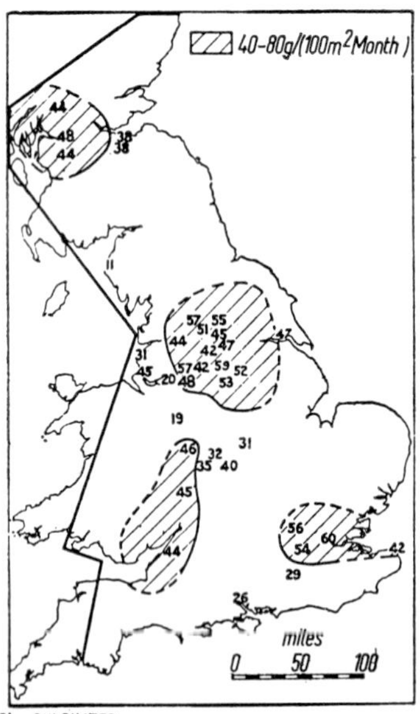


(3) SULPHATES

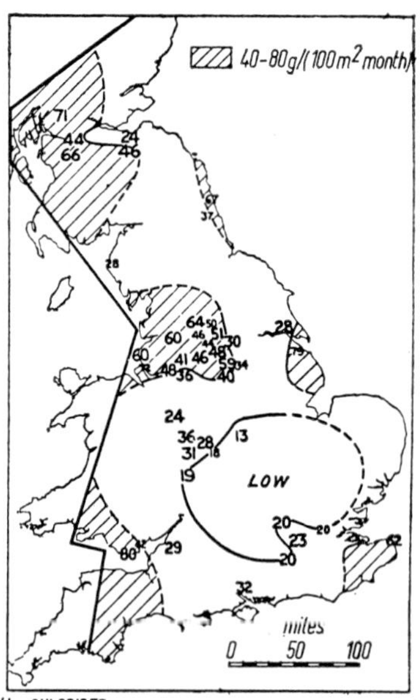


(4) CHLORIDES

D.3.02/5

*Distribution of insoluble and dissolved matter in country areas well away from large towns. (From: Meetham, A. R., 'Atmospheric Pollution, its Origins and Prevention', rev. 3rd Edn., Figs. 87–90, p. 190, Pergamon, 1964)*

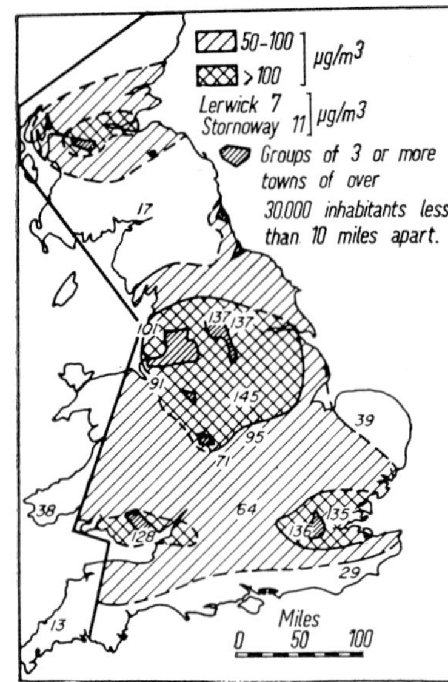


(1) SMOKE mg/(1000 m$^3$)

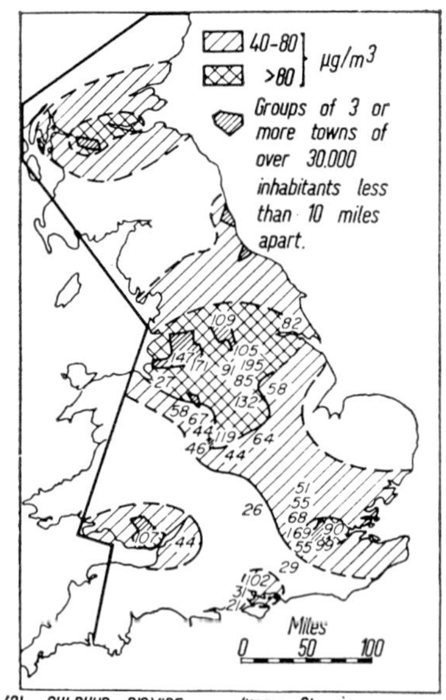


(2) SULPHUR DIOXIDE mg/(1000 m$^3$)

D.3.02/6

*Winter mean (1) smoke and (2) sulphur dioxide in country air (units: mg/1000m$^3$). (From: Meetham, A. R., 'Atmospheric Pollution, its Origins and Prevention', rev. 3rd Edn., Figs. 91–92, p. 194, Pergamon, 1964)*

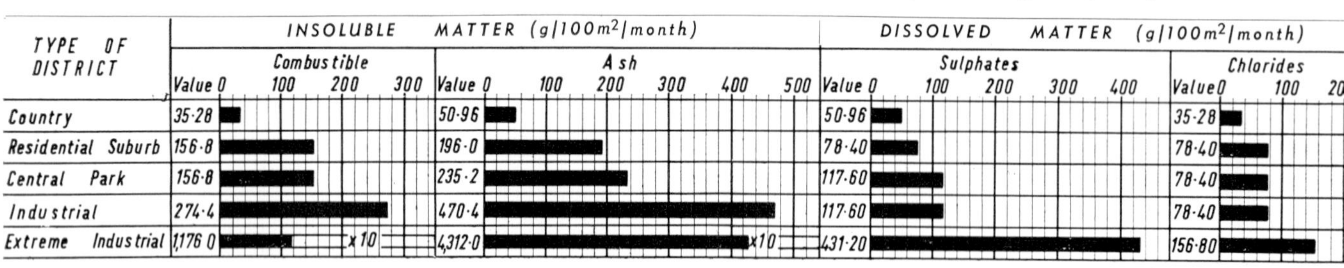


C.3.02/8

*Average values in g/100 m$^2$ per month of pollution deposited in Great Britain (compare with maps 1–4, D.3.02/5) (Values from: 'Investigation of Atmospheric Pollution', 31st Report, Table 30, p. 193, Warren Spring Laboratory (DSIR), 1959)*

which may be obtained from local authorities and others has been mentioned under paragraph (b).

*Country areas.* Despite the lack of measurements of the main pollutants in all areas, an attempt has been made to show the distribution of pollution, both insoluble and dissolved matter, in country areas well away from large towns or some miles to the west or south-west of the nearest source of pollution. The results of the attempts are shown in maps (1) to (4) in diagram D.3.02/5. The diagram should be read with the accompanying comparative chart C.3.02/8, which gives average values for various types of district. It should be noted that the maps have been prepared without information for Wales, S.W. England, Sussex, Kent, East Anglia and the Scottish Lowlands and Highlands. The distribution of chlorides are due more to sea spray than from chimneys. Despite the inherent limitations of the information contained in the maps, they do illustrate, in association with diagram D.3.02/6 in which maps (1) and (2) show the winter mean smoke and sulphur dioxide in surface country air, the fact that pollution may be carried away from the source of emission to other areas, particularly the dissolved matter, as most of the insoluble matter is usually deposited near the point of emission.

*Chlorine and fluorine compounds*

These compounds are formed from the combustion of coal, the amounts involved being small (the concentrations are usually too small for chemical measurement) when compared with sulphur dioxide. However, when associated with water the compounds form hydrochloric acid (HCl), hydrogen fluoride (HF) and silicon tetrafluoride ($SiF_4$), all of which can do harm to materials.

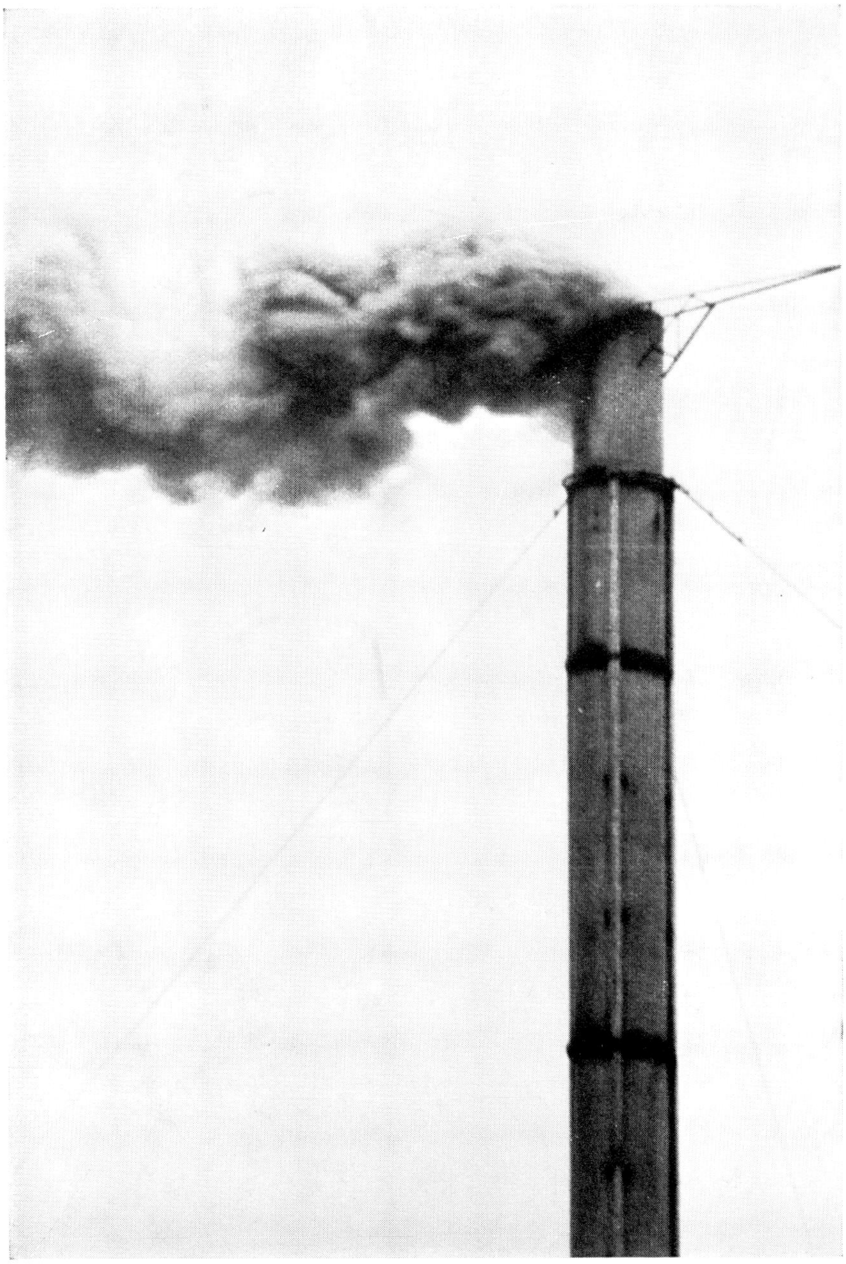

*Entrainment of smoke in eddies downwind of the chimney (Downwash) (Courtesy: Warren Spring Laboratory (Crown Copyright))*

*Downdraught in the wake of a building bringing down smoke to ground level (Courtesy: Warren Spring Laboratory (Crown Copyright))*

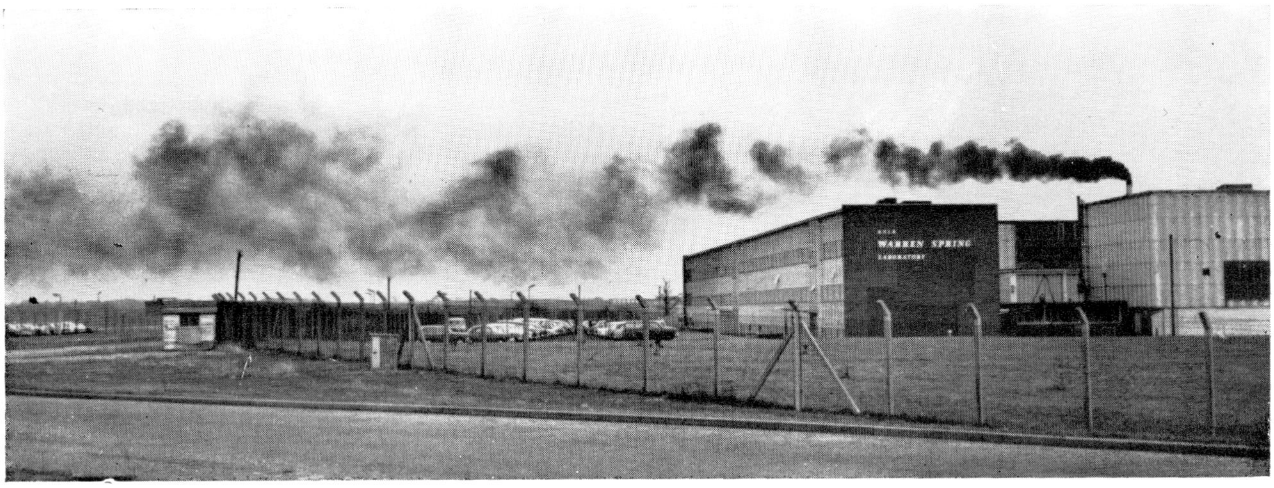

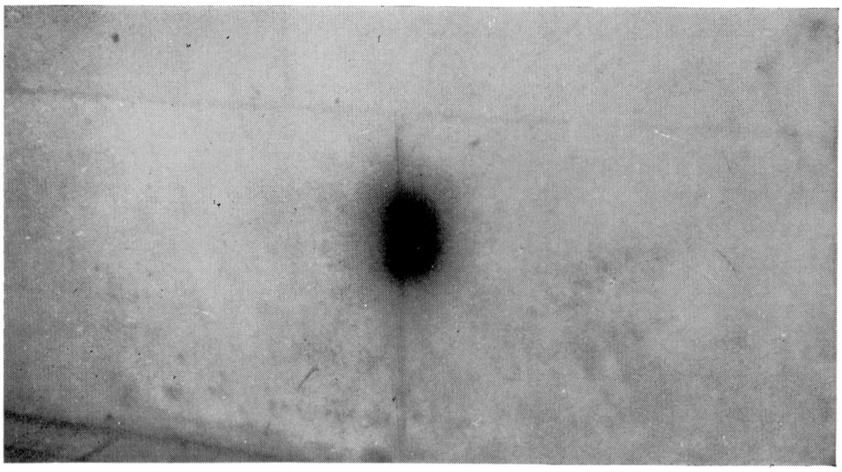

*Stain from a motor car exhaust pipe on a new Portland stone wall*

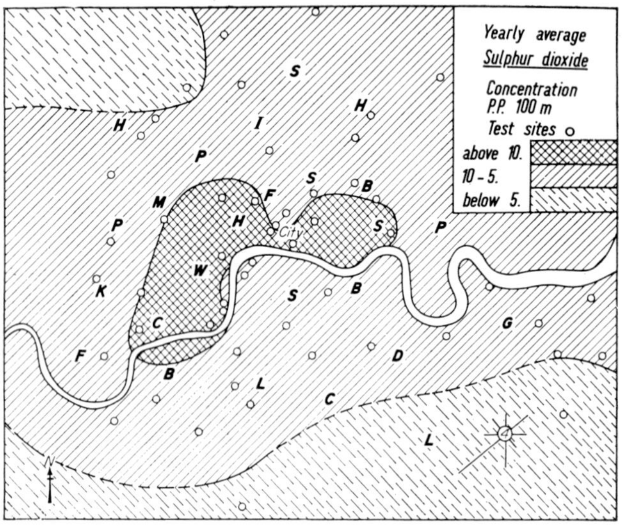


1 SULPHUR DIOXIDE

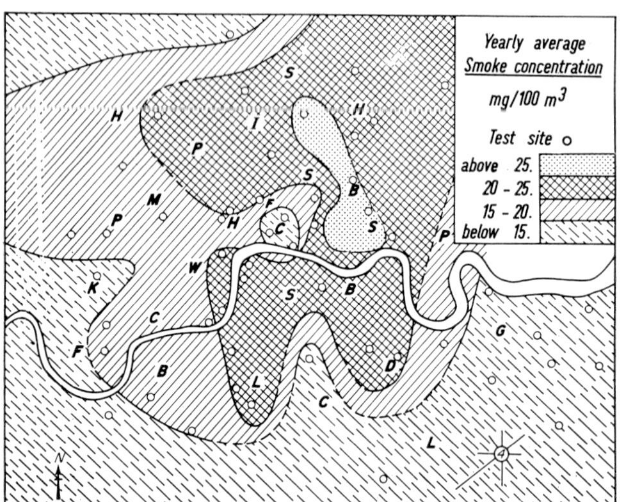


2 SMOKE

*D.3.02/7*
*Yearly average distribution of (1) sulphur dioxide and (2) smoke in London 1957–58. (From: Meetham, A. R., 'Atmospheric Pollution, its Origins and Prevention', rev. 3rd Edn., Figs. 94, 95, p. 198, Pergamon, 1964)*

*Carbon monoxide*

Carbon monoxide is mainly associated with the burning of petroleum products, particularly in motor vehicles. The concentrations are usually high in busy streets. The black smoke from diesel engines is of an oily nature and dirt deposited on buildings is often difficult to remove. In general, carbon monoxide is more harmful relative to human health than to building materials.

(d) *Impurities from other sources*

Although fuel burning is always regarded as the main source of pollutants in general, other sources, essentially industrial, contribute significantly to what can best be termed localised pollution. In terms of the effects on buildings *near* the source of emission they cannot be discounted. In some cases their proximity may be of extreme importance in the selection and use of materials. The concentrations of any of the pollutants will be dependent on the same variables as those concerned with fuel burning. However, each case should be treated separately.

The main impurities from *industrial sources* are:

(i) Paint particles and solvent odours as would be emitted, for example, from motor car works.

(ii) Gases from chemical works resulting in oxides of sulphur; sulphuretted hydrogen; carbon bisulphide; nitrogen oxides; chlorine and hydrogen fluorides. Various other substances may also be involved. Industrial processes other than chemical works also produce corrosive substances. Thus, for instance, fluorine compounds are emitted from aluminium works and brick and pottery kilns. In the case of lime works, carbonates of calcium or magnesium are burnt through the agency of coal.

(iii) Grit and dust may also be emitted in large quantities from certain industrial processes. In the comparative charts C.3.02/4 and 5 it has been noted that an additional quantity of some 0·5Tg of grit and dust is due to industrial processes. Cement works, amongst others, are notorious emitters of grit and dust. Demolition of buildings may also cause a local temporary nuisance.

Smoke control has only recently been possible since the passing of the Clean Air Act, 1956. However, the Alkali, etc. Works Regulation Act. 1906 has for some considerable time controlled the amounts of pollutants allowed to be emitted from industrial processes. This act resulted from the uncontrolled escape into the atmosphere of hydrochloric acid which caused damage to vegetation and property in the early days of the alkali industry when sodium carbonate was made by the strong heating of sodium chloride and sulphuric acid (the Leblanc process). It may also be noted here that many corrosive substances may be discharged from industrial processes into rivers or other water courses.

(e) *Distribution of pollution*

As already noted, the total amounts of the pollutants discharged over the country as a whole (comparative charts C.3.02/4 and 5) do not give any indication of the concentrations of the pollutants at ground level in any particular locality. Furthermore, the totals do not give any indication of the variations due to season or the fact that the dispersion of the pollutants, especially those which are finely divided or gaseous, from the point of emission is materially affected by many factors including chimney height (or any other point of emission), the velocity and amount of emission, the velocity and direction of the wind and other meteorological and topographical conditions. It is not intended to discuss all these factors in detail, but to deal with some of these aspects. An indication of the variation in distribution in London during Winter is given in Diagram D.3.02/7.

*Seasonal variations*. It is perhaps axiomatic that there will be a greater amount of pollution during the winter than during the summer in this country. The range of variation of seasonal average pollution from place to place is given in the comparative chart C.3.02/9. From the point of view of the damage to building materials, the cumulative effect of pollution is, in general, of more significance than the seasonal variations or, for that matter, the daily variations which can be considerable. However, the latter cannot be necessarily overlooked as they are indicative of the severity of conditions which prevail during a period when it is in any case wetter than in the summer. An increase in the degree of severity of conditions is, in turn, indicative of possible accelerated destruction of materials.

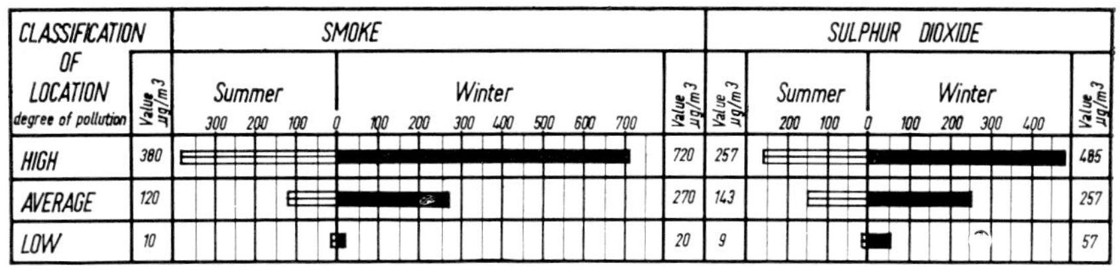


C.3.02/9
*Smoke and sulphur dioxide in Great Britain ($\mu g/m^3$). Range of variation of seasonal average pollution from place to place. (Values from: 'Investigation of Atmospheric Pollution', 31st Report, Warren Spring Laboratory (DSIR), 1959)*

(f) *Changes in atmospheric pollution*

For convenience, and by way of a summary, the causes of changes in the amount of atmospheric pollution are illustrated in the chart C.3.02/10. The basic causes are divided beween human activity and the weather. The control of smoke by the Clean Air Act, 1956, is a human activity aimed at reducing the amount of pollution. Although smoke control will reduce the amount of smoke emitted, that is one of the major pollutants, it is often considered that there will not be a corresponding decrease in the amount of sulphur dioxide emitted. In some quarters it is often felt that the amount of the latter may well be increased rather than decreased. The Warren Spring Laboratory, Note 4 on Air Pollution (revised April 1963), considers both these views to be incorrect, and states that the introduction of smoke control would be expected to cause a decrease in the emission of sulphur oxides by anything up to 25 per cent depending on the proportion of coal used for domestic heating.

Among the reasons given for the estimated reduction are chiefly the major change of fuel, that is from coal to coke, used for domestic heating with its corresponding lower sulphur content and the fact that many householders change to other types of fuels, such as electricity, gas or oil in order to meet the requirements of the Smoke Control Order. The use of these fuels when replacing coal yield reductions in the emission of the sulphur compounds of 100 per cent, 97 per cent and 95 per cent respectively.

A final reason, and an important one at that, is that the removal of smoke from the air lets through more of the sun's heat which sets up convection and so increases the dispersion of the other pollutants harmlessly in the upper air. Thus in the absence of smoke there is much less danger of high concentrations of sulphur dioxide building up than when smoke is present.

These changes in the concentration of atmospheric pollution at ground level may, in the long run, cause important and, in a sense, welcome changes in the selection, use and maintenance of building materials. It would appear, however, that greater consideration may have to be given to

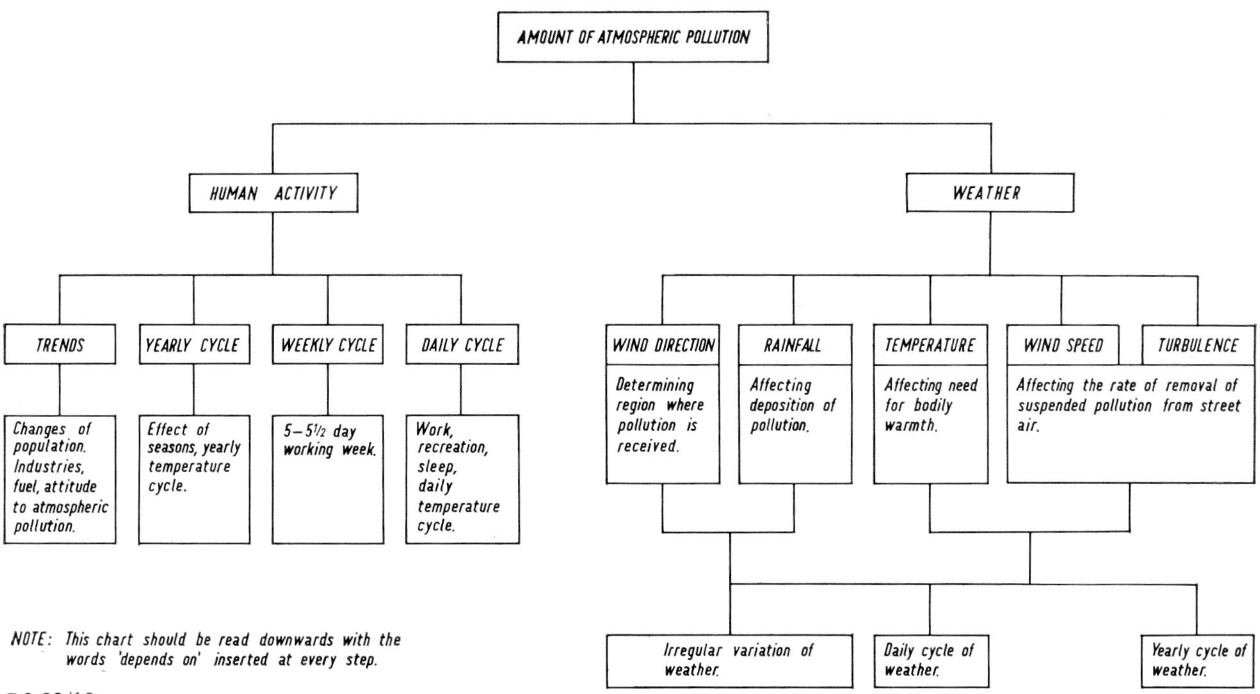


C.3.02/10
*Chart shows causes of changes in atmospheric pollution (From: Meetham, A. R., 'Atmospheric Pollution, its Origins and Prevention', 3rd rev. Ed., Table 333, Pergamon Press, 1964)*

the systematic measurement of the pollution of rainwater in smoke control and other areas.

### 2. Ground

Rainwater is one of the primary agents which result in pollutants found in groundwater. Chief among the corrosive agents which occur in rainwater are free carbon dioxide or sulphur dioxide. These, together with others, react with the constituents of rocks, soils, etc., with the result that groundwater may contain a variety of chemical compounds. Of those which are important relative to materials buried in or in close contact with the ground are the carbonates, sulphates, nitrates and chlorides of calcium, magnesium, potassium or sodium. In addition, groundwater may be corrosive due to its acidity, and this must also be taken into account. The pollution of groundwater may be related to specific problems or materials. A convenient subdivision is: (a) Sulphate attack; (b) Efflorescence; and (c) Acidity.

(a) *Sulphate attack*

Sulphate attack is confined mainly to cement based products. In solution sulphate salts cause considerable expansion and loss of strength. The sulphates of magnesium (Epsom salt) and sodium (Glauber's salt) are the chief destructive agents; calcium sulphate (gypsum or selenite), although also harmful, is less soluble. Although clay and other soils may contain any or all of the sulphates, it must be noted that these may also be derived from other materials used, directly or indirectly, in association with the ground, such as bricks or hardcore. The major areas of the British Isles known chemically and geologically to contain sulphates are indicated in diagram D.3.02/8.

In conditions other than those encountered relative to the ground, sulphate attack may be controlled by ensuring that the elements or materials concerned do not remain damp for long periods of time. Other factors are also relevant, but these are discussed more fully in *3.06 Chemical attack*. Apart from damp-proofing, the solution to the problem may, subject to the concentration of sulphates, lie in the suitable selection and use of cements, such as sulphate resisting, blast furnace slag, or high alumina, which are specifically made to resist or otherwise have special characteristics which resist sulphate attack. The degree of resistance provided by the various special cements available covers a fairly wide range. In addition the quality of the product is significant.

In the case of concrete work, greater resistance is generally provided by precast rather than cast *in situ* members.

The severity of conditions can be obtained by a measure of the concentration of sulphur trioxide either in groundwater (measured in parts $SO_3$ per 100 000 parts of water) or in clay (measured in per cent $SO_3$ or as grams $SO_3$ per litre of water extract). A classification of sulphate soil conditions affecting concrete is available and is given in Table 3.02/3. Only the basic classification is given. The related precautionary measures have been omitted but are included as appropriate in *3.06 Chemical attack* under 'Sulphate attack'. The classification is intended to act as a *guide*; groundwater analysis is the preferred basis of classification.

**Table 3.02/3**

*Classification of sulphates in soils and groundwater affecting concrete*
*(In ascending order of pollution)*

| Class | In soil: Total $SO_3$ % | In soil: $SO_3$ in 1 : 1 water extract (g/litre) | In groundwater (parts/100 000) |
|---|---|---|---|
| 1 | Less than 0·2 | — | Less than 30 |
| 2 | 0·2–0·5 | — | 30–120 |
| 3 | 0·5–1·0 | 2·5–5·0 | 120–250 |
| 4 | 1·0–2·0 | 5·0–10·0 | 250–500 |
| 5 | Over 2·0 | Over 10·0 | Over 500 |

*Reference: Concrete in sulphate-bearing soils and groundwater,* BRS Digest (2nd Series) No. 90, HMSO, February, 1968.

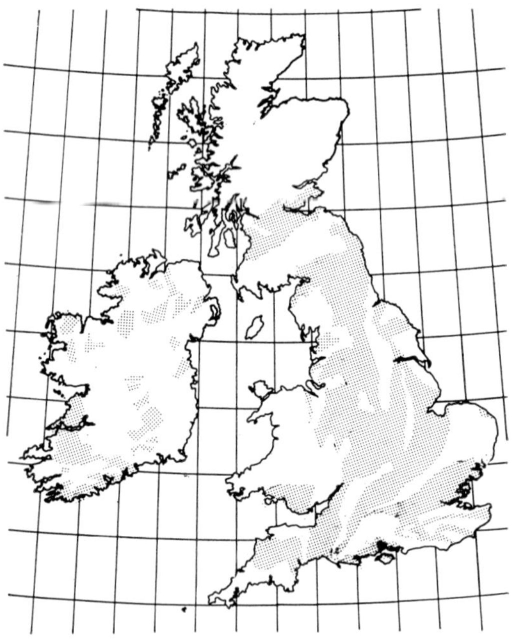

*D.3.02/8*
*Sulphate conditions in the British Isles. Note: the shaded portions of the map indicate major areas known chemically and geologically to contain sulphates in the soil or water. Unshaded portions, however, are not necessarily free from sulphates. Local conditions must be taken into account and each site examined accordingly. (Based on a map produced by Cement Marketing Co. Ltd.)*

(b) *Efflorescence*

On the whole the crystallisation of soluble salts on the surfaces of materials such as brick are not destructive. As in the case of sulphate attack, salts may be derived from the materials themselves. However, the presence of nitrates and chlorides is usually indicative of some contamination from groundwater. Although the damp-proof course is the 'line' above which there should be no transfer of water, the use of unsuitable materials or the physical bridging of the d.p.c. does very often allow the soluble salts to be eventually deposited in uncontrollable positions, thus in some ways negating one of the principal reasons for using a d.p.c. Some examples of the formation of efflorescence due to the use of unsuitable materials in association with the ground or to physical bridging of the d.p.c. are given in the accompanying photographs. (Efflorescence is covered fully in *Section 3.05*.)

(c) *Acidity*

The metals are the chief materials to be affected by the acidity of the ground in which they may be buried or with which they may be in close contact. The acidity or alkalinity of water or soils is measured by the pH value; a value below 7 indicates that the water or soil is acid while that above 7 that either is alkaline. The method of measurement and a broad classification of both acidity and alkalinity relative to metals in particular is included in full in '3. Water supply'.

In addition to metals, lime and particularly cement may be adversely affected by acids. As in the case of sulphate attack, the most successful means of reducing acid attack is by choice of suitable cements relative to particular conditions. Although emphasis has been given to the possibility of the deterioration of the concrete itself, due regard must be taken of the fact that reinforcing steel is vulnerable to the corrosive effects of acids and other substances which occur in the ground. Adequate protection of the steel is important and in this, quality control of the concrete itself is extremely important.

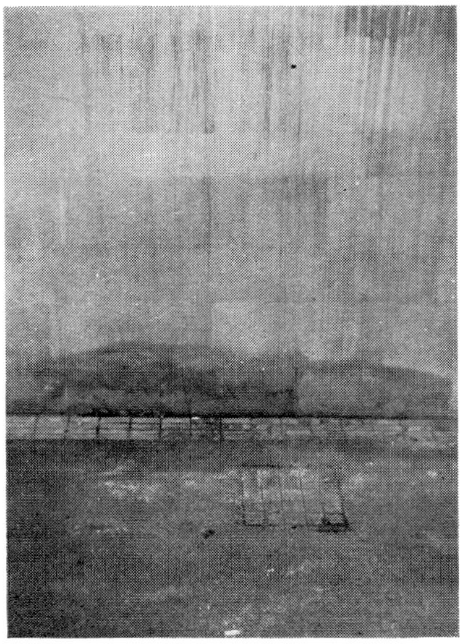

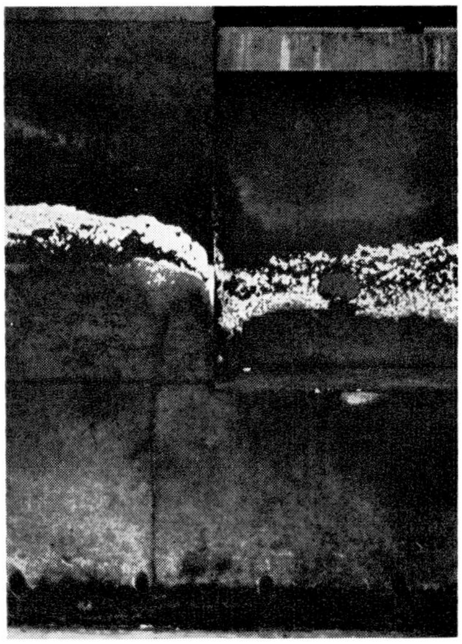

*Some examples of the formation of efflorescence due to the use of unsuitable materials in association with the ground or to physical bridging of the d.p.c. Below, mortar jointing between essentially impervious units allowing transfer of salts in solution.*

*Above left, efflorescence commencing at base of Portland stone wall facing. Above right, efflorescence in advanced state at base of Portland stone wall. Holes at bottom are for silicone injection to form damp-proof layer*

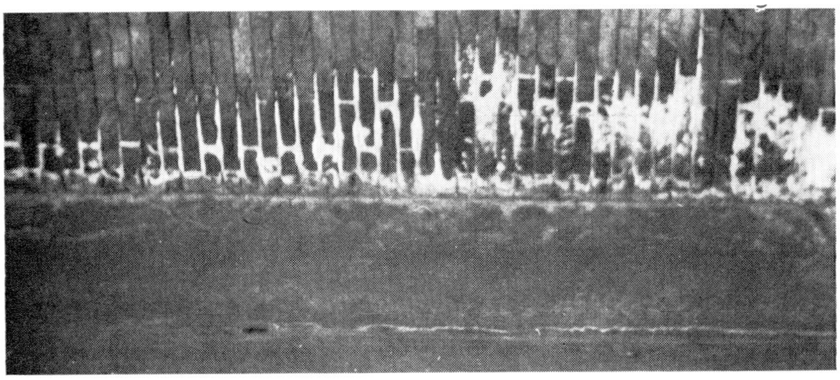

### 3. Water supply

The significance of the corrosive agencies which contribute to the pollution of water supplies is mainly concerned, human factors apart, with the effects of such pollution on materials with which the water will come into contact during its passage through the piped network.* In adition to piping, as such, consideration of the effects of any particular corrosive agents present must also be given to related 'accessories' such as taps, valves, tanks and cisterns and, where relevant, to all the component parts of heating and ventilation systems. Metals of various kinds have, in the main, been used for the greater proportion of all these items (if not for the whole of the items, then at least for those parts with which water comes into contact). Accordingly, some classifications of water supplies have been related to their effects on metals, albeit in general terms. Lack of sufficient experience with the fairly wide range of plastics pipes and other component parts now available has not enabled any of the existing classifications to be suitably, or better reliably, amended. However, many of the plastics do appear to offer greater resistance to some of the corrosive agencies against which metals have, on the whole, proved weak.

There is a fairly wide range of substances to be found in all water supplies. Treatment of 'raw' water by a water authority is primarily directed at meeting human needs (health and taste), rather than the specific requirements of the durability of materials in general and metals in particular. Some consideration is, however, given to the latter. During the treatment processes, and there are many of them, substances other than those occurring in the natural water prior to treatment may be added; on the other hand some substances may be reduced in concentration or removed completely. Thus, there is likely to be a wide variety in the 'quality' of water which can be expected in any particular area of the country. The range becomes even wider if those supplies which make direct use of 'raw' water from wells, catchment tanks and underground sources are included. It is, therefore, essential that the precise chemical nature of any water supply, whether from a water authority or other source, be ascertained prior to the selection of materials to be used in association with the water supply. The quality of any particular water supply serves as a useful, albeit not conclusive, guide on the probable behaviour of metals most commonly used.

When dealing with the use of materials relative to a particular water supply it is also necessary to give consideration to the possibility of the water becoming contaminated during its passage through the piped system. This may be particularly significant in composite systems, that is those in which more than one material is employed, even if each of the materials is resistant to the corrosive agencies contained in the basic water supply when used in isolation. In a composite system traces of one of the materials (usually metals) may provide the required corrosive agency to deteriorate one of the other materials. (This particular point, which is primarily associated with the *juxtaposition* of metals of different kinds, is dealt with in greater detail in *3.07 Corrosion of metals.*) Contamination of the water supply by the component parts of a piped system do, therefore, increase the range of the quality of water which can be anticipated. Thus it is necessary to distinguish between the quality of water as supplied (ascertained from an analysis) and the quality of the water after it has passed through the piped supply system (this has to be anticipated from known facts). Where necessary the quality of the water as supplied is referred to, in

*The emphasis here is on pollution relative to the piped system. However, it should be noted that quality of water is also important in building processes and particularly those in which lime or cement are used. Generally, the water used should be fit for drinking or taken from an approved source, as generally demanded in concrete specifications. In short, the water must be reasonably free from such impurities as suspended solids, organic matter and dissolved salts. A method for checking the effect of any given water on concrete is described in BSS 3148 *Tests of water for making concrete.*

**Table 3.02/4 Significance of some substances found in water**

| *Substance* | *Source/Cause* | *Occurrence* | *Significance* |
|---|---|---|---|
| 1. Aluminium | (1) Use of aluminium products, e.g. cooking utensils, tanks and pipes. (2) Excess use of aluminium sulphate in treatment works. | (1) Seldom found in natural water. (2) Should not occur in direct water supply (limit of aluminium 0·15 ppm). (3) May occur in indirect water supply due to source/cause (1). | (1) Corrosion of aluminium products from copper-bearing waters. (2) Occasionally alkaline waters or waters containing sodium carbonate cause corrosion of aluminium — pitting takes place. |
| 2. Calcium | Action of free carbon dioxide, $CO_2$, a weak acid in rainwater on calcium strata. | (1) Present as (a) bicarbonates (causing temporary hardness) and (b) chlorides and sulphates (causing permanent hardness). (2) Waters from chalk or limestone areas. | (1) Cause of hardness. (2) Calcium bicarbonate one of the most usual causes of alkalinity. Notes: (1) Calcium carbonate is soluble in water, i.e. settles out or held in suspension. (2) Calcium bicarbonate (often present in large quantities) is soluble and predominant cause of hardness. |
| 3. Carbon dioxide | Normal constituent of atmosphere; usually mixed with rainwater. | Often present in large quantities in waters from iron-bearing formations and in moderate quantities from moorland and shallow well waters. | (1) Significance when present as free $CO_2$, i.e. uncombined with other substances such as calcium or magnesium. (2) One of the main causes of acidity of water. (3) Waters containing more than 20 ppm of free $CO_2$ are likely to be corrosive. Note: The free $CO_2$ content of water is significantly reduced by (1) the presence of calcium which helps to absorb the $CO_2$ or (2) aeration of water—a simple means of reducing the $CO_2$ content. |
| 4. Copper | (1) Copper products, e.g. piping, tanks, etc. (2) Use of copper sulphate to reduce algae growth in reservoirs. | (1) Seldom found in natural waters. (2) May occur in direct water supply; more likely to occur in indirect water supply due to source/cause (1). | Causes corrosion, pitting of aluminium or galvanised products, e.g. pipes, tanks, cisterns, etc. |
| 5. Iron | (1) Underground formations. (2) Use of iron piping. | Frequently found in raw waters. | (1) Often corrosive. (2) Brown staining of sinks, baths, basins, laundry. (On exposure to air, water takes up oxygen; iron may precipitate and the deposits cause the brown stains.) |
| 6. Lead | Lead piping in distribution systems by the action of plumbo-solvent waters. | Acid waters; frequently waters from upland and moorland gathering grounds; some well waters. | (1) Lead is a cumulative poison—not more than 0·1 ppm should be present. (2) Each water authority should check its water supply for plumbo-solvency and forbid the use of lead piping if necessary. |
| 7. Magnesium | Action of free carbon dioxide, $CO_2$, a weak acid in rainwater on magnesium strata. | Present as bicarbonates (causing temporary hardness) or chlorides and sulphates (causing permanent hardness). | Most waters which are hard contain a proportion of magnesium compounds, but this is usually less than the proportion of calcium compounds. |
| 8. Potassium | Sulphate: Indirectly from sulphur content of polluted atmospheres. | In 'sulphated water' together with sodium and magnesium sulphate. | Potassium sulphate, a salt, usually only significant compound in water supply. (Potassium nitrate usually associated with sewage pollution.) |
| 9. Sodium | Chloride: Pollution by sea water or sewage. | Some salt found in most 'pure' waters (quantities of 10–20 ppm). | — |
| | Sulphate: Indirectly from sulphur content of polluted atmospheres. | In 'sulphated water'; sodium sulphate chief constituent. | — |
| 10. Zinc | Use of galvanised iron piping and tanks. | (1) Rarely found in natural waters. (2) Direct water supply from hard chalk waters carried in galvanised piping—up to 3·0 ppm of zinc in solution. (3) In indirect water supply. (4) Collection of drinking water from galvanised iron roofs for isolated supplies. | (1) Some waters readily take up zinc, especially in cooking processes. (2) Formation of loose deposits of zinc carbonate as a result of action of hard chalk waters on galvanised products. |

*Reference:* Twort, A. C., *A textbook of water supply*, Chapter 6, Arnold, 1963. Part I—'The significance of various substances found in water', pp. 153–65.

*Definitions:* 'Direct water supply' used under 'Occurrence' means water as supplied by a water authority to a building.
'Indirect water supply' used under 'Occurrence' means water in the distribution system of a building after it has been taken from the water authority's main. Thus the effect of the materials of tanks and piping is taken into account.

this section, as the 'direct water supply', that is the water which reaches the commencement of the piped system of a building; the quality of water after it has passed through the piped system is referred to as the 'indirect water supply'. (Pollution of water which discharges into wastes and drains is better included under '5. Processes and cleansing agents'.)

Although there is a wide variation in the substances to be found in water supplies, together with the variable factors involved which cause this variation, water supplies may be classified into three broad groups according to their degree of (1) hardness, (2) acidity and (3) alkalinity. (Acidity and alkalinity are more conveniently considered under the heading of pH value.) The main aspects of these three groupings are outlined here, with particular emphasis on the substances involved and methods of measurement. Some indication is also given, in Table 3.02/4, of the significance of some of the substances found in water. Only those substances which normally affect the metals used in water supply systems are included. Where possible some reference is made to those broad geological areas in the British Isles in which waters of a particular class are likely to be encountered.

Finally, the limitations of any broad classifications of water supplies, particularly in relation to the effects of such supplies on metals, must be emphasised. None of these classifications can take into account variations due to local conditions. Accordingly, advantage should always be taken of local experience; where necessary, as in the case of new supplies, suitable tests for corrosive effects should be carried out.

### (a) *Hardness*

The term 'hardness' when associated with water is, in some senses, indicative of the 'feel' of the water. However, the term is more commonly associated with the soap-consuming power of water. Soap reacts with certain minerals in water. This reaction causes a precipitation which appears as a scum or curd on the surface of the water. No lather can be formed until all the minerals have reacted with the soap. Waters which behave in this way are said to be 'hard'. (As synthetic detergents do not behave like soap, that is they do not cause a precipitation, the inconvenience of hard water is not felt so keenly.) In addition to the problem of soap lather, precipitation of the hardness compounds causes a hard scale on the surfaces of boilers and the interior of pipes in heating systems. This has been put forward as a further reason against the use of hard waters.

#### *Measurement*

Water may then be classified according to its degree of hardness, covering a range from soft to hard. The measure of the hardness can be obtained by the 'soap-consuming power' of a water, but this may not, however, be very precise. A more precise method would be to measure the total of the hardness producing constituents. Use of the latter method has resolved itself into the expression of these constituents in the chemically equivalent amount of calcium carbonate ($CaCO_3$). The amount of calcium carbonate may be measured in different ways, two of which are:

(i) Grains of calcium carbonate per gallon of water. These have been termed degrees of hardness or, more precisely, 'degrees Clarke'.

(ii) Parts of calcium carbonate per 1 000 000 parts (ppm) of water. This method of measurement appears to be more generally favoured than the previous one. (As grains per gallon=parts per 70 000, a hardness of 100 ppm=7 degrees Clarke.)*

The degree of hardness as experienced by the consumer in relation to the ppm equivalent amount of calcium carbonate is given in Table 3.02/5. The table also includes, for convenience, degrees Clarke, calculated from the formulæ given in (ii) above† Table 3.02/6 indicates the usual range of natural hardness of raw waters.

*Types of hardness*

There are two types of hardness, namely *temporary* and *permanent*. Temporary hardness is destroyed by boiling while permanent hardness is unaffected by boiling. The compounds causing either type of hardness are given in Table 3.02/7. From this it will be seen that calcium and magnesium are the main cause of hardness, with the bicarbonates causing temporary hardness, and the chlorides and sulphates causing permanent hardness.

In the case of temporary hardness the bicarbonates may decompose slowly at ordinary temperatures. The rate is much more rapid when the water is heated. Decomposition results in the formation of carbonates which are insoluble and deposited on surrounding surfaces—boilers, pipes, etc. Although the coating or scale so formed may result in some protection of metals, waters of moderate temporary hardness may contain, in appreciable amounts, other additional substances such as sodium bicarbonate, sulphate and chloride which may pit galvanised products, especially hot water storage tanks. In general, the loss in performance due to the reduction in the bore of pipes, for instance, is probably far more significant than the liability of the system to corrosion. The latter, of course, cannot be overlooked.

*As 'degrees Clarke' is not measured in SI its use is likely to be completely discontinued. However, it has been considered useful to retain values of 'degrees Clarke' in the tables.

†A Classification based on degrees and describing a range from 'very soft' to 'very hard' is included in *Durability*, BS Code of Practice, CP3—Chapter IX, p. 31 (1950). The classification used in Table 3.02/5 has been used in preference as it is from a more recent work (1963). In practice the variations between the two may not be significant.

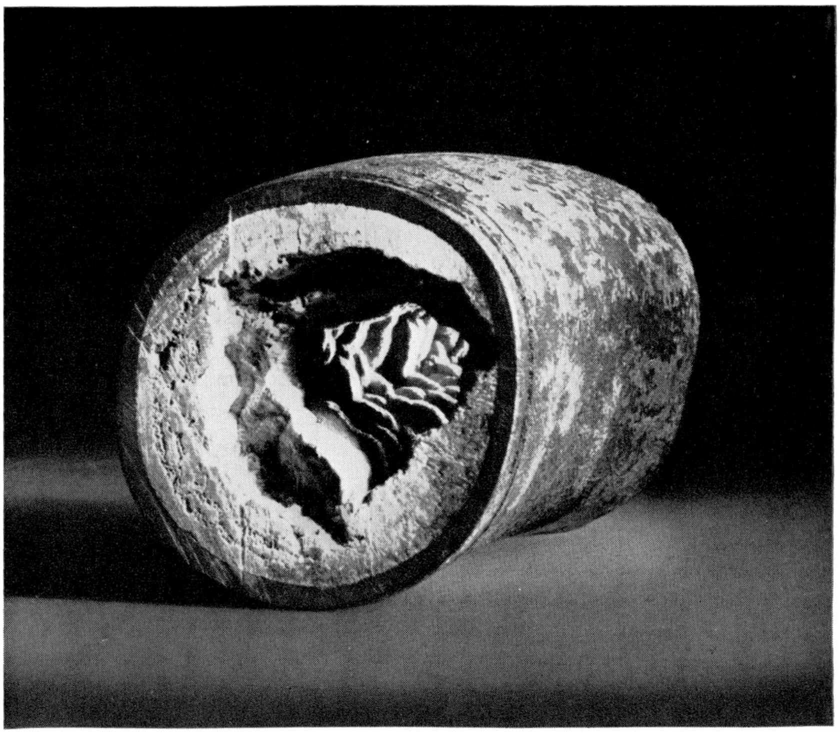

*A section of pipe from an hotel's hot water system showing the build-up of scale caused by using hard water (Courtesy: Permutit Co. Ltd.)*

**Table 3.02/5 Classification of water hardness**

| *Description* | *Quantitative limits (equivalent amount of $CaCO_3$)* | |
|---|---|---|
| | *measured in parts per million (ppm)* | *measured in degrees Clarke* (grains/gallon)* |
| Soft | 0–50 | 0–3·5 |
| Moderately soft | 50–100 | 3·5–7·0 |
| Slightly hard | 100–150 | 7·0–10·5 |
| Moderately hard | 150–250 | 10·5–17·5 |
| Hard | over 250 | over 17·5 |

*Reference:* Twort, A. C., *A textbook of water supply*, Arnold, 1963.6. 19 Hardness, pp. 158–59, for description and related ppm measurements.

*Values of *Degrees Clarke*, a common method of measurement in the past, have been added for convenience from 7 degrees Clarke = 100 ppm. (Degrees Clarke are grains/gallon or parts per 70 000.)

**Table 3.02/6 Usual range of natural hardness of raw waters**

| *Source of water* | *Range* | | *Classification** |
|---|---|---|---|
| | *ppm* | *degrees Clarke** | |
| Moorland catchments | 10–50 | 0·7–3·5 | soft |
| Shallow clays and gravels | varying | varying | varying |
| Sandstones | 100–300 | 7·0–21·0 | moderately soft–hard |
| Chalk | 200–300 | 14·0–21·0 | moderately hard–hard |
| Oolitic and carboniferous limestones | 200–400 | 14·0–28·0 | moderately hard–hard |
| Magnesium limestones | 400–500 | 14·0–35·0 | hard |

*Reference:* Twort, A. C., *A textbook of water supply*, Arnold, table 14, p. 212, 1963.

*'degrees Clarke' and 'Classification' have been added for convenience.

**Table 3.02/7 Substances causing hardness**

| *Temporary hardness* | *Permanent hardness* |
|---|---|
| Calcium bicarbonate. $Ca(HCO_3)$ | Calcium carbonate. $CaCO_3$ (to a limited extent) |
| Magnesium bicarbonate. $Mg(HCO_3)$ | Calcium sulphate. $CaSO_4$ |
| | Calcium chloride. $CaCl_2$ |
| | Magnesium sulphate. $MgSO_4$ |
| | Magnesium chloride. $MgCl_2$ |

*Reference:* Twort, A. C., *A textbook of water supply*, Arnold, table 13, p. 211, 1963.

The largest portion of the hardness in the majority of waters is temporary. However, a high percentage of permanent hardness is usually the cause of water being excessively hard.

In general, and as can be seen from Table 3.02/6, most of the hard waters in the British Isles are to be found in chalk and limestone areas. Both calcium and magnesium are constituents of chalk and limestone. The hardness compounds are primarily formed when rainwater containing free carbon dioxide (forming a weak acid) percolates underground through the chalk or limestone. (See also 'Weathering—limestone' in *Section 3.01.*) The deeper the water is drawn from underground the harder it is likely to be. On the other hand, waters are always soft when they are obtained from surface-run off from impermeable catchments, where there is little or no contact with chalk or limestone. (Soft waters should always be checked for *plumbo-solvency.*) It may be noted that, although calcium and magnesium bicarbonate both cause temporary hardness, it is calcium bicarbonate which is often present in large quantities in water and

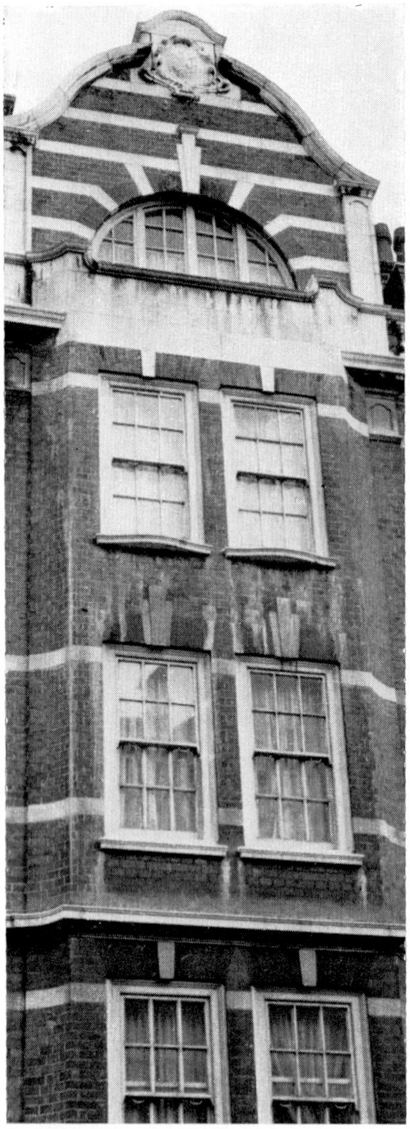

*Some examples of the results of solution of building materials*
*Lime washing from Portland stone*

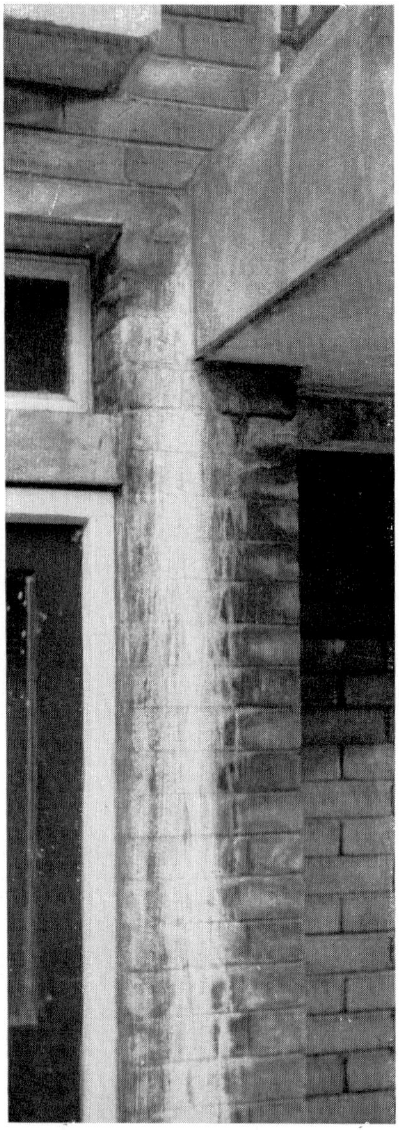

*Lime washing from concrete*

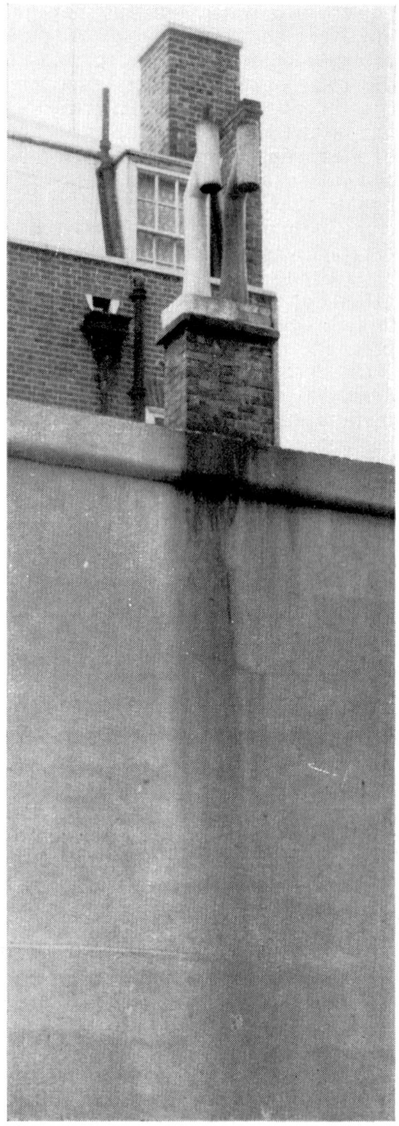

*Staining from rusting steel*

accordingly is regarded as the predominant cause of hardness.

*Removal of hardness*

Removal of hardness by a water authority may be done by (i) chemical means, in which case the hardness compounds are removed, or (ii) 'base-exchange' method—the hardness compounds are changed. Hardness may also be removed by the consumer as part of the distribution system of a building. Various methods are available.

*(b) pH Value (Acidity and alkalinity)**

The pH value is a measure of the acidity or alkalinity of water (also applicable to soils).

*Measurement*

Pure water, $H_2O$, also consists of a relatively small number of positive hydrogen ions, $H^+$, and a relatively small number of negative hydroxyl ions, $OH^-$. The concentration of hydrogen ions in 1 litre of pure water is:
1 / 10 000 000 ($1/10^7$ or $10^{-7}$) of a gramme, which is found by electrical measurement. For convenience the pH value is expressed as:

$$\text{pH value} = \log \frac{1}{1/10^7} \text{ or } \log \frac{1}{10^{-7}}$$

$$= 7 \text{ for pure water.}$$

Generally, when the concentration of hydrogen ions *exceeds* the concentration of hydroxyl ions, the solution has *acid* characteristics, and the pH value of such a solution would be *below* 7. On the other hand, waters are described as *alkaline* when the pH value is *above* 7, that is, there is an excess of hydroxyl ions.

*Neutral waters,* implying non-corrosive qualities, are generally those with a pH value within the range 6·80–7·20.

Natural waters seldom have an acidity below a pH value of 5·50 ; a range of 6·00–7·00 is generally applicable to soft waters from moorland areas, although the value may be lower when peat is present. For comparative purposes it may be useful to note that hydrochloric acid has a pH value of 3. Alkalinity is often associated with waters which have much carbonate hardness but with little free carbon dioxide. These waters may have a pH value of 8 or over. A strong alkali such as caustic soda, when dissolved in water to form an alkaline solution, has a pH value of 14.

*Causes of acidity*

There are three main causes of acidity. These are:

(i) Free carbon dioxide ($CO_2$). This excludes any carbon dioxide which may be combined with other substances, such as the carbonates. The carbon dioxide is picked up from the atmosphere during rain. Most natural waters contain some carbon dioxide.

*Reference: Twort, A. C., *A textbook of water supply*, Arnold, pp. 153–54 and 161–62, 1963.

(ii) Decomposing organic matter. The origin of the organic matter may be vegetable, but peat is of particular significance. A number of different acids are produced. Most *moorland* waters are acid.

(iii) Sulphates. These are formed either as a result of the action of rainfall in polluted atmospheres (sulphur dioxide content important) or during the transfer of groundwater through soils of high sulphate content, such as some clays and some iron-bearing formations. Sulphuric acid is normally produced in the water.

Most acid waters are corrosive (see 'Corrosive quality' below).

*Causes of alkalinity*

Alkalinity is caused mainly by the presence of bicarbonates, carbonates and hydroxides of calcium, magnesium, potassium and sodium.

Calcium and magnesium bicarbonate are the most usual constituents of waters which are alkaline. The same constituents are also one of the primary causes of temporary hardness. Thus, when alkalinity and hardness figures are equal, temporary hardness is known as *carbonate hardness*. On the other hand, where the total hardness figure is less than the alkalinity, then the presence of potassium and sodium salts are indicated.

*Corrosive quality*

Although there are many variable factors to be considered in assessing the corrosive quality of water relative to metals commonly used in connection with water supplies, the following three characteristics of water are normally indicative of the possibility of consequential corrosion:

(i) A low pH value, that is acidity. (ii) A high free carbon dioxide content —in itself a cause of acidity. (iii) An absence of temporary hardness or alkalinity.

Waters, frequently corrosive, are normally derived from the following sources: moorland waters; shallow well waters of low pH value, little temporary hardness but much permanent hardness; water from iron-bearing formations; chalk and limestone waters having a high $CO_2$ content; waters from greensands; waters from coal measures; waters having a high oxygen content or a high chlorine content.

From the point of view of health, it is always imperative that water is checked for its *plumbo-solvency*. Lead is a cumulative poison and, above all, is, when in solution, essentially colourless and thus difficult to detect visually. Where a water is plumbo-solvent, then it is normal for the use of all lead piping to be prohibited in any distribution system.

**4. Solution of building materials**

In this context solution of building materials is intended to imply the 'leaching' of pollutants from a material as water flows over it. This form of pollution is mainly related to the problems associated with the *juxtaposition* of materials of different kinds. Although the results of the incorrect juxtaposition of materials are usually manifest externally, in which rainwater as a source is important, they may also occur within the thickness of a structure or internally from either condensation, maintenance or usage. Accordingly, the range of pollutants and their corrosive quality are wide. Each situation must be considered on its own merits. Some indication may, however, be given of the materials which are likely to provide sources of pollution.

Traditionally stonework and particularly Portland stone is notable for the staining and sometimes deteriorating effects of limewashing on brickwork and other types of stone such as sandstone. Limewashing may also originate from cement based products. The alkaline nature of these products is also capable of causing leaching of oils from bituminous products. When wet, cement and lime have a corrosive effect on some of the non-ferrous metals, such as lead and aluminium.

On the whole, the surfaces of most metals are dissolved to some extent. Copper and copper alloys are notorious for green staining of many materials. This only occurs when the water first flows over the metal. The oxidised surfaces of metals are also capable of being dissolved and later deposited over other materials. Rust staining is a notable example.

Finally, certain types of timber, such as oak and western red cedar for example, are capable under damp conditions of exuding acids which may be harmful to metals.

**5. Processes and cleansing agents**

As in the case of solution of building materials, there is an extremely wide range of pollutants which may be derived from various processes and the use of cleansing agents. Each particular condition must, therefore, be considered on its own merits. However difficult it may be to establish the precise degree of severity of conditions which are likely to prevail, cognisance must be made of any circumstances which are likely to lead to 'special' conditions so that suitable precautionary measures may be taken.

The most vulnerable processes are usually those associated with various types of industry in which highly corrosive acids or alkalis may be produced. Many materials are affected by either of these. However, some mention might be made of the care required in the selection and use of metals and cement based products. Both are important as they are common materials for either carrying the corrosive agents or for the enclosing structure and general fabric. Mention has already been made of the effects of acids on cement. It should also be noted that some industrial processes may provide a source for sulphate attack from spillage or splashing of materials containing sulphates.

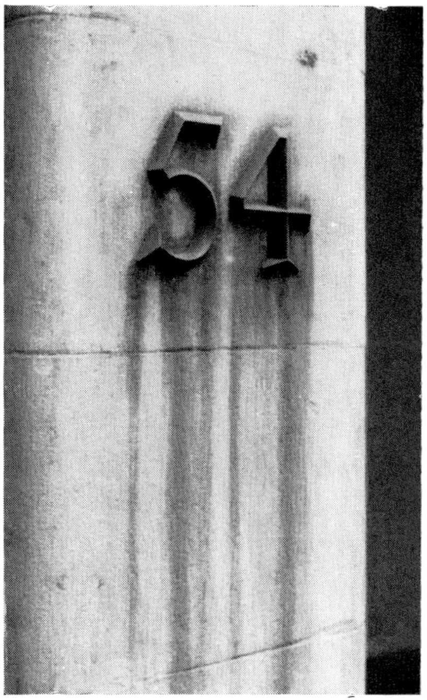


*Staining from bronze (copper alloy)*

Waste water may be highly contaminated in buildings other than industrial, such as hospitals, laboratories, etc. A certain amount of contamination may also occur in waste water from domestic and other similarly apparently harmless sources. The latter do not, on the whole, constitute severe conditions of exposure, nevertheless some consideration must be given to the suitability of materials which may be used.*

Among the building processes which require due consideration are all those which use cement. Cement slurry, which may exude from concrete formwork or wet cement mortar, does stain other materials, notably brickwork, if allowed to dry. Attempts at cleaning off the stains, using a weak acid treatment, are usually less successful than immediate removal of the wet cement with clean water. Ideally, adequate protection to the vulnerable materials should be provided during the progress of work.

Cleaning of stonework, particularly sedimentary stones, is most effectively, albeit more laboriously, carried out by using clean water. The use of alkaline detergents, although quicker, often leads to subsequent efflorescence or decay of the stone.

General cleaning of surfaces of building materials also requires special consideration if cleansing agents are to be used. Many of these may contain substances which may be corrosive relative to a particular material; on the other hand, the inclusion of abrasives may have erosive effects.

*The note on the suitability of materials for wastes and drains, even in those circumstances when the water to be carried away is unlikely to be severely contaminated, has been included in order to emphasise the importance of checking the likely performance of the newer materials. This performance may then be usefully compared with the materials traditionally used.

# 3.03 moisture content

In building practice it is more common to associate changes in the moisture content of materials with the physical rather than the chemical effects which result when there is an interaction between water and the solids of which materials are composed. This interpretation is adopted in this section, although it should be noted that the factors which are included are also relevant in other problems, such as the 'Exclusion of water' (*Section 3.04*), or in gaining an understanding of such phenomena as 'Efflorescence' (*Section 3.05*), 'Chemical Reactions', including corrosion of metals (*Sections 3.06 and 3.07*) and 'Frost Action' (*Section 3.08*).

Although moisture content may affect the mechanical properties of materials (generally the higher the moisture content the lower the strength of a material), changes in the moisture content which result in dimensional fluctuations, that is movement of materials, are far more significant, as restrained movement may result in cracking. This on the whole is one of the commonest, if not the most difficult, problems to be faced in practice. The effects of restrained moisture movement and possible methods of dealing with the problems involved have already been considered in *2.03 Cracking in buildings* and are, therefore, excluded here. Thus, this section is mainly confined to a detailed examination of the *causes* of dimensional fluctuations due to changes in moisture content. In addition to a consideration of the 'mechanisms' involved relative to the properties of materials, the extent of the movement likely to be encountered, together with the practical significance of these, are included.

Moisture content changes and the related movements may take place in some of the non-porous materials, such as plastics (they never take place in metals). However, the extent and, more important, the effects of changes are more pronounced in the *porous materials*. Thus, these materials are primarily considered here. In order to take into account the special, if not acute, problems under 'normal' exposure conditions in buildings which are associated with *timber* and *cement-based products*, special emphasis is given to these materials.* This emphasis should not, however, detract from the fact that due consideration must also be given, in practice, to the movements which are likely to occur with other porous materials (and where relevant, non-porous materials) in extreme cases of exposure.

In order to deal with Moisture Content on a broad basis but at the same time concentrating on the *dimensional fluctuations* which take place when changes occur, some overlapping is inevitable. A further difficulty is the fact that so many of the factors involved are closely interrelated. However, it has been considered convenient to use the following general headings: (1) Basic definitions; (2) General influences; (3) The presence of water in materials; (4) Exposure; (5) Movement in timber; (6) Movement in cement-based products; and (7) Precautions in use.

## Basic definitions

Definitions of (1) moisture content, (2) moisture movement, (3) moisture gradient, and (4) moisture transmission are fundamental in this study. It is more convenient to include their definitions here, although the terms have been (and will be) used elsewhere. Advantage is also taken to include, where relevant, detailed consideration of some aspects of these terms which are necessary for a general understanding of the problems involved.

It may be noted that the definitions commonly used are derived from timber technology, as it was in this field that the greater part of the early work on moisture content changes was undertaken. As the field of study has broadened to include all the other porous materials, and more recently some of the non-porous materials, the definitions now cover all materials. For this reason the word 'timber' has been omitted from the definitions.

### 1. Moisture content

Moisture content is the amount of moisture which a material contains at a given time and is expressed as a percentage of its dry mass (strictly speaking 'oven-dry' mass, that is after all moisture has been expelled from the material) and may be written in formula form as:

$$\text{Moisture content} = \frac{\text{Mass of water present}}{\text{Dry mass of material}} \times 100$$

The moisture content is commonly found by the oven-dry method* as follows:

$$\frac{\text{Initial mass of sample} - \text{dry mass of sample}}{\text{Dry mass of sample}} \times 100$$

The initial mass of a sample is the actual mass at the time of test, and the dry mass of the sample the mass after all the moisture has been expelled.

A visual comparison of the amount of moisture contained in an oak furniture square with moisture contents of about 90 per cent (when freshly sawn) and 12 per cent (after drying) is given in diagram D.3.03/1.

### 2. Moisture movement

Moisture movement is very often mistakenly, although understandably, interpreted as the movement of moisture in and about a material. It is, in fact, concerned with the movement of the material itself, that is the alteration

**Main references:**

(1) Stradling, R. E., *Effects of Moisture Changes on Building Materials*, Building Research Bulletin No. 3, HMSO, 1928. (2) Schaffer, R., *Weathering of Natural Building Stones*, Building Research Special Report No. 18, HMSO, 1932. (3) *Principles of Modern Building* Vol. I, 3rd Ed., HMSO, 1959, and Vol. II, HMSO, 1961. (4) BRS Digests and references included in charts, diagrams, etc. (5) See also *Movement in Timber* and *Movement in Cement-based Products* later.

*Many of the detailed considerations included with these classes of materials should help to clarify many of the inter-related factors which are outlined in general terms only elsewhere in the section. Furthermore, timber and cement-based products represent not only extremes of movement relative to other materials, but also completely different behaviour during movement. Timber is, in terms of moisture movement, anistropic and thus movement is not the same in all directions, while cement-based products, like most other materials, are isotropic, in which case the extent of movement is roughly the same in all directions.

*For details of the method used for timber see *Moisture content Determination by the Oven-drying Method*, FPRL Leaflet No. 7, HMSO, July, 1949.

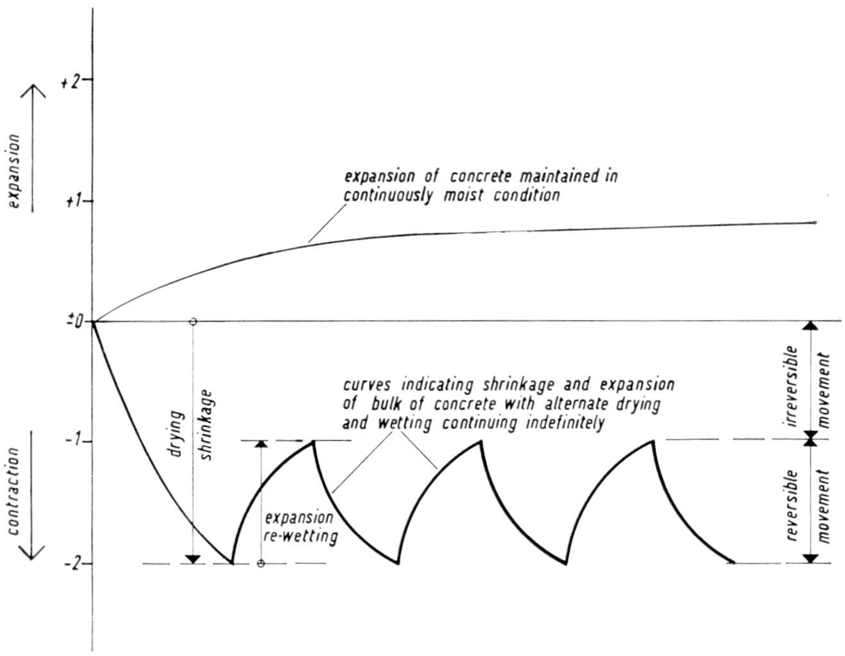


*D.3.03/2*

*Illustration of irreversible and reversible moisture movements in concrete*

in its physical dimensions due to changes in its moisture content. Moisture movement may then be defined as the change in unit dimension of a material due to changes in its moisture content and expressed as a percentage of its original dimension. It is usual to refer to length of a material. Moisture movement may be written in formula form as:

$$\text{Moisture movement} = \frac{\text{Change in length}}{\text{Original length}} \times 100$$

The original length, even in drying shrinkage tests, is usually indicative of the dry length, so that the formula may be re-written as:

$$\text{Moisture movement} = \frac{\text{Wet length} - \text{dry length}}{\text{Dry length}} \times 100$$

(a) *Types of movement*

Values of moisture movement may indicate either an expansion or a contraction of a material. However, a distinction has to be drawn between two types of movement, one of which is irreversible and usually, though not always, implies a contraction, while the other is reversible and implies movement in either direction. Cement-based products are good examples to use of materials which undergo both types of movement. These are shown diagrammatically in diagram D.3.03/2. (This diagram, although previously used in *Section 2.03,* is repeated here for convenience.)

*Irreversible movement.* This movement is concerned entirely with those materials requiring water for their use or manufacture and most, though not all, of it takes place during the drying out period.* Thus the movement only takes place once during the life of the material, and is of particular significance in all the wet trade processes undertaken on a building site. Precautionary measures are always advisable so as to avoid undue shrinkage cracking. In those cases where materials, such as clay- or cement-based products, are made off the building site, the drying shrinkage should be complete before the products are built into a building.

*Reversible movement.* This movement may occur in all materials. Reversible movement is closely related to the moisture content of a material and thus expansion takes place when water is taken in and contraction when water is given off. In general, and taking into account practical application, the extent of movement in either direction is roughly the same. Any significant departures from this should be stated.

(b) *Interpretation of values*

Practical application, in terms of allowing for movement, are restricted mainly because of the complexities of the inter-relationship of the many factors involved, plus the fact that the laboratory tests necessary to evaluate the extent of movement in any material usually employ, as a basis, moisture content extremes, while comparatively small samples of a material are used. In many cases these tend to give exaggerated movements, which may seldom be encountered in practice. This is probably more significant with re-

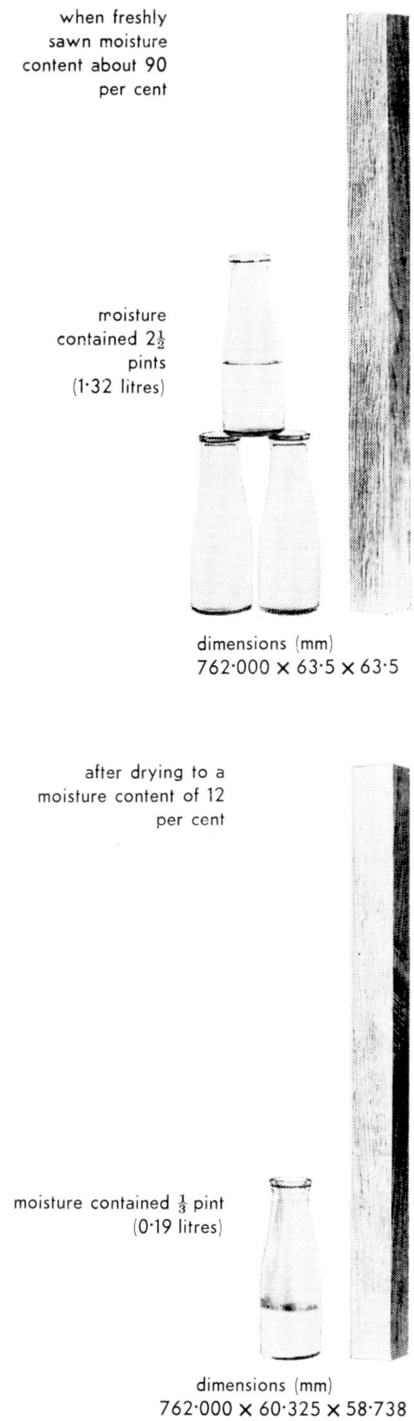


*D.3.03/1*

*Comparison of moisture contained in an oak furniture square when freely sawn (moisture content about 90 per cent) and after drying (moisture content 12 per cent)*

versible rather than irreversible movements. As far as the latter are concerned, it is normal to measure the total drying shrinkage of a material (wet to oven-dry) which, although this may include some reversible movement, is a valuable guide when assessing precautions which should be taken.

In the case of reversible movements, the oven-dry condition is often used as the condition upon which the original length would be based. Thereafter, the

*Timber may be said to undergo irreversible moisture movement during its own initial drying out process. However, in practical building this is of little significance.

material may be totally immersed in water for a sufficient period of time to cause complete saturation, or exposed to controlled temperature and humidity conditions for a specified period of time. Thus, unless the range of moisture content or the method of calculation is stated, values may be misleading, particularly for detailed design application.

The comparative chart C.3.03/1 illustrates the general range of moisture movements in various materials based on a variety of calculation methods and moisture content extremes. It is intended to serve as a comparison of the behaviour of the range of materials in terms of moisture movement and not for detailed design application. There are available values of movements for timber (given later) which can be applied in design for particular circumstances. Generally speaking, rule-of-thumb methods must still be used in the majority of cases. (See also 'Precautions' given later.)

Despite the lack of comprehensive design guidance, some reliance may often be placed on reasonable interpretation of available values. In order to do this, the importance of the relative humidity of the air surrounding a material, as opposed to the amount of liquid water absorbed by a material, together with the relationship between the two, must be understood. In practice both are important.

For the maximum moisture movement over a given range of moisture content to take place, the moisture involved must be associated with the maximum amount of the solids of which the material is composed. (The nature of this association and the conditions under which it will persist are discussed in 'Presence of water; 3. Sorbed water' later.) In general, it is extremely difficult to ensure that the desired association between water and solids takes place if a material under test is, for example, only allowed to absorb sufficient liquid water after immersion to correspond to the range of moisture content required. The reasons for this are complex but, in the main, they are connected with the porosity characteristics of the material which may not readily allow water to permeate throughout the material. On the other hand, if a material is immersed for long enough, saturation can occur, in which case it is then possible for the maximum amount of solids to be associated with water. This, of course, implies, as already stated, the extreme moisture content range for the material and is indicative of the situation that is likely to occur to materials which are used in positions (exposure to the weather, for example) where saturation may take place. However, even in these cases it is unlikely that, in practice, the material would have started off, so to speak, in an oven-dry condition before saturation, so some allowance would have to be made for this. Thus, the movement is unlikely to be as great as the values normally given. It may be noted here that, where partial saturation of a material occurs, there will be a certain amount of differential movement between the wet and dry zones. This may be important in some situations (see '3. Moisture Gradient').

All materials capable of taking in or giving off water will adjust their moisture contents according to the moisture content, that is the humidity, of the air surrounding them, until moisture equilibrium is attained. Thus, depending on conditions, materials may absorb moisture from the atmosphere or vice versa. The process is, however, not instantaneous, the length of time required for equilibrium to be reached is primarily dependent on the nature of the material concerned. This particular aspect is important because *momentary changes* in the humidity of the atmosphere are unlikely to have very much, if any, moisture movement effect on a material.

The adjustments which materials make in their moisture contents so that equilibrium with the surrounding air may be attained has an important bearing on the moisture contents of materials saturated by liquid water. Saturation, whether partial or complete, can only persist while environmental conditions of humidity so allow. In other words, materials exposed to air will not 'tolerate' an imbalance between their moisture contents and that of the surrounding air. The rate at which the adjustment of moisture content takes place when materials are saturated will be dependent on those factors which influence evaporation. Thus, under unfavourable conditions, equilibrium moisture content may only be achieved after a considerable time.

As all materials are not necessarily exposed to liquid water, range of movements based on exposure to specified relative humidities can provide useful guidance. Again it should be noted that most values computed on this basis do, however, use original length based on oven-dry conditions. Some allowance must, therefore, be made for this. On the other hand, the magnitude of movement may not necessarily be the same for all increments in moisture content. Such differences may not always be relevant, but nevertheless detailed values of each material should be considered.

#### 3. Moisture gradient

Moisture gradient is defined as the variation of moisture content between the outer and inner part of a piece of material. The gradient is of particular significance in timber, as its existence may cause stresses to be set up within the material which, if of sufficient magnitude, may eventually lead to rupturing or distortion. (Compare, by way of a useful analogy, the effects of either heating or cooling a material in diagrams D.2.03/5 and 6 in *Section 2.03*.) The gradient is 'set up' during the seasoning process if the moisture from the outer layers is allowed to evaporate at a rate which does not allow moisture from the interior to reach the surface. When the outer layers set in a stretched condition due to the moisture gradient, which in this instance would be steep, the piece of timber is said to be *case-hardened*.

Similar gradients may also be set up when wet-trade products dry out. Stresses may also be set up, but the defects are normally not as pronounced as in the case of timber, although cracking of the surface may take place.

#### 4. Moisture transmission

Moisture transmission, or transfer as it is also sometimes known, may be defined as the movement of water in and through a material or combination of materials. The water may be in either the liquid or vapour state.

The mechanisms involved in moisture transmission, together with the factors which influence it, are of particular importance when considering the drying out of materials. It is also useful in gaining an understanding of the significance of the transfer of water between two adjoining materials relative to such phenomena as efflorescence.

## General influences

There are a number of properties of materials and factors which generally influence moisture content or are often referred to in connection with some of the phenomena involved. These are:

#### 1. Capillarity

Capillary action has been described in *Section 1.11*. The capacity of water to rise in narrow channels is extremely important in porous materials which, by their nature, may contain a variety of channels, including many which are narrow. The functioning and the moisture content of virtually all the porous materials is partly dependent upon capillary attraction. Size and arrangement of the pores within a material, as outlined in *1.12 Porosity*, must be associated with the formation of capillaries, and thus influence both the amount and rate of moisture transmission in and out of a material.

The importance of capillarity may be underlined by considering the mechanisms and factors involved in (a) The drying out of a porous body, and (b) The Transmission of water between two adjoining materials.

(a) *Drying out of a porous body*

Two interrelated factors govern the drying out of a porous body. These are:

(i) *The environmental conditions* surrounding the body and made up of the temperature and humidity of the atmosphere and the velocity of air flow past the surface. All these are concerned with Evaporation (see *Section 1.11*).

(ii) *The structure of a material* which controls the transmission of water to the surface of the material.

A porous solid of appreciable thickness will only dry out if water is evaporated from the surface. Thus, water must travel, in one form or another, from the interior to the surface before it can escape as *vapour* into the surrounding air. The water lost by evaporation from the surface may be replaced by water flowing under the action of capillary forces or the evaporating surface may fall *below* the surface of the solid, in which case the water must 'jump across' a certain length of pore space before it can escape at the surface.

The rate at which evaporation of surface water of a *saturated* material initially takes place is solely dependent on the environmental conditions and is thus the same for any free surface water exposed to the same conditions. Provided compensating water is brought to the surface so as to maintain it in a *wet* condition, evaporation will continue at a constant rate. If, however, the amount of water brought to the surface is insufficient to keep the surface wetted, then there will be a fall in the rate of evaporation. Thus, in materials in which water can move easily, most of the drying out takes place readily at the surface. However, in a dense material the initial constant rate only persists for a short period of the total drying out time. The surface may, therefore, be dry long before all the pores have been emptied, with the result that at some point *below* the surface the material may still be saturated. For the significance of surface dryness in practice see *Section 3.01* 'Dampness'.

The effect of the density of a material or surface relative to two building applications may be noted. In brickwork having dense cement mortar pointing, such as a 1 : 3 cement : sand mix, little transmission of water can occur through the pointing ; thus practically no drying out takes place from the mortar joints. On the other hand, trowelling finishes to renders, etc., may produce dense surfaces which will impede evaporation.

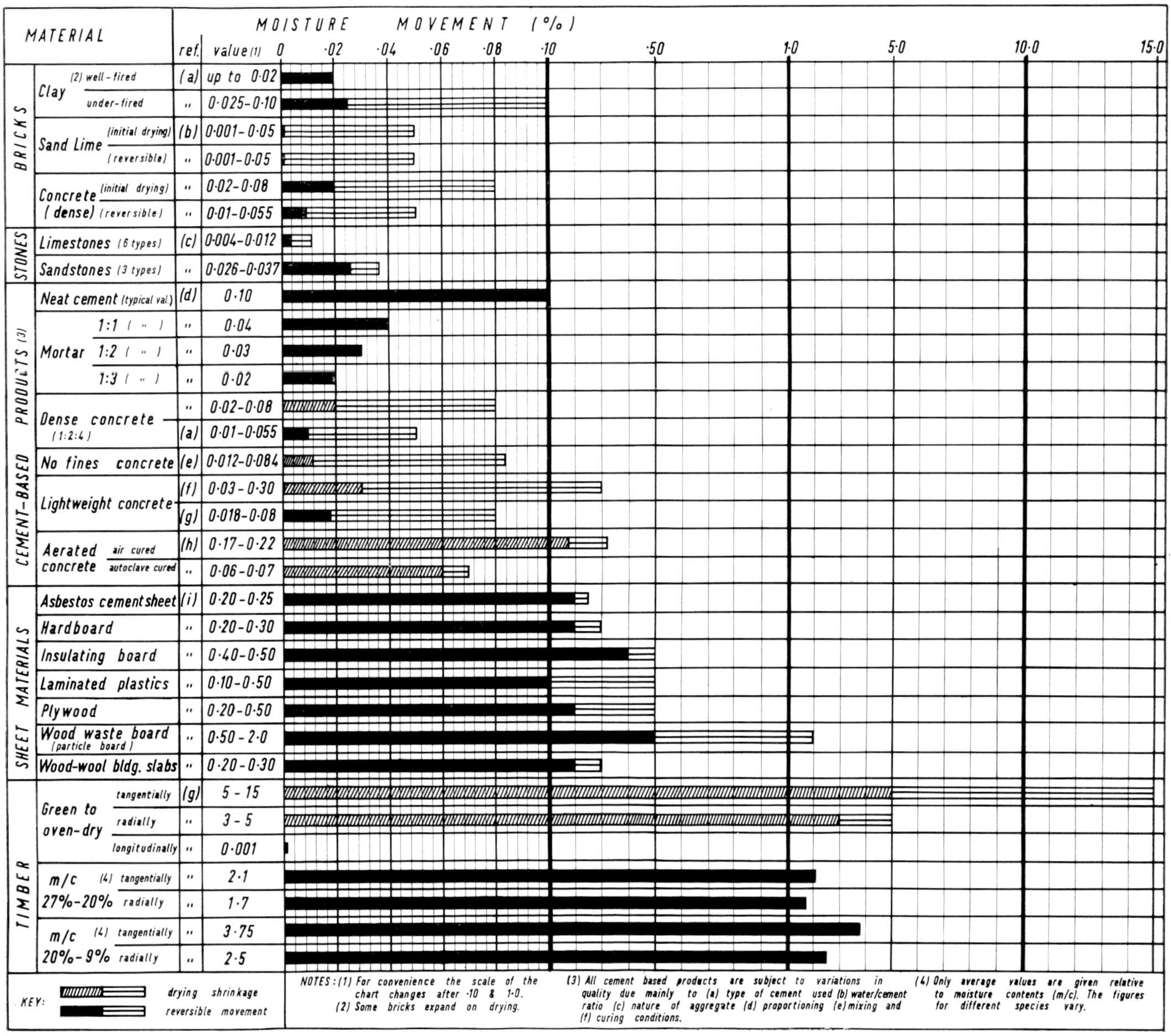


C.3.03/1

*Comparative chart of the range of moisture movements in various materials [References: (a) Butterworth, R., 'Clay Building', NBS Bull. No. 1, HMSO, 1948. (b) 'Sand-lime and Concrete Bricks', NBS Bull. No. 4, HMSO, 1948 and Bessey, G. E., 'Sand-lime Bricks', NBS Special Report, No. 3, HMSO, 1948. (c) Schaffer, R. J., 'The Weathering of Natural Building Stones', Building Research Special Report, No. 18, HMSO, 1932. (d) Lea, F. M., 'The Chemistry of Cement and Concrete' (revised edition of Lea and Desch), Arnold, 1956. (e) 'Shrinkage of Natural Aggregates in Concrete', BRS Digest (2nd Series), No. 35, June 1963. (f) 'Lightweight Aggregate Concrete—1. Materials and Properties', BRS Digest (2nd Series), No. 35, Aug. 1962. (g) 'Principles of Modern Building', Vol. 1, 3rd Ed., HMSO, 1959. (h) 'Aerated Concrete—1. Manufacture and Properties', BRS Digest (2nd Series), No. 16, Nov. 1961. (i) 'House Construction', Post-war Building Studies, No. 1, HMSO, 1944]*

(b) *Transmission between two adjoining materials*

The capillary properties of materials influence the suction force which is exerted to draw water from within a material to the surface. They also control the transmission of water, which may include soluble salts for instance (important for Efflorescence) from one material to another.

Capillary suction is greater in *uniformly* fine-pored materials than in *uniformly* large-pored materials. Thus, if different materials are placed in contact with one another, a uniformly fine-pored material will draw water from a uniformly large-pored material. However, materials normally contain pores of various sizes and so the suction force which is developed will depend on *moisture content*. Thus, subject to the relative pore structure, the *direction* of moisture transmission between two particular materials alters with a change in the degree of saturation. This will, in part, be influenced by capillary attraction, particularly if the material concerned faces on to a source of water. In general, it is extremely difficult and complex to predict the direction of transmission of water between any two materials because the capillary suction of a material varies with its moisture, while the rate of change of moisture content under wetting and drying conditions varies with different materials.

### 2. Absorption

Absorption is the property of permitting water (or any other liquid) to enter the *pores* of materials. (The significance of pore size and arrangement is covered in *Section 1.12*.) In this sense, absorption does not imply any particular association between the absorbed water and the solids of which a material is composed, although a particular association may occur. The amount of water absorbed is expressed as a percentage of the mass of the material.* It may be written in formula form as:

$$\text{Absorption} = \frac{\text{Mass of water absorbed}}{\text{Mass of material}} \times 100$$

Absorption of some materials, together with porosity, is given in the comparative chart C.3.03/2.

In practice, the rate of absorption is usually far more significant than the amount actually absorbed. Usually the rate of drying out is the same as the rate of absorption. It may also be noted that dry porous materials initially absorb water rapidly by capillary action—known as suction—but the rate soon decreases until saturation is reached. The rate of absorption may be increased significantly if the source of water is under pressure (see '4. Permeability' below).

### 3. Saturation coefficient

The saturation coefficient is the ratio of the volume of water absorbed and the total volume of voids in a material.

*Absorption may also be computed on a percentage volume basis.

It may be written in formula form as:

$$\text{Saturation Coefficient} = \frac{\text{Volume of water absorbed}}{\text{Total volume of voids}}$$

Thus, when all voids are filled with water the coefficient equals 1·0. Few materials have coefficients of 1·0 (coefficients for some materials are included in the comparative chart C.3.03/2) which partly supports the theory that not all voids in a material are necessary filled when a material is saturated.

Saturation coefficients are sometimes considered to give some guidance as to frost resistance of materials (see *Section 3.08* later).

### 4. Permeability

Permeability may be defined as that property which permits the passage of a liquid *through* a material and is thus distinct from the penetration of moisture into a substance by means of absorption due to capillary action. In some senses permeability only commences after a material has been saturated.

The passage of water may be caused by (a) capillary action and (b) pressure due to force of gravity, driving-rain, head of water, or thermal expansion of water already absorbed at a lower temperature. Until water has penetrated through a material the rate of flow results from combined pressure and capillary action, but when penetration is complete the rate of flow is entirely dependent on pressure.

The rate of flow is a measure of the permeability of a material. Thus, permeability must be due to the existence of continuous passages *right through* the material. Permeability may, of course, also be applicable to composite elements, in which case water may penetrate at the interface of joints between units making up the element. This implies breakdown of adhesion. Joints in brickwork, for example, often provide through routes for the complete penetration of water, and such penetration usually occurs at the interface of the jointing medium, i.e. the mortar and the bricks.

## The presence of water in materials

Water can be present in building materials in three ways, namely (1) in chemical combination, (2) as free water, and (3) as 'sorbed' water, each of which may influence moisture content but not moisture movement. To understand the significance of these relative to moisture movement they are discussed separately.

### 1. Water in chemical combination

The chemical combination of various materials to form compounds, with properties peculiar to the compounds, requires specific equi-molecular proportions of the individual materials. (*See 1.09 Chemical equations*.) When water is essential to the existence of the compound, it is said to be in chemical combination, and can only be removed by breaking down the compound under certain definite conditions.

Thus, for example, one molecule of calcium hydroxide ($Ca(OH)_2$), slaked lime, can only be formed when one molecule of calcium oxide (CaO), quicklime, unites with one molecule of water ($H_2O$). This may be written as:

$$CaO + H_2O = Ca(OH)_2.$$

Unless the fixed proportions of quicklime and water are present, slaked lime cannot be formed. However, slaked lime can still be formed, and this is important, even if the quantities of water present *exceed* the fixed amount required. Such excess water is not then in chemical combination.

It may be noted here that the reaction of water with cement, although following the same principle, is extremely complex as, among other things, water reacts with the individual constituents of which the cement is composed.

### 2. Free water

Water in a material is said to be free when it is associated with a solid in such a way that its properties still remain, for all practical purposes, unchanged. In general, such water wets the material and remains in association with the material only during external conditions which maintain complete moisture saturation. As an example, consider a good quality brick saturated with water. Almost all the water is 'free' and the association is maintained by keeping the brick either immersed in water or surrounded by air saturated with water vapour.

### 3. Sorbed water

In building materials, 'sorbed' water in association with a solid is a condition intermediate between chemically combined water and free water. Such water is held more firmly to the solid than free water, but is not held so as to form a definite chemical compound. The most important factor regarding 'sorbed' water is that the *association* with the solid material depends entirely upon external humidity conditions. Provided sufficient time is allowed (this is extremely important) the amount of water 'held' changes as the humidity changes. However, the moisture equilibrium of the solid, that is the amount of water in equilibrium with the solid, is dependent on both temperature and humidity of the surrounding air. As previously stated, in practice, relative humidity is usually of greatest value. In addition, different materials have different moisture equilibria.

(a) *Gels*

Sorbed water is associated with *gels* as generally discussed in *Section 1.06*, 'Colloidal solutions, 4. Gels'. Those encountered in building materials are non-rigid gels, which, among other things, means that they do not go into solution but have definite saturation levels. In timber, fibre saturation point is reached when the *cell walls* contain between 25 and 30 per cent of their dry mass.

When water is sorbed by the gels there is an increase in the volume of the material, while there is a corresponding decrease when the moisture is liberated. Thus, the presence of gels makes materials hygroscopic.

The evidence available suggests that the expansion (and corresponding contraction) which takes place may often be ascribed to the swelling (or contraction) of colloidal constituents in the material. However, it is also thought that the action of surface tension forces in the pores may also be of some significance. Thus, it is possible for moisture movements to take place when water is held in the pores of materials, whether the presence of such water implies complete or partial saturation. On the other hand, under certain conditions, some of the water held in the pores may be sorbed into the hygroscopic solids of the material. Water sorbed in this way can only remain in association with the solids for as long as the environmental conditions allow.

(b) *Colloidal constituents in some materials*

The presence of colloidal constituents is more commonly associated with timber and cement. In the case of *timber* and other natural fibrous materials, the gels are 'incorporated', so to speak, during growth and are in a sense an integral part of the material. With *cement* the products of the chemical combination of water and the cement are present as gels. *Clay bricks* (and other clay products for that matter) are formed of typically colloidal material, clay. However, the colloidal character is destroyed by firing and so bricks do not exhibit appreciable moisture movements. It is for this reason that thorough firing must be ensured during manufacture—underfired bricks are liable to large expansions on becoming wet. *Sand-lime* bricks, which are manufactured by heating mixtures of sand and lime with steam under pressure, have fairly high moisture movements. This may be due to the presence of colloidal silicates of lime. Finally, *sandstones* show the most pronounced moisture movement of the natural building stones. This may be accounted for due to the presence of colloidal minerals acting as the cementing medium between the silica grains. Such movement may be significant when sandstone is used as an aggregate in concrete, particularly during initial drying out.

(c) *Drying out*

In general, the water held freely in the capillaries or pores of materials are not regarded as important as sorbed water in considerations of moisture movement. Such free water will, of course, contribute to the moisture content of the material.

During the drying out process it is usually the free water which is first liberated. Once this water has been removed by evaporation, then it is the sorbed water which is given off into the atmosphere until moisture equilibrium is reached. Thus initial, and perhaps substantial, drops in moisture content may not always indicate corresponding contractions in a material.

| MATERIAL | | | POROSITY (% volume) ref. | value | ABSORPTION (% weight) ref. | value | SATURATION COEFFICIENT ref. | value |
|---|---|---|---|---|---|---|---|---|
| BRICKS | CLAY | –handmade (range) | | | (a) | 9-28 | (a) | 0·3-0·8 |
| | | –machinemade ( " ) | (a) | 18·5-48·9 | " | 1-37 | " | 04-0·85 |
| | | Facings london stocks | " | 48·9 | " | 22-37 | " | 0·45 0·65 |
| | | Facings white gault | " | 38·5 | " | 22-28 | " | about 0·85 |
| | | Facings keuper marl | " | 24·6 | " | 12-21 | " | 0·75-0·9 |
| | | Facings flettons | " | 34·8 | " | 17-25 | " | 0·7-0·85 |
| | | Common-london stock | | — | " | 27-38 | " | 0·6-0·75 |
| | Sand–lime | | | | (d) | 10-18 | (d) | 0·6-0·8 |
| | Concrete | | | | | | | |
| STONES | Limestone | –all types | (b) | 14·7-30·8 | (c) | 2·45-13·5 | | |
| | | –portland stone | " | 20 | " | 6·8-7·5 | | |
| | | –bath stones | " | 26-33 | " | 6·2-11·6 | | |
| | Sandstone | –all types | | | " | 2·10-10·4 | | |
| | | –red mansfield (av) | (c) | 14·98 | " | 4·58 | | |
| | | –york stone (av) | " | 11·94 | " | 4·70 | | |
| SHEET MATERIALS | Asbestos | –cement | | | (e) | 20-28 | | |
| | | –wood & wallboard | | | " | 52-53 | | |
| | Hardboard | –medium | | | " | 15-30 | | |
| | | –ordinary | | | " | 15-120 | | |
| | | –super | | | " | 15-20 | | |
| | Insulating board | | | | " | 30-100 | | |
| | Laminated fibreboard | | | | " | 130 | | |
| | Plasterboard | | | | " | 40-50 | | |
| | Plywood | | | | " | 25-35 | | |
| | Wood-waste board (particle board) | | | | " | 10-100 | | |

*C.3.03/2*
*Comparative chart of porosity, absorption and saturation coefficient of some materials [References: (a) 'Clay Building Bricks', NBS Bull. No. 1, HMSO, 1948. (b) Schaffer, R. J., 'The Weathering of Natural Building Stones', Building Research Special Report No. 18, HMSO, 1932. (c) Warnes, A. R., 'Building Stones', Benn, 1926. (d) 'Sand-lime and Concrete Bricks', NBS Bull., HMSO, 1948. (e) 'House Construction', Post-war Building Studies, No. 1, HMSO, 1944]*

(d) *Irreversible movement*

The considerations dealt with above have all been concerned with changes in moisture content which are reversible. However, the behaviour of rigid-gels, formed under super-saturated conditions, is significant when considering initial drying shrinkage, particularly in cement-based products.

When, for example, water is added to cement, it is at first free, then some water enters into chemical combination with the cement; some of the products of this reaction are present as gels. When gels are formed in the presence of excess water, it is thought that more water may initially be associated with the gel structure than is necessary for equilibrium even under conditions of water storage.

The excess water is gradually forced out from the gel and may hydrate further particles of cement which have previously not been reached by water, or may leave the whole mass and pass out into the surrounding atmosphere. As this water cannot be replaced, a shrinkage of the mass occurs when the excess water passes out. Thus, the greater the amount of excess water, the greater the shrinkage.

After equilibrium conditions have been reached, the cement is in the condition previously described, that is capable of undergoing reversible moisture movement.

## Exposure

Emphasis has already been placed on the importance of relative humidity of the air surrounding materials as regards both moisture content and moisture movement. The main factor in this being the ability, if not the 'desire', of all materials liable to movement to adjust their moisture contents to that of the surrounding air until moisture equilibrium has been attained. However, at the same time the rate at which this adjustment takes place when water is being given off to the surrounding air will not only be dependent on the structure and size of the material, but also, and this is important, on the prevailing environmental conditions which encourage evaporation and include temperature and air movement in addition to relative humidity. Thus, it is necessary to take into account the importance of moisture content changes and moisture movements which may result from saturation (complete or partial) by water in the liquid state. Under unfavourable conditions of evaporation (implies either high relative humidity, low air temperature, or low rate of air movement, separately or in combination), materials previously saturated by water in the liquid state may undergo fairly extensive movements. At the same time, the maintenance of high moisture contents may be undesirable for reasons other than movement and chemical action in particular is relevant.

The purpose of this part is (1) to outline the practical significance of saturation by water in the liquid state; (2) to develop certain aspects of the practical significance of relative humidity previously excluded; and (3) to draw attention to the interaction of thermal and moisture movements.

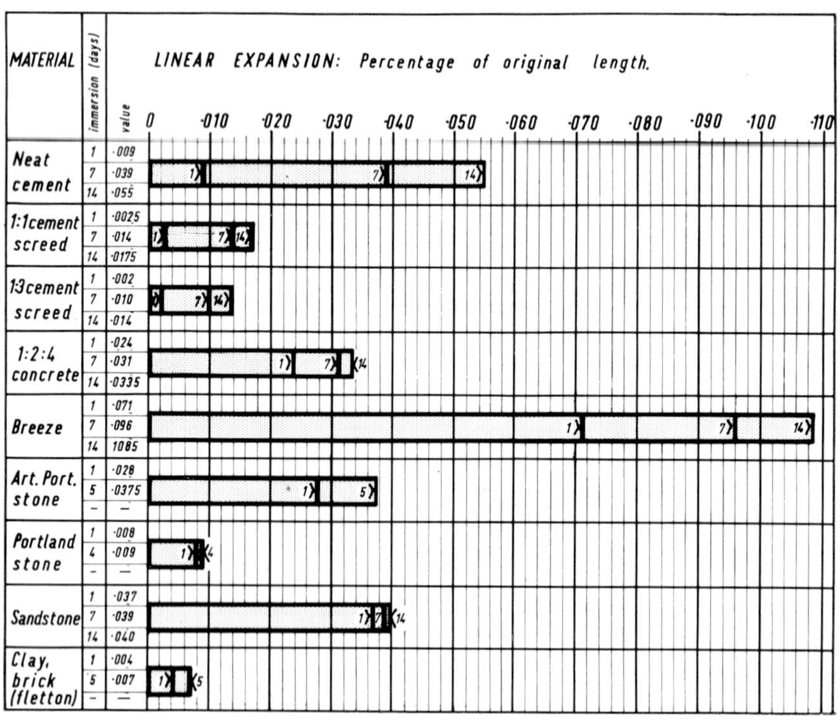


*C.3.03/3*
*Comparative chart of linear expansion in some materials on immersion in water. Note: all specimens immersed in water after drying at 50°C.*

*Samples, except clay bricks, were 152·4 × 152·4 × 76·2 mm (6 × 6 × 3 in) prisms (From: Stradling, R. F., Building Research Bull. No. 3, graphs in Fig. 9, p. 11, HMSO, 1928)*

### 1. Water in the liquid state

All the sources of water outlined in *Section 3.02* are capable of causing materials to become saturated. In general, rainwater presents severe conditions for most external elements; water introduced during construction is particularly relevant for initial drying shrinkage in the wet trade processes, while condensation may present rather severe conditions internally. The other sources, such as water supply, faulty services and maintenance and usage require individual assessment. Finally, groundwater usually implies perennial saturation and the materials used in association with the ground are, therefore, specially selected for this condition.

The extent of the linear expansion which can be expected in a material as a result of saturation will be dependent on two factors. These are: (1) the nature of the material and (2) the length of immersion or exposure to water. The comparative chart C. 3.03/3 illustrates the linear expansion of some materials commonly used externally when small samples of each (except for the clay brick) were immersed in water over a period of days. In all cases the longer the period of immersion the greater the expansion. However, what is significant is the fact that the rate of expansion varies quite considerably with the various materials. Expansions *approaching* the maxima shown on this chart and also on C. 3.03/1 may, within limits, be attained in external elements exposed to rainwater. In this account has to be taken of the prevailing wet and dry conditions (see *Section 3.01*, comparative chart C.3.01/1). In winter, for example, external elements can be expected to be saturated over a long period of time. Drying out will commence during the spring and generally dry conditions will normally prevail during the summer.

From available information, it would appear that materials with movements of 0·04 per cent and above require special design consideration in terms of allowing for expansion, providing sufficient restraint, or providing complete impervious protection which will prevent the ingress (and egress too!) of water. If reference is made to comparative chart C.3.03/1 it will be seen that, in addition to some of the more 'traditional' walling materials such as certain types of sand-lime bricks and various types of concrete, timber, timber-products and most sheet materials have expansions well in excess of 0·04 per cent. In general, the latter materials require special consideration if they are intended to be used in exposed external situations. Although joint design and restraint may offer some solution to the problems involved, it is usually imperative to ensure that as little movement as possible takes place by the provision of an impervious coating. The success of such a coating in reducing changes in moisture content will largely be dependent, in addition to its own characteristics, on complete continuity of the coating. Thus edges, often neglected, must also be protected. At the same time it should also be remembered that the 'backs' of these materials, although not exposed to rainwater, may 'draw' water from backing materials, while cavities behind the material may provide sources of high humidity if not condensation. All these reasons would seem to underline the necessity for ensuring that 'all-round' protection is provided. Care must also be taken to ensure that excessive quantities of water are not trapped within the material during the application of the coating.

The principles outlined above in connection with rainwater are also applicable to other sources of water, although many of these will usually be of a localised nature. Thus, special consideration may only have to be given to the selection and use of certain sheet materials, for example, where there is a risk of excessive condensation.

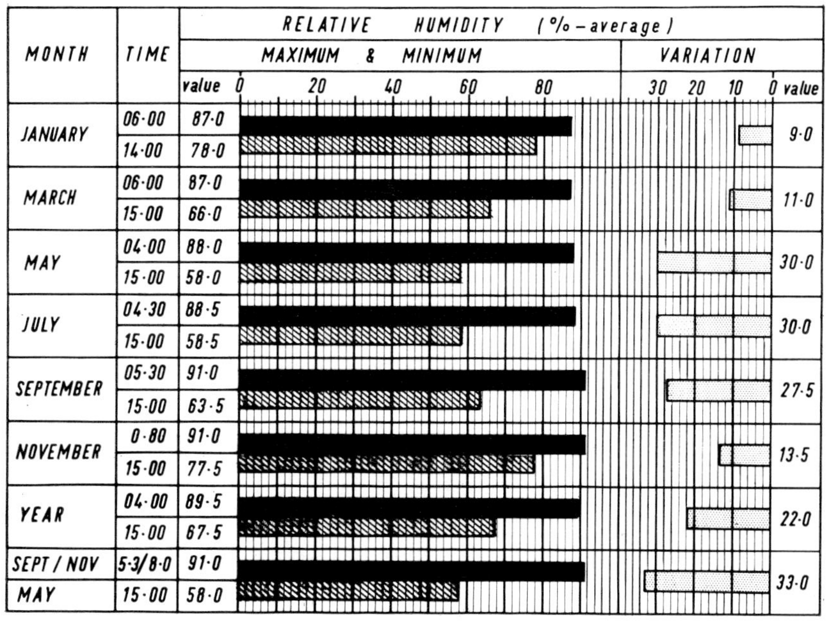


C.3.03/4
*Comparative chart of range of average maximum and minimum relative humidity at various months of the year observed at Kew, London 1901–30*

(*From: 'Climatological Atlas of the British Isles', p. 115, graphs of average hourly relative humidity, Met. Office, HMSO, 1952*)

**2. Relative humidity**

External elements may not necessarily be exposed to rainwater, but will be exposed to prevailing relative humidity. Internally, the relative humidity will approximate to that prevailing outside, except when central heating is used, special humidity control is exercised or excessive quantities of vapour are produced, such as may occur in kitchens, bathrooms, laundries and certain industrial processes. All these present special cases which must be considered on their merits and are, therefore, outside the present scope. However, whatever the condition, the range of relative humidities likely to be encountered in practice are important.

Once the moisture equilibria of materials are known, and provided these can be related to moisture movement, then it is possible to assess the range of movements which are likely to occur due to either diurnal or seasonal variations in relative humidity (see 'Definitions of terms, 1. Moisture movement (a) Interpretation of values'). Comparative graph C.3.03/5 gives moisture equilibria for some materials. The values given, it should be noted, are average and do not take into account variations which do occur within one type of material.

Observations of relative humidity are made at various stations throughout the country. As an example, the average diurnal and seasonal variations of observations made at Kew Observatory over a number of years are given in the comparative chart C.3.03/4. From this it will be seen that the diurnal range is approximately 78–87 per cent (a difference of 9 per cent) in January, rising to approximately 58·5–88·5 per cent (difference of 30 per cent) in July. The annual range is approximately 67·5–88·5 per cent (a difference of 22 per cent). After making due allowances, the maximum ranges of relative humidity, whether diurnal or seasonal, are unlikely to cause movements of the magnitude of those given in C.3.03/1. In fact, the actual movement will be significantly less. This, however, would be the situation in general. The special cases mentioned before could make very important differences (continuous exposure to a heat source may cause excessive drying; continuous exposure to water vapour producing sources may cause excessive wetting), in which case the magnitude of movements given in C.3.03/1 could be attained.

**3. Interaction between thermal and moisture movements**

A somewhat complex situation does arise when materials with significant moisture contents are exposed to solar radiation. In cases such as these, movements caused by temperature and moisture changes may often—perhaps usually—act in opposition, and thus hold a fortuitous balance. This tends to act as an additional safety measure against trouble due to extreme dimensional fluctuations.

## Movement in timber*

When compared with other materials for building, timber presents some special problems. Most of these are derived from the fact that timber is a natural product, with a complex cellular structure (see *Section 1.06*), and cut down while still 'alive'. Furthermore, there are a wide variety of species available, each with its own characteristics. Not only are there variations in the properties and behaviour between the species, but also between samples from the same species. As regards moisture movement in particular, which is in excess of that for any other material, there are significant differences between tangentially and radially cut timber whatever the species. Variations in moisture movement are accounted for by the fact that different species have different fibre saturation points, while hygroscopicity also plays an important part.

The Forest Products Research Laboratory in Leaflet No. 47 (Revised August, 1961), *The Movement of Timbers,* quotes values of moisture movement for over 180 different species. Very few of the values are exactly the same, although in some cases the differences may not be of practical significance. However, in order to attempt to classify timbers according to their degree of movement and so form some *method of comparison,* three classes have been arrived at using as a basis the *sum* of the percentage tangential and radial movements. Thus, Class I—timbers with small movement values—includes timbers where the sum of the movements is *less* than 3·0; in Class II—timbers with medium movement values—are included those where the sum of the movements is *between* 3·0 and 4·5, while in Class III—timbers with large movements—are included all those where the sum of the movements *exceeds* 4·5. A selection of the species

*References
(1) Desch, H. E., *Timber, Its Structure and Properties*, 4th Ed., MacMillan, 1968. (2) Leaflets, Reports, etc. issued by the Forest Products Research Laboratory (FPRL), Princes Risborough, Aylesbury, Bucks.

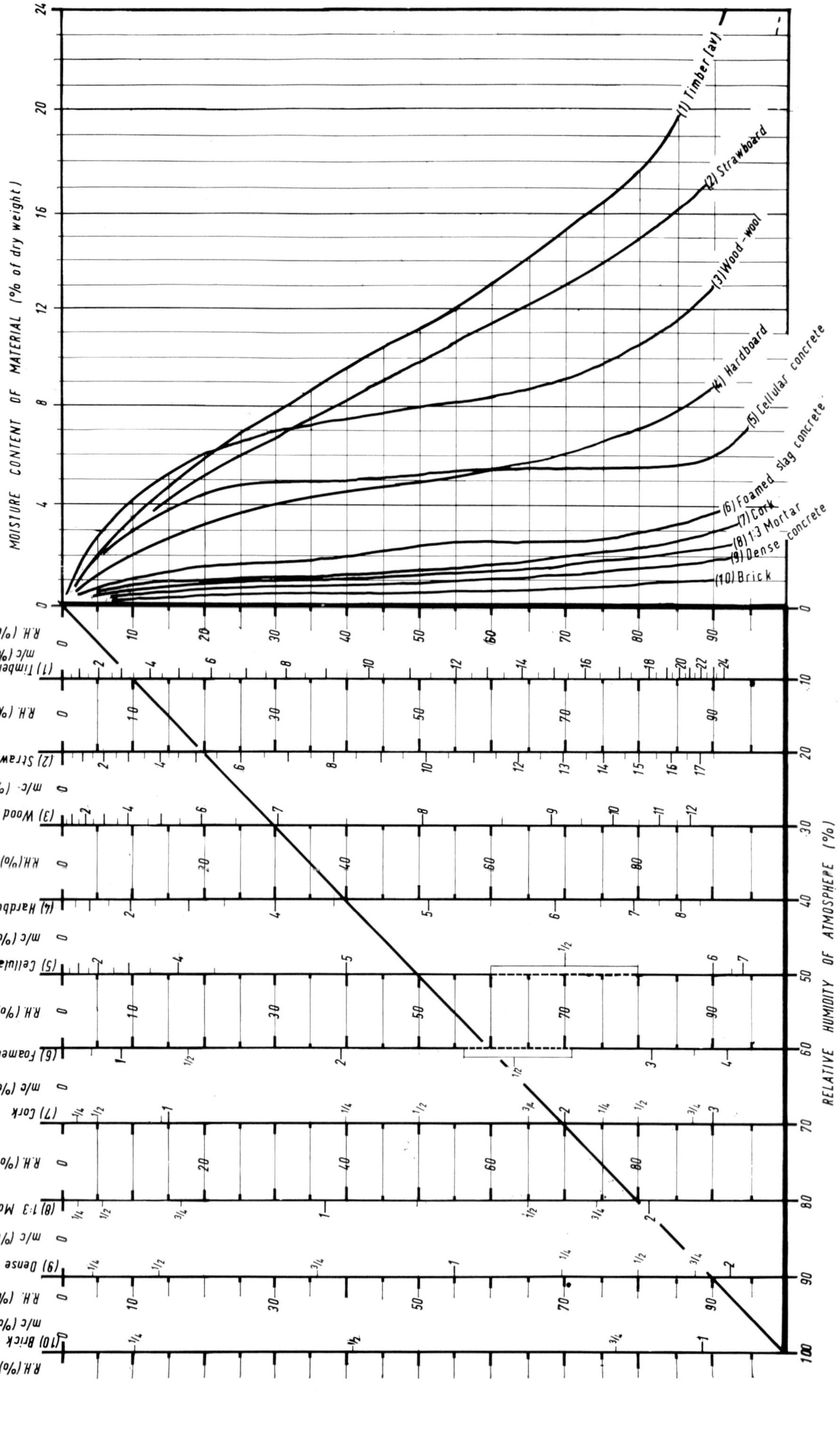

MOISTURE CONTENT OF MATERIAL (% of dry weight)
RELATIVE HUMIDITY OF ATMOSPHERE (%)
(1) Timber (av)
(2) Strawboard
(3) Wood-wool
(4) Hardboard
(5) Cellular concrete
(6) Foamed slag concrete
(7) Cork
(8) 1:3 Mortar
(9) Dense concrete
(10) Brick
R.H. (%)
m/c (%)

quoted in Leaflet No. 47 is included in the comparative chart C.3.03/6 and illustrates the variations between species *and* type of conversion referred to in the preceding paragraph.

Examples of variations in moisture content in living trees may also help to underline the fact that timber cannot really be considered as one material but rather as a group of materials, the individual members of which have characteristics which differ from one another. The moisture content in living trees may vary from 40 to 200 per cent, while further variations in the content of sapwood and heartwood, particularly in softwoods, do occur. For example, the sapwood in long-leaf pitch pine has a moisture content in excess of 100 per cent, while the heartwood ranges from 30 to 40 per cent.

Because of the detailed differences in properties and behaviour of all the available species of timber, it would be virtually impossible to consider every one. In any case, a certain general pattern can be extracted which is useful in any understanding of the special problems involved in the use of timber, while the pattern serves as a basis upon which variations can be assessed. Thus, in this study, *average values* or typical behaviour patterns are used.

Many timber products now available, such as plywood, blockboard, laminboard, laminated construction, many of the fibreboards, particle boards, etc., have, in some respects, been developed in an attempt to overcome many of the inherent weaknesses of timber, not least of all moisture movement. In general, these products do not have moisture movements of the same magnitude as is found in normally converted timber. Accordingly, and despite some notable exceptions, the factors which affect movement in normally converted timber are primarily considered here under the following headings: (1) Effects of conversion; (2) Moisture equilibrium; (3) Control of hygroscopicity; and (4) Precautions.

## 1. Effects of conversion

There are a number of different ways in which a log may be sawn so as to provide sections of timber convenient

| CLASS | TIMBER | MOISTURE MOVEMENT (% original length range 90% – 60% R.H.) TANGENTIAL value | RADIAL value |
|---|---|---|---|
| I – small movement values | African Walnut | 1·3 | 0·9 |
| | Afrormosia | 1·3 | 0·7 |
| | Agba | 1·8 | 0·8 |
| | Balsa | 2·0 | 0·6 |
| | Cedar, South American | 1·5 | 1·0 |
| | Douglas fir | 1·5 | 1·2 |
| | Hemlock, western | 1·9 | 0·9 |
| | Iroko | 1·0 | 0·5 |
| | Mahogany, African (Khaya ivorensis) | 1·5 | 0·9 |
| | Mahogany, Central American | 1·3 | 1·0 |
| | Obeche | 1·25 | 0·8 |
| | Opepe | 1·8 | 0·9 |
| | Pine, yellow | 1·7 | 0·9 |
| | Rosewood, Indian | 1·0 | 0·7 |
| | Rhodesian, teak | 1·6 | 1·0 |
| | Spruce, European | 1·5 | 0·7 |
| | Teak | 1·3 | 0·8 |
| | Western red cedar | 0·9–1·9 | 0·45–0·8 |
| | Whitewood | 1·5 | 0·7 |
| II – medium movement values | Ash | 1·8 | 1·3 |
| | Elm, English | 2·4 | 1·5 |
| | Jarrah | 2·6 | 1·8 |
| | Keruing | 2·5 | 1·5 |
| | Mahogany, African (Khaya grandifoliola) | 1·9 | 1·5 |
| | Oak, English | 2·5 | 1·5 |
| | Parana pine | 2·5 | 1·7 |
| | Pine, Carribean pitch | 2·6 | 1·4 |
| | Pine, Scots | 2·2 | 1·0 |
| | Poplar, Black Italian | 2·8 | 1·2 |
| | Red wood | 2·2 | 1·0 |
| | Sapele | 1·8 | 1·3 |
| | Spruce, Serbian | 2·3 | 1·3 |
| | Sycamore | 2·8 | 1·4 |
| | Utile | 1·8 | 1·6 |
| | Walnut, European | 2·0 | 1·6 |
| III – large movement values | Ash, Japanese | 3·5 | 1·5 |
| | Beech | 3·2 | 1·7 |
| | Birch, Canadian Yellow | 2·5 | 2·2 |
| | Gurjun | 3·3 | 2·0 |
| | Oak, Turkey | 3·3 | 1·3 |
| | Olive, East African | 2·9 | 1·7 |
| | Tasmanian Oak | 3·4 | 2·0 |
| | Wattle, black | 3·5 | 1·2 |

C.3.03/5 (opposite)
*Comparative graph giving equilibrium moisture content of some materials at various humidities. Note: all values taken from graphs [References: (1) 'The Moisture Content of Timber', FPRL, Leaflet No. 9, HMSO, revised Nov. 1963. (2), (3), (4), (6), (8), (9) and (10) Ragsdale, L. A., and Raynham, E. A., 'Building Materials Practce', Fig. 26, p. 96, Arnold, 1964. (5) and (7) Billington, N. S., 'Thermal Properties of Buildings', Fig. 5.3, p. 117, Cleaver-Hume, 1952]*

C.3.03/6
*Comparative chart of the tangential and radial moisture movements in a selection of timber species (From: 'The Movement of Timber', FPRL Leaflet No. 47, HMSO, revised 1961)*

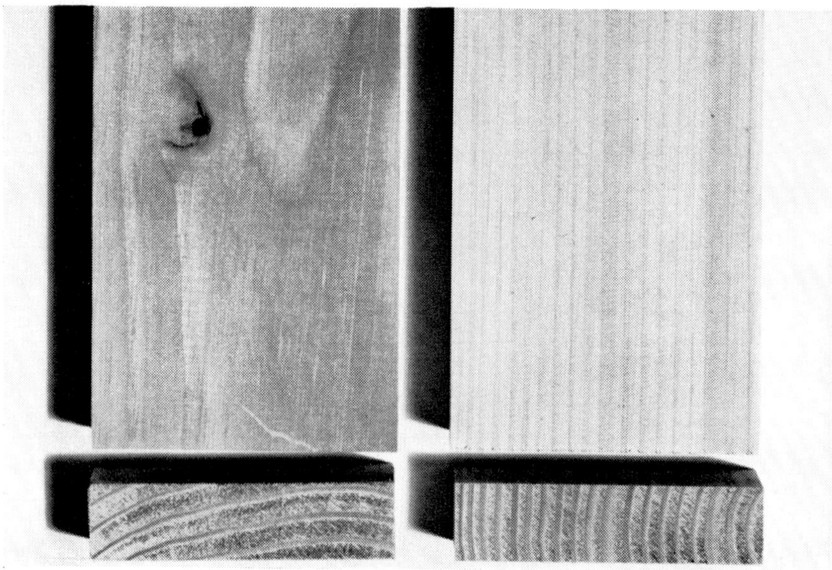

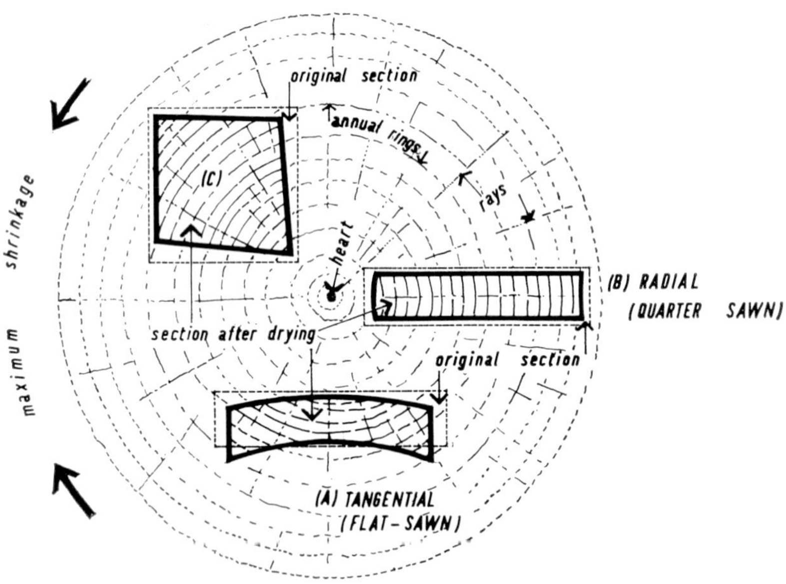


*D*.3.03/3
*Shrinkage of timber cut radially and tangentially. The accompanying photograph from the FPRL illustrates radially cut timber (right hand) and tangentially cut timber (left hand). (Based on: 'Principles of Modern Building', Vol. 1, Fig. 11.3, p. 123, HMSO, 1959)*

and suitable for building and other uses—the process is known as conversion.* However, there are basically two different sections or types of 'cut' which may result. One is *tangential* (derived from cutting basically at right angles to the rays and producing what is commonly referred to as flat-sawn or through and through sawn timber) and *defined* as timber converted so that the annual rings meet the face at an angle of *less* than 45 degrees ; the other is *radial* (derived from cutting basically parallel to the rays and producing what is commonly referred to as quarter- or rift-sawn timber) and *defined* as timber converted so that the annual rings meet the face at an angle *greater* than 45 degrees. Tangential and radial sections of timber are illustrated in the accompanying photograph and diagram D.3.03/3. The diagram also shows the manner in which both types will shrink after drying. Not only is the shrinkage greater in the tangential direction, that is in the direction of the annual rings (see also diagrams at the end of *Section 1.06*), but there is also notable distortion because the annual rings tend to bend away from the heart. Thus, the wide faces of the rectangular tangential section (A) deform with a noticeable curvature, while the narrow end faces of the rectangular radial section (B) are, by comparison, only moderately curved and, although the magnitude of shrinkage is still greatest in the tangential direction, the section does not distort. In the case of the square section (C), the net result of the tendency of the annual rings to bend away from the heart is to cause significant uneven shrinkage on the two 'radial' faces. These are probably the most important effects of conversion in terms of movement, although other types of distortion in the length of a section, which are excluded here, may also result.

The precise differences in the magnitude of movement in the tangential and radial direction have already been included in the comparative charts. However, as radially cut timber is far more stable, in terms of distortion particularly, than tangentially cut timber, it is important to note the practical implication of the distortion of tangentially cut timber. In this the relationship between the curvature of the annual rings and the backgrounds to which timber may be fixed are relevant. Possible results which may occur when tangentially cut timber is used in such situations as skirtings, cover fillets and floors are illustrated in diagram D.3.03/4. It should be noted that, in order to illustrate the principle involved, the examples have been *greatly exaggerated,* while the effects of restraint by any fixings which, within limits, could mitigate the bending effect, have been generally disregarded.

## 2. Moisture equilibrium

The comparative chart C.3.03/7 illustrates the way in which both relative humidity and temperature affect the moisture equilibrium of timber. In general, the relative humidity has a greater influence than temperature, although it can be seen that there is a significant difference between the temperature range 15° – 40°C and 70°C. For practical purposes equilibria based on a temperature of 15·6°C and related to a range of relative humidities has been considered most convenient. This is the basis used for the conversion chart C.3.03/8 which gives values of moisture contents determined in a number of environments. The headings do not include all uses of timber included in Leaflet No. 9, but conditions for a particular case can be estimated by analogy or reference to more comprehensive headings in the original (and those related to it). The chart, it must be stressed, gives *average* values for timber as a whole, while no account is taken of the effects of previous treatment of timber (see '3. Control of hygroscopicity'). The extent of the variations in some timbers may be obtained by making allowances based on the equilibrium moisture content values included in the comparative chart C.3.03/6 given previously. For most practical purposes the moisture

*Conversion takes place prior to seasoning. Subsequent sawing or shaping of converted and seasoned timber is more commonly known as 'manufacture'.

**Table 3.03/1 Moisture Content of Timber for Various Positions**

| *Position of timber in building* | *Average moisture content attained in use in a dried-out building (per cent of dry mass)* | *Moisture content which should not be exceeded at time of erection (per cent of dry mass)* |
|---|---|---|
| Framing and sheathing of timber buildings (not prefabricated) | 16 | 22 |
| Timber for prefabricated buildings | 16 | 17 for precision work, otherwise 22 |
| Rafters and roof boarding, tiling, battens, etc. | 15 | 22 |
| Ground-floor joists | 18 | 22 |
| Upper-floor joists | 15 | 22 |
| Joinery and flooring | | |
| (*a*) in buildings slightly or occasionally heated | 14 | 14 |
| (*b*) in continuously heated buildings | 11–12 | 12 |
| (*c*) in buildings with a high degree of central heating, e.g. hospitals | 10 | 10 |
| Wood flooring over heating elements | 8–9 | 9 |

*Reference: Home-grown softwoods for Building*, BRS Digest (II) No. 72, HMSO, July 1966.

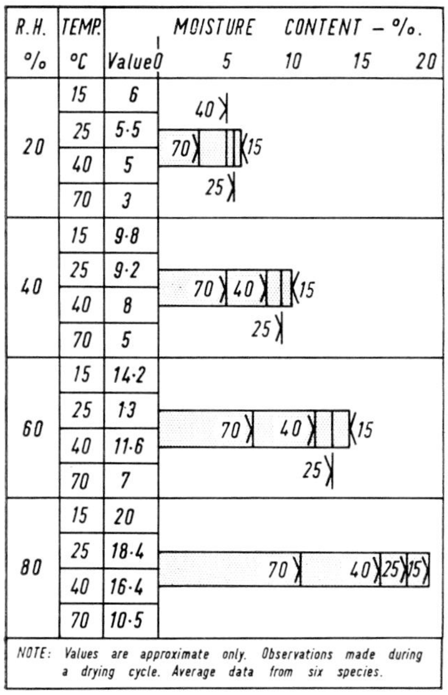


*C.3.03/7*
*Comparative chart of the effect of both relative humidity and temperature on the moisture equilibrium of timber. Moisture content—humidity equilibrium at four relative humidities and temperatures. (Interpolated from graphs supplied by FPRL)*

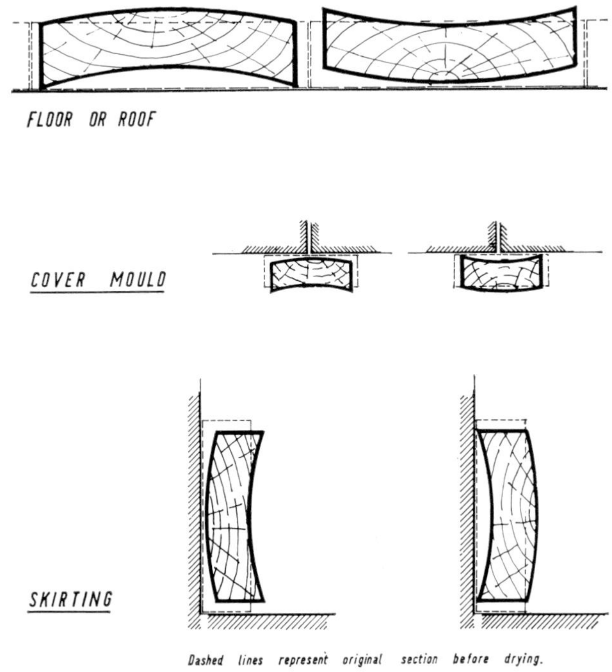


*D.3.03/4*
*Distortion due to drying in timber used in three common ways. Compare with D.3.03/3*

content of timber for various positions given in Table 3.03/1 is a useful guide.

The relationship between moisture content and the *average shrinkage* of timber (mm/m) *in drying* for both tangential and radial sections is given in the conversion chart C.3.03/9. For most practical purposes the amount of swelling which will take place during increases in moisture content can normally be taken as the same as those given in the chart.

For design purposes, the significance of fluctuations in moisture content which are bound to occur should be noted. Some examples may help to illustrate this.

(a) *During service*

During service, timber furniture in a well heated living room will have an average moisture content of 12 per cent.* In the autumn, the moisture content would be about 14 per cent, falling, when the room is heated, to about 10 per cent at the end of the winter. From C.3.03/9 a change in moisture content from 14 to 10 per cent would result in a movement of 8·3mm/m and 13·3mm/m in radial and tangential sections respectively.

In connection with light cladding, the Building Research Station† has recommended that in protected conditions internally an average of 13·3mm/m should be allowed. This value is based, after making allowances, on the probable variation in moisture content of 15 per cent in late autumn before heating commences to 8 per cent in mid winter in a well-heated building. On the other hand, variations externally are likely to be in the range from 15 to 22 per cent (as between summer and winter), in which case an average allowance of 16·7mm/m should be made. It should be noted that thin boards and shingles may reach moisture contents as low as 10 per cent in very hot weather.

(b) *During and after installation*

In general, the fluctuations in moisture content in timber during service, particularly internally, are, in some respects, not as important as the fluctuations which may occur during or soon after initial installation. Small variations in moisture are unlikely to

**The Moisture Content of Timber in Use*, FPRL Leaflet No. 9, p. 1, HMSO, revised November, 1963.

†*Light Cladding—Part II*, Materials in Detail, BRS Digest (1st Series) No. 99, p. 8, HMSO, June, 1957.

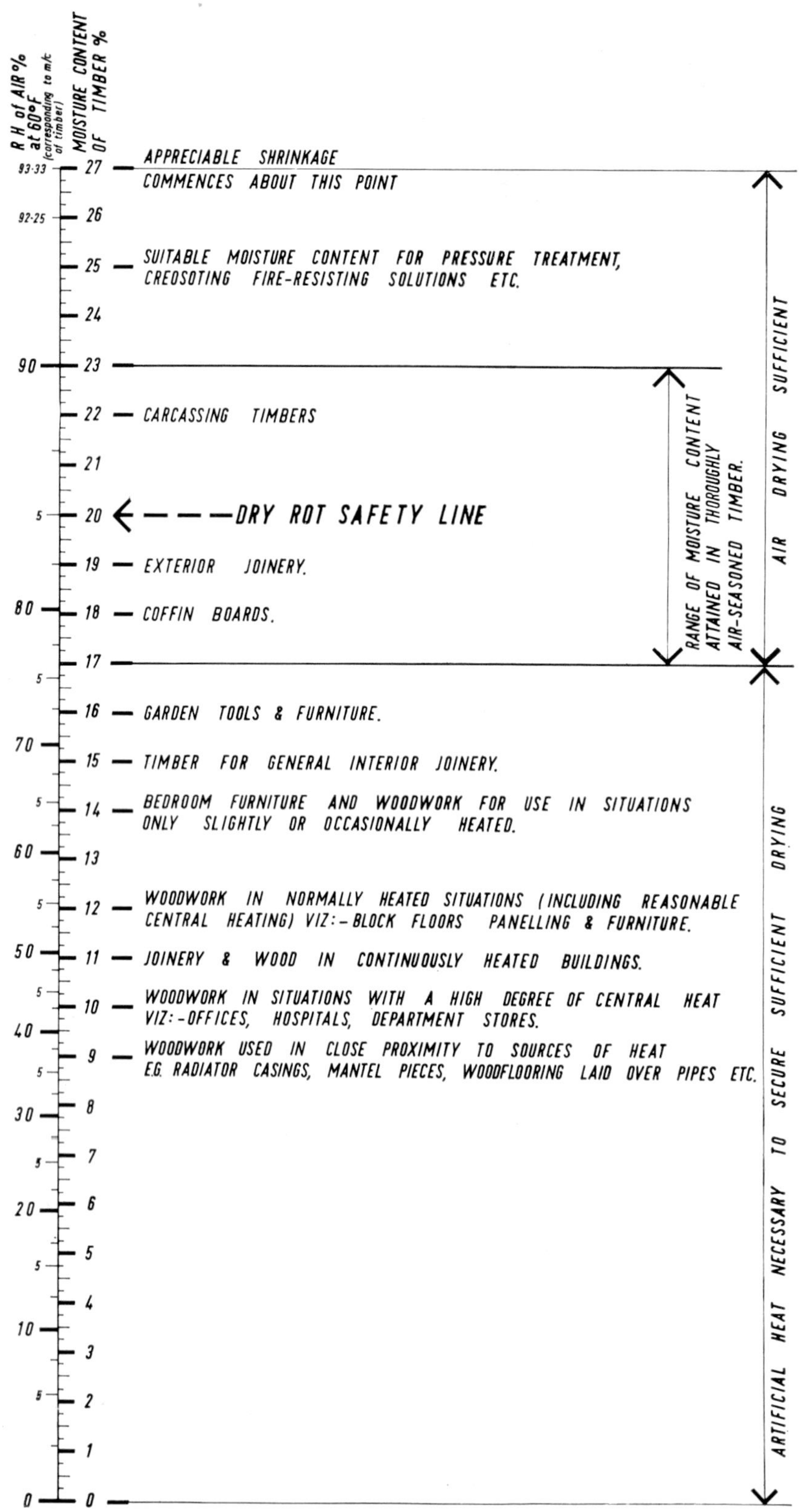


*C.3.03/8*
*Conversion chart giving equilibrium moisture content of timber for various uses. Note: values for different species vary and the chart gives average values (From: 'The Moisture Content of Timber in Use', FPRL Leaflet No. 9, HMSO, revised 1963)*

lead to significant movements. However, this does not detract from the fact that timber should be seasoned to moisture contents likely to be achieved in service, although precise 'matching' is not always essential and, perhaps more important, not easily attained in practice. Thus, in addition to ensuring correct seasoning for the expected service environment, further allowance by way of expansion joints is also necessary. Expansion joints may be advisable even for service conditions. A selection of traditional joints are illustrated in diagram D.3.03/5.

As an example of the moisture content fluctuations which may occur after installation, consider joinery dried to 12 per cent moisture content (equilibrium for the service environment) and installed in a new building before the drying out process has been completed. During drying out of the fabric of the building, the timber will absorb moisture and probably reach moisture contents of 16 per cent or 18 per cent. This will inevitably lead to expansion. As important, of course, is the likelihood of timber seasoned to low moisture contents absorbing excessive quantities of water if left unprotected after manufacture and before installation.

(c) *Safety line*

The dry rot safety line has been included on C.3.03/8. It is important to note that, irrespective of position, dry rot cannot develop in timber at moisture contents at or below 20 per cent.

(d) *Fibreboards*

Fibreboards, and particularly hardboard, normally require to be moisture conditioned before being fixed in a building. During this process, as in storage generally, they require special methods of handling and storage.

### 3. Control of hygroscopicity

In view of the fact that the hygroscopic nature of wood is responsible for causing variations in moisture content and resultant movements in timber, attempts have been made to eliminate this inherent 'disadvantage'. It has been shown that, although it is not possible to eliminate hygroscopicity completely, it may be permanently reduced by certain treatments. Briefly these are: (a) High temperature treatments, in which care has to be taken to ensure that the timber is not damaged; (b) Boiling and steaming, with boiling more effective than steaming: and (c) Certain chemical means, including methods of impregnation with waxes and synthetic resins. None of these methods, except impregnation which is still being studied, are generally regarded as effective commercial methods for reducing shrinkage or subsequent moisture movements.

In many ways a more practical method of reducing the moisture movement in timber, other than the drying

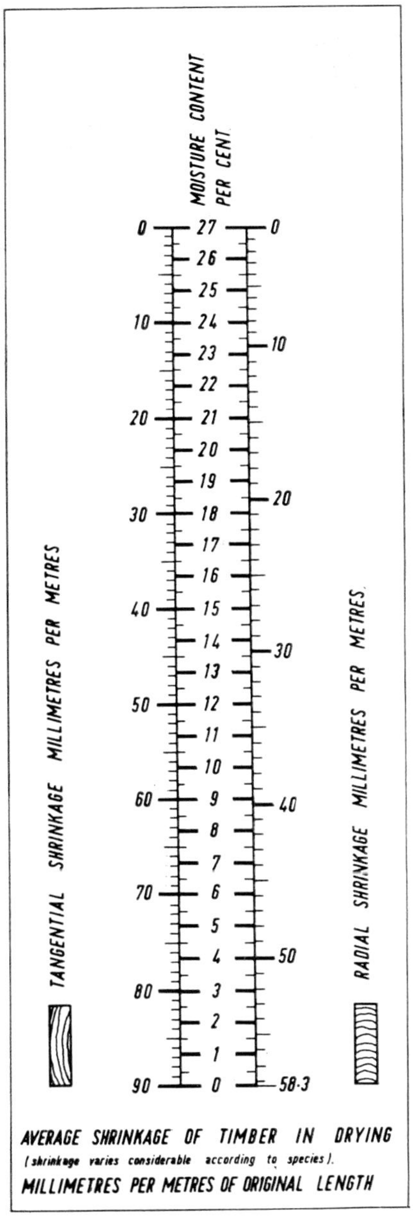


*C.3.03/9*
*Conversion chart giving the shrinkage movement of timbers relative to moisture content. Note: values for different species vary and the chart gives average values only (From: 'Principles of Modern Building', Vol. 1, Fig. 11.2, p. 122, HMSO, 1959)*

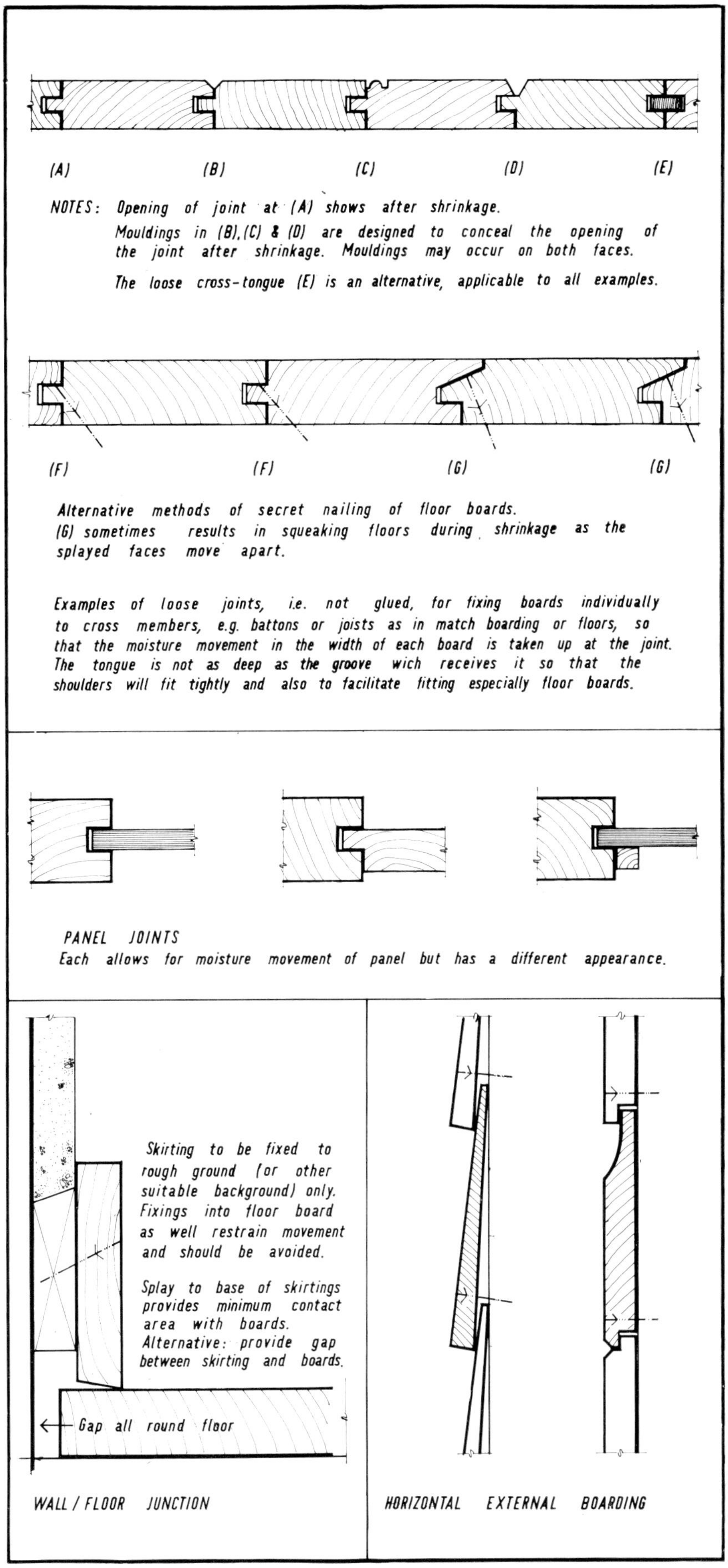


*D.3.03/5*
*Some traditional methods of jointing so as to provide for movements in timber*

F

shrinkage which takes place during seasoning, would be to prevent the wood from absorbing moisture by enveloping the timber with a protective coating. One of the main requirements of such a coating would be to reduce, to negligible amounts, the transmission of water vapour. Tests* carried out on the relative effectiveness of protective coatings against moisture absorption of dry wood exposed to a saturated atmosphere for 17 days have shown that considerable reductions in absorption may be obtained. The coatings used in the tests ranged from a variety of paints and varnishes to metal leaf coatings, including electroplating. The metal leaf coatings provided the greatest degree of protection, while it was shown that the selection of suitable paints and varnishes is important.

The success of coatings of any kind require that the selected coating completely envelopes the timber. In the long term, on the other hand, there should be no breakdown in the vapour resistance of the coating. In a great many building applications it is often difficult, if not impractical at the present time, to ensure that there is no eventual breakdown in the coating. Among other things, a great deal of joinery is actually affixed to other elements, thus at least one face is concealed. The use of protective coatings is thus most useful in reducing the magnitude of moisture movements during the drying out period of a new building. To gain the maximum advantage it is important that all joinery, and particularly that to be affixed to other building elements, should be completely primed soon after manufacture, while concealed faces should be undercoated and topcoated before fixing. Such procedure may not be possible with joinery which is to be left unpainted. However, it is common for unpainted joinery to receive some other form of coating, such as varnish, wax or synthetic resin, in which case application of the coating to concealed faces prior to fixing should be of some advantage.

The provision of some form of protection would seem to be advisable to the concealed faces, particularly those in juxtaposition with materials capable of allowing water transmission—external conditions are significant. In these situations other types (mainly chemical) of protection against decay may in any case be employed, but such protection does not normally limit moisture movement.

### 4. Precautions

The interaction of the many conflicting factors involved in fluctuations in moisture content usually makes it extremely difficult to effect all the desirable precautions in everyday practice. The essential aim should always be to ensure that timber has the moisture content required to maintain equilibrium with its service environment, and that the requisite moisture content is maintained until normal conditions have been established in the building in which it is installed. (See Table 3.03/1.) The precautions which should be taken to minimise the magnitude of changes in moisture content are*:

1. Careful storing after manufacture.
2. Protection during delivery to site.
3. Careful storing on site, before and after fixing, avoiding conditions of exposure which are materially different from those expected in service.
4. Delaying delivery of joinery (or other timber, as relevant) to site until it is needed.
5. Priming of joinery to be painted immediately after manufacture and prior to leaving the joinery works. Such protection will delay, but not prevent, absorption of water by the timber, if it is exposed to damp conditions for a long period of time.
6. All protective coatings must completely envelope all faces of the timber (concealed faces may require additional protection).

## Movement in cement-based products

Unlike timber, cement-based products, which include concretes, both dense and lightweight, cast *in situ* or precast for panels, planks, bricks or blocks, screeds, mortars and renders, are manufactured. The magnitude of their moisture movements is primarily dependent on the quality of the individual constituents (essentially cement, which is the root cause of the movements, aggregates in a variety of shapes and sizes, which basically restrain the movement of the cement, and water, which is basically required for chemical reaction but also for workability) and the quality of control exercised during the *whole* process of manufacture. However, like timber, cement-based products exhibit a wide range of movements, even when strict quality control is exercised in selection and manufacture, because there are significant differences in the properties of the types of cement and aggregate available, which may, among other things, be combined in a variety of proportions in which the quantity of water is also very important.

One of the most important factors related to the moisture movements of cement-based products is the comparatively large initial drying shrinkages which occur. In general, the initial drying shrinkage, most of which is irreversible (see diagram D.3.03/2), is about 50 per cent *greater* than any movement due to wetting and drying of the matured product. Restriction of drying shrinkages (they cannot be entirely prevented) is, therefore, of paramount importance if cracking is to be prevented. However, this does not mean that the reversible movements must be entirely neglected, even if these are more or less constant. Cement-based products rarely attain a stable condition as there will be periodic changes in moisture content of the environment. The periodic moisture movements of those products which are exposed to the weather (see 'Exposure' previously included in this section) must, therefore, be taken into account.

As quality control plays such an important part in the magnitude of the initial drying shrinkage of all products*, it has been considered advisable to deal with this aspect, relative mainly to concrete practice, in detail under the following general headings: (1) Type of cement; (2) Mix proportioning; (3) Type of aggregate; and (4) Curing. All these, in addition to precautions required in placing and compaction, which are excluded here, not only influence movement but are also important in the strength properties of the product. This usually receives particular attention in concrete work, but is equally important in all the other products. Consideration is given, where relevant, to the significance of moisture movement in composite elements such as brick or block walls, in which cement-based products are used as 'adhesives'.

Before dealing with the four individual factors, it is important to note that they are all very closely interrelated. In practice they are all important if drying shrinkage is to be controlled. Again, it should be emphasised that the values of movement quoted under any of the factors have been obtained from comparatively small samples tested under controlled conditions. The latter, of course, rarely obtain in practice. However, this does not detract from the fact that the information can provide a useful guide on the effects of the factors on movement in general. They do illustrate clearly the pattern which can be expected. When related to practical conditions, the laboratory information may be an under-estimation, that is movements may be greater, in many cases and this needs to be taken into account.

### 1. Type of cement

The magnitude of moisture movements quoted are normally for ordinary Portland cement. Shrinkage of different types of Portland cements varies by as much as 50 per cent.

### 2. Mix proportioning

If the type of aggregate (see 3 below) is excluded, then two aspects of mix

*Koehler, A., *The structure, properties and uses of wood*, McGraw-Hill Book Co., New York, 1924, quoted in Desch, H. E., *Timber, Its Structure and Properties*, 4th. Ed., MacMillan, 1968.

*The precautions given here are specifically related to moisture movement in timber. However, it is important to note that, although for different reasons, similar precautions are also necessary to reduce the likelihood of fungal attack in timber as outlined in *Section 3.06*.

*Shrinkage may also be restrained by special reinforcement, as discussed in *2.03 Cracking in buildings*. This aspect is excluded here.

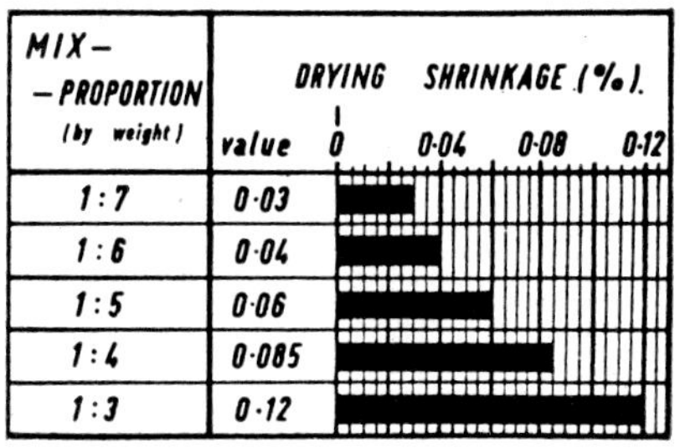


*C.3.03/10*
*Comparative chart of the variation of drying shrinkage with cement content of concrete or mortar. Values are for specimens 127 × 127mm (5 × 5in) section, water/cement ratio 0·5 and after 6 months in air at 21·1°C and 50 per cent R.H. (Abstracted from C.3.08/11)*

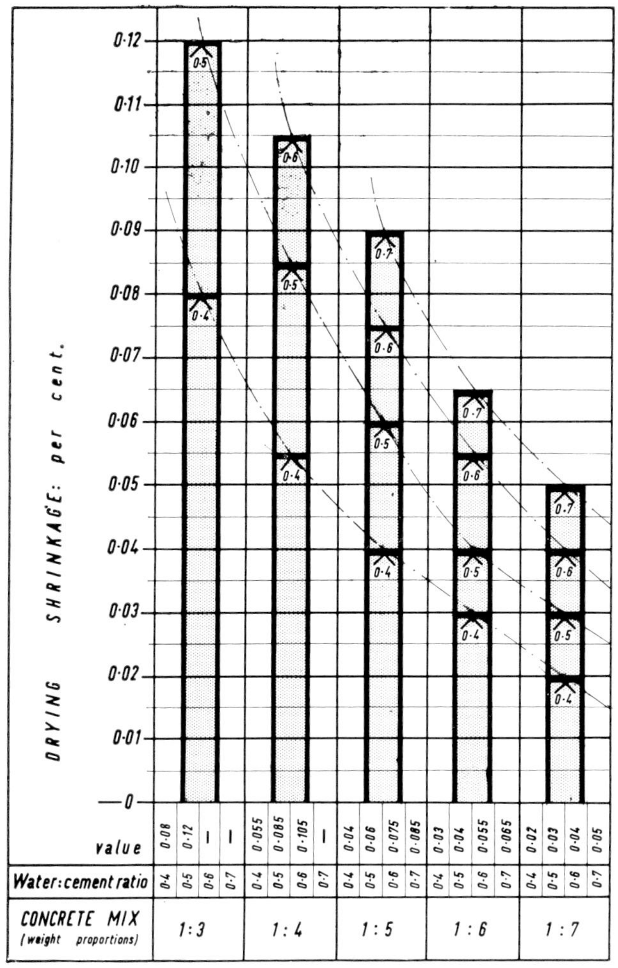


*C.3.03/11*
*Comparative chart of the variation of drying shrinkage with cement/water ratio. Values are for specimens 127 × 127 mm (5 × 5in) section, after 6 months in air at 21·1°C and 50 per cent R.H. (From: Lea, F. M., 'The Chemistry of Cement and Concrete', revised edition of Lea and Desch, Table LIV, p. 253, Arnold, 1956)*

proportioning will influence drying shrinkage. These are:

(a) *Quantity of cement.* In view of the fact that it is the cement which is basically responsible for movement, it follows that the greater the amount of cement used, the greater the movement. The comparative chart C.3.03/10 illustrates the drying shrinkage for five mix proportions and it will be seen that the shrinkage increases significantly as the cement content is increased.

(b) *Quantity of water.* The quantity of to the quantity of cement used in what water used in a mix is usually related is known as the water/cement ratio. Theoretically, only sufficient water which will allow the necessary chemical reaction of the cement to take place should be used. However, for practical purposes, it is necessary to use more water than the theoretical minimum. The effect of the excess water in terms of shrinkage has already been covered under 'Presence of water, 3. Sorbed water, (d) Irreversible movement'. It was stated that the greater the excess water, the greater the shrinkage. The comparative chart C.3.03/11 illustrates the effect on drying shrinkage of different water/cement ratios in concretes of different concrete mixes. It should be noted that this chart includes values of the 0·5 water/cement ratio for all mixes shown in C.3.03/10.

Although it is not intended to discuss the manner in which the correct water/cement ratio is obtained in practice (among other things, allowance has to be made for water contained in the aggregate), it is important to note that additional quantities of water may be introduced during brick or block-laying, if the units are wet prior to use or become wet immediately after use. For this reason it is also advisable to ensure that bricks and blocks are no wetter than is required to avoid excessive absorption of water from the mortar (the same holds true when plaster or render is applied). This means that bricks and blocks must be protected from wet weather at all times.

### 3. Types of aggregate

In general, the aggregate acts as a restraint to the shrinkage of the cement. Grading and shape may have an indirect effect on the magnitude of shrinkage due to the quantity of cement and water/cement ratio. However, some aggregates may themselves have significant drying shrinkages which will increase the shrinkage due to the cement, while all aggregates do not provide the same degree of restraint. There are notable differences in behaviour between (a) dense aggregates and (b) lightweight aggregates. It is convenient to deal with these separately.

(a) *Dense aggregates.* Rigid dense aggregates, such as crushed rock and gravels, do not expand or shrink on wetting and drying and, therefore, are able to restrain the shrinkage of cement significantly. On the other hand, some natural aggregates, such as dolerite, exhibit appreciable changes on wetting and drying, which may lead to shrinkage of concrete made with them being, in the extreme, nearly four times that normally encountered with non-shrinkable aggregates. The comparative chart C.3.03/12 compares the shrinkage of three different rocks and two different types of concrete made with them.

(b) *Lightweight aggregates.* There are a variety of aggregates available for use in lightweight concrete—aerated concrete employs fine aggregate with lightness created by the formation of minute voids or cells during manufacture and are, therefore, usually treated separately. Accordingly, a wide range of properties are obtainable. However, all the aggregates do, in varying degrees, expand and shrink on wetting and drying or provide less restraint

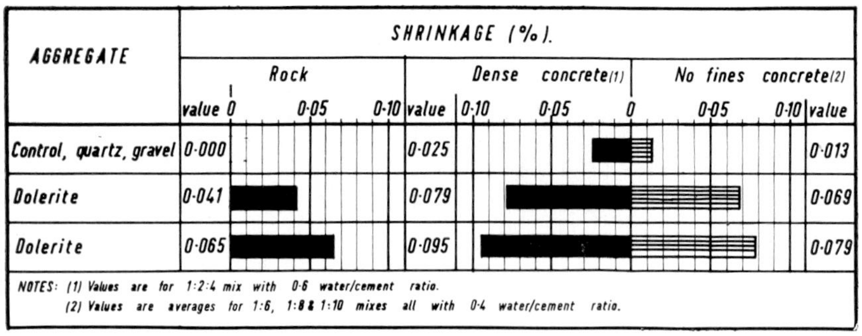


C.3.03/12
*Comparative chart of shrinkage of natural aggregate in concrete (From: 'Shrinkage of Natural Aggregates in Concrete', BRS Digest (2nd Series), No. 35, Table 2, p. 4, June 1963)*

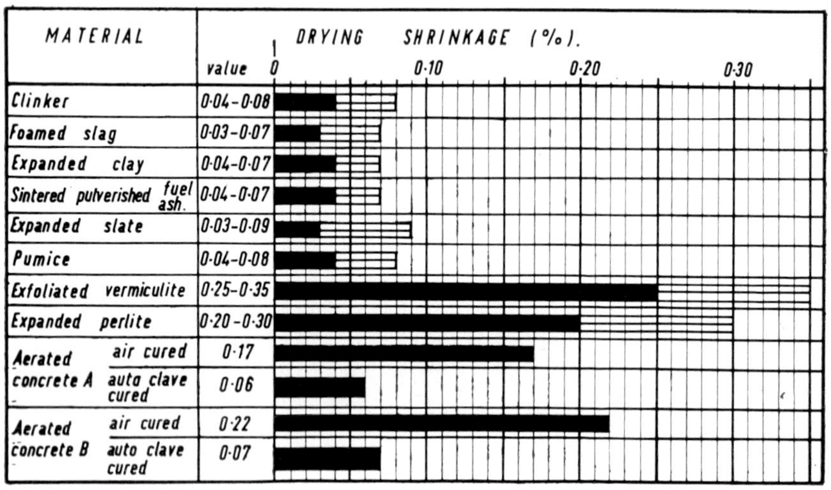


C.3.03/13
*Comparative chart of the drying shrinkage of concretes made with lightweight aggregates. [References: (1) Clinker to expanded perlite: 'Lightweight Concrete Aggregates—Materials and Properties', BRS Digest (2nd Series) No. 25, Table 1, p. 3, Aug. 1962. (2) Aerated concrete: 'Aerated Concrete—1: Manufacture and Properties', BRS Digest (2nd Series) No. 16, Table 2, p. 2, Nov. 1961]*

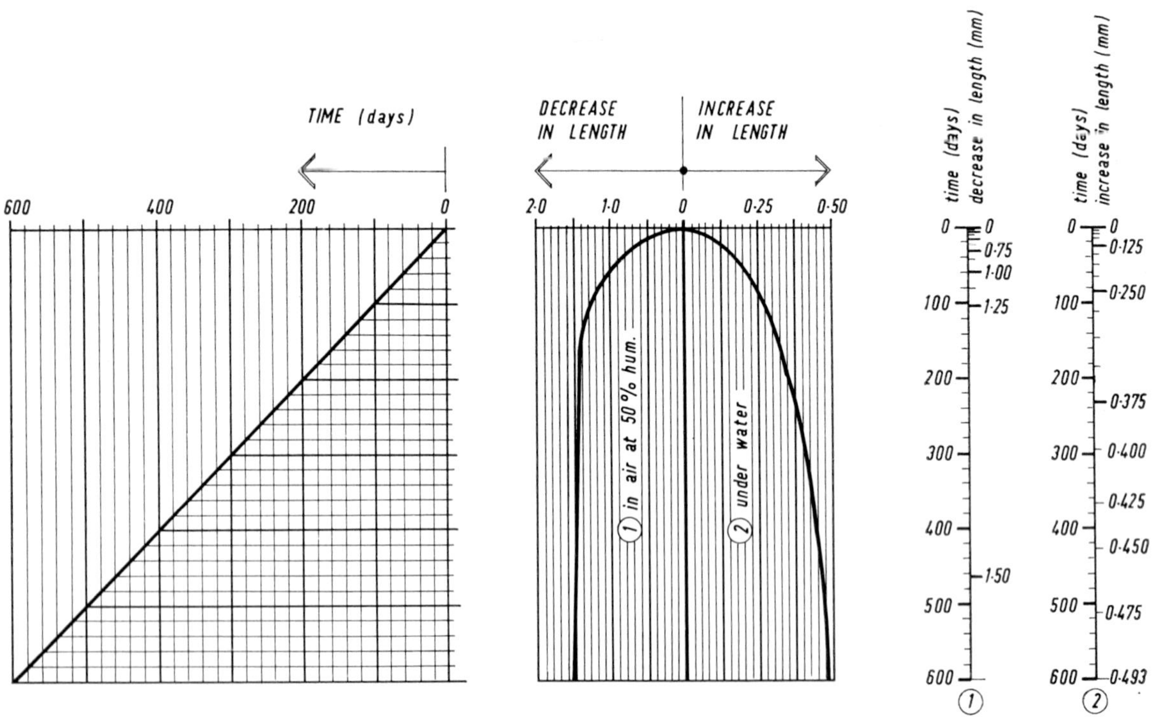


C.3.03/14
*Comparative graph of changes in length of 1:5 crushed granite concrete, 76·2 × 76·2mm (3 × 3in) sections, under different conditions of curing, (1) Dried in air at 50 per cent R.H. and (2) under water (From: Lea, F. M., 'The Chemistry of Cement and Concrete', rev. ed. of Lea and Desch, based on graphs on Fig. 109, p. 352, Arnold, 1956)*

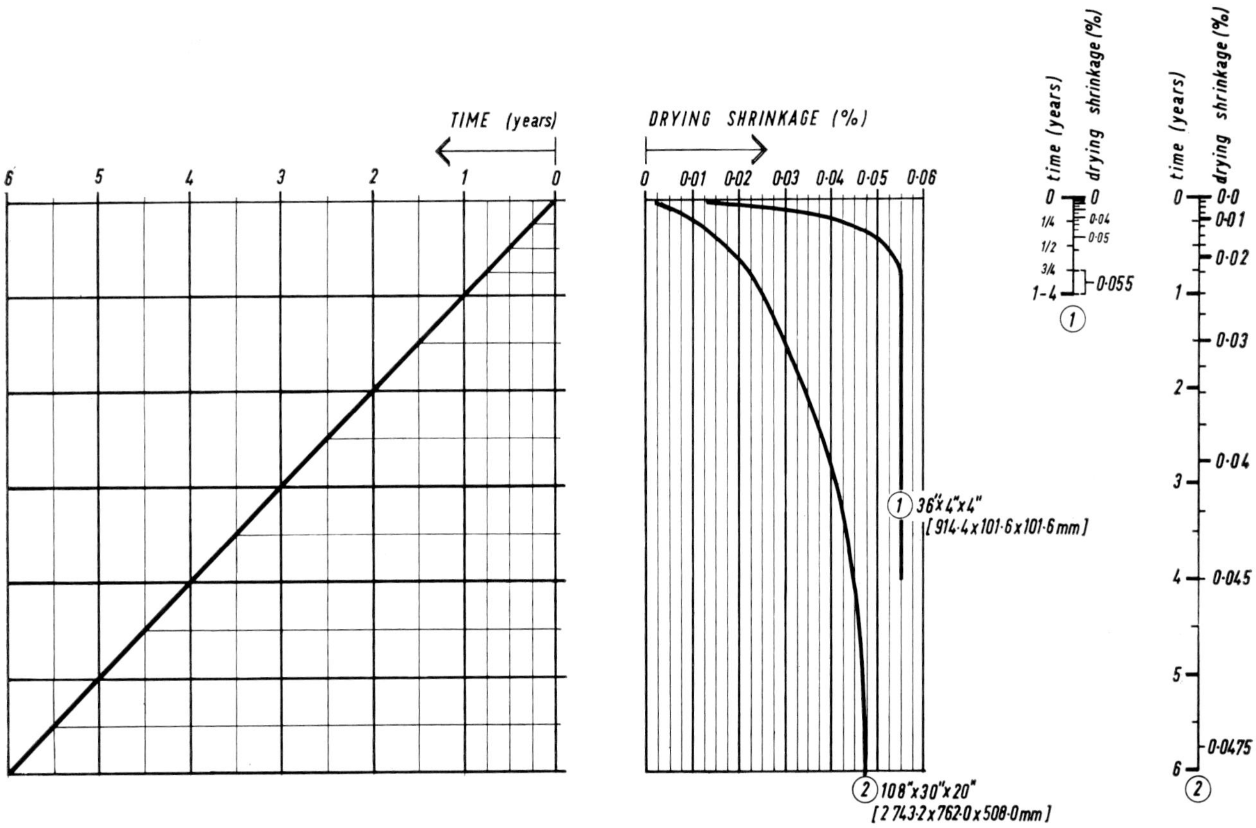


*C.3.03/15*
*Comparative graph of the effect of size on drying shrinkage. 1:2:4 concrete specimens exposed to air at 17·8°C and 65 per cent R.H. (From: Lea, F. M., 'The Chemistry of Cement and Concrete', rev. ed. of Lea and Desch, Fig. 110, p. 353, Arnold, 1956)*

than aggregates for dense concrete. In addition, the porous aggregates used absorb water during the mixing process and thus high water/cement ratios are required to obtain workable mixes. Consequently, not only are their drying shrinkages generally greater than dense concrete, but also their subsequent reversible movement. It is for this reason that particular attention must be given to control of movement, both during manufacture and use. As regards the latter, protection from the weather so as to avoid excessive wetting is again important.

The magnitude of the drying shrinkage of concretes made with lightweight aggregates is illustrated in the comparative chart C.3.03/13. Also included are some aerated concretes.

**4. Curing**

The *conditions* under which concrete is cured will affect the magnitude of shrinkage. When drying takes place in air there is a progressive *increase* in shrinkage as the relative humidity of the air is *decreased*. Drying in an oven at 10°–38°C produces even greater shrinkage. However, if the concrete is cured *under* water, then an expansion takes place. The comparative graph C.3.03/14 illustrates the changes in length, over a period of time, of concrete specimens, 76·2mm by 76·2mm in section, dried in air and under water. For air drying the relative humidity was 50 per cent. In addition to conditions, the *time* during which curing takes place also influences the magnitude of shrinkage, both initially and in the long term.

The importance of *size* relative to the magnitude of drying shrinkage and the period over which this takes place is illustrated in the comparative graph C.3.03/15. It will be seen that, not only is the magnitude of movement greater with the smaller section, but also the movement takes place far more rapidly.

With reference to the comparative chart C.3.03/11 some further points regarding the effects of both conditions during the time of curing and size may be noted. The sections of concrete used were 127mm by 127mm, dried for six months at 21·1°C and 50 per cent R.H. If the R.H. had been between 65 and 70 per cent, the values would have been *decreased* by about two-thirds; on the other hand, they would have *increased* by about one-third if the exposure had been prolonged with no change in the humidity. For a smaller cross section the *maximum* value would be obtained in six months.

The excessive drying shrinkages which occur with air-cured aerated concrete can be overcome in precast units by steam-curing or autoclaving, as will be seen in the comparative chart C.3.03/13. In addition, significant reductions in subsequent expansion is also effected.

Finally, it is necessary to draw a distinction between precast and cast *in situ* concrete, in terms of practical application. If damage to the structure of a building is to be reduced when precast units are built-in, then it is essential that the units are completely cured before use. This means that no irreversible movement should take place after the units have been positioned. Some further drying out and related movement may, of course, still take place and this should be treated as reversible movement.

**Main reference:**
Lea, F. M., *The Chemistry of Cement and Concrete*, rev. ed., of Lea and Desch, Arnold, 1956.

## Precautions in use

In practical terms it is usually more important to ensure that precautions are taken to reduce the risk of cracking due to moisture movement. At the outset it must be realised that it is not normally possible in building practice to ensure that no cracking takes place at all. For this reason, it is often argued that it is not necessary to take all possible precautions (they all add to the cost of building) and that such cracks as may occur can be filled or made good as necessary. On the reverse side, of course, it can be argued that filling and making good may not always be successful and the trouble

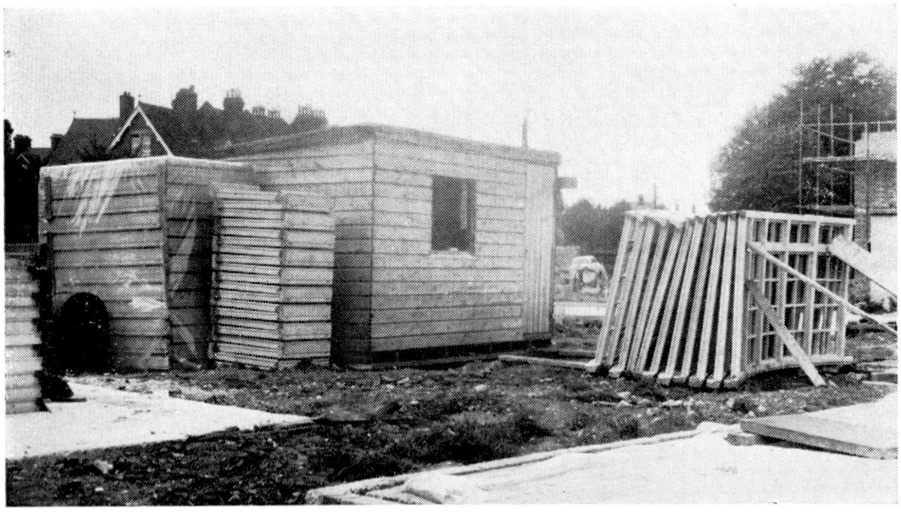

*Timber window frames stored in the open although an attempt has been made to protect some of them. Note that all ends of frames have not been primed. Below, storage of lightweight concrete blocks in a position which encourages high moisture contents with little or no possibility of drying out*

*An attempt to store precast concrete members so as to allow ventilation. The attempt has not been carried through properly while the protection used is only a 'token'*

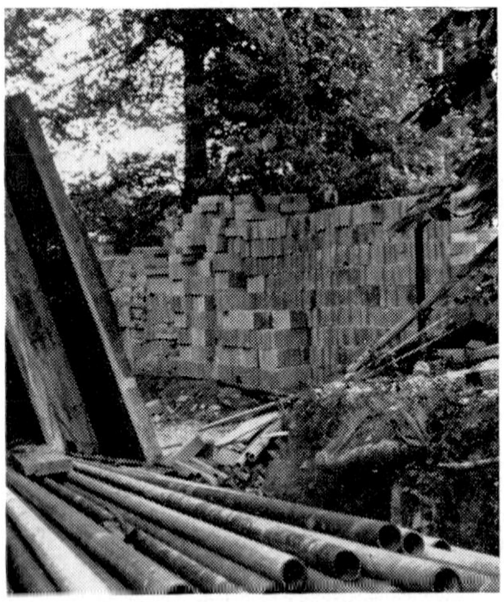

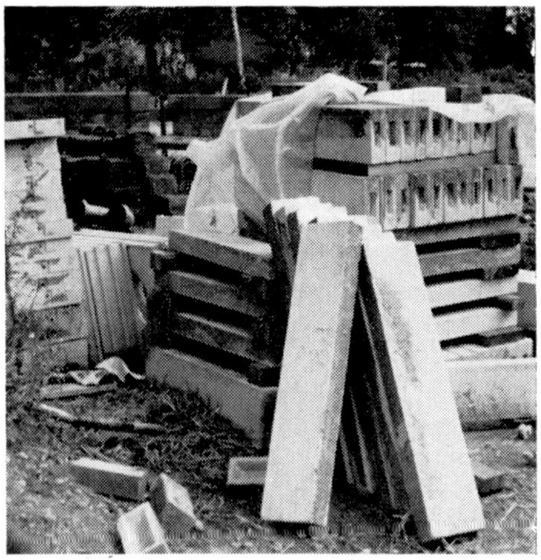

*Below, in addition to the lack of any form of protection to the bricks or timber frames which are fully exposed to the weather, the bricks are stacked, mostly untidily, directly on the ground*

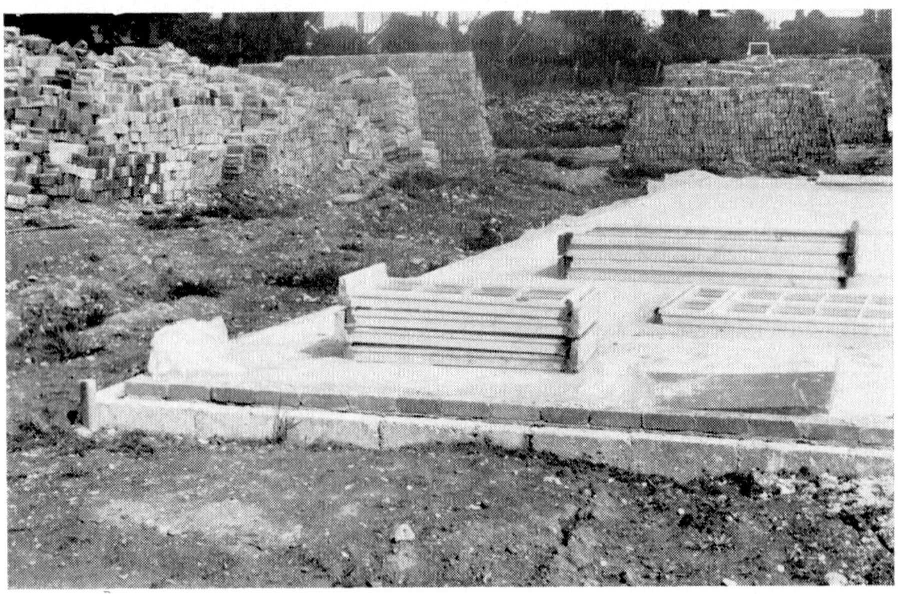

*Amongst the most obvious precautions which could be taken on a building site (or at the works for that matter) to avoid materials attaining excessively high moisture contents before, during or after use in construction is to protect them from undue exposure during wet weather. The unreliability of weather conditions in this country almost points to the advisability of affording some form of protection at all times. Protection may, of course, be desirable during hot weather in order to control the drying-out of cement-based products and thus reduce the possibility of shrinkage cracking.*
*For a number of different reasons there seems to be a general reluctance to adopt even the most elementary forms of weather protection, particularly while materials are being stored on sites. Storage is usually in the open air and in addition to lack of weather protection, materials such as bricks and blocks, for example, are seldom stacked so that drying out may proceed rapidly during good weather. Provision for through ventilation would greatly assist.*
*The group of photographs on this page illustrates some of the less desirable methods often used for storing materials on sites during wet weather.*
*With the advent of polythene and other waterproof sheets, now obtainable in specially strengthened varieties, there are greater opportunities for providing shelter not only for materials but also for the site operatives.*
*The second group of photographs on the next two pages illustrates some of the methods, and in a sense the trends, of affording protection from wet weather. In many cases protection from cold weather is also intended. Also illustrated are some of the methods, sometimes elaborate, which may be used under factory conditions for curing concrete*

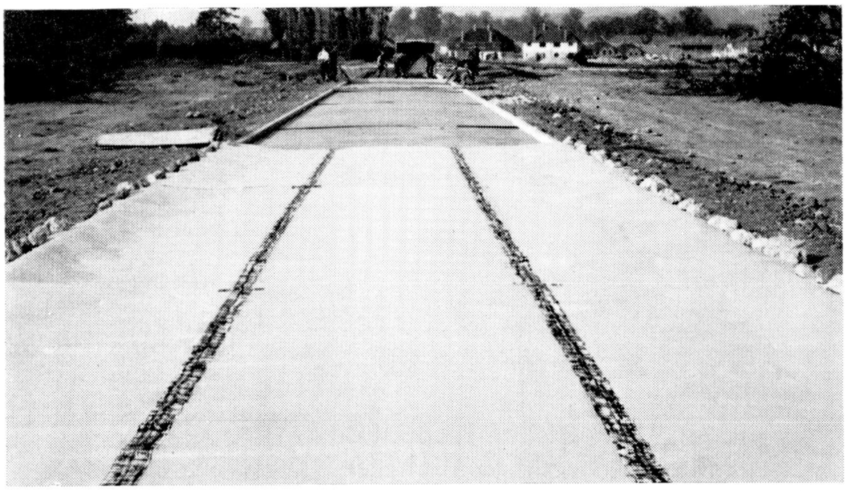

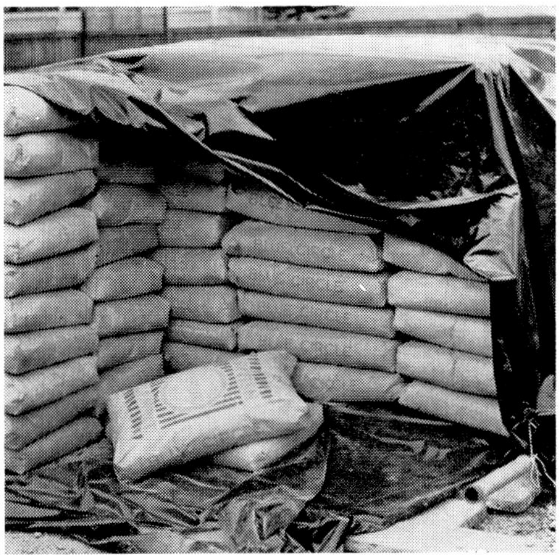

*'Sisalkraft' prefabricated concrete cooling blankets being used to control the drying out of a concrete road (Courtesy: Cement and Concrete Assn.)*

*Bags of cement covered with heavyweight black polythene sheeting which has also been laid underneath to prevent hardening of the bottom layer. Below, cast in situ concrete beams and columns 'bandaged' with lightweight polythene sheeting to control drying out and to keep the members clean (Courtesy: British Visqueen Ltd.)*

*Below, polythene sheeting used to completely protect a stack of bricks. The bottom picture shows the protection of timber frames with polythene sheeting. Although not clear in this photograph the sheeting is carried under the frames so that they are not in contact with the soil—an extremely important point (Courtesy: British Visqueen Ltd.)*

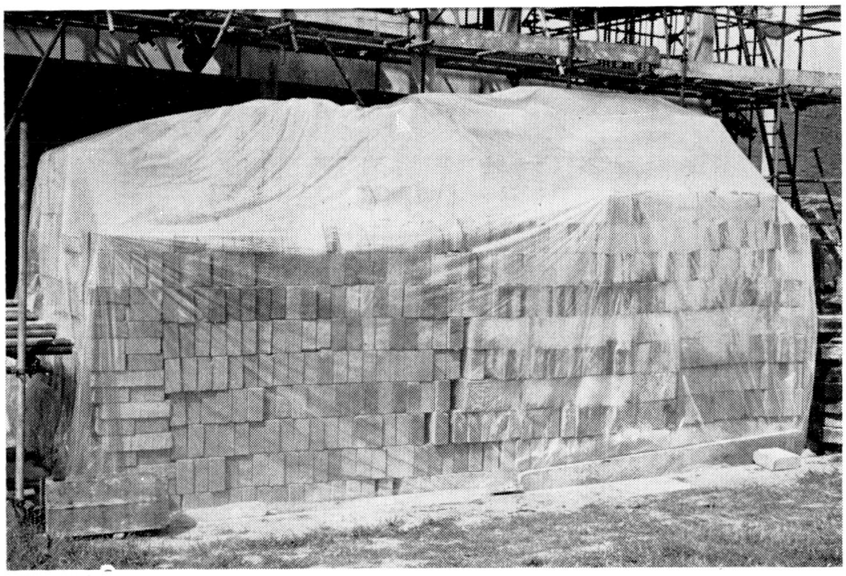

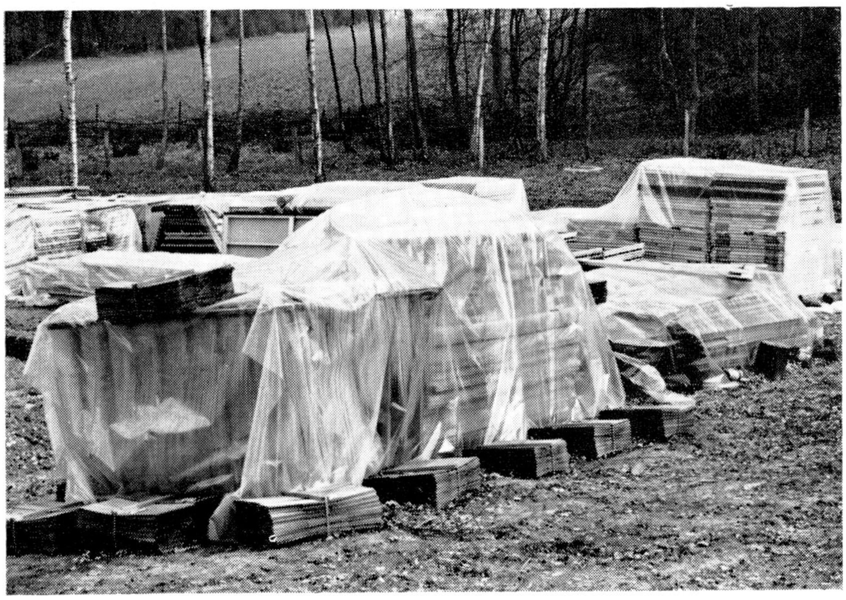

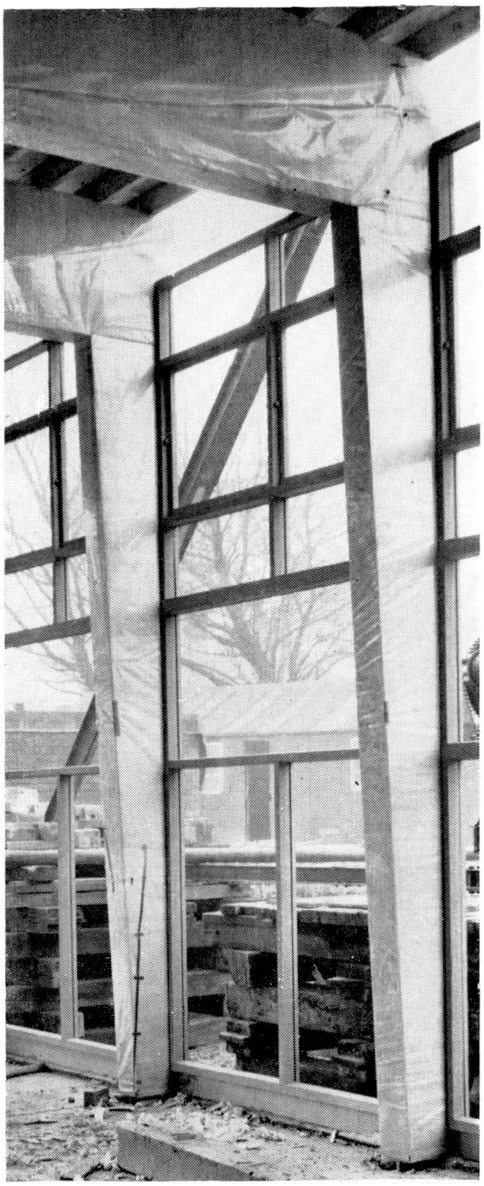

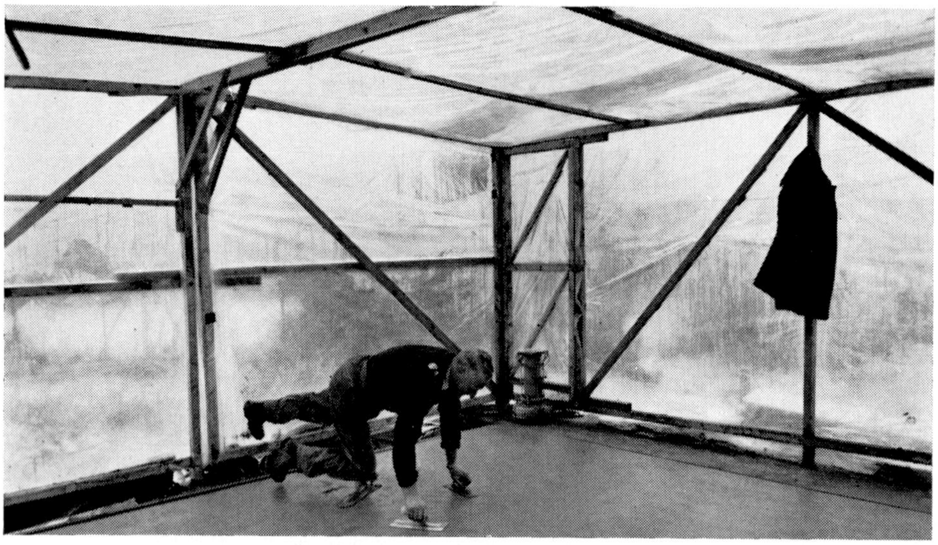

Below, a highly sophisticated example of providing weather protection during construction. Flats in Coventry being built by the 'Jackblock' system. Work, which continued unhampered even by snow and ice, was carried out within a four-storey heated polythene tent, while successive floors built at ground level were jacked up. Architect: Arthur Ling, Coventry city architect and planning officer. Contractors: Richard Costain (Construction) Ltd. Engineer: Felix Adler (Courtesy: Cement and Concrete Assn.)

Portable timber shelter clad with heavyweight olythene sheeting affording protection to the site operative and to the granolithic floor finish he is laying (Courtesy: British Visqueen Ltd.) Below, steam curing concrete in a factory (Courtesy: C & CA)

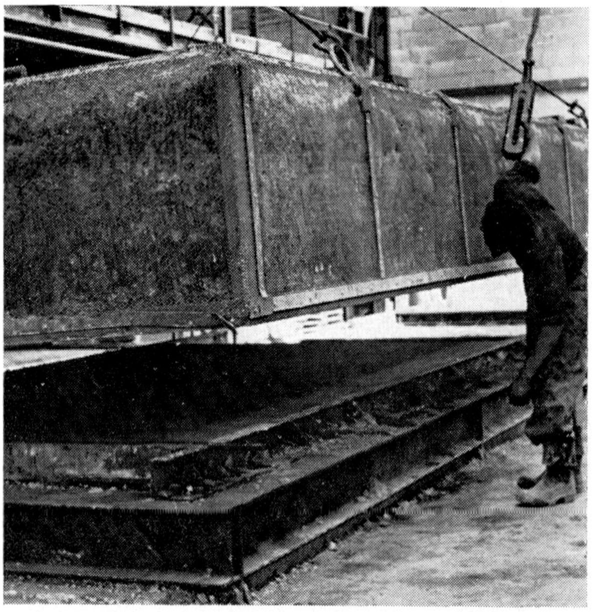

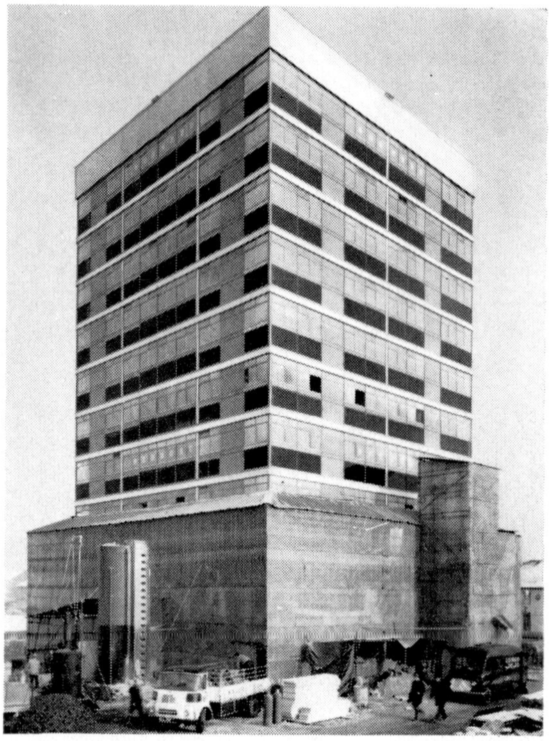

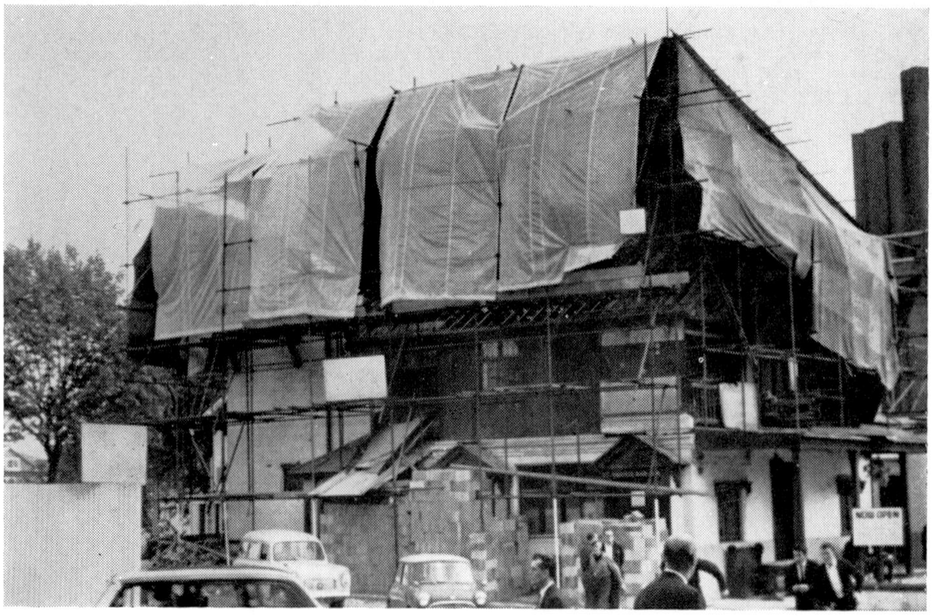

Left, reinforced polythene sheeting (front) being used with 'traditional' canvas sheeting (sides) for weather protection while alterations are proceeding in an existing building

**Table 3.03/2**
**Precautions to reduce the likelihood of shrinkage cracking with various materials due to changes in moisture content**

| *Material* | *Magnitude of Moisture Movement* | *Precautions in Use* |
|---|---|---|
| Well-fired clay bricks, blocks and terra-cotta | Very small | 1. Preferably do not lay fresh from kiln—should be either wetted or exposed to the air for a week or two before use.<br>2.* Avoid excessive wetting prior to laying or rendering so as to reduce large drying shrinkage of mortar and render. Protect from the weather.<br>3.* Do not use strong mortars unless absolutely essential |
| Concrete bricks | Appreciable | 1. Discrimination in choice of bricks.<br>2. INSIST on fully matured units prior to laying—first drying shrinkage must occur before erection.<br>3. Protect from wet weather during storage and progress of the work.<br>4. Do not use strong mortars |
| Sand-lime bricks | Appreciable; may vary with different types of brick | 1. Discrimination in choice of bricks.<br>2. Protect from wet weather during storage and progress of the work.<br>3. Do not use strong mortars |
| Limestones | Generally very small | None called for |
| Sandstones | Appreciable; may vary with different types of stone | 1. Discrimination in choice of stone.<br>2. Do not use a very strong mortar.<br>3. Protect work in progress in very wet weather.<br>4.* Special drying shrinkage precautions may be required with some types used as aggregate in concrete work |
| Cast stone and dense concrete products | Appreciable | 1. INSIST on fully matured precast units—for cast stone provide details to manufacturer in ample time.<br>2. Do not use very strong mortar.<br>3. Protect work in progress during very wet weather |
| Rubble masonry and flint work | Very small for the rocks but, because volume of mortar in a wall is great, shrinkage of mortar is important | 1. Do not use very strong mortar.<br>2. Protect work in progress during very wet weather |
| Lightweight concrete blocks | Moderate, varying with composition and mix —with aerated concrete* method of curing is important | 1. Ensure that material complies with BSS 2028 (Type B for external walls; Type C for internal walls).<br>2. Do not use very strong mortar.<br>3. Do not allow blocks to become wet before, during or after laying.<br>4. Allow to dry before plastering |
| Wood-wool slabs | Considerable, but readily restrained | 1. Avoid use in external panels, except in short-life buildings or* if protected by impervious lining.<br>2. For internal partitions ensure that shrinkage is restrained by suitable joint treatment.<br>3.* Protect from wet before use in dry construction.<br>4.* Allow to dry before plastering, particularly when used as permanent shuttering |
| Most building boards, plywood | Considerable, but readily restrained | 1.* Complete sealing of *all* surfaces (include edges) may permit external use, otherwise confined to internal use, humidity conditions permitting.<br>2. Fix at all edges.<br>3.* Condition boards to environment before fixing, particularly hardboard |
| Plaster blocks and slabs | Small | 1. Use internally only, unless specially protected.<br>2. Build dry and keep dry |
| Plastics | Very small | None called for |
| Timber* | Considerable | 1. Ensure correct moisture content for environment, and maintain at all times.<br>2. Allow movement joints.<br>3. Do not rely entirely on restraint to control movement |

Reference: Table has been based on Table 13.5, *Principles of Modern Building*, Vol. 1, 3rd Ed., p. 196, HMSO, 1959. * denotes a material alteration or addition to the reference.

Note: The precautions suggested are general in nature and are mainly for reversible movements (see text).

may become perennial, particularly if the failure is due to reversible movement. Furthermore, there is always the inconvenience and expense of having to return to a job to make good the defects. This alone may outweigh the initial cost of the necessary precautions. These are opinions and each case must be treated on its merits. There is, unfortunately, no panacea.

If the risk of cracking due to moisture movements is to be reduced, then the precautions given below, which are essentially related to reversible movements, should be taken. These do not cover all materials, and so Table 3.03/2 sets out, by way of a summary, precautions in use for a number of materials. This table, it must be stressed, is of a *general* nature. The precautions suggested are, mortars apart, mainly related to reversible movements and do not advise when, for example, expansion joints should be incorporated or additional restraint provided. These aspects must be related to specific problems. Similarly, there is no guidance given on drying shrinkage of cement-based products, particularly those cast *in situ* or manufactured and used on site, as so much depends on control of quality.

1. Where precast concrete products are used they should meet the relevant requirements of BS, as these include limits for drying shrinkage and so serve as a valuable safeguard.

2. All precast concrete products should be well matured before use ; in general, they should not be use for at least one month after being made.

3. Keep materials under cover, particularly in wet weather. Wet winter weather, it should be remembered, makes it difficult for products to be properly dried out. Protection from wet should be maintained both during storage of materials on site, that is prior to being built-in, and during the progress of the work.

4. Allow all backings and undercoats to dry and shrink before finishes are applied.

5. Strong mixes (1 : 3, cement : sand) for mortars, plaster undercoats or renders should be avoided. Sand should be clean.

6. Reduce warping of structural timber in floors, roofs, etc. by using adequate binders and struts.

7. Where practical, timber units should be conditioned approximately to the moisture content they will attain in normal use and should be maintained at that content before, during and after fixing. Condition fibreboards, particularly hardboard, before fixing.

8. Conceal cracks by use of cover moulds or specially designed joints.

9. Where practicable, provide movement joints.

10. Materials with large moisture movements should be avoided for external use where seasonal changes in moisture content are likely to be severe. Similar precautions may also be necessary internally where there are likely to be fluctuations in relative humidity, as, for example, in kitchens, bathrooms, some industrial processes.

11. Ensure that impervious protective coatings used to reduce moisture content changes *completely* envelop the element or material concerned—and that these are applied *prior* to fixing.

12. Avoid the use of excessive heat to ensure a rapid dry-out. This includes the running of central heating plant to capacity before occupation. In a rush-job selection of non-shrinking materials would be desirable.

# 3.04 exclusion

It is not normal in building practice to expect that all materials used will, or can, be maintained in a state of complete dryness, that is containing no moisture at all, at any time but particularly during the life of a building. Porous materials may, in terms of quantity, have significant moisture content values under normal environmental conditions in buildings (see *Section 3.01*, 'Dampness'). Materials used externally, on the other hand, may, particularly in the British Isles, be exposed to long periods of wet weather and thus, porous materials, may, at times, be completely saturated.

Water introduced during construction, including absorption of rainwater (see *Section 3.02*, '3. During construction', p. 43), accounts for high initial moisture contents in porous materials, but this water generally evaporates in a comparatively short period until the materials reach their normal dry state for the prevailing external and internal environmental conditions (see *Section 3.03*, p. 66). There may be, as will be seen later in this section under 'Entrapped Water', some very important exceptions to this general rule, when construction water is prevented from evaporating freely and so becomes entrapped within the construction often, and this is important, for excessively long periods of time.

*Exclusion of water* is, therefore, primarily concerned with what may best be termed *precautions* which should be taken during the construction of a building, including by implication initial choice, design and application of materials (referred to in this section as 'design and construction'), which will ensure that materials will be maintained in a requisite state of dryness during the life of a building. Looked at in another way, this means ensuring the exclusion, for a predetermined time, of that portion of water which is likely to cause dampness sufficient to lead to deleterious effects on the properties of materials. In this respect, present-day functional requirements of buildings necessitates the inclusion of thermal properties as well. In addition to the effects of water, held within or on the surfaces of either materials or constructions, on the properties of materials, consideration must also be given to the exclusion of that portion of water which is likely to have ill-effects on the occupants of buildings. Thus it may be essential, in particular circumstances, to restrict the retention of certain quantities of water within or on the surface of materials or constructions, not because such quantities are likely to lead to deleterious effects on properties of the materials concerned, but because of the probable ill-effects of the water involved on the health of the occupants. It is perhaps axiomatic that exclusion of water in the liquid state also implies that water is not allowed to penetrate the complete thickness of a construction, whatever the nature of the materials used. In certain cases, however, the arrangement of layers of materials of different vapour transmissions may require the inclusion of special internal drainage systems to allow condensed vapour to escape harmlessly. (See *4.00 Heat and its effects*.)

Although exclusion of water is primarily concerned with precautions to be taken during design and construction so that materials used in a building may be maintained in a dry condition during its life, this should not detract from the fact that it is equally important that precautions should be taken to ensure that materials dry out as quickly as possible after construction of part or the whole of a building.* The rate at which drying out may be allowed to proceed, environmental conditions apart, will be dependent on the structure and general characteristics of materials and their moisture contents prior to drying out. The problem is related essentially to porous materials and particularly to the restriction of shrinkage cracking as outlined previously in *Section 3.03*. It may be noted that surface dryness of impervious materials may be important in certain cases as, for example, when finishes, such as paint, have to be applied.

In this section the main emphasis is placed on the precautions which are necessary during design and construction for the exclusion of water during the life of a building from the building fabric. The chief sources of water taken into account are: rain, ground and atmosphere. The one important exception to this concerns the special problems now associated with both constructional water and water formed as a result of interstitial condensation in flat roof constructions. In order to understand the problems involved and thus the precautions which may be necessary in particular circumstances it is essential to examine the general function and behaviour of both porous and non-porous materials. At the same time the problems involved are closely interrelated with factors previously outlined under *3.01 General considerations* (particularly 'Flow'), *3.02 Exposure* and *3.03 Moisture content*.

With rain, ground and atmosphere taken as the chief sources of water which must be excluded from the building fabric, the elements of a building which are more commonly involved are: (1) The building envelope, that is external elements such as walls above ground and roofs. These are associated with exposure to rainwater and vapour in the atmosphere, particularly that within heated buildings during winter. (2) Walls and floors in contact with or near the ground, which are exposed to groundwater. All the elements, that is both (1) and (2) could form the basis for examination. However, in practice, exclusion of water can, perhaps better does, require, sometimes only in localised zones, the use of a combination of materials* with differing properties

*Drying out of part of a building while other parts are still under construction may be necessary, if not essential, in order to allow following trades to be progressed.

*The use of a number of materials to form a composite element of a building may arise initially from other functional requirements. Nevertheless, in situations such as these the presise positioning of the various 'layers' of material, including cavities, may, in the final analysis, be strongly influenced by factors associated with the exclusion of water.

relative to the transmission of water. At the same time there is the extremely important, albeit complex, problem of joint design, which, in addition to exclusion of water, must take movement into account. For these reasons, and perhaps particularly because the building fabric is usually made up of a variety of different materials or elements, it is more convenient to divide this section into different headings, each of which deals with a specific aspect(s) of the whole problem. Thus, with the exception of 'Entrapped Water', the aspects covered in the individual headings are, for the most part, closely interrelated. Furthermore, it is necessary to include, in far greater detail than is the general intention of this study, properties and techniques of the use of materials such as damp-proof courses, membranes, flashings, water vapour barriers and mastics.

For convenience, the following general headings are used:

(1) *Permeability of materials*. The degree to which materials are permeable (some are, of course, completely impermeable) to water in both liquid and vapour states is fundamental in any study of the exclusion of water. Under this heading the significance of permeability, including what may best be termed partial penetration of water, is discussed.

(2) *External walls*. The general problems of the exposure of external walls above damp-proof level to rainwater are outlined. Specific problems and detailed examination of joints and junctions are excluded.

(3) *Roofs*. The general problem of both sloping and flat roofs are considered relative to rainwater exposure. An examination of the jointing problems between the units commonly used, particularly in sloping roofs, is included. However, detailed examination of the problems of junctions between roof and other elements such as parapets, chimneys, etc., is excluded.

(4) *Damp-proof courses and membranes*. This heading includes the materials and the principal techniques used in walls and floors below or near the ground, and also in the special junction problems at (a) openings in walls, (b) walls and roofs, and (c) roofs and other projecting elements such as chimneys, etc., which may also necessitate the use of flashings.

(5) *Water vapour barriers*. The need for water vapour barriers arises from problems associated with condensation. The mechanics of condensation are covered in *4.00 Heat and its effects*. Thus materials only generally used are included here.

(6) *Joint Design*. Under this heading a detailed examination of joint design relative to walling units is included, together with a consideration of the general properties and uses of mastics.

(7) *Entrapped Water*. As previously mentioned, problems of entrapped water are chiefly associated with flat roofs which arise either from constructional water or the formation of interstitial condensation or, as is often the case, from both sources. The problems involved and possible solutions are covered in detail.

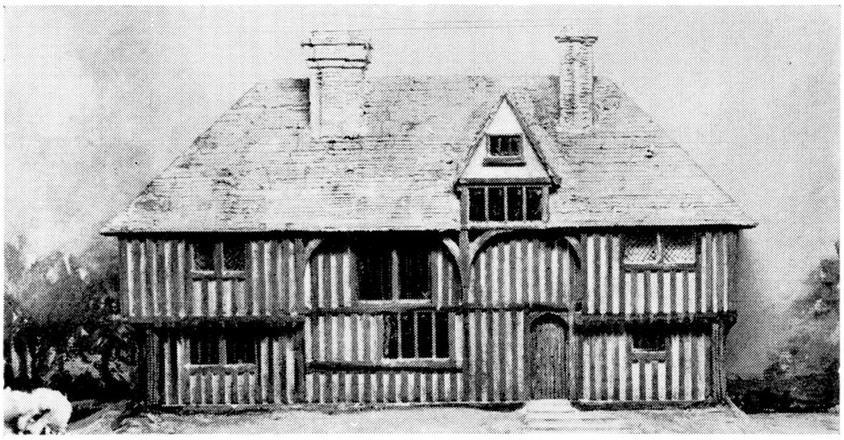

*The photograph shows an example of wattlework in medieval construction in which the infill panels were composed of porous materials. In present-day terms infill panels may be composed of either impermeable or permeable materials (Courtesy: Radio Times Hulton Picture Library)*

## Permeability of materials

In some ways it is a little misleading to analyse the function and behaviour of materials according to their degree of permeability or their degree of imperviousness because, in the final analysis, water penetration must be related to complete structures. This means that methods of jointing, together with the effectiveness of the joint, are also important. However, if the relevance of permeability of a complete construction is accepted at the outset, then it is possible to examine the significance of permeability under interrelated headings. In this part the following general headings are used: (1) Background, (2) Complete impermeability, (3) Lateral and downward penetration, (4) Wetting and drying cycle, and (5) Thin applied coatings.

### 1. Background

There are a number of different reasons why, even in present-day buildings, materials which are completely impermeable to water, in both liquid and vapour state, have not been used as the chief barrier to water, and particularly rainwater in the building envelope. Among other things, most of the available impermeable materials are thin, require support and the inclusion of other materials to make up a composite element which will also meet, for example, thermal, acoustic or fire requirements. It is, in building practice, extremely difficult, if not impractical, to provide the building envelope with a continuous impervious 'raincoat', even though this would seem to be the most logical solution to the problems of excluding rainwater.

Historically the development of the whole fabric of buildings has, in general, been based primarily on the structural use of essentially porous and on the whole permeable materials, with the available impermeable materials reserved for special conditions within the structure, for windows (often small in size anyway) or, to a limited extent, for roofs. Even in timber-framed buildings (in some ways the fore-runners of many contemporary steel or reinforced concrete framed buildings, prefabricated or otherwise) the infill panels were also composed of porous materials (wattlework in medieval construction, for example).

The importance of historic example is that it has not only produced a tradition, but has also shown that it is not necessarily essential for completely impervious materials to be used when dealing with problems of water exclusion. On the other hand, it has also shown what limitations must be imposed when permeable materials are considered for use. In contrast to this, the more recent increased use of impermeable materials on the external surfaces of the building envelope has shown that, jointing problems apart, these materials also have certain limitations which require consideration, among other things of drainage, particularly when there is a risk of the formation of interstitial condensation.

### 2. Complete impermeability

The combined effect of both types of experience (historical and contemporary) has demonstrated fairly conclusively that permeability of materials must be considered in its widest context. Thus, it must include its traditional meaning of the ability of a material to allow the passage of *liquid water* right through it (see *Section 3.03*. 'General Influences, 4. Permeability', p. 70) and the ability of a material to allow the passage of *water vapour* through it. The latter, which is derived from thermal considerations (see *4.00*

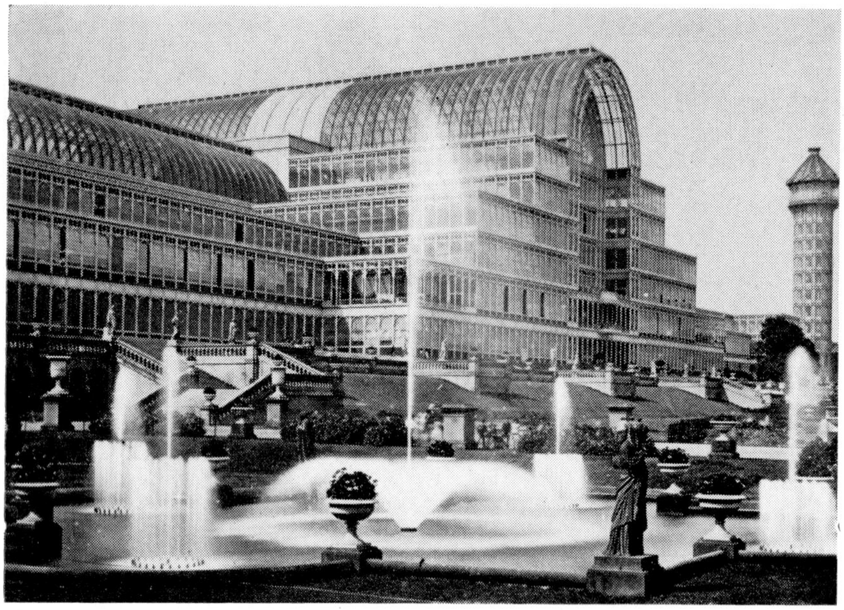

*'It is, in building practice, extremely difficult, if not impractical, to provide the building envelope with a continuous impervious "raincoat", even though this would seem to be the most logical solution to the problems of excluding rainwater.' Various attempts have, however, been made to apply the raincoat principle. Initially this meant the use of impermeable materials in comparatively small units and incorporating joints. The Crystal Palace 1851 Exhibition Building (top picture) was an early example of the complete use of impermeable materials (glass in a cast-iron frame) on a large scale (Courtesy: Radio Times Hulton Picture Library). With the development of plastics attempts have been made to reduce the number of joints in the envelope. The reinforced plastics vehicle washing tunnel by Mickleover Transport Ltd. (bottom picture) shows the structural use of plastics where not only are the number of joints reduced but where there is no intermediate frame for jointing (Courtesy: Mickleover Transport Ltd.)*

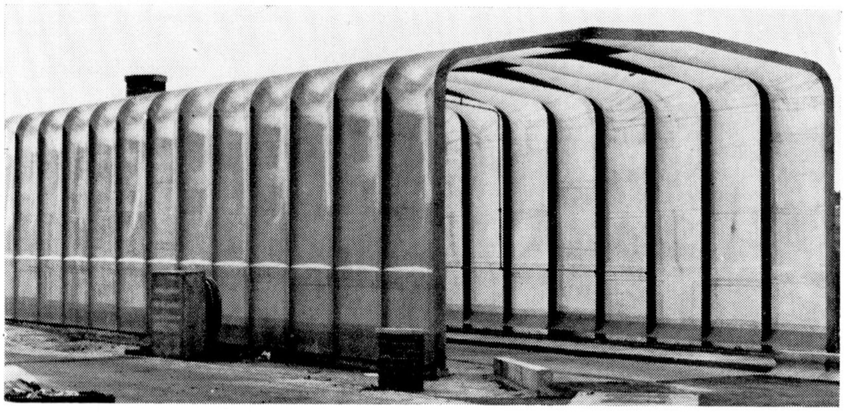

*Heat and its effects*), is more commonly referred to as the diffusion of water vapour through a material and may be given quantitatively by vapour diffusivity per unit thickness) or diffusance (stated thickness) of a material.* The implication of treating permeability† so as to include both liquid and vapour states is to render some materials inadequate as *perfect* barriers. Thus, for example, paint films, bituminous emulsions and dense cement products may be impermeable to liquid water, but nevertheless permeable to water vapour. Other reasons, such as comparatively rapid deterioration and cracking, may render many of these inadequate even as barriers to liquid water (see '5. Thin Applied Coatings' later).

*Available values are included in detail in *4.00 Heat and its effects*.

†The use of the term 'permeability' to include water in both liquid and vapour states is restricted to this part only, so as to draw attention to the overall problem of water exclusion. Elsewhere, permeability is used in its traditional sense, that is as applied to liquid water, while the transmission of water vapour is referred to as 'vapour diffusion'.

Materials which may, with safety, be regarded as being *completely impermeable* to water in both liquid and vapour states are restricted to metals, glass, hot-poured asphalt or bitumen and some synthetic resins (plastics). All these are, within the context of building practice, non-porous. The efficacy of these materials, it should be stressed, is entirely dependent on freedom from cracks through the material or other weak points, such as joints between units.* The importance of the latter cannot be overlooked. At the same time it may be noted that other non-porous materials, such as slates, marble and granites cannot strictly be regarded as being *completely* impermeable even to liquid water due to the fact that they are not necessarily free from cracks or fissures. However, many of these, and other non-porous materials, may be impermeable *enough* for particular applications and, therefore, cannot be regarded in the same way as porous materials.

*In order to emphasise the importance of the complete construction insofar as water penetration is concerned, there is repeated reference to the significance of imperfections and cracks either in the materials themselves or in the joints between units.

**3. Lateral and downward penetration**

All porous materials will, in varying degrees, absorb water. On the other hand, not all porous materials are permeable to liquid water, while some are more permeable than others. For example, timber may generally be regarded as impermeable and has, in the past, been used successfully as cladding (weather or shiplap boarding) to exclude rainwater from vertical surfaces. However, cracking, general weathering and also jointing usually require the use of additional precautions behind the cladding or the application of a protective coating on the exposed surface. More recently, *good quality* dense concrete, which may also be impermeable to liquid water, has been used, particularly in precast 'sandwiched' panels, with the core consisting of an insulant, such as one of the expanded plastics. Here

*Monsanto House* (*right*), *is also an example of the structural use of plastics in which the raincoat principle is almost achieved to perfection. The new forms which are evolving in structural plastics are significant* (*Courtesy: Monsanto Chemicals Ltd.*)

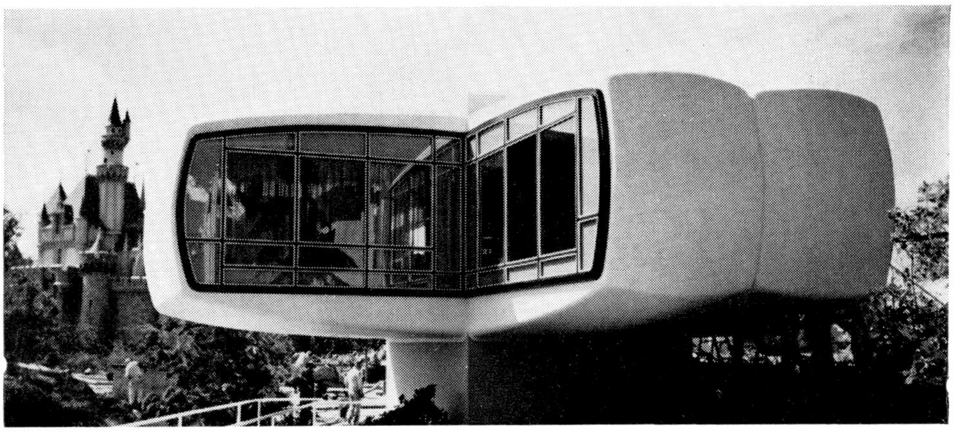

again, joint design and freedom from cracks, often more easily prevented in precast than in *in situ* concrete, are important if the impermeability is to be maintained.*

When assessing the probable use of a permeable material for a particular condition of exposure it is important that cognisance is taken of the method and intentions used in tests to determine permeability. The permeability of a material is measured, *after* saturation of the sample under test, by *forcing* water through it, with the pressure obtained by maintaining a suitable static head and finding the rate of flow in absolute units, for example, cubic centimetres per second. The flow is, in fact, measured whilst the sample is in a horizontal position. The pressure used is 200mm, and this is deemed to be equivalent to the pressure produced by the strongest gust of wind blowing on to the *rain-covered* face of a wall. Thus, permeability is mainly, though not entirely, concerned with the lateral penetration of water through vertical elements. (Roofing units, such as clay tiles, may be subjected to permeability tests.) It is, therefore, important to note that, for any given material, downward penetration of water, as in parapet walls or horizontal surfaces (flat roofs and projections) with slow water run-off, is generally far more considerable than it would have been laterally if the same material had been used in a vertical element. Standing water, whether retained as in a parapet wall or 'free' as on a flat surface, creates a head of water and increases the extent of the downward penetration. Once again, failures at joints will be significant. Accordingly, it is essential that a distinction is made for any given material between the flow of water laterally, as in vertical elements, and downwards, as in horizontal elements, including exposed horizontal surfaces in vertical elements (tops of parapets are always important). For all intents and purposes it may be assumed that, once the source of water ceases, the pressure aiding lateral flow also ceases. This, of course, does not occur with downward penetration as the head of water may persist long after the source of water has ceased. The length of time during which the head of water will be 'operational' depends on the rate at which the retained water evaporates. In general, therefore, it is unwise to attempt to use even relatively impervious materials, such as concrete for example, for flat roofs, canopies and other horizontal surfaces, without a complete impervious barrier to the exposed surface. As will be seen later under 'Roofs', this precaution is not necessary when permeable materials are used on a slope.

*Although it is still a little too early to judge conclusively whether the concrete will remain impermeable in the long term, available evidence suggests that there is a greater risk of water penetration at faulty joints than through the material itself. At the same time there is a risk, subject to the positioning of the insulant, of interstitial condensation which must be taken into account (see *4.00 Heat and its effects*).

## 4. Wetting and drying cycle

In general, the principle upon which the use of porous materials exposed to rainwater is primarily based relies on the interrelationship of *either* the amount of absorption *or* the rate of penetration of water relative to the rate at which water can be evaporated. In a sense this may be regarded as a wetting and drying cycle. Thus, provided a material is not, for a given intensity of exposure to water, permeable,* reliance is placed on the fact that the absorbed water will eventually evaporate after the source has ceased. A time-lag is involved and in many instances evaporation, complete or as complete as is required, may only take place long after the source of water has ceased. During the winter period, for example, there are usually long periods of saturation due to unfavourable environmental conditions for evaporation, with drying out accelerated during the spring. (See *Section 3.01*, 'The Water Cycle', particularly C.3.01/1, p. 10). On the other hand, if penetration of water through a material or construction is to be allowed, then the penetration must not only be slow but must also be accompanied by evaporation at the penetrating surface with the water carried away by evaporation. There must, therefore, be a *balance* between the rate of flow of liquid water and the rate of evaporation of this water, so that a state of dryness is attained after the source of water has ceased. Little or no harm, except for the possibility of efflorescence (*Section 3.05*) will occur *provided* the water is not allowed to collect behind the surface of the material furthest away from the source of water. When used in either way, it is more realistic to regard the absorptive or permeable porous materials used as 'sponges' than complete barriers to the penetration of water. In all cases the *degree* of absorption or the *degree* of permeability, together with the *rate* of evaporation are the criteria to be used for the choice of materials for particular conditions of exposure.

*It should be noted that the severity of exposure is extremely important. Materials which may be found to be impermeable in practice under one condition of exposure may be permeable when the exposure is increased. Some caution is, therefore, necessary when comparing familiar and unfamiliar conditions, as previously noted in *3.02 Exposure*.

## 5. Thin applied coatings*

Absorption of water by a porous material takes place when the 'open ends' of the capillaries formed by the arrangement of the pores in the material occur at the exposed surface. Permeability, on the other hand, can only take place if there are *complete* through routes, sometimes devious, from the exposed to the unexposed surface. If, therefore, an absorptive material is to be rendered impermeable, then one of two basic methods may be employed. Both these are illustrated diagrammatically in diagram D.3.04/1. (1) The open ends of the

*References: (1) Gratwick, R. T., *Dampness in Buildings*, Vol. 1, Crosby Lockwood, 1966. (2) *Colourless waterproofing treatments on damp walls*, BRS Digest (1st Series) No. 90, HMSO, July, 1956. (3) *Principles of Modern Building*, Vol. 1, 3rd Ed., HMSO, 1959.

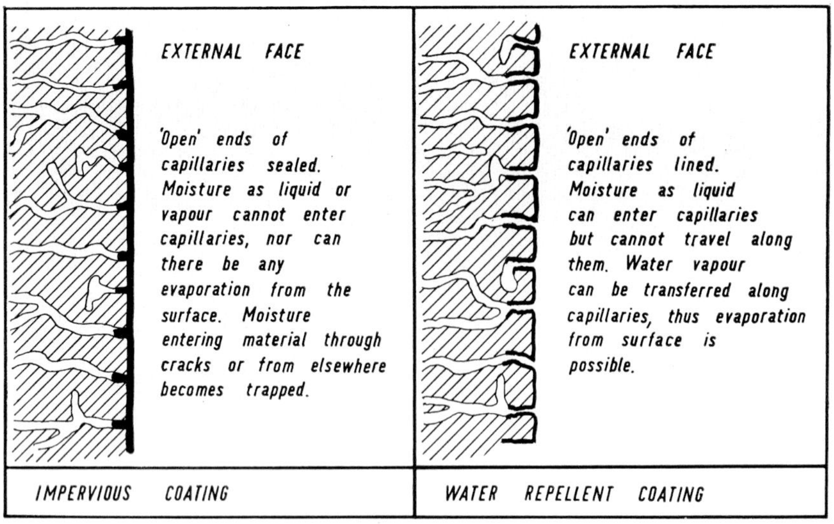


*D.3.04/1*
*Two basic methods of making absorptive materials impermeable by the application of thin coatings*

capillaries may be sealed by the application of a thin liquid coating, such as paint, which eventually solidifies and becomes impervious, or (2) the walls of the capillaries may be lined with a clear water-repellent substance which will prevent water from being transmitted by capillary action. In the latter case the water-repellant acts in a way analogous to grease on a glass surface which prevents the water wetting the surface. (See *Section 1.11,* 'Surface Tension' and 'Capillary Action.') Water-repellants also cause shedding of water from the treated exposed surface. However, it is important to note that liquid water under pressure may be driven along the through-routes even if these are *completely* lined with the water-repellant. Particular circumstances must, therefore, always be taken into account, especially as it is uncommon for the lining to penetrate the complete volume of material treated.

Despite differences in behaviour (noted later) of paint and water-repellent treatments relative to liquid water and water vapour, there are two important factors common to both treatments. Firstly, there is *increased run-off* of rain water from the treated surfaces which immediately increases the risk of water penetration through cracks, defective joints and other weak areas and, secondly, *periodic renewal* of the applied coating is necessary (partial deterioration may, of course, cause local penetration). As regards maintenance of the coatings, a great deal will depend on the properties of the coating relative to conditions of exposure. Among other things, coatings to horizontal surfaces need to be renewed more frequently than similar coatings to vertical surfaces. Some may only last two or three years, while others, such as masonry paints based on chlorinated rubber, styrene/butadiene or isomerised rubber, may not require renewal for 10 years.

The restriction imposed by the necessity for periodic renewal of the applied coatings has, in general, discouraged their use as the *primary* means of defence against exclusion of rainwater. In many cases they have been used as an additional precaution or for purposes of appearance. Consequently, one of the widespread uses of coatings is to be found in the treatment of the external fabric of existing buildings where dampness or water penetration has occurred due to the failure of the materials concerned, including the effects of incorrect detailing.* Experience in this respect has shown that treatments may be effective for moderate or intermittent dampness. Thus, where new buildings are concerned, they should not be regarded as alternatives for taking precautions during design and construction. In general, treatments cannot be expected to seal cracks or to be effective on cracked walls. It may be noted here that opinion is divided on the use of so-called 'preservative' treatments, usually water-repellent, for the exposed surfaces of natural stone. The Building Research Station generally discourages their use.†

(a) *Paints*

The surfaces of absorptive materials may be sealed by a wide variety of paints, including oil paints, plastics based emulsions, bituminous emulsions, masonry and other paints based on chlorinated rubber.* Because of their poor appearance (perhaps better restricted to black) bituminous paints are more commonly used in concealed positions, where their high resistance to both liquid water and water vapour have additional advantages.

Most paints have a high resistance to liquid water and can be regarded as impervious in this respect. Some plastics based emulsions do allow some condensed water to be absorbed into the porous background. Resistance to water vapour is, except for most plastics based emulsions, high enough to prevent entrapped water from evaporating, but not necessarily high enough, except for bituminous emulsions, to act as complete vapour barriers.

Plastics based emulsions do, on the whole (the exceptions are usually those with semi-gloss, glazed or high-gloss finishes), have high porosity to water vapour. In new work this is an advantage as there is an opportunity for certain quantities of water contained in the background to evaporate after the paint has been applied without causing breakdown of adhesion of the paint film. Because of their 'breathing' potential, emulsions may be applied to backgrounds which may otherwise be too wet for successful application of oil paints.† This does not, however, mean that excessive dampness arising from other sources during the life of a building will evaporate 'through 'the emulsion film.

(b) *Water-repellents*

Under the general heading of water-repellents are a number of colourless solutions or emulsions, more commonly known as 'waterproofing' liquids, which in the past have been formulated from waxes, oils, resins or fats or from metallic soaps. However, more recently there has been a notable increase in the range of waterproofers consisting essentially of solutions of silicones in an organic solvent such as white spirit. Colourless solutions do have the advantage of not obscuring to any noticeable extent the appearance of the background—thick coats of some products may darken the tone of the surface or form a film that encourages the retention of dirt.

Cleaning of treated surfaces requires care including the avoidance of detergents which tend to nullify the water-repellent properties of the treatment.

The best of the colourless treatments used on walls can produce a hundredfold reduction in the rate of absorption of rainwater, but at the

*It is not the intention of this study to include methods by which existing buildings may be treated to overcome faults or failures which have developed. Although the principles outlined for new work are also applicable when the problems of remedial work to existing buildings are being considered, it may be noted that solution to the latter may justify the use of coatings or other measures not normally acceptable in new building work.

†References: (1) *The weathering, preservation and maintenance of natural stone masonry, Part 2,* BRS Digest (1st Series) No. 21, HMSO, August, 1950. (2) *Colourless waterproofing treatments for damp walls,* BRS Digest (1st Series) No. 90, HMSO, July, 1956.

*The term 'oil paint' is used here to include those paints which may include significant proportions of synthetic resins in place of traditional 'oils'.

†See *Painting walls: 1,* BRS Digest (2nd Series) No. 55, p. 6, Table 1, HMSO, February, 1965, for quantitative methods of determining dryness for application of various paints.

same time there is a fivefold reduction in the rate of evaporation from the wall. In general, this relationship between the rate of absorption and the rate of evaporation produces a sufficiently favourable balance. This explains why it is important that water does not find its way behind the film. Once entrapped, it will tend to migrate to the inner surface of the construction.

## External walls

Lateral penetration of rainwater through or into external walls to satisfy the requirements of the exclusion of water may, in principle, either be prevented or controlled. *Prevention* implies the use of completely impermeable materials, while *control* implies the use of permeable materials. Techniques of building have been developed which include the use of either type of material in single or multiple 'layers', with or without cavities, but nevertheless employ the principle of prevention or control. The materials used also vary in their degree of permeability, including complete impermeability. Thus, among other things, the first or main 'lines of defence' may occur in a range of positions, from the outer face to any position within the thickness of a construction. On the other hand, parts of the external fabric may consist of materials which rely on the application of control and other parts on the application of prevention (windows are an obvious example, but sheet metals and other impermeable claddings must also be included).

It is, therefore, difficult only to discuss the two basic principles because these can be broken down into three basic principles. On the other hand, one of three basic techniques may be employed, but these do not necessarily follow either principle in any chronological or obvious order. For example, impermeable materials may be fixed to framing or solid walling made up of permeable materials. The latter may, of course, be used adopting the principle of the control of water penetration. Some materials, such as concrete, which are basically permeable may, by suitable quality control, be made more or less impermeable for most practical purposes, in which case their use (so far as the material itself is concerned, that is joints apart) must be considered in relation to the principle of prevention. This is important in large panel concrete construction, particularly prefabricated precast work. Thus it is more convenient, and in some ways a little more realistic, to consider the three basic principles first and then to deal, in general terms only, with the three basic techniques separately. To this end the following four general headings are used: (1) Basic principles; (2) Light cladding; (3) Solid walling; and (4) Cavity walling.

### 1. Basic principles

The three main principles which may be employed to exclude water were shown diagrammatically in *Section 1.11* under 'Capillary Action' and may be summarised as follows:

(a) *Complete prevention*

The transmission of water may be completely prevented by using a skin of material that is completely impermeable, or impermeable for practical purposes, either at the outer face or at some predetermined position within the thickness of a construction. In general, completely impermeable skins are used at the outer face of a construction in the form of claddings or finishes. The use of impermeable skins within the thickness of a construction is usually restricted to specific or local problems related to the exclusion of water, either to supplement the external skin or to control penetration of water through permeable material. This restriction normally implies those positions in which a damp-proof course or membrane is required.

Examples of thin impermeable skins would include sheet metals, some plastics, glass, paint on woodwork and other surfaces and, to a limited extent, bituminous products such as asphalt and felts. (The limitation of these for walling surfaces is due more to appearance than to performance relative to water—their most widespread use is as roofing or damp-proof coursing materials.) Tiles, slates and sheet materials such as asbestos cement may, within limits, be included as examples of thin materials which are impermeable for practical purposes.

(b) *Controlled penetration*

The penetration of water through permeable materials may be allowed, *provided* the water is prevented from reaching the inner face of the wall or some other harmful position within the thickness of the construction before favourable environmental conditions allow the absorbed water to evaporate. The essential requirement is that penetration should be slow. The term 'slow' should be interpreted as the rate at which water may reach a particular position or 'line of demarcation'. Thus, for any given permeability of a material and, taking constructional techniques into account, the thicker the wall the longer it will take for water to penetrate to the inner face, for example. The same principle can be applied to any other distance from the inner face. Subject to the permeability of the materials used and conditions of exposure, control will largely be dependent on overall thickness.

Severity of exposure is critical when techniques incorporating permeable materials employ the principle of controlled penetration. This is not to say, of course, that conditions of exposure are not relevant or important when the two other principles are employed. However, the latter are in a sense specifically designed to deal with severe conditions of exposure. In the case of controlled penetration the effects of shelter, for example, and particularly that provided by projecting elements of building design, can be significant.

The success of any particular technique is very often dependent on the effects of shelter (implying here decrease in severity of exposure) provided by such 'traditional' features as projecting eaves or cornices, particularly on relatively low buildings (two-storey housing, for example). A similar technique used without these or other sheltering elements may, therefore, prove inadequate. In this respect tall buildings should be treated with a good deal of caution. In addition to the effect of height relative to wind which generally increases the severity of exposure (*3.02 Exposure*), tall buildings may lack adequate protection from projecting elements (even where these do exist), particularly at or near the top of the building.

(c) *Breaking capillary paths*

The capillary paths along which water may be transmitted in permeable materials may be broken by incorporating suitably designed air spaces or cavities. Capillary paths may, of course, be deemed to be broken by the incorporation of an impermeable skin within a construction. However, this method would be included under the first principle, namely complete prevention, and is particularly relevant in those situations where damp-proof courses or membranes are required.

Traditionally the method employed is to provide a continuous cavity behind an outer skin of permeable material which is then allowed to become completely saturated. In order to form a cavity, an inner skin is required. The latter, however, does not have to have any particular resistance to water transmission so far as rainwater is concerned and may, therefore, be selected on the basis of other requirements (strength, thermal insulation, etc.). Although the 'split' wall has its own special problems regarding design and construction (outlined later under '4. Cavity Walling'), it has proved that, *when properly executed,* it does offer one of the most efficient methods of providing complete resistance to penetration of walls by rainwater. In many ways it can be regarded as a certain safeguard. In saying this it should be appreciated that success is dependent on the complete adherence of the fundamental principles required in cavity construction. In practice these are, unfortunately, often difficult, though not necessarily impossible, to achieve. The oft encountered unwillingness to overcome the difficulties can, however, usually be attributed to a general lack of understanding of the importance of the precautions contained in the fundamental principles.

More recently attempts have been made, particularly by the BRS, to develop clay bricks which contain within their thickness carefully designed cavities. One type, known as the

double frogged solid brick

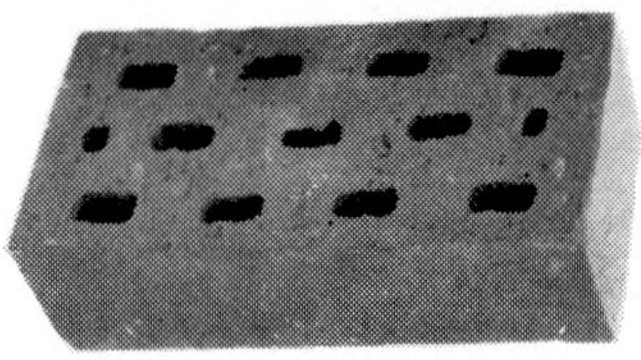

perforated brick 16 per cent voids

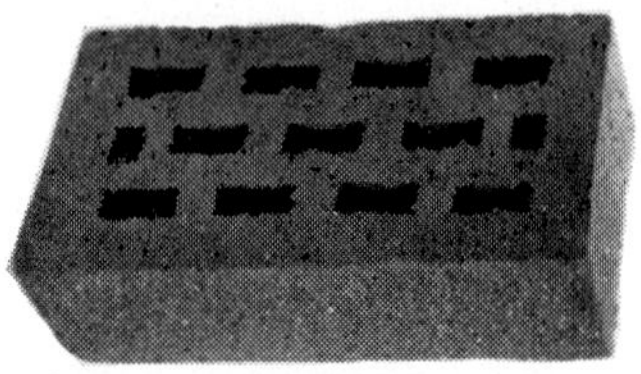

perforated brick 25 per cent voids (Courtesy: National Federation of Clay Industries)

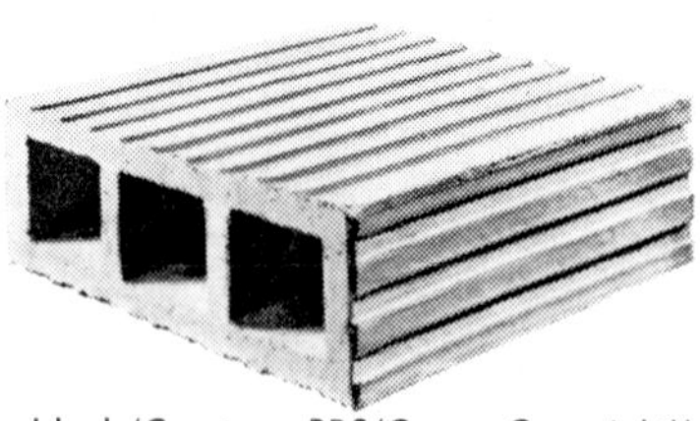

hollow block (Courtesy: BRS (Crown Copyright))

*Illustration of the fundamental differences in the cavity design of some perforated bricks (the top three include for comparison a solid and two types of perforated brick and hollow blocks with that of the BRS V brick (below). Unlike the perforated bricks and blocks, the mortar for the V brick is restricted to the outer voids as shown, thus allowing the larger voids in the centre of the brick to break capillary paths*

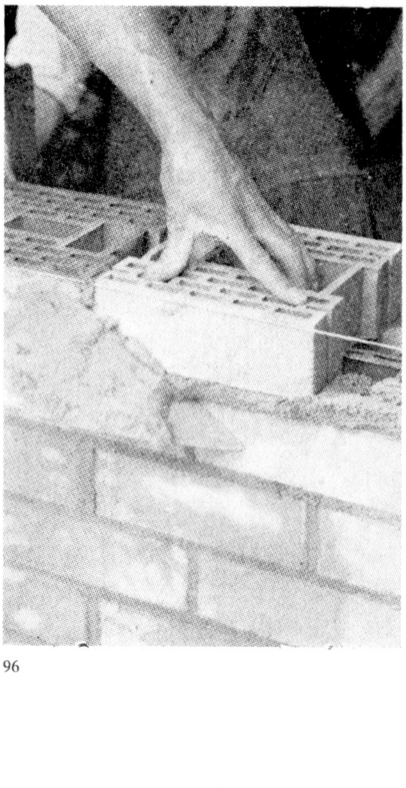

V-brick (the letter 'V' indicating that it is vertically perforated), is now commercially available.* Like many other innovations, sufficient time has not yet passed for an assessment to be made on the practicability of these special bricks or of their economic viability relative to the cavity wall which they are intended to replace†—the size of the brick is nominally 229mm by 229mm by 76mm including joint tolerances and weighs roughly the same as a conventional 229mm by 114·5mm by 76mm brick. Laboratory tests, it should be noted, have proved successful insofar as resistance to penetration by rainwater is concerned. Some confusion sometimes arises between the performance of the V-brick and other perforated or hollow clay or concrete bricks and blocks. The latter are usually made in widths more or less similar to the standard brick, namely in the region of 114·5mm,‡ and should therefore be used as the outer skin in cavity walling in the same way as solid bricks or blocks of a similar width. The perforations or hollows may reduce the permeability of the individual units,** but the permeability of the wall as a whole is still dependent as much on the joints as on the units themselves. Joints may be regarded as the 'weak link' and, in general, are more important than the units. The V-brick, on the other hand, has been specially designed so that walls built of them act in the same way as cavity walling insofar as the mortar joint is concerned. The accompanying photographs illustrate the fundamental differences in the cavity design of some perforated and hollow bricks and blocks with that of the BRS V-brick.

The incorporation of cavities, particularly relatively narrow (not more than 51mm) also helps to increase thermal insulation (see *4.00 Heat and its effects*). This is significant in the 279·5mm cavity wall, for example, as the increased thermal insulation is provided without the use of additional material (bricks, that is). The essential function, it should be noted, is still, however, to break capillary paths and so it is important that some caution is exercised when filling of the cavity with insulants to increase thermal insulation is being considered. (See '4. Cavity Walling', later.)

*A programme of research to develop big hollow and perforated bricks to replace traditional solid brick and, by implication, the cavity wall was commenced at the BRS in 1954. An account of the development, which includes some of the early 'H-bricks', is given in Butterworth, B., *The Resistance of Single-Leaf Walls to Rain Penetration*, in a paper to the Sixth International Ceramic Congress (Reprints from BRS). *The Use of the BRS V (Vertically Perforated) Bricks*, Note No. A.82 (Revised), August, 1961, issued by the BRS (November 1965) has been revised. (see *Building with BRS V-Brick*, Miscellaneous Papers, No. 5 (BRS) ). This note also includes an introduction giving some ideas behind the development of the BRS V-brick. Reference to a larger brick (V-7) measuring 13¼in by 3in (including joints) is given in *Building Research 1959*, HMSO, 1960.

†The weight of the V-brick does allow it to be handled by one man. Until special bricks are made to deal with corners and other junctions, the use of the V-brick is restricted to relatively simple and straightforward runs of walling.

‡It is appreciated that hollow bricks may be obtained in thicknesses from 50·8mm to 229mm, but this does not materially affect the points being made.

***Perforated Clay Bricks*, BRS Digest (1st Series) No. 53, p. 53/3, HMSO, April, 1953, and BRS Digest (1st Series) No. 114, p. 114/2, HMSO, September, 1958, *Hollow Clay Blocks*.

## 2. Light cladding*

At the outset it is necessary to clarify what is implied by the use of the term 'light cladding'. The relatively thin non-structural 'skin' used on the outer face of the building envelope has been (and still is) known by a number of different terms including 'curtain walling', 'cladding', 'panelling', 'wall panel', 'sheath wall', 'window wall', etc., etc.

In his excellent analysis R. Michael Rostron (reference (2), p. 45) has defined 'cladding' as 'that part of the building envelope which carries no loading beyond its own dead weight and imposed horizontal forces such as wind and cleaning loads'. This definition is implied in *this* study.

The criterion upon which the same author has based the use of the term 'light' has been related to methods of fixing, which provide the secondary means of support (relative to the main structure that is) for the cladding. Such support may consist of light framework erected between or over the structural frame, a light bracing contained within the cladding or a fixing device attached directly to the structure. For the present purposes this definition is considered too wide. Thus, in *this* study the term 'light' is primarily intended to imply the use of relatively thin materials which are light in terms of their normally usable thicknesses as claddings. (The significance of density of materials per stated thickness as normally used rather than in kg/m³ was discussed and shown in *Section 1.07*. See comparative chart C.1.07/2, Vol. 1, p. 46.) All the materials dealt with here are, in addition to being thin and light, completely or relatively impermeable to rainwater and usually fixed to light framework Other claddings which vary in their degree of permeability, including impermeability, such as brickwork, rendering, glazed tiling, stonework (natural and reconstructed), precast concrete panels (large and small), etc., which may or may not be fixed with fixing devices or to a framework, are more conveniently included under '3. Solid Walling' see p. 100).

(a) *Range of materials*

The range of materials which may be included under light cladding are: sheet metals (aluminium, copper and copper alloys, steel including stainless steel); cast metals (cast iron was used

*References: (1) *Light Cladding*—Parts I and II, BRS Digests (1st Series) Nos. 98 and 99, HMSO, May and June, 1957; (2) Rostron, R. M., *Light Cladding of Buildings*, The Architectural Press, London, 1964.

quite extensively as a cladding material but is not generally used nowadays); glass (transparent, translucent and opaque); plastics (thermo-plastics and thermosetting plastics); timber and timber products; asbestos compositions (mainly asbestos cement); tiling (clay and slate similar to roof tiling).

The sheet metals (and cast metals where applicable), glass and plastics are completely impermeable. Slate tiles can, within certain limits, also be included with the latter. The remaining materials, and taking into account the positions in which they are normally used, can for most practical purposes be regarded as impermeable. Except for the tiling, all the materials are used in relatively large sheets or units.

(b) *Distinguishing feature and exposure*

The fact that all the materials used are, for all practical purposes, impermeable to rainwater means that the principle of their use is entirely related to prevention of lateral penetration of water (1 (a) previously). This is their most distinguishing feature when compared with other techniques of walling. None of the materials can be literally stretched over the envelope in one piece and so *joints* between sheets or between units, as the case may be, or between sheets or units and other elements of external fabric (columns, beams, walls, etc.) are fundamental. Exposure of all joints is greatly increased as there is little or no absorption of rainwater by the materials themselves.* In this account must also be taken of the cumulative effect, in terms of quantity, of the water flowing down the face of a building. Height is, in this context, far more important than length and so the higher the building the greater the cumulative effect.† Taking as a basis a run-off equal to 15 litres/m²/h (see *3.02 Exposure*, p. 38), the run-off during *fifteen minutes* of rain on a building 10m high would be 75 litres/m length. Each increment of 1m in height would contribute a further 3·75 litres. The quantities quoted would all occur at the base of the building. From this it will be seen that the duration of rain also plays an important part.

So far as joints and other features are concerned, the basic exposure indicated above is further aggravated by the effects of wind. Again, the greater the height of the building the greater the deleterious effects of wind. One of the main effects of wind is to

*The absorptive capacity of most traditional walling techniques (brick, stone, etc.), which results in less run-off of rainwater over the faces of a building, has often been said to account for their success in terms of resistance to rain penetration when compared to the early uses of impermeable materials over the greater part of the face of a building.

†Where the run-off is to be drained, the total area of the building face exposed to rainwater will be important. However, in terms of exposure of the claddings and particularly joints and junctions, cumulative run-off relative to height is still significant.

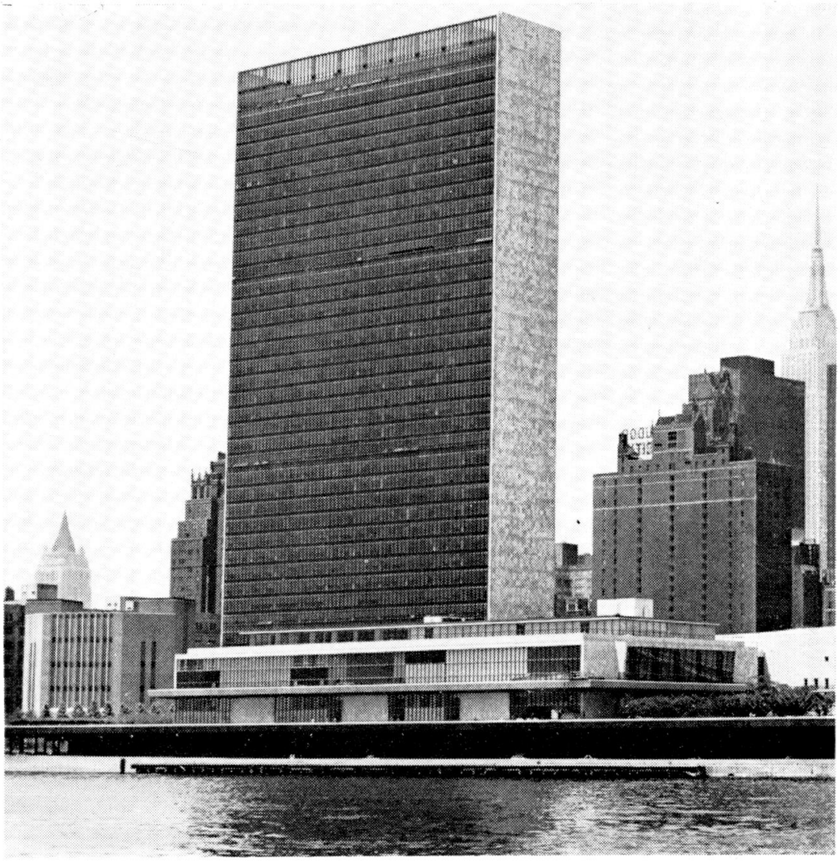

*The riverside façade of the United Nations Secretariat Building in New York provided an early and worthwhile warning of the combined effects of height and exposure which resulted in leakage of weep holes, etc., in the impervious sheath wall (Courtesy: United Nations Information Centre)*

*Below left, traditional horizontal timber boarding has provided the basic appearance motif for impervious claddings made of aluminium and plastics. The picture illustrates the use of a relatively new vinyl cladding, Marley Shiplap Siding, as used on the Colt timber house. (Courtesy: Marley Tile Co. Ltd.) Below right, horizontal timber boarding. The boarding has been treated with a thin applied coating, some of which has deteriorated*

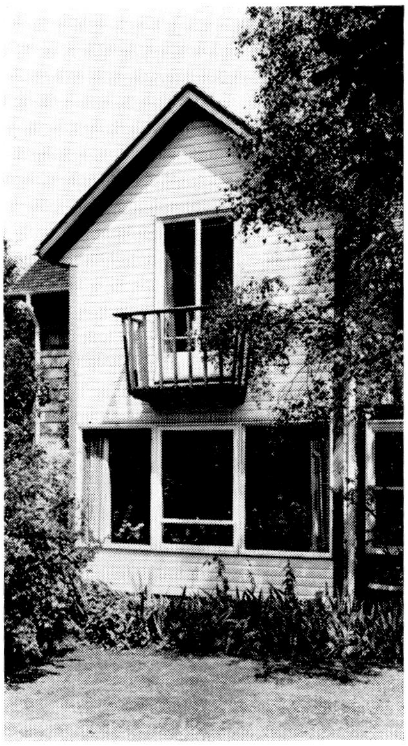

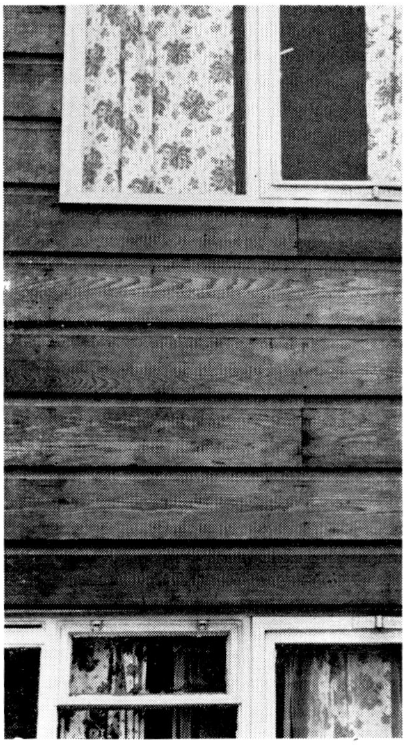

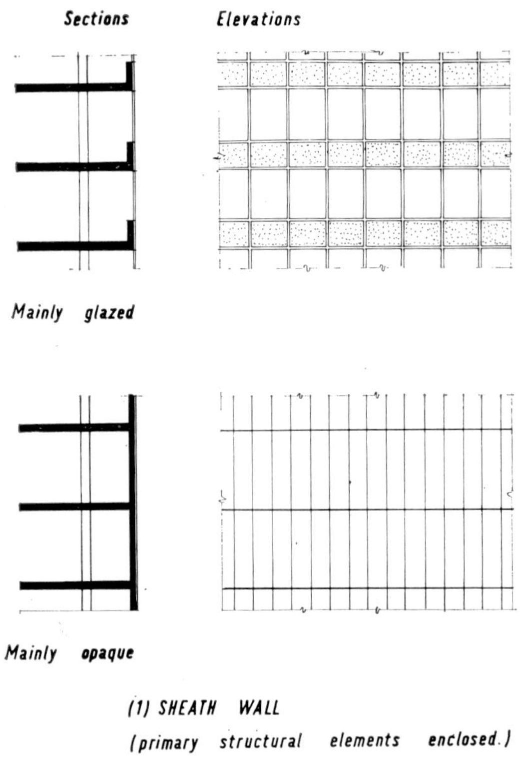


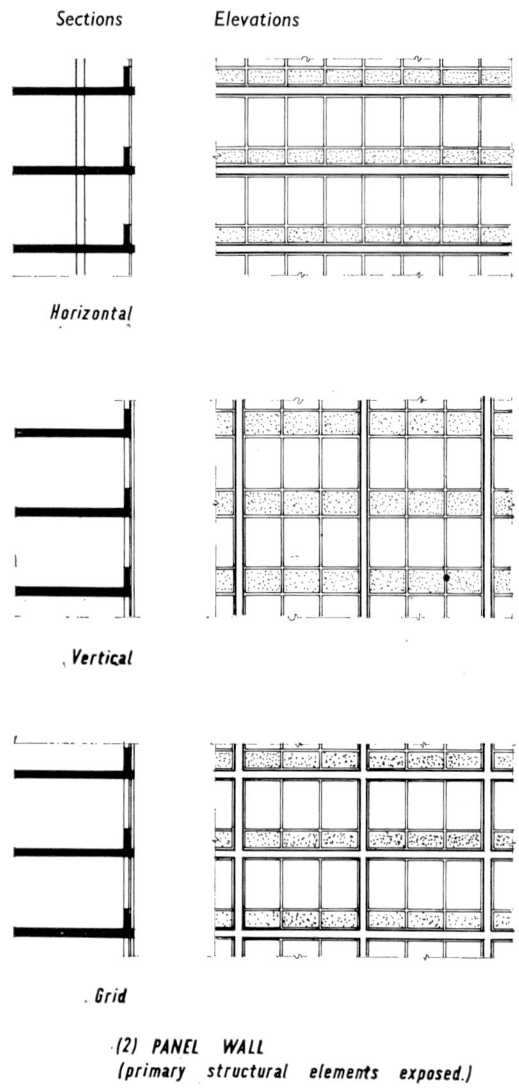


*D.3.04/2*
*Two basic forms of light cladding related to primary structural elements. (From: Rostron R. M., 'Light Cladding of Buildings', The Architectural Press, 1964)*

cause rain to be blown through joints. In some cases (unsealed joints are notable) wind may cause *snow* to be troublesome. Another is to cause rainwater to be blown *up* the face of the building. When this is likely to happen, then it is most important that care is taken in the design of weep holes or other drainage outlets. The bitter experience of the United Nations Secretariat Building in New York, where the combined effects of height and exposure to the openness of the river resulted in leakage of weep holes, etc., on the riverside façade, should serve as a worthwhile warning. This particular example is notable as New York is not unaccustomed to erecting high buildings. At the time the latter were either 'secluded' in terms of exposure or did not employ impervious cladding. Finally,* wind, when accompanied by abrasives (dust, ash, etc.), may result in surfaces being scoured. Although most claddings are likely to remain unharmed, mastic jointing materials and other sealants may be seriously affected. In view of the fact that most, though not all, cladding 'systems' rely on mastics of one kind or another to effect resistance to rain penetration at the joints, the scouring effects of wind cannot be overlooked, particularly when the mastic jointing is exposed. When considering this particular aspect, account should also be taken of the fact that joints between cladding and other elements of the fabric (the junction of windows with other elements are notable) present problems similar to those of the cladding as a whole. Thus, the problem of the scouring of joints needs to be considered when impervious claddings are used in conjunction with absorptive materials. Windows are always important.

(c) *Forms*

Where cladding is used as the primary means of external enclosure, irrespective of the size of the units used, two basic forms may be employed. Rostron (reference (2)) has classified these as:

*Form* (1): *Sheath wall.* The cladding is placed outside the main structure so that no primary structural elements appear on the wall surface. The cladding is used literally as a skin enveloping the outer surface of the fabric.

*Form* (2): *Panel wall.* The structural elements are exposed or well defined and the cladding is erected between these elements. Thus the panel wall may be *horizontal* when it occurs between beams or floor slabs; *vertical* when it occurs between columns or cross wall; or as a *grid* when it occurs between a combination of horizontal and vertical elements.

These basic forms are shown diagrammatically in diagram D.3.04/2. Of the two, the sheath wall is less capable of variation in terms of its relationship with the primary structural elements. Variations in terms of its 'patterning' or modelling are, of course, possible. With the panel wall, however, the situation is somewhat different. Either of the primary exposed horizontal or vertical elements may be varied until in the extreme condition the cladding forms no more than a small infill element. The realization that even such small infills still obey the principles implicit in panel wall forms is important. Whereas the joint problems of the sheath wall are universally applicable over the whole area of the cladding and are, in a sense, more or less

*The aspects of wind included here are mainly those associated with rainwater penetration. It may be noted that wind must also be considered relative to structural stability of the cladding, while the problems of air, including dust, infiltration through joints must also be taken into account.

*Right, illustration of the sheath wall (form (1), diagram D.3.04/2) to office buildings. (Architects: Gollins, Melvin, Ward and Partners). Although built within a short time of each other the building on the right-hand of the photograph was completed first and represents one of the earliest examples in London of the application of the sheath wall. Far right, tile hanging. (Architect: Eric Lyons)*

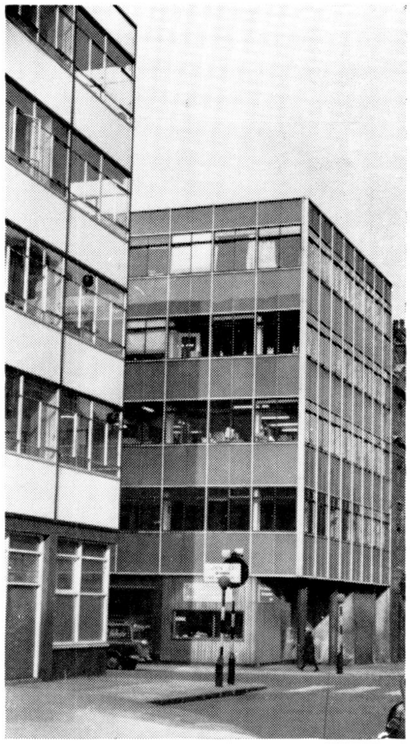

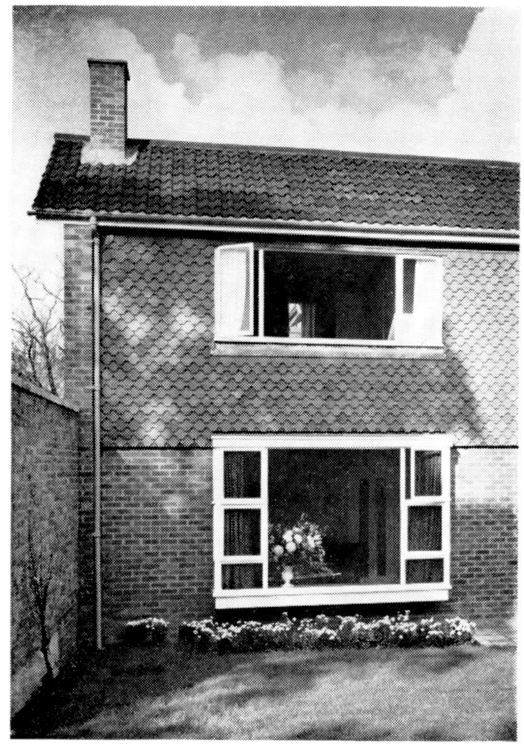

of one kind, this is not completely true of the panel wall. The latter, in addition to the jointing problem between the cladding units (the solution may be the same as for the sheath wall), also has the special problem of the joint at the junction between the cladding and the exposed primary elements, as already noted earlier. The solution of these problems may require the use of additional impermeable materials behind the cladding, in the form of damp-proof courses, or the use of impermeable coverings in the form of flashings. The principles upon which these must be based are discussed later under 'Damp-proof courses and membranes'.

(d) *Type of joint, cavities and drainage*

From the point of view of resistance to rain penetration, joints in any light cladding system are the weak links. The larger the cladding unit the fewer the joints but, at the same time, the problem of solving the joint becomes more critical due mainly to increased exposure in terms of the quantities of water which have to be resisted. Joints, on the other hand, also provide a means for allowing for movement of the cladding. Looked at in another way, it could be said that joints are necessary in order to allow for movement. Again, the larger the unit the greater the amount of movement which has to be accommodated. The interaction of the requirements of rainwater resistance on the one hand and allowance for movement on the other are indicative of the problems associated with joint design.

Although there are a number of detailed variations possible, joints fall into one of two categories, namely (1) overlapping, and (2) butt* The type of construction, that is whether the framing is essentially behind the cladding, or forms exposed horizontal or vertical members (or a combination) or is incorporated within the cladding prior to erection will, to a large extent, influence the type of joint used. The joints may be left *open* or completely *sealed* by means of mastic, gasket or other joint sealing techniques. Open joints are a common feature of traditional tile or slate hanging, which employ overlapping joints and where, among other things, the units are small. Movement of the units is automatically taken care of, unlike the sealed joint when movement must also be accommodated by the sealing compound, without loss of adhesion or other failure. Timber boarding may also be used in a way similar to tile or slate hanging, that is by simple overlapping, but in some cases joints may appear to be sealed when tongue and groove techniques are employed. Such sealing is not always effective so far as resistance to rain penetration is concerned and a secondary line of defence behind the cladding is necessary.

By virtue of the basic method by which claddings are fixed, namely to a system of framework attached to the primary structure, cavities are formed behind the claddings. For large unit claddings advantage may be taken of such cavities so that they form a drainage system whereby water which may leak (or be allowed to leak) through joints may be discharged at some convenient point to the outside, thus preventing any transmission of water into the body of the fabric or allowing the water to be trapped. Specially designed cavities, as in the case of patent glazing (virtually a traditional cladding system but restricted essentially to horizontal rather than vertical elements), may be considered so as to design 'dry' joints. Where it is proposed to use cavities for drainage purposes, care must be taken to ensure that the framework or other obstructions behind the cladding do not restrict the flow of water to the outlet points. The latter may, of course, have to be designed to prevent the ingress of updriven water caused by wind. A system of drainage intended to deal with penetration of rainwater may act equally well for drainage of condensed water, particularly during the winter period. On the other hand, under some conditions drainage may be more important for carrying away condensed water than penetrating rainwater.

Whether or not it is necessary, when open joints are used, to provide a secondary line of defence, other than drained cavities that is, against penetration of rainwater behind the cladding depends to a large extent on the nature of the background to which the claddings are fixed. *Tile and slate hanging* provide a useful, albeit traditional, example. Many of the principles outlined may, within certain limits, also be applied when larger cladding units are being used in similar ways. The units may be fixed to

*Rostron has noted a third type, namely the mated joint. This is essentially a sophisticated form of an overlapping joint, with a mechanical interlocking basis. For simplicity, and because this part is not primarily concerned with joint design, it has been excluded.

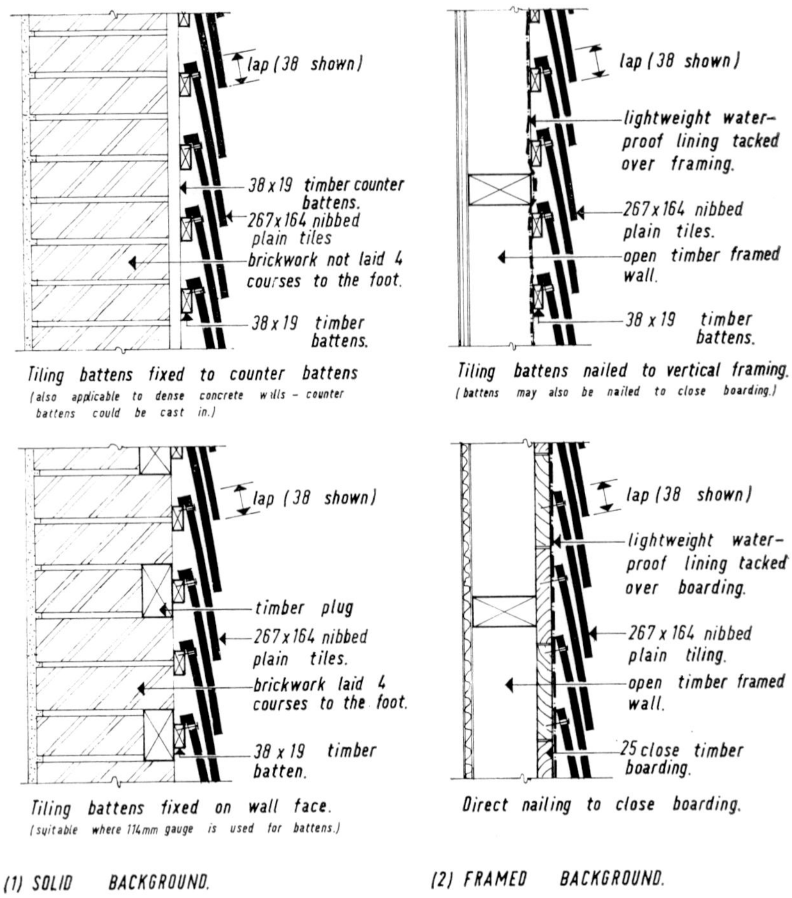


D.3.04/3

*Methods of fixing tile cladding to solid and framed backgrounds. Note: the illustrations are not intended to be exhaustive but do show the basic principles. The lap of the tiles will be dependent on exposure (see text). The gauge of battens is for the lap and size of tiles illustrated only. (From: 'Cladding of Vertical Surfaces', The Clay Tile Bull., Vol. 1, No. 11, which also includes recommended details for junctions, openings, etc.) —Dimensions in mm*

framing (tiling battens) which may either be fixed to a solid background, such as brick, block or concrete* (diagram D.3.04/3 (1)) or form part of a framed secondary structure (diagram D.3.04/3 (2)). In the first case the background itself is sufficiently weathertight to exclude air penetration, while any water (usually a small quantity anyway) which may leak through the joints in the cladding will, depending on the absorptive characteristics of the background, either be absorbed (and subsequently evaporate as air movement behind the cladding is possible) or simply 'flow out' through the joints. In the second case there is a possibility of air penetration to the interior, significant loss in thermal insulation, while water may find its way into the body of the construction. A second line of defence must, therefore, be provided behind the cladding. This may be a lightweight waterproof roofing felt, stout waterproof paper or lightweight polythene sheeting, fixed over the structural framing. In some cases the framing may be covered with boards. The boards may be used to resist air penetration or provide added thermal insulation. They may, therefore, dispense with the need for battens. However, the waterproof lining should be fixed over the boards. Similar requirements are also necessary when *timber boarding* is used, even when apparently sealed joints are used (e.g. tongue and grooved).

The use of horizontal battens for fixing may in any of the cases quoted above provide ledges along which water may collect. It is important, therefore, to ensure that the water can drain away and not be absorbed into the background or cause decomposition of the battens which are more commonly of timber. In the case of vertical timber boarding, for example, water drainage may be effected by suitable joint design, as shown in diagram D.3.04/4. In other cases where this is not possible the battens may be suitably notched.

The waterproof lining behind the cladding will also act as a vapour barrier. Care must, therefore, be taken to ensure that condensed water is allowed to drain away, when there is a risk of interstitial condensation forming.

It should be noted that the use of any waterproof lining behind the claddings is only intended as a *secondary* line of defence. The cladding itself must still provide the *primary* resistance to lateral penetration. The extent of the lap in tile or slate hanging must, therefore, be sufficient to prevent water being blown in by a strong wind. The BRS has suggested* that the lap may be calculated from the expected wind pressure (see Table 3.04/1) which can be readily translated from N/m$^2$ to head of water in mm by dividing by 11·3. Thus, if the wind pressure is likely to attain 574·56 N/m$^2$, the vertical lap will need to be at least 50·8mm. It will be seen from the table that the conditions of exposure affect the pressure which can be expected. In diagram D.3.04/3 a lap of 38·1mm (pressure up to 430·92N/m$^2$), generally considered adequate for most two-storeyed housing, has been shown. The use of this lap is, taking the formula into account, inadequate for Exposure D or, where the effective height exceeds 6·096m, in Exposure C. The table does not, however, give any guidance as to whether there is any likelihood of rain being driven upwards during wind†

### 3. Solid walling

Solid walling would seem, at the outset, to imply that the principal method of dealing with the lateral penetration of water is by control. This is, however, not necessarily the case. The basic materials commonly used in the majority of cases for what may be termed the structure of the wall are mostly porous. Granite blocks are an obvious exception. To some extent, glazed bricks or glass blocks could also be included in this category. Nevertheless, many of the basic porous materials, such as concrete, for example, may, subject to quality control, be regarded for practical purposes as impermeable, in which case the principle of prevention would have to be used. The same principle also has to be used whenever the basic structure, which may very well be absorptive, is faced externally with essentially impermeable materials. This is a common occurrence. Brickwork, for example, may be faced with renders, glazed tiling, faience (a facing material which has generally declined in application since the war), glass or ceramic

*In some cases tiles or slates may be fixed directly to brickwork without the use of framing. The mortar joints would be used. However, departures such as these do not materially affect the considerations being outlined. For a fairly intensive coverage of details of methods for fixing tiles to vertical surfaces see *Cladding of Vertical Surfaces*, The Clay Tile Bulletin, Vol. 1, No. 11. (Reprints obtainable from the National Federation of Clay Industries, Drayton House, 30 Gordon Street, London, W.C.1.)

*Reference: *Principles of Modern Building—Vol. 1*, HMSO, 3rd Ed., p. 199, 1959.

†The values given are for guidance only. Wind pressure for use in structural calculations has in recent years been modified in the light of advances in knowledge. See Note to Table 3.04/1.

mosaics, and granite, slate or marble facings. The use of surface coatings as outlined under '1. Permeability of materials' may also render a wall impervious, albeit only for a limited time when compared with the facings already quoted.

Because of the wide variations possible it is more convenient to deal firstly with general considerations and secondly with some specific applications of solid walling. All materials commonly used are not intended to be covered in detail. The coverage included should be sufficient to serve as a guide to the principles which should be adopted.

(a) *General considerations*

As in all building problems, *joints* between units are an important consideration. In the case of solid walling units may be small or large, the degree of permeability in either case being immaterial. A construction made up of stones, bricks or blocks (generally small units with the possible exception of some traditional stonework) is commonly known as masonry,* and may for convenience here be termed solid masonry walling. This type of walling is characterised by a substantial number of joints which occupy a fairly large proportion of the wall area. *Large panel construction,* on the other hand, which at the present time appears to be restricted to precast concrete walling units could, within the present context, include monolithic walls of reinforced concrete. This type of walling is then characterised by comparatively few joints. Monolithic walls may in theory have no joints. (In most practical applications it is usually impossible to avoid any joints at all. Those that do occur have to be carefully designed.)

Although the number of joints† is important in any consideration of the penetration of rainwater, the effect of the nature of the units being joined on the joint itself is, in the first instance, more important. The size of the unit is important relative to the amount of movement which may occur due either to moisture or thermal effects. The permeability of the unit will influence the quantity of water to be resisted at each joint. Again, the larger the units and the greater their impermeability, the greater the exposure of the joint to water. Furthermore, once water has gained entry through joints (or cracks for that matter) between impermeable materials, it is likely to become entrapped.

Unlike light claddings and with the possible exception of large precast concrete panels, the *jointing medium* in solid walling consists of *mortar.*

*Glossary of General Building Terms*, BS 3589 : 1963, p. 19. The standard advises that 'if necessary, the term *masonry* should be qualified by a reference to the material used, e.g. stone masonry, brick masonry, glass masonry'.

†In brickwork the surface area of the mortar jointing is equal to nearly one-quarter of the total wall area.

**Table 3.04/1.—Basic wind pressure (p)**

| Effective height of building* (metres) | Wind Pressure p ($N/m^2$) | | | |
|---|---|---|---|---|
| | Exposure A ($V = 20\ m/s$) | Exposure B ($V = 24\ m/s$) | Exposure C ($V = 28\ m/s$) | Exposure D ($V = 32\ m/s$) |
| Up to 3 | 188·50 | 282·76 | 377·01 | 471·26 |
| 6 | 235·63 | 329·88 | 424·13 | 565·51 |
| 9 | 239·63 | 377·01 | 518·39 | 659·76 |
| 12 | 282·76 | 424·13 | 565·51 | 754·02 |
| 15 | 329·88 | 471·26 | 659·76 | 848·27 |
| 18 | 377·01 | 518·39 | 706·89 | 942·52 |
| 24 | 424·14 | 565·51 | 801·14 | 1036·77 |
| 30 | 424·14 | 612·64 | 848·27 | 1131·02 |
| 36 | 471·26 | 659·76 | 895·39 | 1178·15 |
| 42 | 518·39 | 706·89 | 989·65 | 1272·40 |
| 48 | 518·39 | 754·02 | 1036·16 | 1319·53 |
| 54 | 565·51 | 801·14 | 1083·90 | 1413·78 |
| 60 or more | 565·51 | 801·14 | 1131·02 | 1460·91 |

* Linear interpolation for intermediate heights.

*Exposure gradings:*
The exposure gradings are based on wind records taken at 10m above ground and do not take into account gusts of wind (see note below)

*Exposure A.* Exceptionally small exposure to wind. To be adopted in rare cases only.

*Exposure B.* Of general use except near the sea coast or estuaries or for altitudes over 152m above sea level.

*Exposure C.* Open country generally, altitudes up to 244m above sea level, but not near the sea coast or estuaries.

*Exposure D.* Exposed sites within 3km of the coast or estuary, or at an altitude over 244m above sea level.

*Reference:* BS Code of Practice CP3—Chapter V (1952), *Loading* Table 3, page 13 and pp. 21–22. Units in table above converted from Imperial units.

*Important Note:* The values given in the table were those used for wind loading. With advances in knowledge of wind loading, emphasis is now given to clearer definition of a specific problem and the use of formulae. *Wind loading on buildings—1, 2 & 3.* BRS Digest 99, 101 & 105, HMSO, Nov. 1968, Jan & May 1969, describe and give examples of the new approach. In so far as driving rain is concerned, the table above is still useful as a guide.

Generally speaking, the mortar should have strength and porosity characteristics similar to those of the units being joined. This is often possible to secure, but the mortar may still differ from the units in terms of moisture or thermal movements. Shrinkage cracking during initial drying out, for example, is almost impossible to avoid completely and so there is inevitably some breakdown in the bond at the interface of the mortar and the units, usually resulting in fine cracks or fissures, and is generally more marked with strong dense mortars than with weak porous mortars. The practical significance of this is that perfection of material and workmanship is essential if relatively impervious units are to remain resistant to penetration by rainwater. Such units require the use of strong dense mortars and, above all, the bond between the units and the mortar must be perfect. Relatively absorptive porous units, on the other hand, with weaker and more porous mortar joints will reduce the load on the joints for as long as the units absorb rainwater falling on them and prevent a continuous film of water flowing down the wall surface. Water is unlikely to penetrate through cracks and fissures in the mortar joint if these are wider than the pores still absorbing water. Thus, where absorptive units are used workmanship and supervision are much less important than in the case of relatively impervious units. In order to emphasise the importance

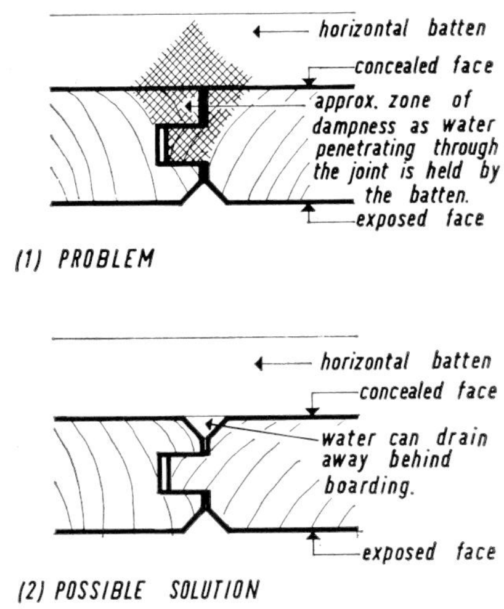


*D.*3.04/4

*Joints in vertical timber boarding to allow for drainage of water behind the boarding*

of the correct relationship, that is compatibility, between the characteristics of the units and the mortar, the effects of the use of a dense mortar with an absorptive unit may be noted. The use of such a mortar may lead to a concentration of water just above the horizontal joints. The likelihood of penetration at the interface of the joint and the unit is thereby increased. The characteristics and possible uses of

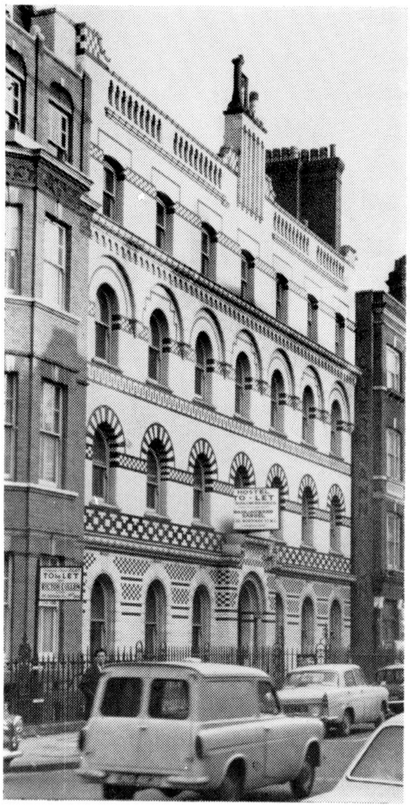

*A rather more imaginative use of glazed bricks in solid walling than is normally associated with the material. Although essentially porous, in common with many of the other materials used in solid walling, glazed bricks do, however, have a relatively impervious outer skin*

mortars of different mixes is included under 'Joint Design' later.

(b) *Specific applications*

*Pointing*

The time at which pointing of brickwork or blockwork is undertaken is sometimes considered to effect the resistance of joints to rain penetration. Far more important than whether the pointing is carried out during laying of the units* (flushing up as the work proceeds) or after completion is the fact that the pointing should not be stronger than the body of the mortar, as the stronger pointing mortar will in time break away. When this happens risk of rain penetration is increased. It is important to note that whenever pointing is carried out the operation must be carried out with care.

*Renderings*

Renderings to brickwork or blockwork have the advantage, if they are properly applied, of filling up cracks in the mortar joint and in other

*Strictly speaking, working of the surface of the mortar joints during laying of bricks or blocks to give a finished face while the mortar is still green is known as 'jointing'. 'Pointing' then refers to the practice of filling previously raked out joints with mortar, the surface of which is worked to give a finished face. This pre-supposes that the mortar in the wall has at least hardened.

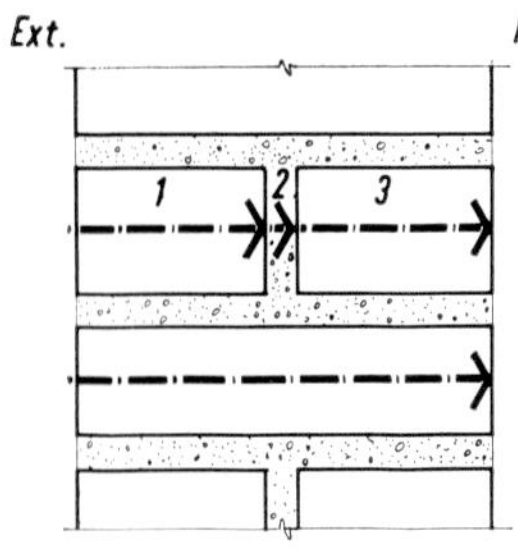


*stretcher bond: rainwater must penetrate (1) outer brick (2) vertical mortar joint (helps to break capillary paths) and (3) inner brick.*

*porous header: no breaks in capillary paths other than that provided by the structure of the brick.*

*D.3.04/5*

*Susceptibility of porous headers in 229mm solid brick masonry to penetration by rain water*

places. Accordingly, they can offer increased resistance to penetration by rainwater. Like mortars, renderings can be strong and dense or weak and porous. Although dense renderings will themselves provide greater resistance to water penetration, this advantage only lasts whilst no cracks develop. Water which gains entry then becomes entrapped. Porous renderings, on the other hand, may still provide some resistance to water penetration even when cracked, as they allow absorbed water to evaporate during favourable environmental conditions.

*Brickwork*

In the less severely exposed and drier parts of Britain 229mm fair-faced brick walls have given satisfactory protection against penetration by rainwater. Projections which throw water clear of the wall below, particularly in low buildings (one- and two-storeyed houses, for example) can reduce exposure considerably. Under severely exposed positions (lack of water throw off or walls at some height from the ground) even 343·5mm or 458mm brickwork have been known to have inadequate resistance to wind-driven rain. In many cases, however, water penetration does often occur via indirect paths through local defects, such as cracked sills, badly designed parapets or other features.*

Porous *headers* have often allowed penetration. Stretcher bond does in general offer far greater resistance. Bricks laid in this type of bond are separated by a layer of mortar and so water entering the exposed brick must be transferred from the brick to the mortar and then from the mortar to the inner brick (see diagram D. 3.04/5).

A more positive key between bricks and mortar, thus reducing the formation of cracks and the risk of water penetration, can be obtained when perforated rather than solid bricks are used. In this, however, the quality of mortar and workmanship are still important.

*It may be noted here that dampness occurring on the internal face of a solid wall may not be due to rainwater penetration by direct or indirect paths, but to condensation. The thermal conductivity of a wall is increased significantly when it is wet. This, in turn, results in a lower internal surface temperature of the wall, which encourages condensation, as explained in *4.00 Heat and its effects*.

*Natural stone masonry*

The principles governing the use of natural stone in solid walling are, in general, similar to those applicable to brickwork. There are, however, some detailed points which should be noted.

The range of building stones offers degrees of permeability very much the same as found in bricks. The sedimentary stones (limestones and sandstones) may be said to resemble some of the permeable bricks, while the granites, slates and marbles the more impermeable bricks (engineering and to some extent glazed bricks). An important difference concerns the size of stone unit generally used. Units of stone are usually much larger. The trend is, in fact, towards larger and larger units. Accordingly, the number of joints in stonework is becoming considerably less than in brickwork.

The width of joints used in stone masonry, unlike those in brick masonry, may vary from 51mm (or more in some cases) to as little as 3mm, depending on whether the stone is laid according to a class of walling known as *rubble work* on the one hand or *ashlar* on the other. Although there are a number of detailed variations (surface patterning, shape, bonding, etc.) possible in each class, the essential characteristics are shown in diagram D.3.04/6, which includes (drawings (3) and (4)) developments of 'traditional' ashlar.

*Rubble work (1)* consists of blocks of stone that are either undressed or comparatively roughly dressed and having wide joints. The units are generally smaller than those used in ashlar. Bonding incorporates some headers or through units. Unlike ashlar, the whole thickness of the wall consists of stone. The problem of obtaining a watertight solid wall is essentially the same as with the brick wall.

*Ashlar (2)* consists of blocks of stone carefully and accurately dressed or carefully wrought with narrow joints. The stone units usually have a larger elevational surface area than in rubble work. Although walls may consist of stone throughout, this is costly and so a practice grew up* of building composite walls. The ashlar

*In general, this method of using ashlar, particularly for the sedimentary stones, has been replaced by methods using fixing devices as described later.

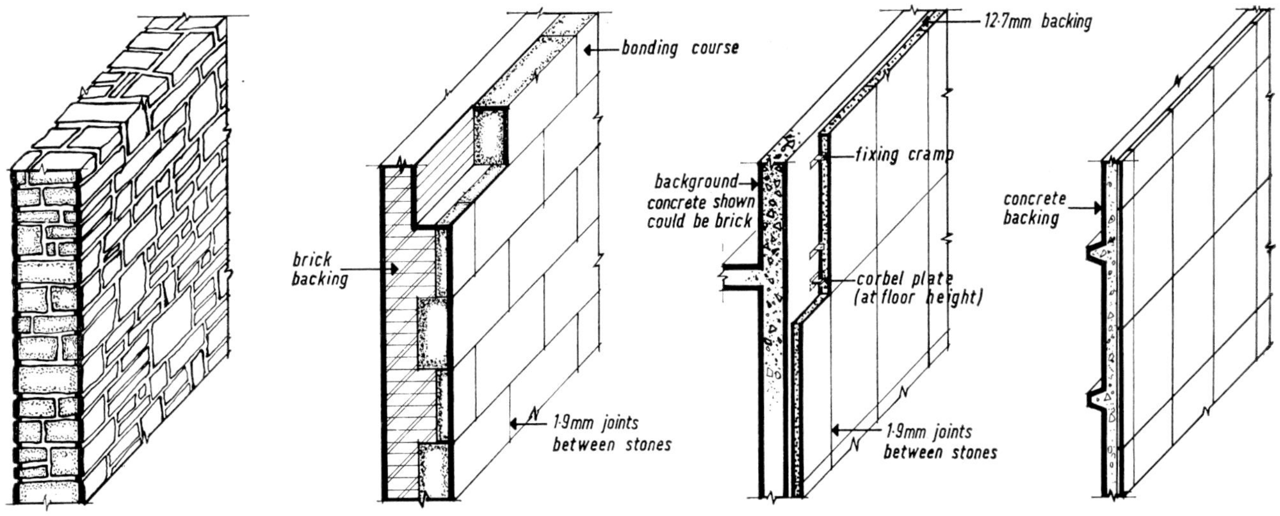


(1) RUBBLE WORK
(random built to courses illustrated – other types possible.)

Scale: 0mm 500mm 1 000 mm

(2) 'TRADITIONAL' ASHLAR
(block bonded to brickwork)
stone min. thickness 63·5mm

Note: Stone in types (2),(3) & (4) assumed to be sedimentary. In (3) particularly, other types of stone may be as thin as 19·0mm

(3) ASHLAR FIXED TO CONCRETE
(using fixing devices
stone min. thickness 63·5mm

(4) ASHLAR CAST ONTO CONCRETE
(precast panel technique – stone min. thickness 63·5mm

*D*.3.04/6
*The essential characteristics of rubble work and ashlar in natural stone masonry. Diagrams* (3) *and* (4) *illustrate developments in traditional ashlar*

is made of minimum thickness (for the particular performance required—intermediate courses 63·5mm minimum with bonding courses about twice as thick) and combined with a less expensive material such as brick, which forms the background. Effective bonding of the ashlar and brickwork is, of course, important.

With the aid of *fixing devices* (now generally of copper or copper alloys such as bronze for durability) it has been possible to 'thin down' the slabs of sedimentary stone and avoid the necessity for block-bonding (3). The stones, now used as a skin and often in larger elevational surface areas, may be fixed to either brickwork or reinforced concrete walling backgrounds. Although a cavity of about 12·7–19·1mm may be left between the back of the stone slab and the face of the background, this is often grouted up. Whether or not the cavity is filled, it cannot be depended upon to provide watertightness. (Even in unfilled cavities mortar 'dabs' used behind each joint in the slab act as 'bridges'.) In order to avoid transference of soluble salts from the background or from the mortar to the stone (relevant when sedimentary stones are used) the backs of the stones are often waterproofed. The efficacy of this precaution against penetration by rainwater has been questioned, as water can still enter the background walling through the joints. Furthermore, subsequent evaporation of water to the outside air is severely retarded as transmission of water through the stone is restricted by the waterproofing which provides an almost impervious coating. In principle, it would seem better to apply a waterproof coating to the background and reduce grouting behind the stone slabs to a minimum. Where this is done (account must be taken of the practical difficulties of providing a continuous waterproof membrane—base of wall and top of openings are important positions—fixings may break the membrane) some form of drainage, similar to that provided in cavity walling, would be advisable.

A more recent development (4)* which allows slabs of sedimentary stone to be used in thicknesses down to 25·4mm, compared with about 76·0–102·0mm where fixing devices are used, embodies precast concrete techniques. Concrete is poured on to the stone slabs which have bronze pins to aid adhesion and are already in the casting mould. Reinforcement is used in the concrete. The complete precast panels which may incorporate a number of slabs may be large in size. Methods of erection and jointing are then similar to those used for other types of large precast concrete units.

Finally granite masonry. In general, it is difficult to obtain a completely dry wall with an impervious material of this kind. Even thick walls of granite have been known to allow penetration by rainwater. Again, joints provide the 'through' routes. Water tends to stream through any cracks or fissures in an otherwise impervious joint, while a porous mortar is unlikely to have sufficient absorptive capacity to hold back penetrating rainwater for any length of time. Where, however, granite or other relatively impervious stone facings, such as slate or marble, are used as 'skins', rainwater penetration at joints can be dealt with by incorporating some form of drained cavity, on the lines described in the text to diagram D.3.04/6 (3).

*Cast or reconstructed stone units*

These are defined* as building materials 'manufactured from cement and natural aggregate for use in a manner similar to and for the same purpose as natural building stone'. The method of use of the units resembles the 'skin' technique (diagram D.3.04/6 (3)) of ashlar described previously. Although the units may be regarded as cement-based products, careful control during manufacture

*Changes in detail of techniques used to ensure bonding between the slabs and the background concrete will no doubt occur as more experience is gained. The illustration and description is deemed sufficient to outline the basic principle employed. Until the results of experience with stone slabs used in this way are better known, advice should be sought from manufacturers. Reference for the details given here is *Stone and the Architect*, issued by *The Stone Firms Ltd.*, 3rd Ed., January, 1965. See also Bird, Eric, *Modern Building in Stone*, Building Materials, pp. 31–34, September, 1965.

*Reference: *Glossary of Terms for Stone used in Building*, BS 2847 : 1957, p. 30. It may be noted that the Standard deprecates the use of the term 'Artificial Stone'.

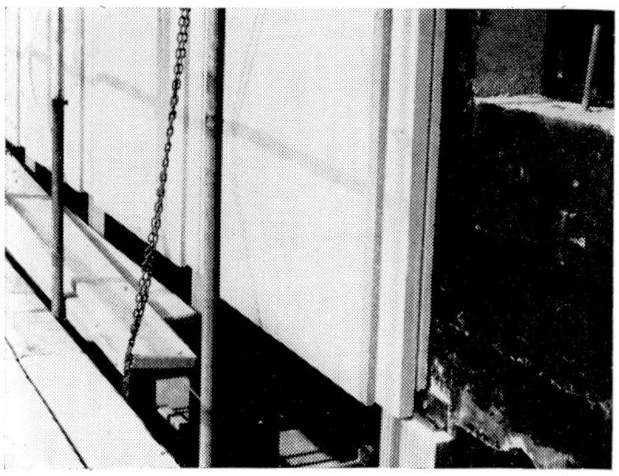

*An example of the use of a waterproof coating to a concrete background which is to receive a precast cladding panel. The coating is provided to prevent the transfer of soluble salts to the panel rather than as a secondary means of excluding water—see text (Courtesy: The Stone Firms Ltd.)*

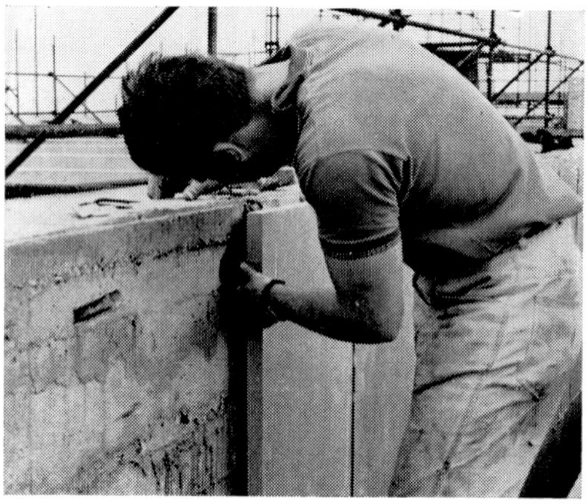

*The use of fixing devices, at one time more commonly associated with relatively thin slabs of slate (shown in the photograph), marble or granite, has enabled sedimentary stones to be used in relatively thin sections without blockbonding as in traditional ashlar. (Architects: Arthur Swift and Partners) (Courtesy: Empire Stone Co. Ltd.) Below, the thickness of sedimentary stones used as facings have been reduced to 25·4mm in essentially precast concrete techniques, some of which may be used as structure (Courtesy: The Stone Firms Ltd.)*

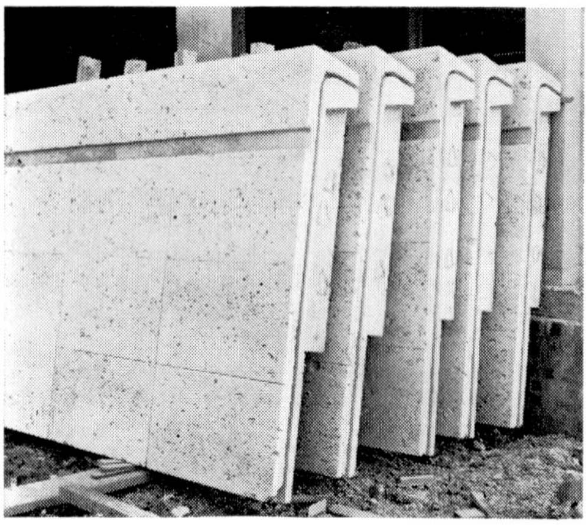

usually ensures that reversible moisture movements are kept to a minimum. However, in some cases (size of unit will be important) possible movements may have to be taken into account to minimise joint failures.

*Precast concrete blocks*

Unlike cast stone, precast concrete blocks are not generally manufactured with appearance in mind, although such appearance as they may have does not necessarily preclude their use (other things being equal) for fairfaced work. The blocks may be either of *dense* concrete made from gravel or crushed rock or of one of the *lightweight* concretes including the aerated varieties. (See the comparative chart C.3.03/10, p. 83.)

One of the basic characteristics of the blocks is their size, which is generally much greater than that of traditional bricks. This is particularly true of the lightweight varieties. Reduced density still allows one-man handling of the increased size. Coupled with size are the appreciable reversible moisture movements which must be taken into account so far as the joints are concerned. In saying this it is assumed that the blocks have been adequately cured before they are built into a wall. Once again, strong mortars should be avoided if cracking of the joint which allows water penetration is to be reduced to a minimum. Although weak mortars are to be preferred, it is still doubtful if weathertightness of a solid fairfaced wall of blockwork can be attained without using cavity construction.

Rendering, properly executed, to the exposed face of a solid wall may provide sufficient resistance to rainwater penetration where exposure is not too severe. It may be noted that one type of dense concrete block which has a porous open texture is not intended to be impermeable. When used externally, therefore, it is intended to be protected by a rendering. The texture of the blocks provides an excellent key.

*No-fines concrete*

The use of no-fines concrete as solid (in the terms implied in this section) walling presents a rather interesting example of a highly porous material in which the pores are large enough to prevent the formation of capillary paths. The large pores are formed as the concrete consists essentially of small stones cemented together at their points of contact. The open texture provides no resistance to wind or to rain carried in the wind. Accordingly, the exposed face must be rendered.

Although the rendering is intended to provide the main line of defence against penetration by rainwater, if water should penetrate then it will trickle down the inner face of the rendering through the interstices of the no-fines concrete. Drainage outlets for this water must be provided at the base of the wall or any other position where there is an interruption of the no-fines structure (lintels to windows, for example). Rain penetration of a no-fines wall is then unlikely if the drainage details are adequately designed.

The principle by which no-fines concrete walling excludes rainwater is in many respects similar to that of cavity walling. Provision of drainage, among other things, is a common requirement. However, it should be noted that the nature of the aggregate used may influence the extent to which water trickling down behind the rendering may gradually drift towards the inner face, particularly at the base or other interrupted area of the wall. Experience has shown that the drift appears to be small with dense aggregates; with porous aggregate penetration can occur more readily.

*Monolithic reinforced concrete*

Dense reinforced concrete properly made is one of the most impermeable porous materials commonly used. Yet use of the material in solid walling presents difficult problems relative to exclusion of rainwater. The problems arise as the result of basically two closely inter-related factors.

First, for any given condition of basic exposure water run-off is at a maximum which means the water runs down the external wall face in a continuous sheet and may, therefore, penetrate into the interior wherever cracks or local defects occur.

Second, monolithic walling implies *in situ* casting so as, among other things, to avoid joints. Practical difficulties makes the avoidance of joints almost impossible. Where it is not possible to cast the whole of a wall at one time it is necessary to incorporate day or construction joints. These may run in either a horizontal or vertical direction, or both. By judicious patterning of the exposed face, as is often accomplished by the use of boarded shuttering, for example, it is possible, from the point of view of appearance, to conceal the construction joints. However, they still exist in the wall and so far as penetration of rainwater is concerned will, unless carefully designed, afford a through route for water. In an attempt to facilitate a solution to this and other similar problems, special waterbars, now usually made of synthetic resins or rubbers, have been developed for casting-in with the concrete. When these are used it is important that they are continuous—treatment of their joints must be carefully considered. On the other hand, cracks may develop as a result of initial shrinkage, in which case additional control of this movement should be provided by properly distributed reinforcement. The area of wall cast at any one time is also significant. Local defects such as 'honeycombing' can only be prevented by careful placing and compaction of the concrete which, in turn, requires careful choice of mix so that workability may be achieved without an excess of water. Shuttering design is also important and consideration should be given to the treatment of bolt holes which, in principle, may also provide through routes.*

*Reinforced precast concrete units*

One, though not the only, advantage of precast concrete work of any kind is that many of the practical difficulties associated with cast *in situ* work can be overcome more easily. Under controlled factory-like conditions quality control is facilitated, thus reducing the likelihood of excessive shrinkage cracking and other local defects. It should, however, be noted that factory-like conditions may take care of such factors as weather protection, but are *not* in themselves substitutes for the care that is still required in the design and application of the concrete mix.

Initially the development of precast concrete units was restricted to comparatively small units, the use of which was (and still is) similar to that used for cast stone described earlier. Recent developments include large-scale precast reinforced concrete panels, sometimes of a composite or sandwiched nature (different types of concrete—dense and lightweight—special types of aggregate for the external face, or insulants—expanded plastics—may be used). The panels may be used simply as cladding or may form part of the basic structure. Storey-height panels are not, therefore, uncommon.

Problems of exclusion of water are mainly associated with the joints. Unlike light cladding, large-scale panels have additional weight and thickness to be taken into account. Thus, although the principles of joint design are basically similar, detailed variations are necessary. The special problems of joint design are covered more fully later.

**4. Cavity walling**

Although cavity walling has been developed chiefly with clay bricks, it may equally well be used with other types of brick and building units, such as concrete blocks, stone, and precast concrete, whether as primary structure or as infill. In many cases it is now common to have the outer leaf of one material, say brick, and the inner leaf of another, say lightweight concrete block. Thus, the nature, including size, of the materials used is not significant. For convenience, reference is made here mainly to walls of brick.

(a) *Basic principle and requirements*

The success of cavity walling is primarily dependent on adherence to one basic principle. *There should be no 'bridge' of solid material capable of transmitting water across the cavity.* It is important to note that water should not be able to be transmitted through or along the surface of the solid material.

Two basic requirements follow from the basic principle and are related to the main function of the outer leaf, namely that it can become saturated and, if necessary, allow water to trickle down its inner face, that is the face fronting on to the cavity. Thus water trickling down the inner face of the outer leaf must (1) not be allowed to splash across the cavity, while (2) adequate provision must be made for its escape to the outside at the base of the wall. Base in this context, as mentioned before, must also include any position in the height of a wall where it is necessary for some solid material (lintel, floor or roof slabs, etc.) to project into or bridge the cavity. The 'weep holes' that should be incorporated to allow water to escape to the outside also appear to have another 'indirect', though important, function, namely allowing an equalisation of the air pressure in the cavity with that on the external face of the outer leaf. This pressure equalisation tends to prevent water being blown under pressure across the cavity. Consequently the sealing of the cavity by the omission of the weep holes in attempts to achieve better thermal insulation is not always wise.

(b) *Practical significance*

Good design, together with conscientious and careful work on site, are imperative if the basic principle and the two basic requirements outlined above are to be satisfied and thus ensuring complete resistance of the wall as a whole to penetration by rainwater. From the practical point of view, precautions may be related to particular procedures or zones of an external wall. These are briefly summarised below.

*Ties*

For structural reasons it is necessary for the two leaves on either side of the cavity to be tied together. From the point of view of water penetration this is an embarrassment. Not only do the ties provide potential bridges which will allow water to run from the outer to the inner leaf, but they also provide obstructions upon which pats of mortar may easily lodge and so form a more efficient bridge than the tie itself.

The design of the ties should, therefore, prevent water from running along them by incorporating a drip in the centre of the tie, while at the same time affording the minimum lodgement for pats of mortar. Three types of tie aimed to satisfy these requirements are specified in BS 1243 : 1964. These are illustrated in diagram D.3.04/7.

When used, the ties must not be allowed to slope towards the inner

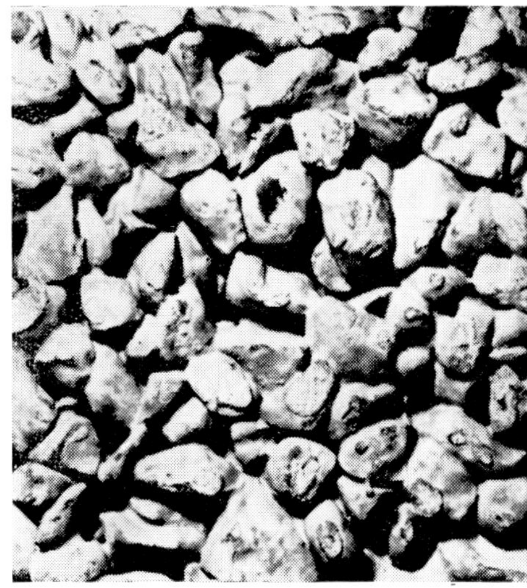

*A close-up view of no-fines concrete illustrating its open texture (Courtesy: George Wimpey and Co. Ltd.)*

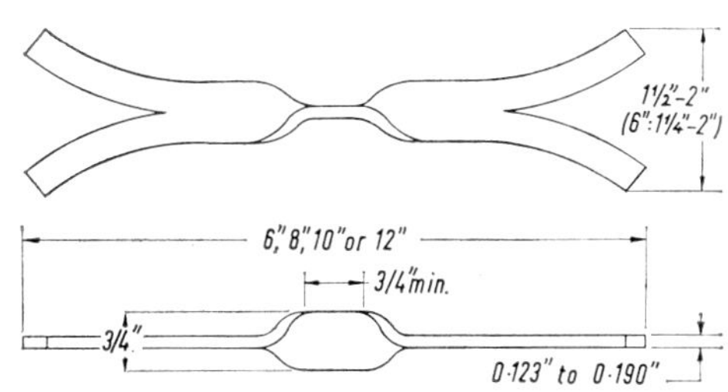


VERTICAL TWIST STRIP TYPE WALL TIE

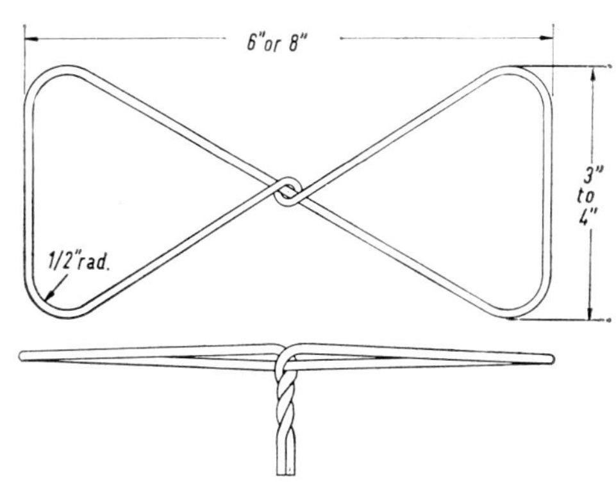


BUTTERFLY WIRE TYPE WALL TIE

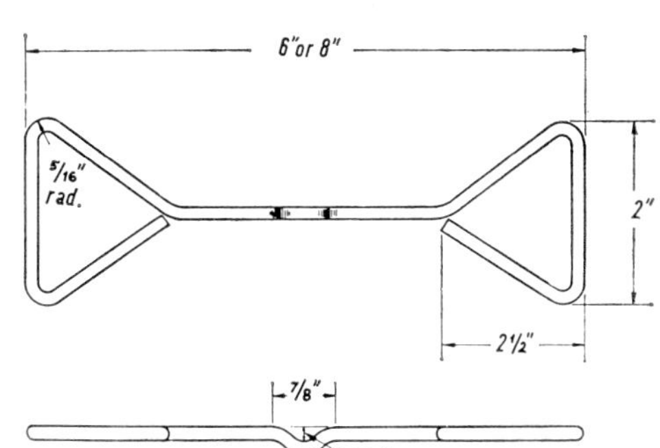


DOUBLE-TRIANGLE WIRE TYPE WALL TIE

*D.3.04/7*
*Three types of cavity wall ties specified in BS 1243: 1964 (It has been considered inappropriate to convert the original imperial dimensions)*

*An indication of the care that should be exercised in both design and construction of monolithic reinforced concrete solid walling which is to be left 'fair-faced' may be obtained from the excellent description of the concrete work and finishes used in the construction of the Wolfson Institute, Hammersmith Hospital, W.12 (Architects: Lyons, Israel and Ellis), published in *Architectural Design*, pp. 355–356, August, 1961. Preceding pages have many illustrations of the walling as executed.

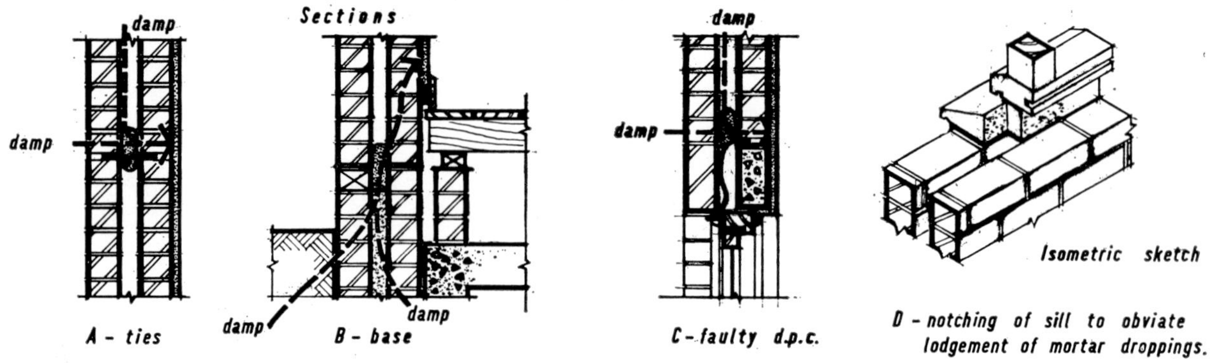


(1) MORTAR DROPPINGS BRIDGING THE CAVITY.

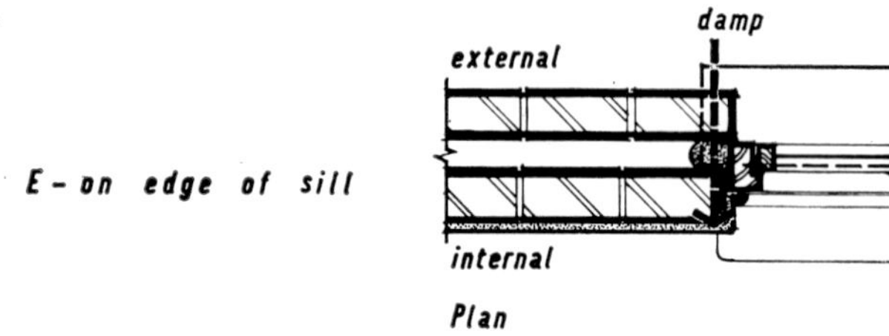


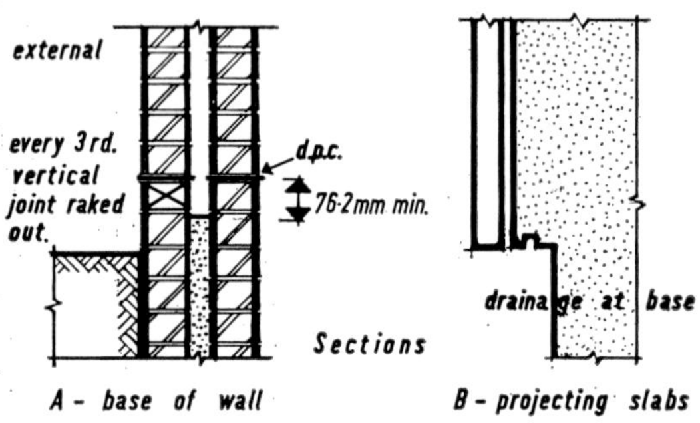


(2) OUTLETS FOR DRAINAGE.

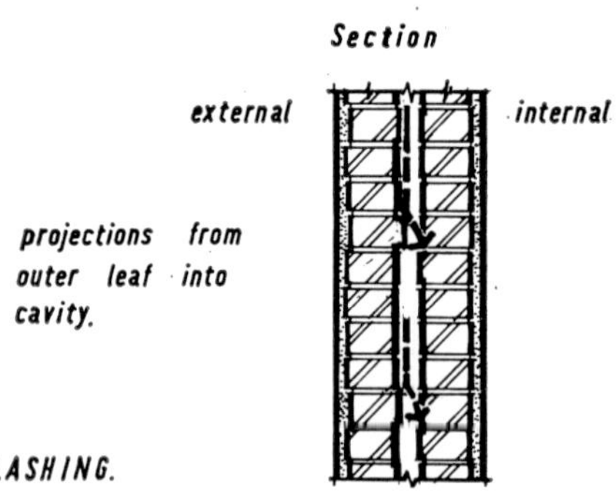


(3) SPLASHING.

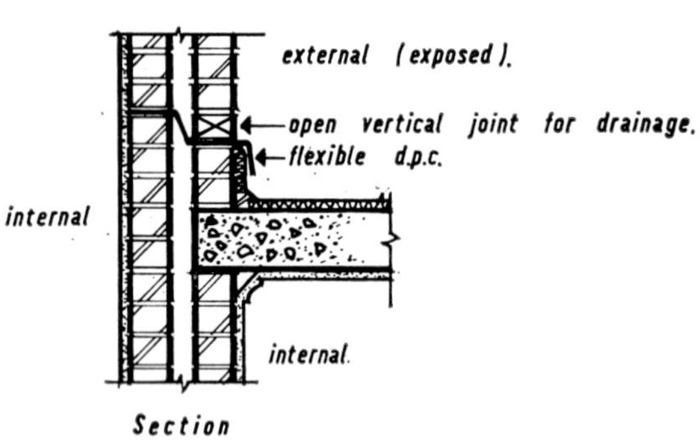


(4) CHANGE OF FUNCTION.

Scale : 0 500 1000 mm.

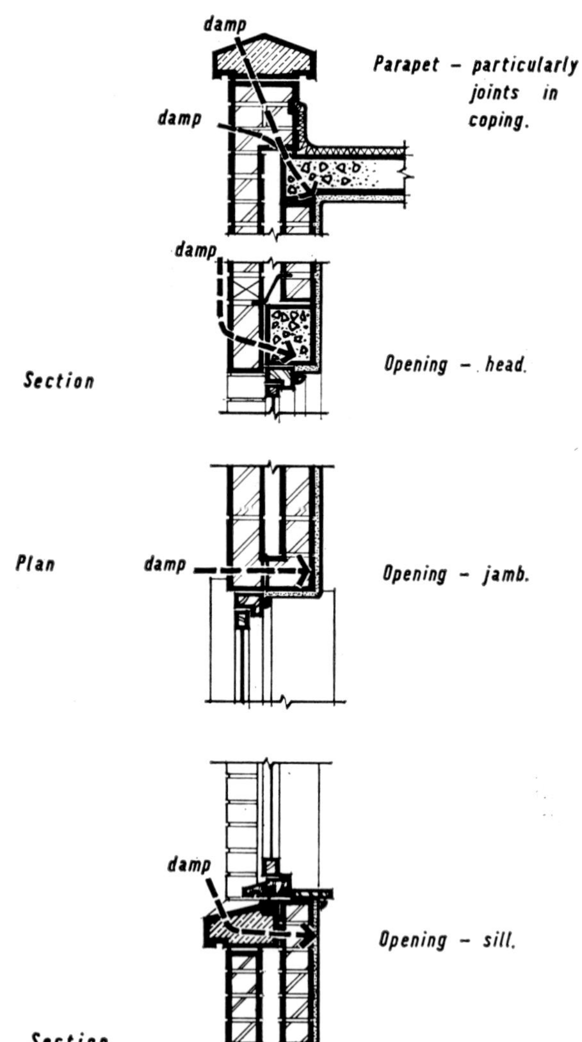


(5) CLOSURE OF THE CAVITY.

*D.3.04/8 (opposite)*
*Basic analysis of the significance of common details in cavity walling. (Read with text (b) 'Practical significance')*

leaf. For durability they should be of non-corroding metal.*

*Mortar droppings*

Mortar droppings may easily cause a bridge across the cavity and commonly occur (see diagram D.3.04/8 (1)) around ties, at the base of the wall or where unsuitable d.p.c. material has been used, resulting in a ledge or catchment area being formed.

During construction, mortar droppings can be reduced considerably by drawing a batten up the cavity as the wall is being built in order to catch the mortar. The use of the batten also prevents other rubbish from collecting at the base of the cavity. For added security, holes may be left in the wall so that the collected mortar can be removed. It is, of course, much easier to remove the mortar while it is still green.

Care is also required in the design of window sills so that they do not provide ledges upon which mortar droppings can collect, as shown in (1) D & E.

*Drainage*

Any water which may collect in the cavity must be allowed to discharge to the outside (diagram D.3.04/8 (2)). In brickwork open vertical joints at approximately 287mm centres, that is every third joint, are usually provided in the outer leaf. The same principle may be used with other forms of masonry. The bottom of the cavity should be at least 75mm below the level of any d.p.c. in the inner leaf. Where overhanging claddings are used it may be possible to leave the bottom of the cavity open for drainage purposes.

*Avoiding projections*

If the inner face of the outer leaf projects into the cavity there is a possibility that such projections will allow water trickling down the face to splash across the cavity (diagram D.3.04/8 (3)). They also provide ledges for collection of mortar droppings. For this reason it is unwise to specify Flemish bond for the outer leaf, as it is difficult to avoid the ends of snapped headers projecting into the cavity. For cavity walling this type of bonding is regarded as inefficient.

The design of the inner face of concrete or other cladding units is also important if splashing is to be avoided.

*Polypropylene wall ties, such as 'Kavi-Tie Type T1' (Rawlplug Company), have received an Agrément Certificate, 69/27. In the Agrément Board's opinion these ties are not subject to corrosion or decay and can withstand satisfactorily loads in excess of those likely to occur in practice.

*Change of function*

Where buildings of different heights adjoin one another a change of function of the outer leaf of the higher building takes place. Above the roof of the low building the outer leaf must perform as already outlined. However, below roof level the same leaf becomes an internal wall. Accordingly, provision must be made for water to be discharged through outlets above roof level. A flexible DPC material can conveniently be bent so as to form a sloping tray which will aid discharge of the water. (Diagram D.3.04/8 (4).)

*Openings, junctions and d.p.c.'s*

Bridging of the cavity by solid material usually presents problems at openings (doors and windows) and parapet walls when it is necessary to close the cavity. In some cases it may be possible to close the cavity of the jamb of the opening without using solid 'bridging' material, but nevertheless the head requires special consideration, particularly as regards drainage as, among other things, a horizontal ledge (base) is formed in the cavity. In the case of parapets special care is required in the detailing of the coping, if this bridges the cavity, as water must not penetrate joints or run along the underside of the coping.

Details of the closure of the cavity which may result in water penetration are shown in diagram D.3.04/8 (5). In nearly all cases solutions require the use of d.p.c. material. The purpose of the drawings is to expose the problem only. The solutions are included under 'Damp-proof courses and membranes' later. Two points may be noted here. Firstly, the d.p.c.'s are usually required to be dressed carefully over at least two bends. If the material is not flexible enough or does not keep its shape, there is a danger of the formation of mortar bridges, as explained earlier. Secondly, as far as openings are concerned, an efficient damp-proof course over the head of the opening is essential.

Finally, it is important that, where either party walls or partitions meet a cavity wall, they should not make contact with the outer leaf.

(c) *Filling the cavity*

From all that has been said so far it would seem that there should be no justification at all for filling the cavity, as such filling would negate the whole purpose of the cavity. At one time attempts were made 'to improve' the rain resistance of cavity walls (presumably failures had been experienced because of poor workmanship) by filling the cavity with dense mortar. More recently, however, the cavity has been seen to be an ideal, if not convenient, space to incorporate additional thermal insulation. The insulation value of the air space is considered by some to be significantly reduced anyway by the ventilation provided by drainage outlets.

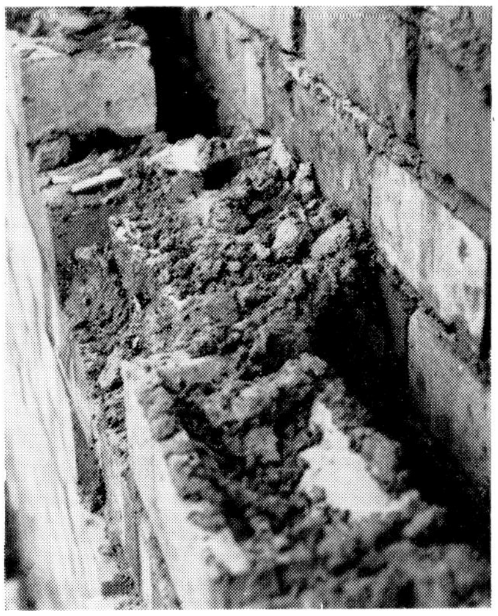

*Examples of bridges formed across a cavity by mortar droppings on the ties (see photographs below) and a partly built party wall (above). The 'column' to be seen in the photograph has been left in order to enable the rest of the party wall to be completed later on. Some fairly excessive projections of mortar into the cavity may also be seen*

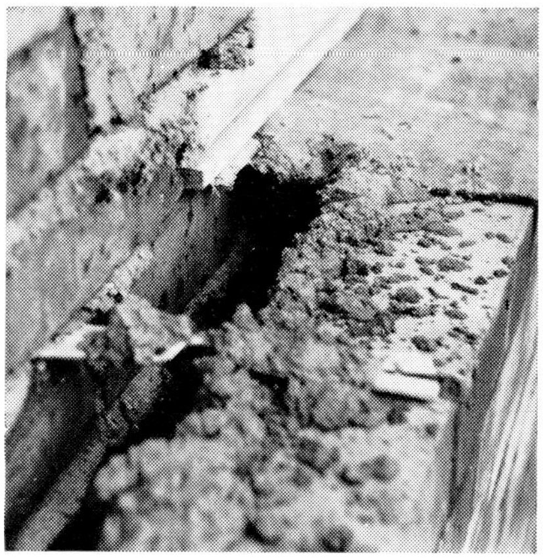

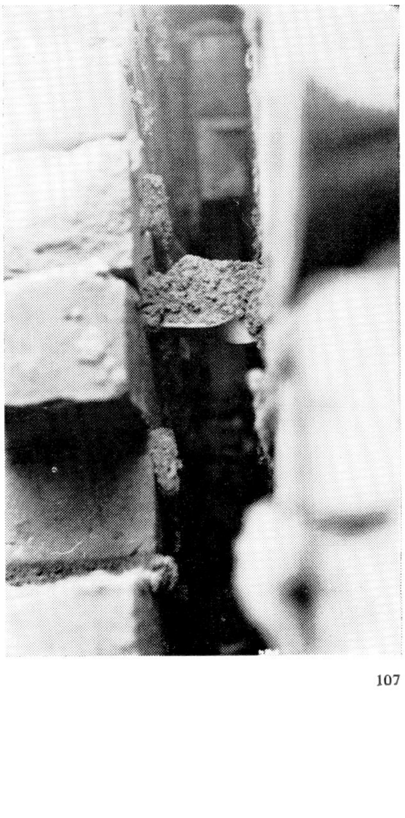

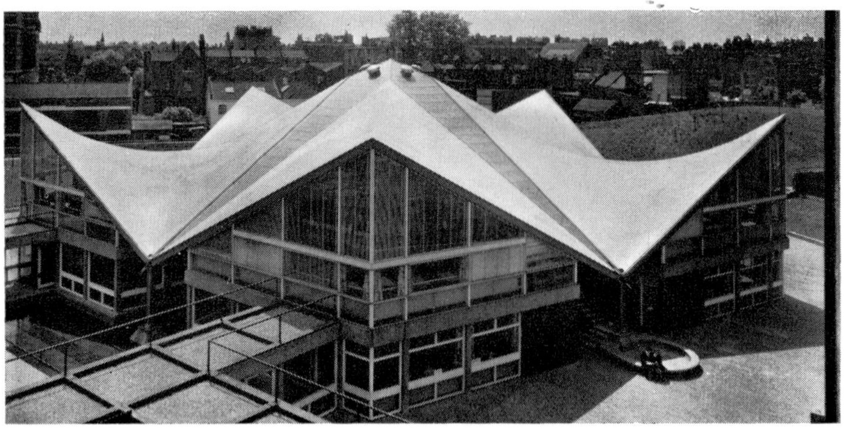

*'The actual external profile of a roof may vary from the relatively simple, as in a flat or pitched roof, to the highly complex, as in one of the many types of hyperbolic paraboloid roofs'. (Assembly hall, girls' school, Southwark, London, S.E.1. Architects: Chamberlin, Powell and Bon)*

Whatever the reasons for wanting to fill the cavity, it is still difficult, in the face of the success as regards resistance to rain penetration of no-fines concrete, the V-brick, etc., to condemn the practice out of hand. However, at the same time, filling of the cavity cannot be recommended unconditionally.

The chief requirement of any material used as a filling is that it should not be capable of transmitting water. Some materials may be treated,* prior to filling, with a water repellent substance, thus preventing any capillary action. Resistance to water penetration can only last for as long as the water repellant remains effective. Long-term durability, say up to 50 years, of substances which may be used is still unknown. The use of foamed plastics, such as urea formaldehyde, for example, which can be injected into the cavity, presents an anomaly. Once the foam has solidified it is greasy in nature and thus provides considerable resistance to capillary action. However, it is possible that fissures may develop through the thickness of the material. If these occur in a downward direction, then the greasy nature of the material cannot prevent penetration by water, when water trickles down the inner face of the outer leaf. It has been stated recently that modern manufacturing techniques have virtually eliminated fissuring of the material.† Apparently the material has also 'given full satisfaction under all conditions'.

While detailed results of investigations are not readily available, it would seem reasonable to assume that the filled cavity, properly executed, is likely to afford satisfactory resistance to rainwater penetration in all but severe conditions of exposure. For other conditions of exposure the wall will probably behave very much in the same way as a solid wall of the same thickness.

*References to laboratory tests of cavity filling, with water-repellent treated nodules of glass silk fibre, is given in *Principles of Modern Building—Vol. 1*, HMSO, 3rd Ed., p. 205, 1959.

†Reference: Diamant, R. M. E., *Thermal and Acoustic Insulation of Buildings*, Iliffe Books Ltd., pp. 121–122, 1965. A description of the properties and method of application of urea formaldehyde foam is given on pp. 214–217.

## Roofs

In simple terms a roof may be defined as a covering to a building. The nature of this covering which, in general terms, would include the exposed finish and the roof structure may, subject to the functional requirements which must be satisfied, be complex in form or require the composite use of materials with differing properties. Among functional requirements which have come to play an increasingly important part is thermal insulation. Composite coverings including an insulant are among recent developments. The actual external profile of a roof may vary from the relatively simple, as in a flat or pitched roof, to the highly complex, as in one of the many types of hyperbolic paraboloid roofs. In fact, the permutations of the planes which roofs may have are innumerable. The associated methods of construction may also vary in their complexity.

Whatever the form or functional requirements of a roof may be, the primary means of excluding rainwater is through the use of *essentially thin coverings* which, if external wall terms were used, would be described as claddings. The main structure, substructure and associated methods of fixing are, of course, important relative to the exclusion of rainwater, insofar as they must maintain the roof covering in position. Unlike external walls, where the whole thickness of a construction, incorporating where necessary internal drainage, may be used to exclude rainwater, roofs must rely on the exposed thin covering to resist rainwater penetration. The employment of a secondary means of defence behind the covering or within the thickness of the structure is generally not possible nor practicable. It may be noted here that the practice of incorporating a waterproof lining behind cladding units, such as tiles or slates, in pitched roofs is aimed to seal the roof against penetration of fine snow through the interstices of the units and is not intended to provide a secondary means of defence. Misunderstanding of the primary function of this lining has often led to the failure of a roof to exclude rainwater. Systems of internal drainage within the construction, particularly in flat roofs, are intended to cope with the problems of entrapped water, including interstitial condensation. These systems, described later under 'Entrapped water', are also not intended as secondary means of defence against the penetration of rainwater.

In the present context the use of the term 'roof' is being restricted to the coverings or claddings used to exclude rainwater and fine snow. The exclusion of condensation is dealt with under *4.00 Heat and its effects*. The nature of the coverings used may vary from completely impervious materials to relatively impermeable porous materials. Although the principles of complete prevention or controlled penetration previously outlined under 'External walls' are also applicable to roofs, the detailed application of these principles is substantially different. Traditional roofing practice has tended to divide roofs into two types, namely flat and pitched, each of which has led to the use of certain materials in specific ways. The flexible, completely impervious materials and liquid applications are generally associated with flat roofs, while rigid tiles or sheets with pitched roofs, although flexible materials may also be used as a covering for the latter. There are certain general aspects which are common to all types of roof. It is, therefore, convenient to deal with roofs under three headings, namely, (1) General considerations, (2) Flat roofs, and (3) Pitched roofs. Under the last two headings the use of specific materials or distinct groups of materials are discussed separately.

### 1. General aspects

Despite the wide variety of materials available as roof coverings, plus the variety of possible inclinations, there are basically two ways in which a satisfactory roof can be produced. In the *first* method an impervious membrane covering can be applied to a flat or nearly flat surface; in the *second* a series of relatively thin overlapping units which may not necessarily be impervious can be laid on a slope.

Flat roofs are usually covered with asphalt, several layers of bitumen felt, sheet metal or, as more recently, several layers of plastics-based felts and applied liquid coatings also plastics-based. A characteristic of flat roofs is that all movement joints and discontinuities are made to stand above the general level of the covering. Furthermore, all the coverings used have to be fully supported.

Pitched roofs may also be covered with the same materials used in flat roofs. However, two groups of units are more commonly encountered, both

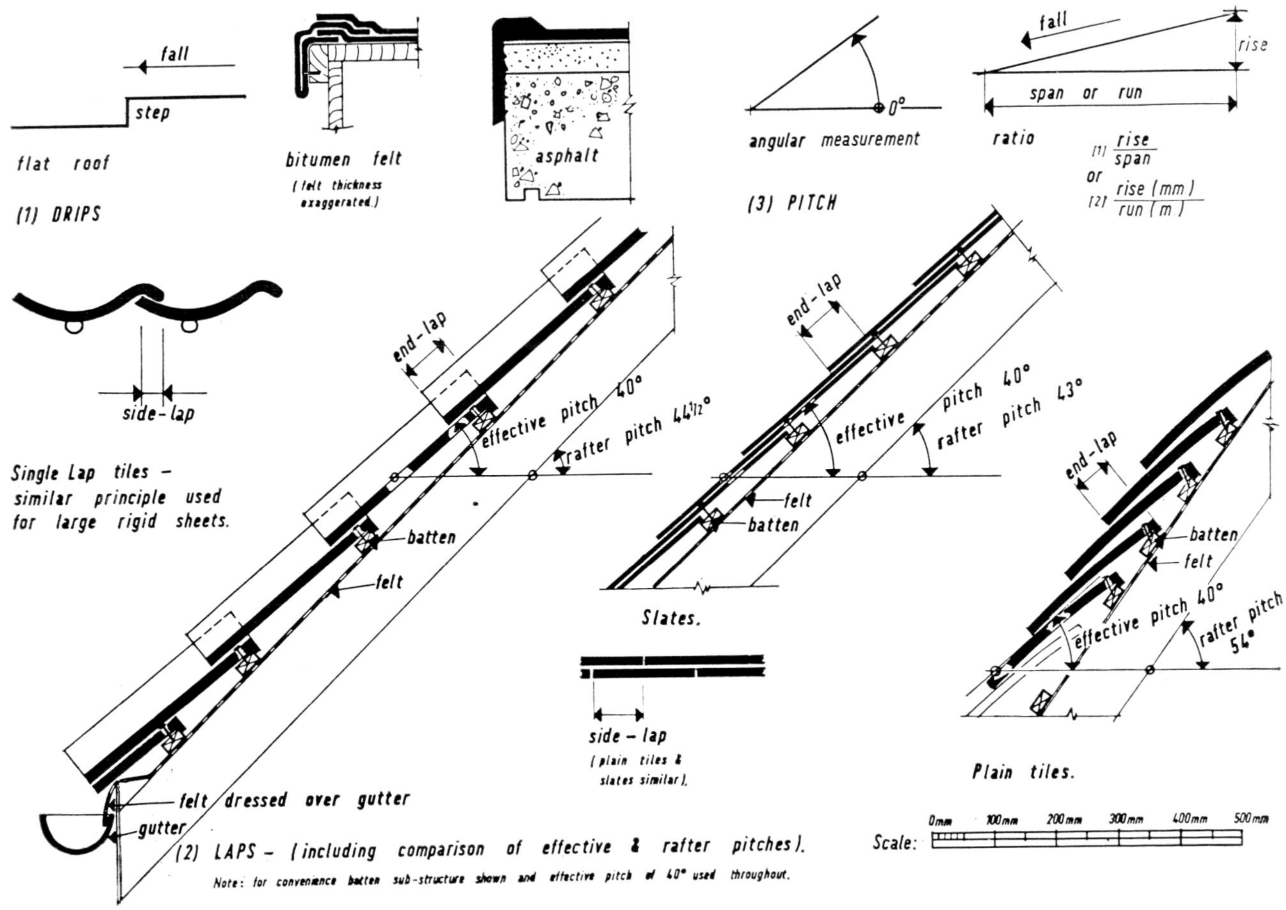


*D*.3.04/9
*Illustrations of some terms applicable to roofs*

of which only require support at predetermined distances.† The groups are (1) the small units such as tiles, slates or shingles, or (2) the large units such as corrugated asbestos-cement or metal sheets. Glass in patent glazing and corrugated plastics sheets may also be used, but are usually restricted for use where daylight through the roof is of particular significance. Among these materials some are completely impervious or very nearly so, while others are porous. The latter which include clay tiles and asbestos-cement sheets are impermeable enough because their fine pore structure does not allow water to pass through them readily under the small pressures that are set up. This takes into account the manner in which they are used.

From these basic principles a number of different permutations in terms of the type of covering and slope, if any, which may be used, can be developed. Some of the more important detailed factors which must be taken into account in the application of these basic principles are discussed separately under various headings below. Also included is a selection of terms.

†Thatch roof covering is not considered in this study at all. Patent glazing, although referred to is not considered in detail, but see 'Joint Design' later.

(a) *Selected terms*
Misunderstanding can sometimes arise when certain terms are applied to roof coverings. Among other things the same term may not have the same meaning for different coverings. Definitions and, where appropriate, descriptions of selected terms are given below. All terms marked with an asterisk (*) have been taken from BS 2717 : *Glossary of terms applicable to roof coverings.*

DRIP—(diagram D.3.04/9 (1) ). Only applicable to flat roofs and gutters, but may have three meanings subject to roof covering.

(i) For flexible sheets other than bituminous felt:— a step formed in a flat roof or gutter across the direction of fall;* (ii) for bitumen felt:— a strip of roofing felt or metal fixed under or between the layers of the roof covering at eaves or verges and turned down;* and (iii) for asphalt:— the undercut edge of an asphalt apron,* i.e. applied vertically to the fascia or overhang of a roof.

FLAT ROOF (known in Scotland as a *platform roof*):— a roof the pitch of which is 10 degrees or less to the horizontal.*

LAP: (diagram (D.3.04/9 (2) ). The term is generally restricted to pitched roofs although it may also apply to flat roofs with asphalt or bitumen felt coverings and gutters, flashings, ridge coverings, etc., in flexible metal sheets. The term generally used in connection with the latter is 'laps' (or passings). In general, lap can be considered as the amount by which a sheet or layer overlaps the sheet or layer below it. The precise method of measuring the effective length covered relative to the disposition of the superimposed sheets or layers varies with the covering being used. The variations which are important are noted below. Despite this, a distinction must first be made between *end-laps* (sometimes also known as 'head-laps') measured in the direction of the slope or fall and *side-laps* measured across the slope or fall. The diagram illustrates these for small units—the principles are also applicable to large units. It should be noted that in trade and other literature the term 'lap' is often not specifically qualified. In these cases 'end-lap' is usually implied.

(i) Slates, plain tiles and shingles: *End-lap:* The amount by which a slate, plain tile or shingle overlaps the course next but one below it.* There are thus three thicknesses at the lap. *Side-lap:* The amount by which a slate, plain tile or shingle overlaps the course below it. There are thus two thicknesses at the lap. (There are some detailed variations in the case of shingles, see '3 Pitched roofs', later.)

(ii) Single-lap tiles: *End-lap:* The amount by which a tile overlaps the course below it. *Side-lap:* As for end-lap, but it should be noted that the amount of the lap is usually dictated by the design of the tile, the ends of which are specially profiled to overlap. For this reason side-lap is seldom specified.

(iii) Corrugated or profiled sheets (large units): *End- and side-lap* as for single-lap tiles. With corrugated sheets it is possible to vary the side-lap; most specially profiled sheets have specific side-laps to suit the sheet.

(iv) Asphalt: The extent by which abutting edges in successive coats of asphalt are staggered.* Qualification of the lap is usually not relevant.

(v) Bitumen felt: A limited range of cover is implied and 'lapped joint' is sometimes used instead of lap. A lapped joint is, therefore, a joint formed by overlapping adjoining widths of felt by about 50mm or 75mm.

PITCH (diagram D.3.04/9 (3) ). The angle of inclination with the horizontal of the rafters or substructure surface on which the roof coverings are laid.* Angular measurements are usually restricted to pitched roofs. For flat roofs the pitch, often known as the 'fall', is expressed either as a ratio of the rise to the span (e.g. 1 : 40) or as a ratio of the rise in millimetres to a 1 metre run (e.g. 25mm/1m). The angular inclination with the horizontal of both the examples given in brackets is the same, namely approximately 1·5 degrees.

It should be noted that with pitched roofs there is likely to be a significant difference, particularly with slates, tiles and shingles, between the pitch of the rafters or substructure and the pitch of the covering, which has been defined as the 'effective pitch'. In general, the effective pitch is *less* than the pitch of the rafters or substructure (see diagram D.3.04/9(2) ). This is due to the tilt which takes place when the units overlap one another. The degree of difference between the two pitches will be governed by the shape, size and method of laying the units. The degree of difference for single lap of tiling is between that for plain tiling (greatest difference) and slating (least difference) for the same effective pitch. Because of the variations which can occur with all these small units, it is far more realistic and safer to regard recommended minimum pitches as the effective pitch. In this account must also be taken, particularly in severely exposed cases, of the reductions in the effective pitch which must occur in particular zones of a pitched roof (eaves which have the greatest accumulative run-off and other abutments). As will be seen later, pitch does play an extremely important part in the prevention of rainwater penetration.

PITCHED ROOF: A roof the pitch of which is greater than 10 degrees to the horizontal.

(b) *Exposure*

It is perhaps axiomatic that the basic conditions of exposure on any particular site will be more severe for roofs than for walls. However, differences in the degree of exposure will also vary according to the inclination of a roof.

In addition to exposure to rainwater, solar radiation with its attendant effects on durability and thermal movement on the one hand and frost action on the other must be taken into account. *Thermal movement,* which is discussed more fully in *4.00 Heat and its effects,* is particularly important. In many instances provision for expansion is fundamental if deformation and/or cracking of the covering is to be avoided. The methods used may at one extreme employ expansion joints through the complete structure, including the covering, or at the other extreme simply allow the covering alone to move. Whatever provision is made, it is, nevertheless, important that special consideration be given to detail so that penetration by rainwater is not possible. Defects in roofs leading to penetration by rainwater, it should be noted, are often caused due to insufficient care having been taken either with the problem as a whole or detail in particular.

As in the case of external walls, exposure of roofs to rainwater implies driving-rain. Unlike external walls which may, in fact, be sheltered, particularly in low-rise buildings, by overhanging eaves or other projections, roofs cannot, to any significant degree, be sheltered by details of building design. Some local shelter may be afforded by chimneys or by parapet walls in flat roofs, but this is hardly likely to make any real difference to the problem in general. In fact, abutments of roofs with projections of this kind (and others may also be included) require special 'sealing' in order to prevent penetration of rainwater at the junction of the two elements.

Conditions of exposure have, as in the case of external walls, been classified into three classes. For roofs these are 'sheltered', 'normal' and 'exposed'. As a guide, the classification of sites as shown in diagram D.3.02/2 (p. 35) is useful for comparative purposes. However, in addition to the driving-rain aspects associated with wind, account has also to be taken, as explained in *3.02 Exposure* (p. 32), of the fact that wind may drive water uphill into joints or over upstands and that it also exerts a pressure. The degree of exposure which should be taken for design purposes is, at present, largely a matter of experience. To this extent *local practice* with any particular covering should always be taken into account. It is recommended that when in doubt manufacturers' advice should be sought. Recommended minimum pitches together with associated laps for particular coverings, it should be noted, are usually given, unless otherwise stated, for normal and sheltered sites. An increase in pitch and/or lap is, therefore, required if the covering is to be used on an exposed site.

The prevailing direction of wind-driven rain may be significant in the determination of the degree of exposure, particularly in pitched roofs. In addition to basic exposure, side-laps will be more secure against rainwater penetration if the 'open ends' of the laps face away from the prevailing direction of the wind-driven rain. As already noted, wind may blow rainwater already flowing over the covering into joints or over upstands (see also '(c) Flow' below).

Although it may be a little misleading to suggest priorities regarding the care which should be taken in establishing as accurately as possible conditions of exposure for any element in a building so that the necessary precautions can be taken to exclude rainwater, it should be emphasised that, in the case of roofs, leakage, even if it is *slight,* can lead to serious damage. In this sense, external walls are not normally as vulnerable.

(c) *Flow*

The flow pattern of rainwater over a roof covering is not only affected by the action of wind, but also by the exposed profile and pitch of the covering.

Roof coverings which present a more or less plain face across the pitch, as in the case of slates, plain tiles or shingles, allow the action of wind to cause rainwater to flow across the units in a diagonal direction. This type of flow has been aptly described as 'diagonal creep.'* The angle of creep widens as the pitch decreases. The wider the angle of creep the more vulnerable the side-laps of the units used to penetration by rainwater. As the side-laps of these particular types of unit may be increased by the use of wider units, wider units and thus wider side-laps are imperative at lower pitches.

Diagonal creep may also occur in other types of roof coverings. However, with such coverings as single-lap types (including corrugated sheets) and flexible metal sheets, regularly spaced ridges are formed, as an integral part of the design of the coverings, in the direction of the fall of the roof. The effect of these ridges is to form channels along which rainwater can flow. Although diagonal creep can still occur within the width of the channel, its effect is reduced, while the vulnerable side of the channel could be the covered side of the lap. Arrangement of the side-lap to suit exposure to wind blown water may not always be possible. Where side-laps cannot be increased nor sealed recommended minimum pitches cannot, without risk, be lowered.

The problem of diagonal creep in

*Gauldie, W. S., *Pathology of pitched roof coverings, The Architects' Journal,* pp. 981–84, May 2, 1962.

flat roofs with coverings of asphalt or bitumen felt (and other types) is not as important as the covering is either continuous or fully sealed. In felt work added security is provided by laps.

(d) *Drainage*

The whole design of a roof must ensure that rainwater is either drained or shed, *clear of the building*, through gutters and downpipes. Gargoyles may, within limits, also be used proided they ensure that water is shed clear of the building. Rainwater run-off from a roof should not, wherever possible, increase the exposure of the external walls beneath it. Hence the emphasis on draining and shedding rainwater clear of the building.

The rate at which rainwater should flow over a roof is largely dependent on the type of covering and/or the nature of the joints used. Porous materials should not be allowed to absorb excessive quantities of water; the rate of flow must be regulated by the pitch. Although rate of flow is not important where completely impervious and jointless coverings, such as asphalt, are used, it is nevertheless advisable to ensure that adequate falls are provided in order to avoid 'ponding', when the rain has ceased. 'Ponding' which is also relevant when felt is used may lead to deterioration of the covering, particularly from solar radiation.

(e) *Jointing*

As in the case of external walls, joints are a significant feature of all roof coverings except asphalt and applied coatings. Joints are primarily necessitated by the limitation of the sizes of units or sheets available, although, as already noted under '(b) Exposure', special joints may be required to deal with thermal movement. However, unlike walls, joint design in roofs has been traditionally developed without the use of mortars or sealants. Special zones such as ridges and hips of pitched roofs with tile or slate coverings are the exceptions. In fact, where mortar has been used to seal the joints between tiles or slates, water penetration has, due to the porosity of the mortar, usually been encouraged rather than resisted. Joints in roofs are, therefore, characterised by their 'dryness'.

The design of these dry joints vary according to the covering used. The lap is the basic method used in pitched roofs, while the upstand and welt which require bending and/or folding down is common in flexible metal sheets used for flat roofs. (The same basic upstands are also employed when flexible sheets cover pitched roofs.) Illustrations of some of the more common joints are included under '(2) Flat roofs' and '(3) Pitched roofs' later.

*Lapped joint*

The effectiveness of the lapped joint in resisting rainwater penetration is primarily dependent on the relationship between the extent of the lap and the pitch.* The nature of the material (permeability is important in porous materials) and the manner in which it may be fixed are also important. *Fixing holes,* particularly when they are concealed may reduce the effective length of the lap. It should be remembered that fixing nails do not completely seal the fixing holes. Although in general terms it is true to say that the greater the laps the less the pitch may be, the actual design of the laps (end and side) is significant. Various types of laps incorporating specially designed grooves for the end-laps and other methods of interlocking for the side-laps have been developed so as to allow lower pitches for slates and tiles. In the absence of collective experience of coverings used at pitches lower than those normally recommended, CP 142 advises that satisfactory behaviour over a period of 15 years or more should be an adequate safeguard.

Lapped joints, it may be noted, are sometimes used with flexible metal sheets, notably lead.

*Upstand*

The size of the upstand and welt associated, in various forms, with flexible metal sheets can be adjusted to suit the effective condition of exposure, in which the fall of the roof will be important.

A feature of the various joints used with flexible metal sheets is that they are virtually air-tight.

*Sealing*

Very few, if any, of the units or sheets used with dry lapped joints are air-tight. On the other hand, some may allow fine snow to penetrate through the joint.

In the case of tiling and slating, the joints should not, except possibly in special circumstances, be sealed† with mortar or, as it is more correctly termed 'torching' (lime mortar containing hair). The principle upon which the roof can be sealed relies on the creation of a pressure barrier behind the units, by lining the underside with an air-tight layer. Traditionally, close boarding was commonly used, but this has now been largely replaced by the use of a layer of sarking felt. Where sarking felt is used it is important to ensure that it is carried over the gutters so

*In another context the amount of laps, both end- and side-laps, affects the quantity of units needed to cover a particular area of roof. Thus, a desire to reduce cost by reducing the laps can seriously militate against the requirements of resistance to rain penetration. In many cases reduction of the laps proves to be a false economy.

†In view of the success of many mortar sealed slate and tiled roofs in preventing penetration by rainwater, opinion is still divided on the desirability of using 'torching'. In the context of present-day functional requirements it would seem to be safer to avoid 'torching' whenever possible. This view is taken throughout this study for small units.

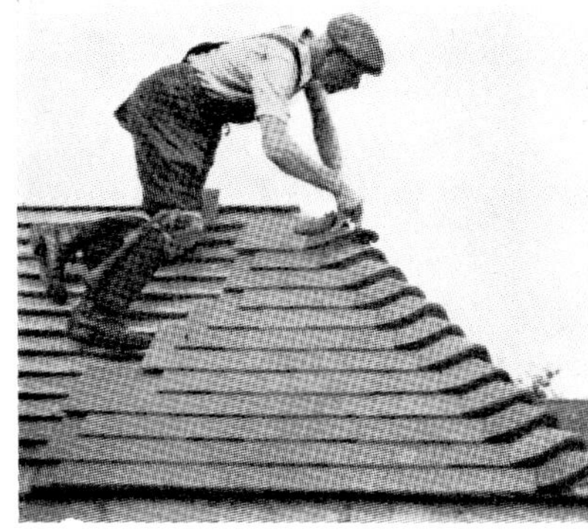

*'Joints in roof coverings are characterised by their dryness'. Special areas or conditions may require a jointing medium or sealant. The photograph above shows pointing of the hip in a plain tiled roof. Valleys require special treatment if they are to remain watertight. The photograph below shows the use of special tiles in plain tiling. In the absence of 'specials', a gutter in flexible or continuous materials is formed at the valley. (Photographs by courtesy of the National Federation of Clay Industries)*

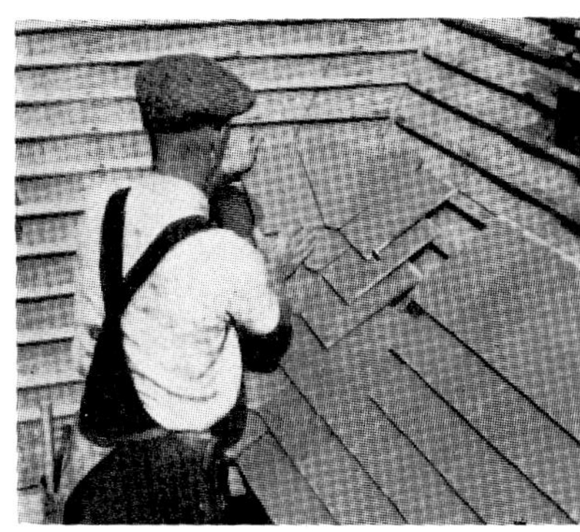

that any snow which may penetrate at the joints may subsequently, on thawing, have an outlet to the drainage system and not drip into the building.

The use of *non-hardening sealants* is, therefore, restricted to the large rigid coverings such as corrugated asbestos-cement, aluminium or galvanised iron. In order to be able to reduce the pitch of these coverings, sealants have been recommended for both end- and side-laps sometimes in addition to increasing the laps. Sealants may, of course be used primarily to ensure dust-tightness.

*Abutments*

Wherever a covering meets an element which projects above the level of the roof, special treatment of the joint at the abutment is required. In some cases this may require the use of a more flexible and impervious material than that used for the general covering. Consideration of these special conditions are included under 'Damp-proof courses'.

It may be noted here that special gutters using flexible or continuous impervious materials are usually re-

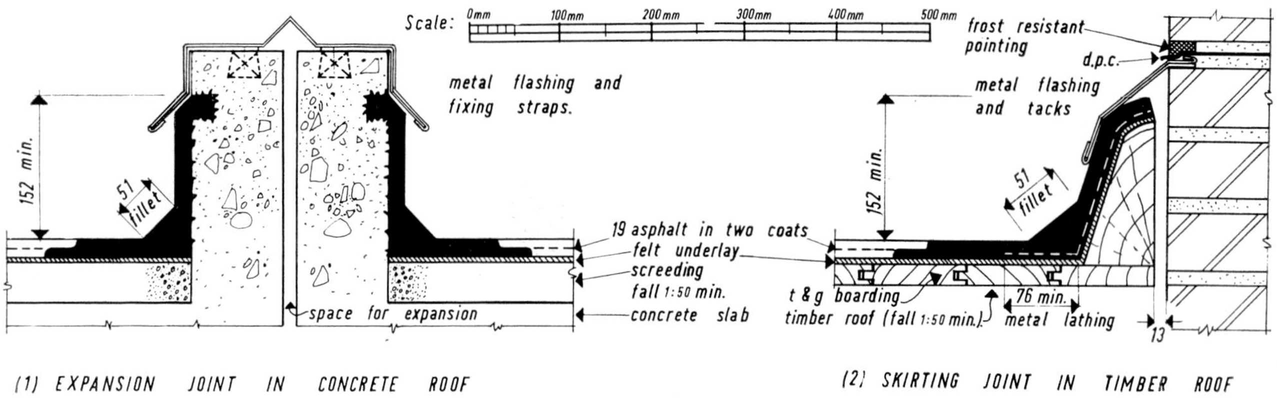


*D.3.04/10*
*Basic methods of sealing an expansion joint in roof with asphalt covering. Similar principles applicable to bitumen felt—dimensions in mm*

quired where two inclined roof surfaces with rigid coverings meet at a re-entrant angle—valley for example.

(f) *Handling and fixing*

In addition to correct detailing, good workmanship, as in all building practice, is important in roof work. Some coverings, particularly asphalt, bituminous and other felts and flexible sheet metal, require the use of experienced specialist firms who have trained craftsmen and the proper tools and appliances. Craftsmen with a different training are required for the rigid small or large units. Nowadays these too may be confined in certain areas to specialist firms.

The relatively thin nature of all the materials used, plus the fact that many of the small and large units are comparatively brittle, requires special care in both handling and fixing. In this it has to be remembered that the material provides the chief means of exclusion of rainwater. Thus, satisfactory joints and other detailed points are of little avail if the coverings is itself cracked or torn through mishandling. Some coverings may not be specifically designed to take foot traffic and may, therefore, have to be adequately bridged during laying or subsequent maintenance.

Excessive bending of some materials during fixing can eventually lead to a delay in the flow of water over the covering and thus increase the risk of penetration at the joints.

**2. Flat roofs**

The minimum pitch for all roof coverings except asphalt should be not less than 1 : 60 (i.e. about 16 mm/m). For asphalt the pitch should not be less than 1 : 50 if 'ponding' is to be avoided.

(a) *Asphalt*

Apart from the more recent liquid coatings based on plastics, asphalt is the only coating applied in the liquid state and which, when solidified, provides a completely continuous impervious membrane. Two separate layers of asphalt which bond together are normally laid; the joints between the sections are, however, laid staggered to effect a lap and thereby to minimise the risk of a leak through both layers. Added security at internal angles (junction of horizontal and vertical) is provided by fillets.

Asphalt should not be in direct contact with the substructure as movement of the latter may crack the asphalt. It is, therefore, important that there is a felt underlay, laid loose and with lapped joints, interspersed between the asphalt and the substructure. Where excessive movement of the substructure is anticipated and an expansion joint used, then the asphalt must be made discontinuous on either side of the joint and taken up a curb which is sealed by a flexible metal capping to prevent penetration of rainwater. A typical detail is shown in diagram D.3.04/10. Similar consideration is also required, when a timber substructure is used, at the junction of the roof and parapet walls, as illustrated in the same diagram.

(b) *Built-up bitumen felt*

Although composed of alternate layers of felt and bitumen, it is the bitumen which effects the waterproofing. In this country, where three layers of felt bonded with a minimum of hot bitumen is typical, emphasis is on the felt with the bitumen regarded as an adhesive. Lapping of the felt is, therefore, important. In the USA and some European countries, on the other hand, the roofing is regarded as one of bitumen with the felt providing layers of reinforcement. Thus five or more thin layers of felt are used, allowing the bitumen to form the major part of the roof covering.

Developments are still taking place in laying techniques. To this must be added the recent introduction of felts which are based on plastics.* Common defects in bitumen felt are either tearing or blistering. Both lead to penetration of rainwater.

Tearing is associated with the movement of the substructure. All felts will stretch a little under load without splitting. Continual movement cannot always be accommodated. Where movement in the substructure is slight, the felt should be left free of the deck for a short distance on each side of the line of movement, as shown in diagram D.3.04/11. Alternatives for moderate movement are also shown. Expansion joints through the structure may require the use of a solution similar to that used for asphalt.

(c) *Flexible sheet metal coverings*

The flexible sheet metal coverings used, namely lead, copper, zinc and aluminium, are all non-ferrous.

None of these coverings, because of their relatively large thermal movements, can be laid jointless. They are, therefore, laid in small sheets. The joint between each sheet must not only accommodate movement, but also prevent penetration by rainwater. Nearly all joints rely on the principle of interlocking. Typical side and end joints are illustrated in diagram D.3.04/12.

(d) *Applied liquids*

Recent developments in roof coverings include plastics membranes consisting of a mixture of vinyls which can be applied in liquid form (two or more coats) either by brushing or spraying. In some cases application is restricted to certain types of substructure. Various colours are available. As yet, the long-term performance of these coatings is not fully known.

**3. Pitched roofs**

Coverings commonly used for pitched roof fall into two categories, namely, (1) small units and (2) large rigid sheets. Both groups are characterised, in contrast to coverings used for flat roofs, by the fact that they only require support at predetermined distances. The size and distance apart of the supports vary basically according to the size/strength relationship of the units being fixed. As already noted, the fully supported roof coverings commonly used on flat roofs may also be used on pitched roofs. Details of joints, particularly with the flexible metal sheets, may be varied to suit the reduced exposure conditions, while other prac-

*Detailed consideration of the plastics-based felts is, in the absence of collective experience of their long-term performance, excluded here. However, the potential of these felts, better known simply as sheets, appears to be encouraging.

tical considerations have to be taken into account. These are noted later (b) (vi) ).

(a) *Small units*

There are three main types, namely, (1) slates (natural or reconstructed stone and asbestos-cement); (2) tiles (clay and concrete); and (3) shingles (oak and western red cedar). The supporting substructure is generally closely spaced. Bitumen felt may be cut into what are known as slates and tiles for use on pitched roofs. They have to be fully supported and are excluded from this part.

Where sarking felt (reinforced if spanning between rafters) is used underneath the units, it is important to note that it must be lapped at joints, carried down to the eaves and dressed over the gutter. This requirement should not detract from the basic reason for using the lining which is to prevent fine snow or air penetration through the interstices of the units. It is *not* intended as a secondary means of defence against penetration by rainwater. No lining should be used with shingles (see (iv) later).

With the exception of some special units and conditions, roof pitches for the small units are generally high, that is from 30 degrees and above. At these pitches *condensation* which may form on the underside of the units tends to run down the soffit of the units rather than drip inside the roof. Provided the joints are not sealed (one of the reasons against torching or other filling of the joints) the condensed water can find its way to the open by 'dropping' to the exposed unit below and then flowing down the external surface of the covering to the rainwater drainage system.

(i) *Slates.* (Diagram D.3.04/9 (2), p. 109. In *natural* slate there are a number of variations possible in both lap and pitch, due mainly to the fairly wide variation in sizes generally obtainable. Sizes are graded from 609·6mm × 254·0mm, the largest which may be conveniently handled, to 254mm × 152·4mm.

End-lap may be varied by the gauge of the battens from the formula

$$\text{Gauge} = \frac{\text{Length of slate—lap}}{2}$$

Side-lap must be varied by the width of the slate, bearing in mind that the side joints (random slating apart) which should be open to facilitate drainage should be placed as centrally as possible over the slate below.

For slates with width *less* than half their length, the end-lap should be not less than 76·2mm with a pitch of 35 degrees. The end-lap should be *increased* by not less than 6·4mm for each 5 degrees *reduction* of pitch.

An adequate side-lap may be provided for roofs of not less than 30 degrees pitch provided the minimum width of the slates is equal to half their length. Below a pitch of 30 degrees the slates should be wider than half their length, the proportion of width to

H

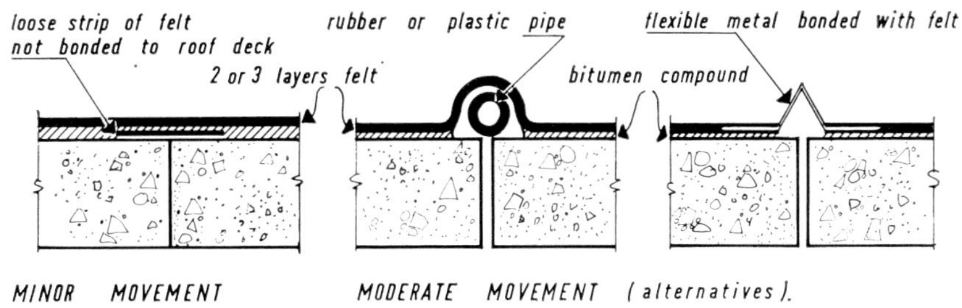


D.3.04/11
*Methods of providing for minor and moderate movements in concrete roofs with bitumen felt covering. See D.3.04/10 for principle to be used to provide for major movements*

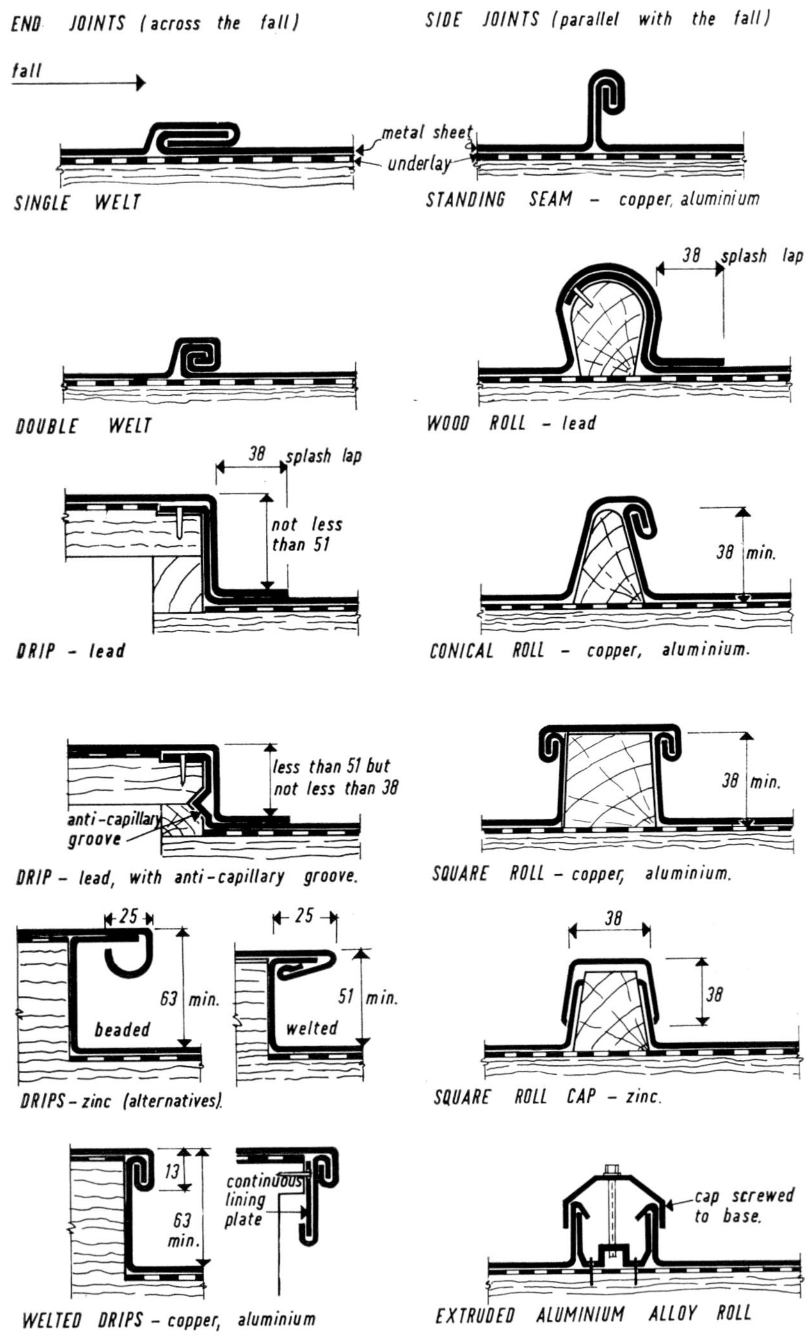


D.3.04/12
*Typical side- and end-joints used with flexible sheet metal roof coverings. Types illustrated are merely intended to indicate the basic principles employed —dimensions in mm*

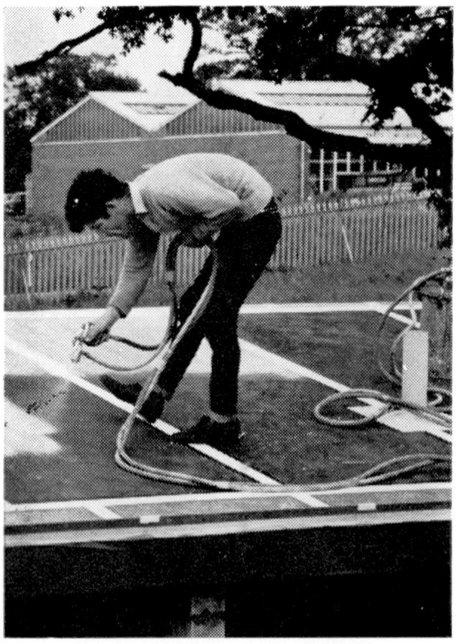

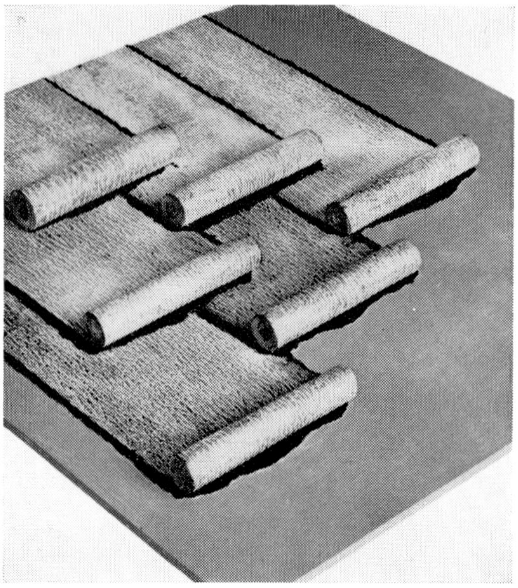

*Far left, applying one of the recent developments in liquid coatings, 'Trinasco' (vinyl copolymer), by spraying onto a 'Stramit' roof deck in an experimental house (Courtesy: ICI Ltd. and the Limmer & Trinidad Lake Asphalt Co. Ltd.). Left, model showing laying of three-layer built-up bitumen felt sheet roofing. Note method of side-lapping (Courtesy: Permanite Ltd.)*

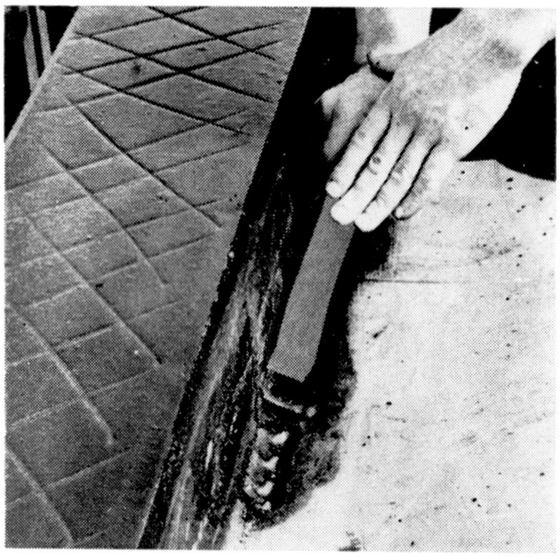

*For added protection against penetration by rainwater, fillets, 50mm wide in two coats, should be provided at all internal angles in asphalt work. The scored surface to the top of the asphalt to the parapet is necessary to increase the mortar bond in subsequent masonry work—or just the coping. Alternative to scoring is to lightly press in sand or grit while the asphalt is still hot (Courtesy: Permanite Ltd.)*

*Below, illustration of the relatively narrow widths used in all forms of sheet metal coverings—short length is, in this case, a design feature. Example shows standing seam in various stages of fabrication. Note staggering of welts which overcomes difficulties of effecting a multiple joint*

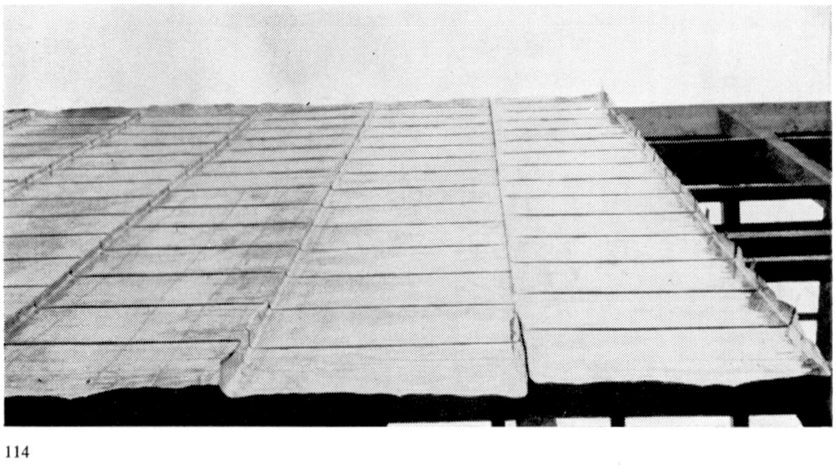

length being increased as the pitch is reduced.

Assuming the appropriate width/length ratios and the important fact that slate sizes need to be reduced as the pitch increases in order not to unduly load the fixing nails, the following can act as a useful guide:

| | | | | | |
|---|---|---|---|---|---|
| 152mm | width | 45 | degrees | min. | pitch. |
| 178mm | ,, | 40 | ,, | ,, | ,, |
| 203-254mm | ,, | 35 | ,, | ,, | ,, |
| 305-356mm | ,, | 30 | ,, | ,, | ,, |

In general, the use of *asbestos-cement* slates follows that for natural slate. Some variations may be required in terms of both lap and pitch for the diamond and honeycomb patterns which are available.

(ii) *Plain tiles.* (Diagram D.3.04/9(2).) Although the method of lapping plain tiles is similar to that used for slates, the pitch in normal conditions should not be less than 40 degrees and the end-lap not less than 63·5mm.

(iii) *Single-lap tiles.* (Diagram D.3.04/9(2).) Special cases apart, single-lap tiles should not be laid at a pitch less than 35 degrees. Unless the end-lap is fixed by the design of the tile, it should not be less than 76·0mm.

A special characteristic of single-lap tiles is that the dimensions of both end- and side-lap are usually fixed by the design of the tile. Some designs available are said to be suitable for pitches below 35 degrees ($17\frac{1}{2}$ degrees being the lowest quoted). As already noted, intending users are advised to satisfy themselves that tiles used at pitches below 35 degrees have behaved satisfactorily for 15 years or more.

(iv) *Shingles.* The detailed application of shingles (usually oak or western red cedar) is somewhat different from that used for the other small units. One of the fundamental differences is that neither boarding nor felt should be used underneath the shingles. The use of such linings prevents air circulation around the units and, if included, could hasten decay of the timber of which they are made. It may be noted here that shingles fit closely together, thus eliminating the likelihood of snow or air penetration.

Other differences are concerned with the method of laying and measuring end-lap. A typical section is illustrated in diagram D.3.04/13. It will be seen that the end-lap is measured through four thicknesses, while the exposed portion of the shingle is known as 'exposure' (sometimes also as 'gauge'). The minimum pitch for 127·00mm exposure (providing not less than three thicknesses in any part of the roof) is 30 degrees; a minimum pitch of 20 degrees may be used if the exposure is decreased to 95·25mm (providing not less than four thicknesses in any part of the roof). Oak shingles, unlike western red cedar, depend on a steep slope for durability—the pitch should not be less than 45 degrees.

Shingles are laid from random widths. The minimum side-lap is 38·1mm. Side joints between shingles should be between 6·3 and 9·5mm wide to allow for swelling.

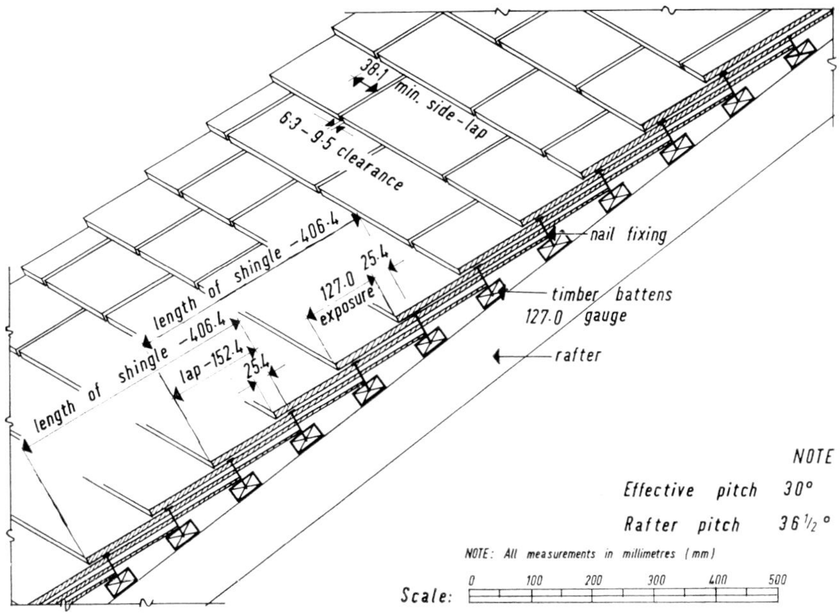


*D.3.04/13*
*Typical section of a pitched roof covered with shingles. Important: neither felt nor boarding should be used under the shingles*

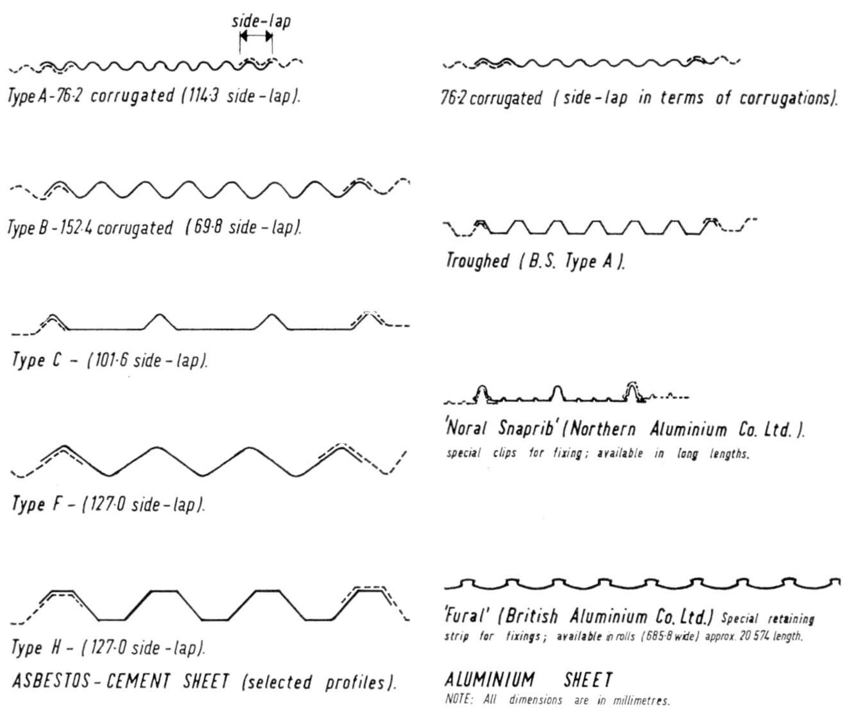


*D.3.04/14*
*Profiles of selected asbestos-cement and aluminium sheets. All sheets have been drawn to the same scale. For clarity, lapped joints have been exaggerated. For comparison, standard widths have been shown. Note that the side-laps indicated are not universally applicable —see text. Asbestos-cement sheet types taken from BS 690: 1963*

(b) *Large rigid sheets*

(See diagram D.3.04/14). The main characteristics of large rigid sheets, when compared to the small units, are: (1) corrugated or troughed sections; (2) light in weight and self-supporting over large spans (substructure is, therefore, comparatively widely spaced); (3) generally available in lengths up to 3·048m, although longer lengths may be obtained, with effective widths ranging from 0·610m upwards; (4) fewer end- and side-laps (with long sheets and short spans end-laps may be dispensed with completely); (5) materials are themselves impermeable; (6) fixing usually, but not always, exposed; (7) flatter minimum pitches (normal range from 15 to 25 degrees); and (8) more suited to covering large plain areas of roof.

The end-lap for pitches between 15 and 25 degrees is normally 152mm. This should be increased to 229mm (sometimes 305mm) for pitches flatter than 15 degrees. For added security, the end-laps should be sealed with a non-hardening sealant. The side-laps may, subject to the profile of the sheet, be varied—it is often specified in terms of the number of corrugations or troughs.

No underlay is required for exclusion of water, but may be provided for other functional requirements, e.g. thermal insulation, sound absorption or providing a level surface for decoration.

Rain penetration may occur at fixing holes as the sheets are usually secured by means of hook bolts or drive screws passed through the crown of the corrugations or troughs to be fixed to purlins below. Thus the holes through the sheeting should be waterproofed by means of bitumen or plastics washers. Breakdown of the fixing holes may also occur during use (metal sheets only) due to *corrosion* or (all sheets) due to insufficient allowance for *thermal movement*. (In practice most of the thermal movement can be accommodated by clearance of the fixing holes.)

Materials commonly used are:

(i) *Asbestos-cement sheets.* A wide variety of patterns are available in both corrugated and troughed sections. A pitch of between 22½ and 25 degrees is common for unsealed laps. Some patterns may be laid at extremely low pitches and may, therefore, be regarded as flat roof coverings. Sheets are normally available in lengths commencing at about 1·2192m and increasing in 152mm steps to a maximum of 3·0480m.

Hips, valleys and other junctions can be made weather-tight with the same material as a comprehensive range of flashing and weathering accessories is available.

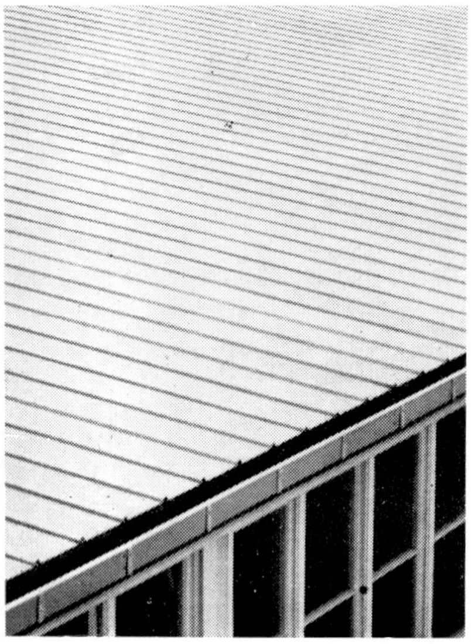

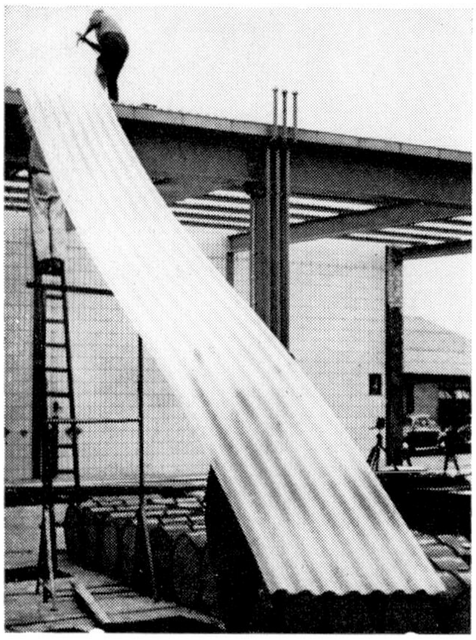

*Far left, 'Rigidal Lokroll', with concealed fixings (characterised by few end-laps. In the example shown there are no end-laps at all) (Courtesy: British Aluminium Co. Ltd.). Left, translucent corrugated PVC roof sheeting being fixed to a roof to a car service station (Courtesy: Marley Tile Co. Ltd.) Various profiles are available to match most profiled and corrugated opaque sheets (asbestos-cement and aluminium) for use as 'rooflights', without traditional rooflight junction problems*

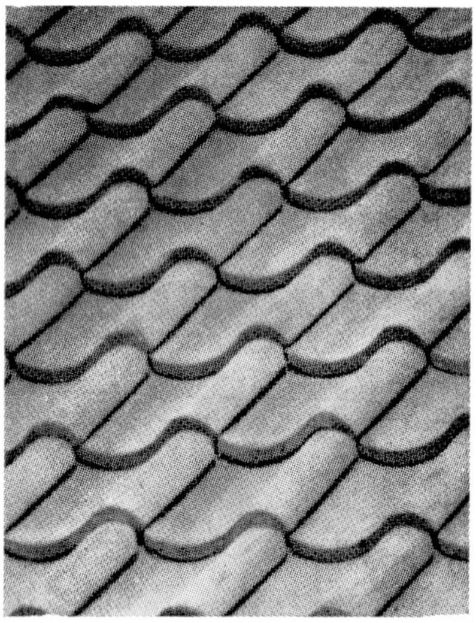

*An example of small unit covering—single lap tiling (Courtesy: National Federation of Clay Industries)*

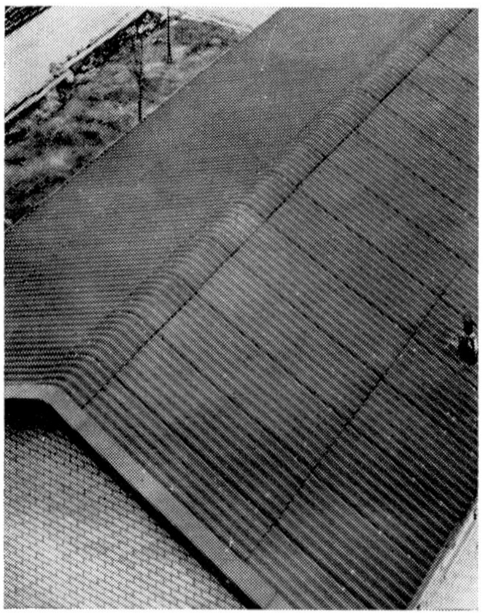

*Big Six asbestos-cement (Courtesy: Turners Asbestos Cement Co. Ltd.)*

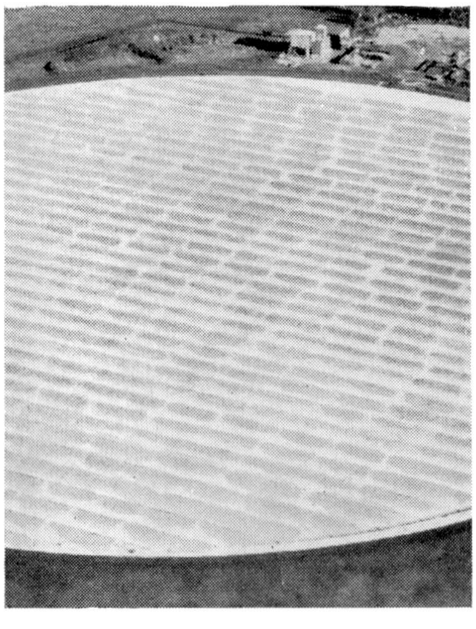

*Curved and slotted Trough Type B aluminium sheet to barrel vaults roof covering 680ft dia reservoir (Courtesy: British Aluminium Co. Ltd.)*

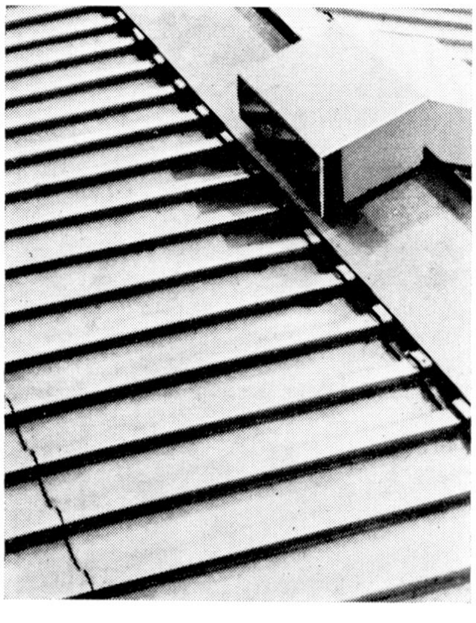

*'Fural' aluminium roofing (characterised by few side-laps) (Courtesy: British Aluminium Co Ltd.)*

Sheets are liable to become more brittle on exposure. This does not affect weather-tightness, but does reduce resistance to impact loads, thus making the roofs dangerous to walk on. Adequate safety precautions (ladders, duckboards or crawling boards and warning notices) are required for workmen having to pass over the roof*.

Cracking of sheets may occur as a result of shrinkage due to slow carbonation of the asbestos-cement from the surface inwards if (1) the sheets are too tightly bolted through holes with insufficient clearance, or (2) one side only is painted and sheets are tightly fixed—shrinkage of one face only may lead to bowing and distortion.

(ii) *Aluminium sheets*. A feature of aluminium sheets is the comparatively long lengths commonly available, which allow long-span roofs to be covered with few (in some cases without) end-laps. Lengths up to 4·8768m and 6·0960m are generally available, although longer lengths may be specially made to order. Some sheets, supplied in rolls up to 9·1440m long, are laid across the slope, thus increasing considerably the distance between side-laps.

The more usual pitch is 15 degrees, although the elimination of end-laps allows pitches as flat as 10 degrees to be used. At these low pitches condensation is likely to drip off the sheets.

A significant development in some proprietary systems is concealment of all fastenings, leaving an unbroken exposed surface. Fixings may be to clips, brackets or strips fastened to the roof structure. The sheets are pressed down to engage with the fixing devices.

(iii) *Steel sheets*. In use, and other things being equal, the effectiveness of corrugated steel sheets relative to the exclusion of rainwater is primarily dependent on the continuing durability of protective coatings. Sheets are thus normally galvanised, but in heavily polluted atmospheres painting may be essential to provide additional protection. Fixing holes, it should be noted, require special care. Corrosion

*See *The Building (Safety, Health and Welfare) Regulations*, 1948, particularly Regulation 31.

as soon as the membrane has been completed to prevent damage before the loading coats are applied.

There are basically two methods by which the membrane may be applied, namely, (i) *externally applied tanking* which is defined* as 'an external application of an impervious membrane to the structural walls' and (ii) *internally applied tanking* which is defined as 'an application of an impervious membrane to the inner surface of walls and the upper surface of floors before placing of structural walls or floors or protecting or loading coats'. It should be noted that the diagrams are not intended to be exhaustive and exclude, among other things, details related to column bases. However, there is no alteration in the principles shown. In externally applied tanking it is necessary to protect the vertical membrane from being punctured during backfilling or subsequent excavation. Such protection may be provided by a wall of either brickwork or blockwork built against the membrane.

(c) *Requirements*

Extrusion of either membrane may take place if the membrane is not fully confined. In cases such as these, it is necessary to limit, at normal temperatures, the design compressive load to 643·5kN/m$^2$ in the case of mastic asphalt and 1 072·5kN/m$^2$ in the case of bitumen sheeting.

Treatment of both internal and external *angles* to avoid any weakness which may result in water penetration is important. Angle fillets, 51mm wide and applied in two coats, should be used with mastic asphalt and angle strips, 305mm wide bonded into the angle, with bitumen sheeting. These are indicated in the diagram.

*Mastic asphalt* should be applied in three coats, 29mm thick on horizontal surfaces and on sloping surfaces not exceeding 30 degrees to the horizontal and not less than 19mm thick on vertical surfaces and sloping surfaces over 30 degrees to the horizontal. All vertical and sloping surfaces must be suitably keyed-raked joints in brickwork or blockwork, or surface of concrete obtained from timber shuttering, for example. Smooth, soft or friable surfaces are to be avoided. Joints in successive coats of asphalt should be staggered at least 152mm for horizontal work and 76mm for vertical work. Finally, the surface of the structure on which the asphalt is to be laid should permit complete uniformity up to d.p.c. level.

The number of layers of *bitumen sheeting* which should be applied to either horizontal or vertical surfaces depends on the weight of the sheeting. Three layers of 3·5kg/m$^2$ and two layers of 5·0kg/m$^2$ should be applied and all bonded with a suitable hot compound. All surfaces to which bitumen sheeting is to be applied must

*Reference: British Standard CP 102 : 1963, p. 27, *Protection of buildings against water from the ground.*

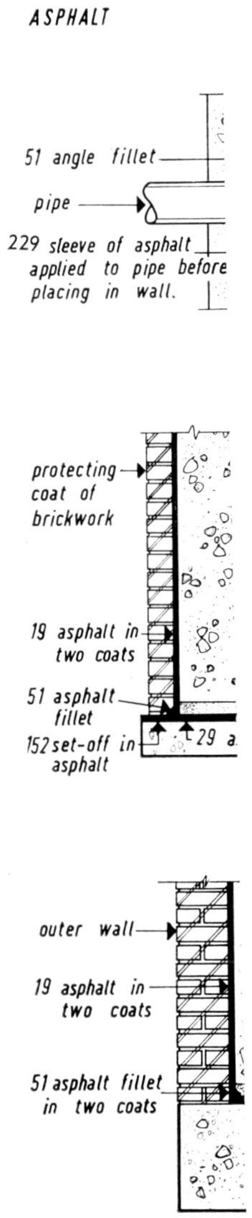


*D.3.04/15*
*Application of masti*
*bitumen sheet in tan*
*in mm*

be true and even fı indentations so as ing of the sheetin surfaces must be c dust, sand and fo requirement is equ the structural base provided by prece Laps between su sheeting should b at the side and 152r

*Openings* in th should, wherever p as these break the membrane used. U ings require spec indicated in the diag


**References**

1. *Protection of buildings ground,* British Standard C

2. *Damp-proofing solid f* Series) No. 54, HMSO, Ja

3. *Materials for damp-p* 1951.

4. *Damp-proof courses,* No. 68, HMSO, July, 1954

5. Various publications fr and Aluminium Developm


*Some examples of joints in flexible metal sheet coverings are given on this page. Right, standing seam and welts in aluminium. Far right, batten roll in aluminium (Courtesy: British Aluminium Co. Ltd.)*

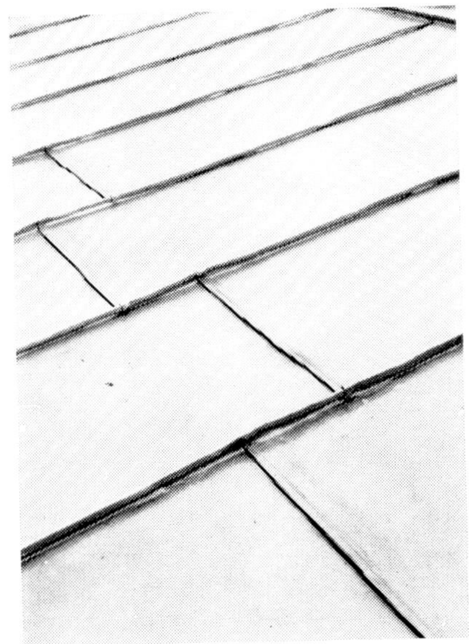

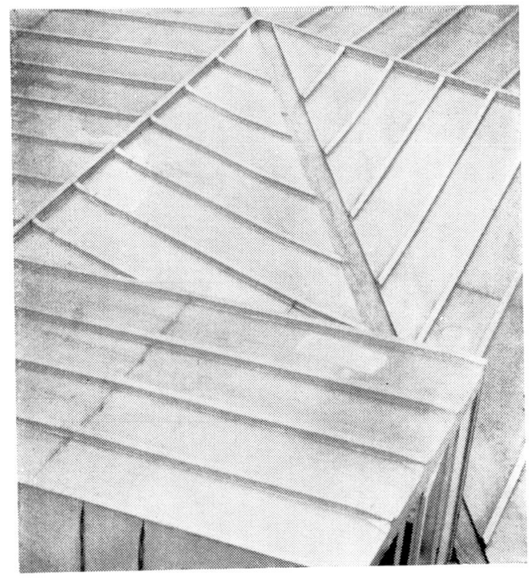

*Right, lead hollow roll with drip (Courtesy: Lead Development Assn.) Far right, zinc roll cap (Courtesy: Zinc Development Assn.)*

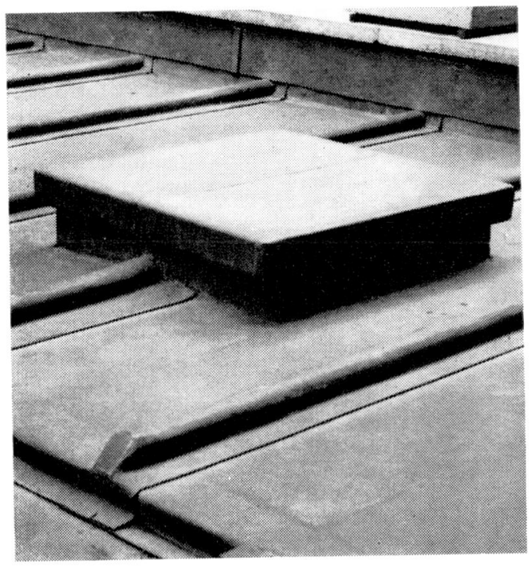

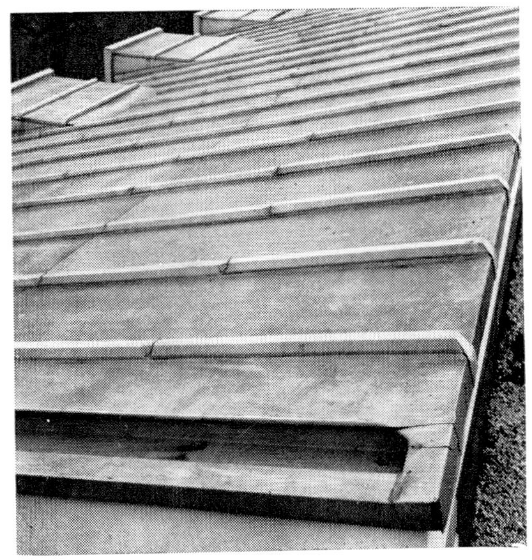

can be hastened if the steel is left unprotected after the holes have been made.

(iv) *Translucent sheets.* A wide variety of standard sheets to match most of the metal or asbestos-cement profiles are obtainable in glass reinforced polyester resin, acrylic resin, rigid vinyls and corrugated glass with wire reinforcement. Although originally intended to allow a means of providing daylight through parts of pitched roofs with opaque coverings, in new and existing buildings, translucent sheets continue to be developed. Departures from matching profiles and the use of the sheets for complete pitched roof applications are already noticeable. Following the example set by manufacturers of asbestos-cement sheeting, a range of special junction accessories are also available.

(v) *Opaque laminated plastics sheets.* Standard corrugated laminated plastics sheets composed of kraft paper impregnated with phenol-formaldehyde resin, and used in a similar way to other 'traditional' corrugated sheets, are also available. A range of junction accessories is available. Developments continue to take place.

(vi) *Fully supported sheets.* When the materials commonly used on flat roofs are to be used on pitched roofs, water exclusion does not present as severe a problem and, among other things, features such as drips in metal sheeting may be eliminated and laps substituted. Practical considerations require a slightly different technique to be employed, particularly with asphalt, bitumen felt and lead, on pitched roofs.

Asphalt requires a good mechanical key on steeply sloping surfaces, that is when the slope exceeds 10 degrees. In multi-layer work bitumen felt the sheets should be laid up the slopes from eaves to ridge; in single-layer work the sheets should be laid across the roof slope. Methods of fixing are the same as for flat roofs.

Lead, because of its tendency to creep, requires to be limited in size, while additional fixings and support other than that provided at the edges is required for pitches exceeding 15 degrees. At roof pitches steeper than 15 degrees the maximum size for a piece of lead should not exceed 2·2m$^2$ nor 3m in length.


**References:**

1. *BS Codes of Practice*: CP 142 : 1958 & 1968 *Slating and tiling.* CP 143 : 1958 *Sheet roof coverings*: Part 1: *Aluminium corrugated and troughed sheeting.* CP 143 : 1961 *Sheet roof and wall coverings*: Part 2: *Galvanized corrugated steel.* CP 143 : 1960 *Sheet roof coverings*: Part 3: *Lead roof coverings.* CP 143 : 1960 *Sheet roof coverings*: Part 4: *Copper roof coverings.* CP 143 : 1964 *Sheet roof and wall coverings*: Part 5: *Zinc.* CP 143 : 1962 *Sheet roof and wall coverings*: Part 6: *Corrugated asbestos-cement.* CP 144. Part 1 : 1968 *Built-up bitumen felt.* CP 144. Part 2 : 1968 *Mastic asphalt.* CP 145.101: 1951 *Patent glazing.* CP 301 : 1950 (amendment added March, 1954) *Building drainage.*

2. BS 2717 : 1956 *Glossary of terms applicable to roof coverings.*

3. *Principles of Modern Building,* Volume II, HMSO, 1961 (reprinted 1963).

4. Clay Tile Bulletin Vol. 2 No. 2, *Roofing tile details,* and No. 3 *Single lap tiling.*

5. Manufacturers' literature.

6. *Built-up felt roofs,* BRS Digest (2nd Series) No. 8, HMSO, March, 1961 and *Developments in roofing,* BRS Digest (2nd Series) No. 51, HMSO, October, 1964, amended 1968.

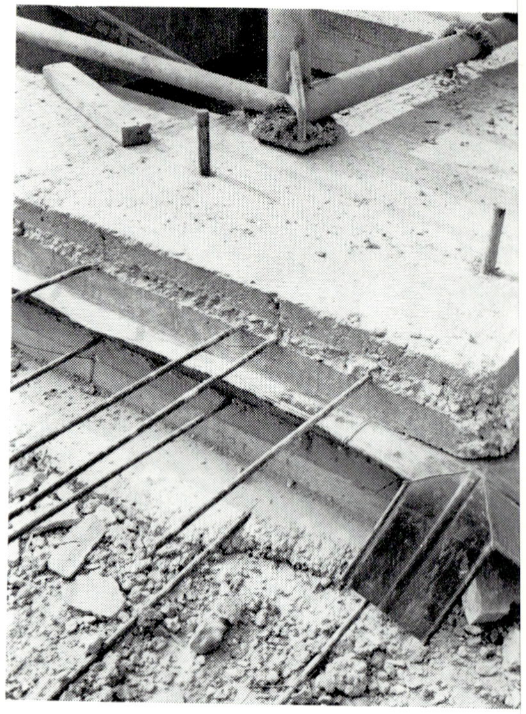

*One type of PVC water bar for use in horizontal and vertical construction joints in concrete to prevent penetration by water (Courtesy: Sealocrete Ltd.)*

## Damp-proof courses and membranes

THERE are a number of specific positions in building construction where it is necessary to use the principle of complete prevention (p. 95) and thus completely impervious materials. Examples of the application of these materials as damp-proofing to a building include the following:

(1) Below ground in basements as tanking to withstand the penetration of water under pressure; (2) at or near ground level to prevent the rise of water, as liquid or vapour depending on conditions, in walls (external and internal) and floors; (3) at openings in external walls to exclude rainwater; (4) in parapets, in chimneys, or in similar positions to prevent the downward transmission of water; and (5) at the junction of different elements or materials, such as cladding and primary structure, horizontal projections from external walls (set-backs, cornices, string-courses, etc.), walls and roofs, projections above a roof covering (chimneys, pipes, etc.) in the form of flashings and weatherings.

*The main function* of the materials used for damp-proofing is, therefore, to prevent the transmission of water either from an external source into a structure or from one part of the structure to another. Apart from flashings and weatherings, the damp-proofing materials are so located within the structure that replacement, although not always impossible, is either impracticable or extremely expensive. Accordingly, it is imperative that every precaution is taken in

selection
ensure
particula
deteriora
settlemer
building.
propertie
requirem
restricted
monly re
proofing
3.04/2.
the range
further
tended t
parison
used with
tors whic
detailed a
materials
has been
to deal v
tions sep
general h
ground; (
flashings
Apart
flashings
common
in other p
term of c
More rece
of using
comparati
material
positions i
damp-proo
the appl
materials
as is comr

*For conveni
two terms, v
used througho



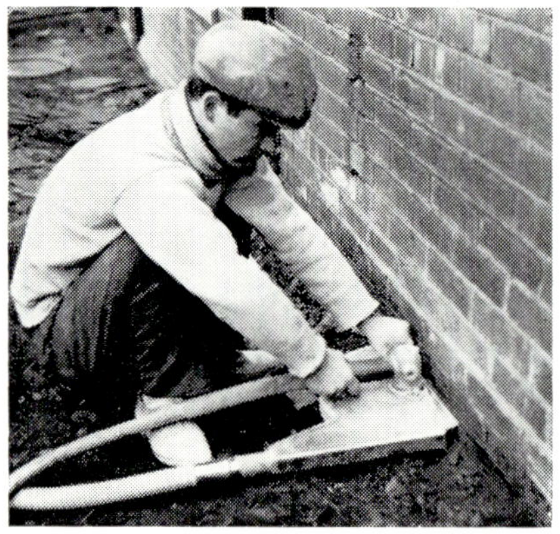

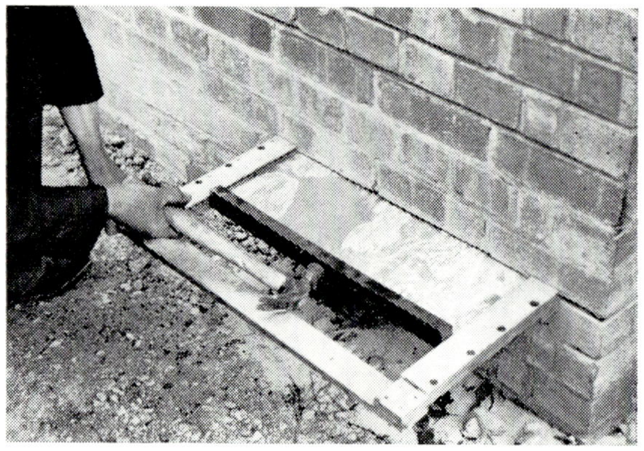

*Inserting a d.p.c. Above left, illustrates the use of a special saw for cutting through the bed joint and right, driving a rigid sheet into the slot with the aid of a special guiding frame.*
*(Courtesy: HMSO, Crown Copyright)*

*Below, injecting a d.p.c. The picture on the left shows the holes drilled at regular intervals along the line of the proposed d.p.c. and right, feeding of the silicone solution by gravity into pre-drilled holes*

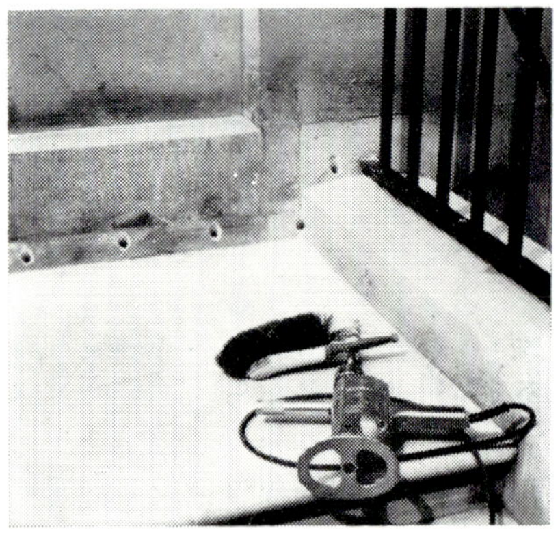

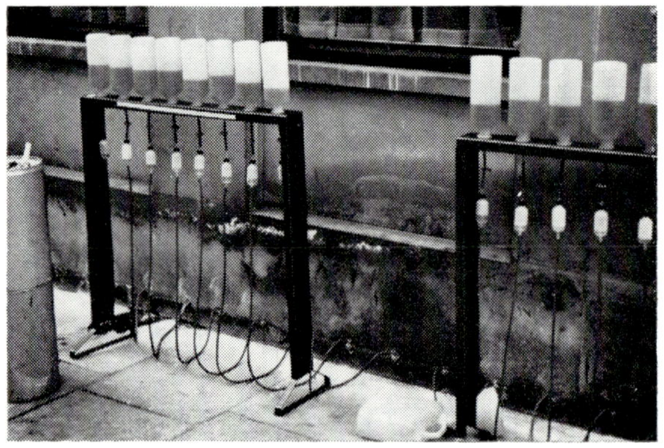

*Below, electro-osmosis—the right-hand picture illustrates the measuring of the voltage between the damp wall and earth and the left-hand picture shows a wall electrode and part of the copper conductor looped into holes previously drilled in the wall (Courtesy: Rentokil Laboratories Ltd.)*

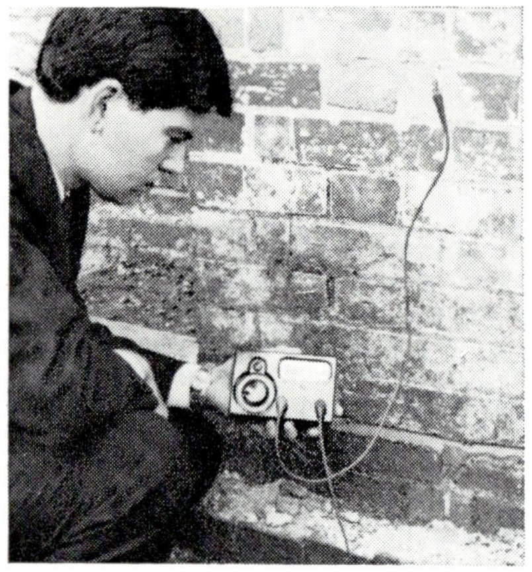

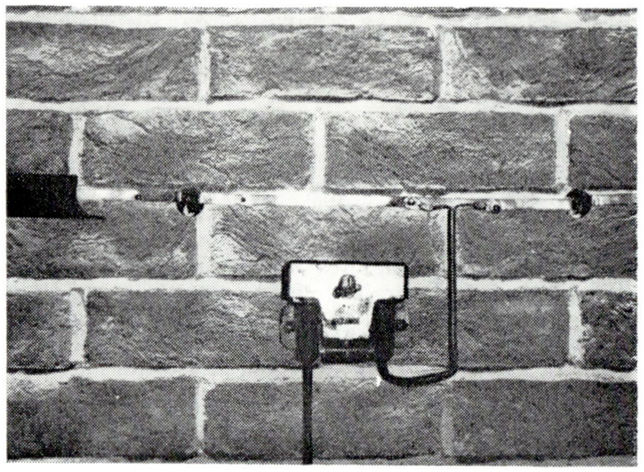

rigid sheets may be simply inserted, although it may be necessary, if the d.p.c. does not fill the slot, to pack the joint with a mortar bed in order to reduce settlement.

(ii) *Injection.* In contrast to the necessity of cutting through the bed joints of a wall, a number of proprietary techniques have been developed which, in principle, involve drilling holes at regular intervals along the base of a wall, into which water-repellant substances may be injected by gravity or under pressure. The substances are intended to penetrate into the wall and once 'set' are claimed to produce a moisture barrier in the wall. The efficacy of such barriers has still not been proved conclusively by the BRS while their durability is still not known with certainty.

Solutions used include silicones, usually with water displacing fluids; an aqueous siliconate/latex mixture; hot wax or setting resins. Among difficulties associated with most of these are injecting the liquid into a wall that is already saturated; ensuring that a continuous membrane is formed for the complete thickness of the wall, while the presence of salts or detergents can impair the effectiveness of the silicone treatment. However, the aqueous siliconate/latex mixture would seem to be the most satisfactory as, among other things, it

*D.3.04/23 (opposite)*
*Examples of some common applications of flashings. The use of preformed flashings such as those now available in aluminium and plastics for use with asphalt and bitumen at eaves have been omitted*

---

the top of the ground or covering and the underside of the joists should not be less than 152mm.

(c) *Board or strip ground floors*
Details of d.p.m.'s applicable to unventilated board and strip ground floors for the prevention of fungal attack in timber are given in diagram D.3.06/1 (Vol. 3, p. 42).

**4. Flashings and weatherings**

The essential function of a *flashing* is to seal the joint between different materials or elements. In this it also maintains continuity between a roof covering and the d.p.c. in an adjoining wall projecting above the level of the roof covering. Unlike d.p.c.'s and d.p.m.'s, the flashing is mostly exposed. Despite the fact that exposure to the atmosphere may tend to increase susceptibility to deterioration, materials such as aluminium and zinc, which are not commonly used as d.p.c.'s, are often employed as flashings. The reason for this may be attributable to the fact that flashings are comparatively easily replaced and, above all, they can be reasonably well inspected. Nevertheless, when materials such as aluminium and zinc are used in close association with deteriorating agencies such as cement or lime they should be adequately protected. The use of bitumen paint is often sufficient.

Apart from durability, flexibility is an essential requirement of flashings. In some cases extremely complicated shapes must be dressed. In these cases lead is often the only suitable material. However, all the flexible materials normally used as d.p.c.'s may also be used, within limits, as flashings. Some common applications of flashings in buildings are, together with appropriate notes, illustrated in diagram D.3.04/23.

The diagram includes the treatment of pipes projecting above roofs which do not necessarily require flashings as such. Other examples are also illustrated in the accompanying photographs.

*Some examples of the use of flashings. Right, stepped flashings in lead (slate roof). Below left, flashings in lead to junction with single lap tiles and party wall. Below right, apron and stepped flashings in zinc (slate roof)*

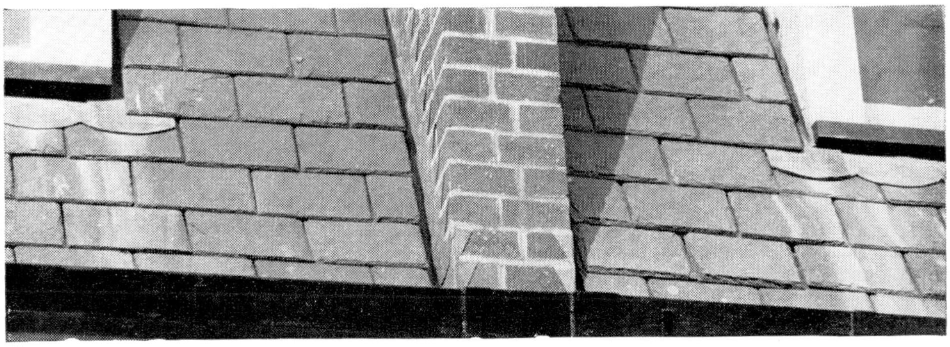

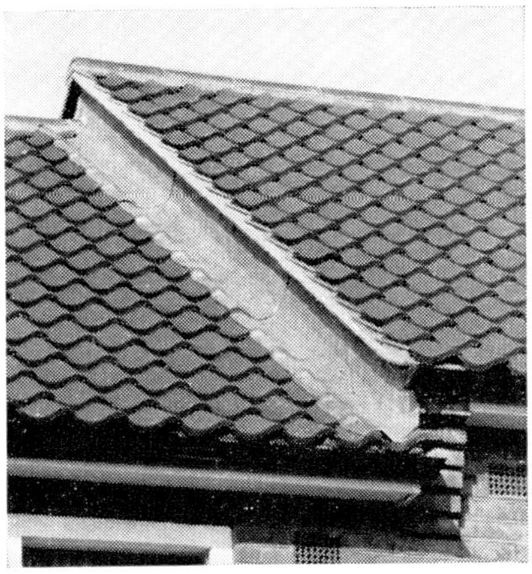

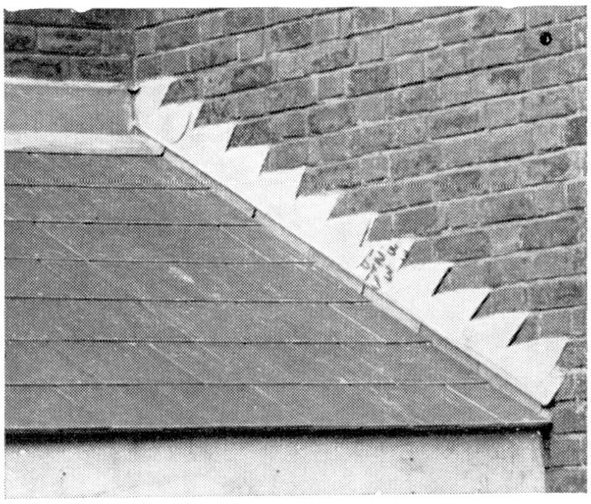

*Right, apron and stepped flashings in zinc (slate roof). Far right, stepped flashing in zinc (slate roof).*

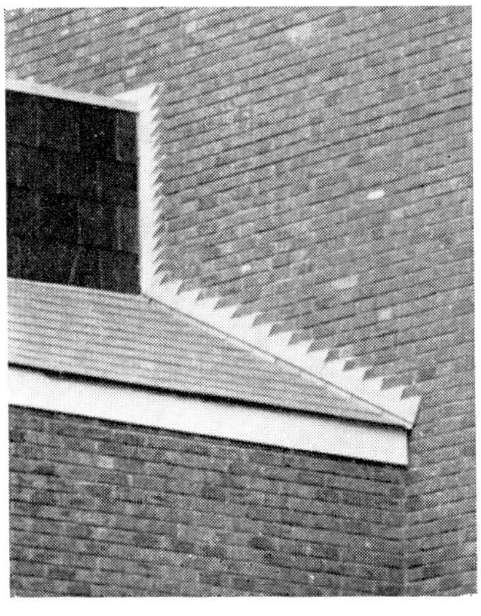

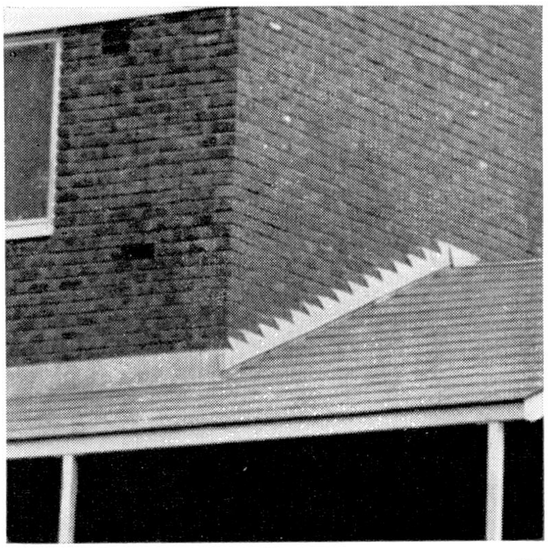

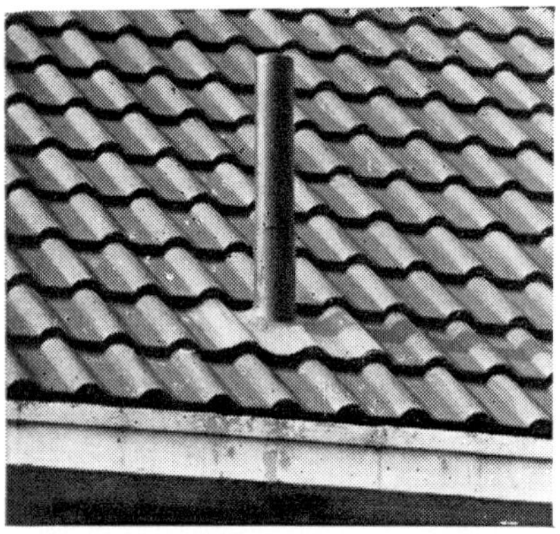

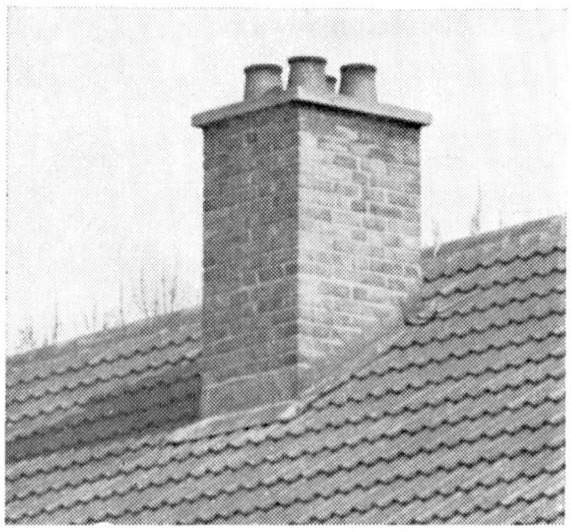

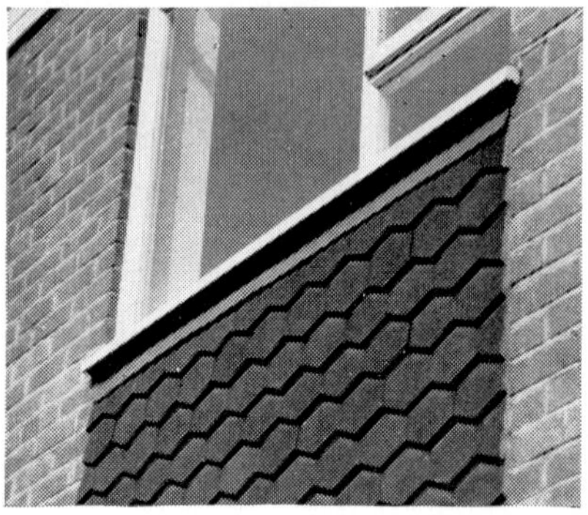

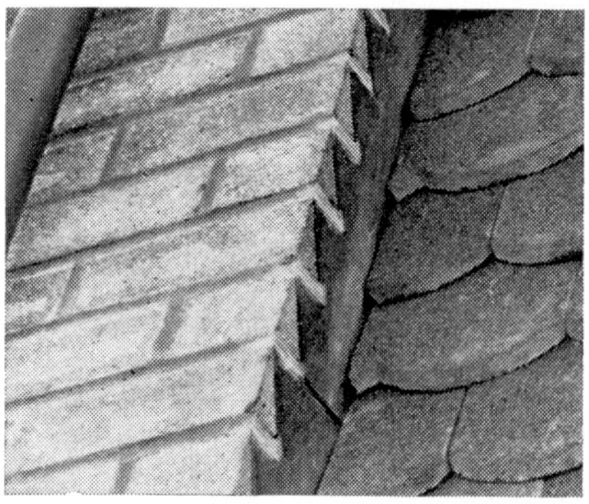

*More examples of the use of flashings. Top left, preformed flashings to pipe (single lap tiled roof). Lower left, flashing under sill and over tile hanging. Top right, flashings to a chimney (single lap tiled roof). Lower right, stepped flashings to brick jamb with tile hanging*

*More examples of weatherings. Below, an integral d.p.c., flashing and weathering, protecting a narrow projection. Right, an interesting example of 'developing experience'. Two similar stepped projections from the same development being carried out in stages. In the top picture the weathering used has not completely solved all the joint problems. A better solution to the problem is being attempted in the photograph beneath*

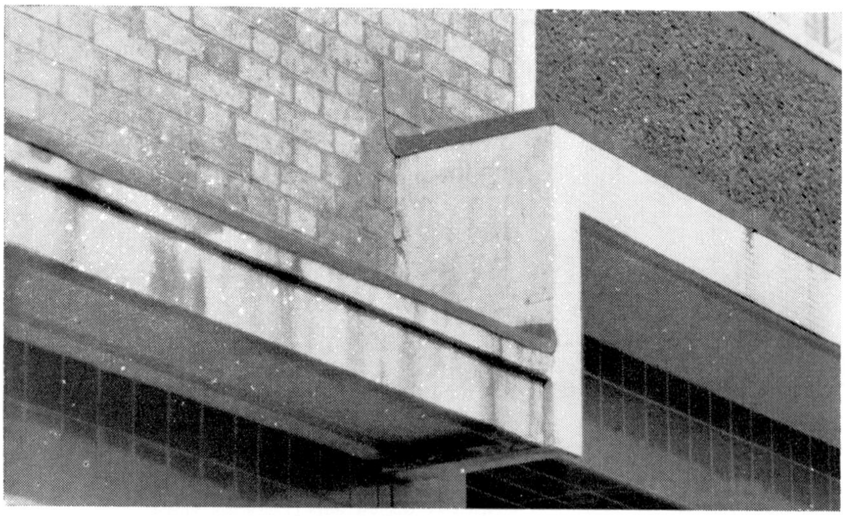

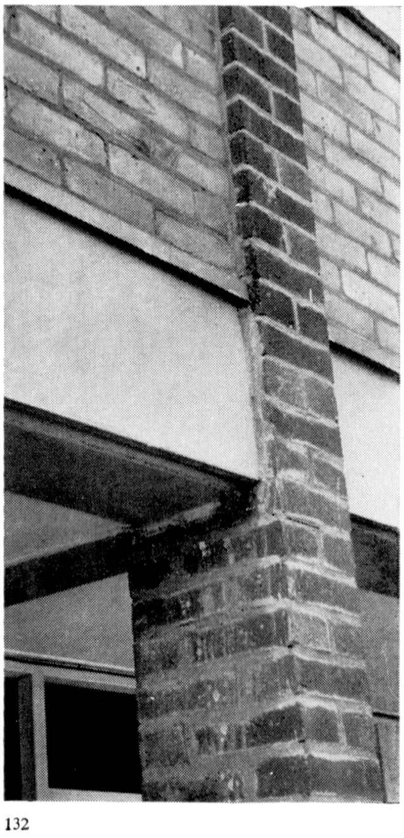

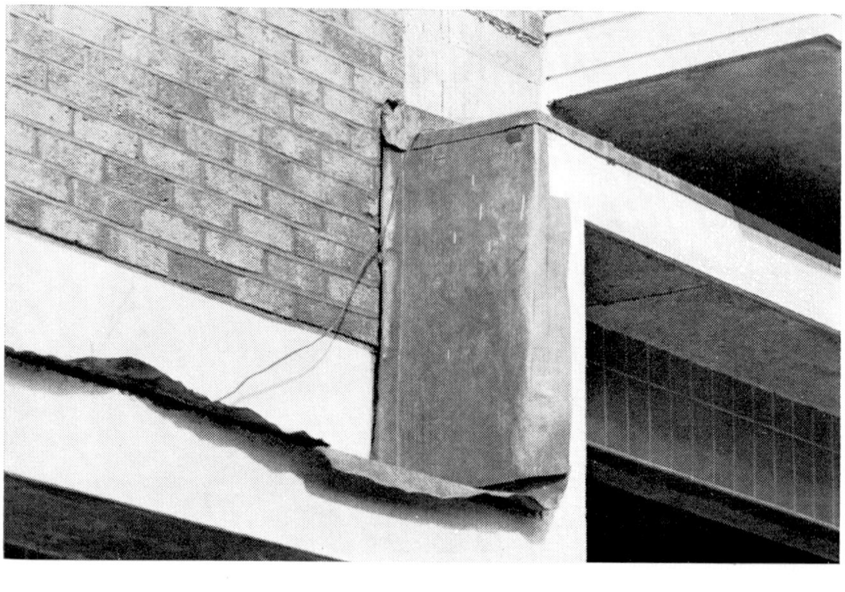

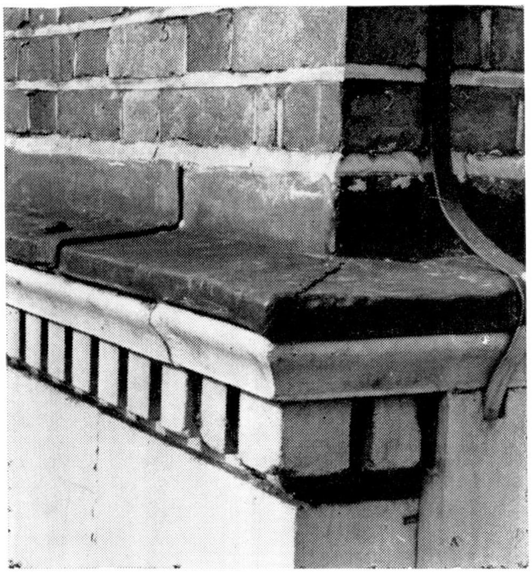

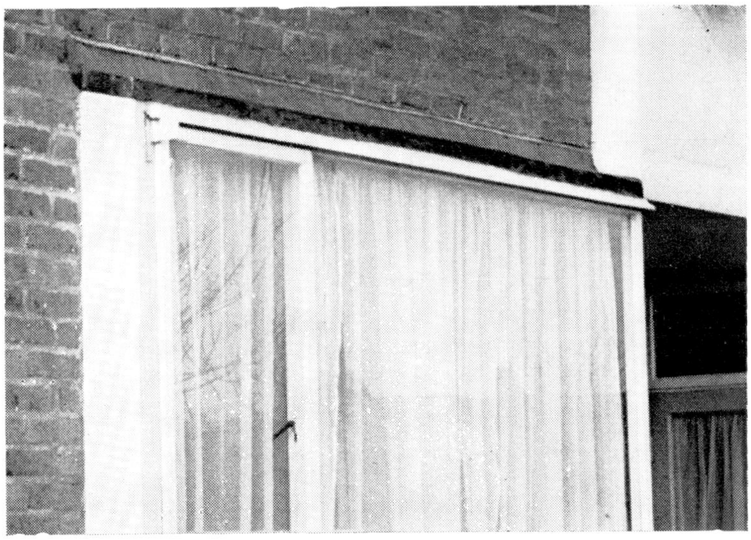

*Above, lead flashing to narrow projection. Above right, protecting the head of a projecting concrete frame*

*Failure to use flashings correctly—note remedial work*

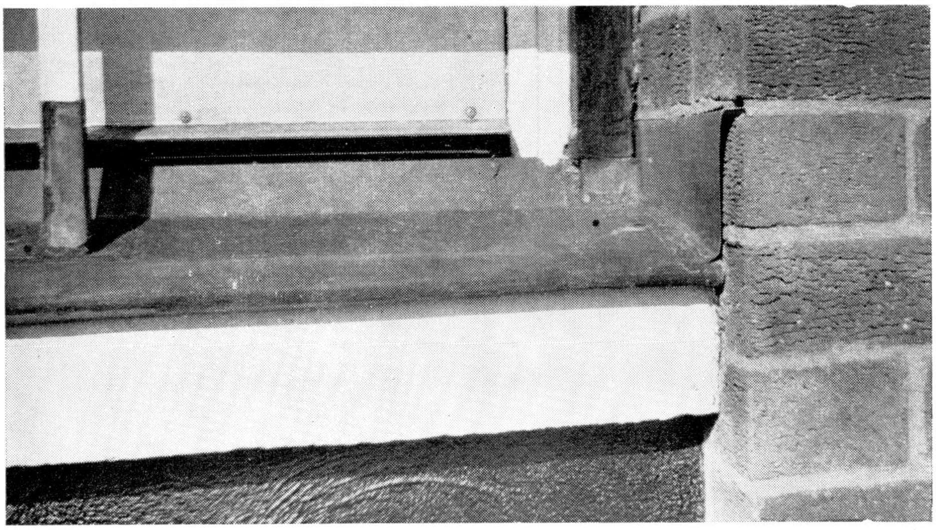

*Use of mortar flaunching in lieu of a flashing (slate roof)—requires vigilant maintenance for success*

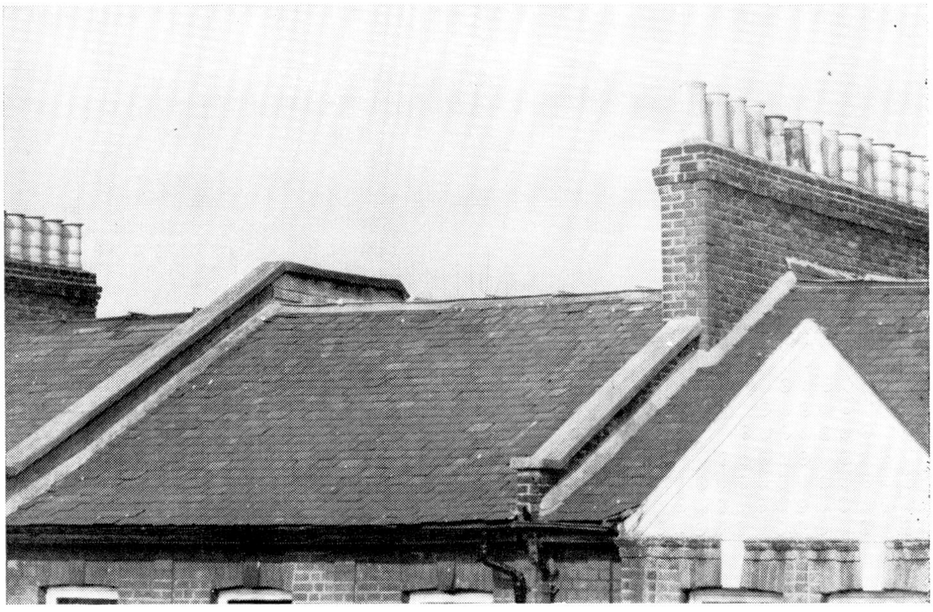

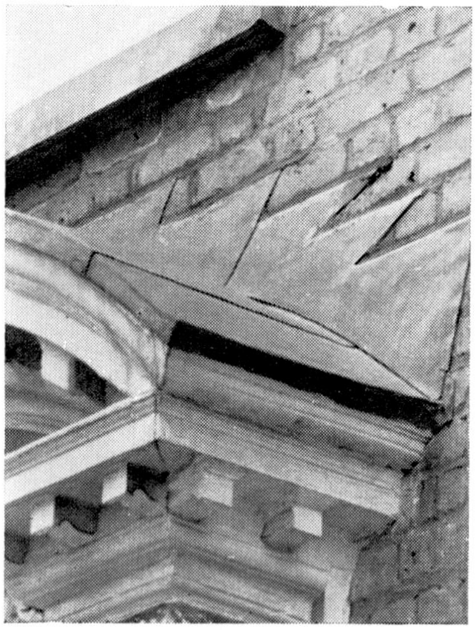

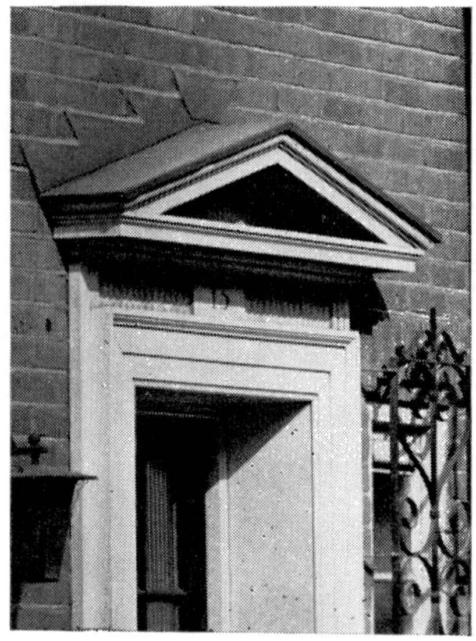

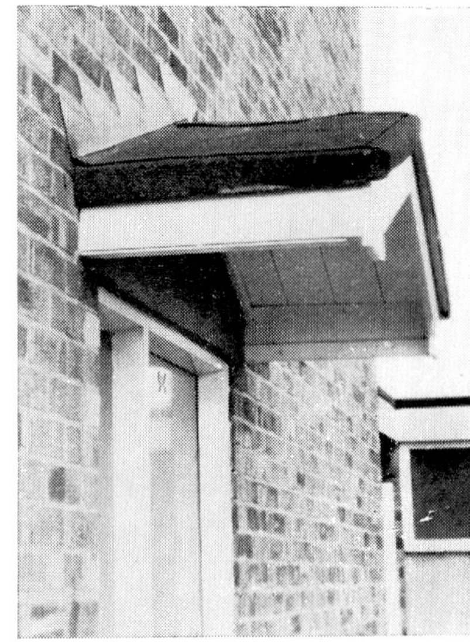

*The photographs show examples of weatherings*

In simple terms *weatherings* can be regarded as miniature flat roofs. They are used to provide an impervious covering to relatively small projections, such as cornices, string-courses, small canopies, etc. Accordingly, materials commonly applied are similar to those used for flat roofs. Some examples of the application of weatherings are illustrated in diagram D.3.04/24.

## Moisture vapour barriers (M.v.b.'s)

In general terms, the need for the inclusion of materials which may resist the passage of water vapour through wall and roof constructions arises chiefly as a result of the heating of buildings, particularly when internal temperatures and humidities (the combination is significant) are high relative to those externally. The whole problem of the use of suitable materials is associated with the prevention of interstitial condensation. This aspect is dealt with more fully in *4.00 Heat and its effects,* and is also referred to under 'Entrapped water' later in this section. Accordingly, only a brief general outline of the problems involved and the materials commonly used is included here.

As already noted previously under 'External walls' and 'Roofs', many constructions may include on their external surfaces cladding materials such as metals, glass, asphalt or bitumen-felt which, in addition to being impervious to water in liquid state, are also impervious to water in vapour state. In these positions, and subject to conditions, water vapour diffusing through the construction may condense behind the claddings. This may be regarded in some ways as a fortuitous use of a moisture vapour barrier, although this does not detract from the fact that suitable precautions (usually by drainage) must still be taken to ensure that the condensed water vapour is eventually able to escape to the air so as not to damage materials used in the construction.

When, however, interstitial condensation risk has been determined, and if, as a result, it is decided to restrict the amount of water vapour which may be allowed to enter any part of the construction, then it is necessary to provide a moisture vapour barrier. Such a barrier may be provided internally, that is on the warmer side, although in some constructions it may be incorporated within the thickness of the construction.

Although termed 'barriers' the materials which may be used are not necessarily, nor do they have to be, completely impervious to water vapour. Accordingly, m.v.b.'s are commonly, though not exclusively, extremely thin sheet materials, such as aluminium foil, impregnated paper and plastics sheet or applied coatings such as paint. In order to be classified as an m.v.b. a material should have a vapour diffusance value not exceeding 0·04692 $\mu$g/Ns.* A comparative chart of the vapour diffusance of various materials is included in *4.00 Heat and its effects.* Values (all in $\mu$g/N s) for some materials are: aluminium foil (0·00013–0·00027); bitumen impregnated paper, Scutan 10 (0·09368); roofing felt, according to type (0·04692–2·67660); 25·4mm expanded polystyrene (0·09368–0·14721); 25·4mm expanded PVC (0·02677); 25·4mm expanded ebonite (0·00267).

As in all problems connected with the transmission of water, joints between sheets or cracks in the coating will affect the performance of the barrier. In sheeting, plain lapped joints are usually not good enough and so welted joints are to be preferred. Sealing the joint (hot bitumen, adhesives, etc.) does provide some additional advantage. It should be noted that even in properly sealed joints there may be some leakage, but the amount is usually negligible. This only helps to reinforce the importance of effecting a good joint.

Finally, a barrier may be rendered ineffective if it contains small holes or imperfections. In this connection it should be remembered that the materials commonly used are even thinner than d.p.c.'s. Accordingly, m.v.b.'s require extremely careful handling. Surfaces to which the barrier is to be applied should be smooth and even and free from any projections which may puncture the material during or after application.

## Joint design

In this part only joints in external walls are considered—the joints between units of the same material, the joints between units of different materials or the joints between different elements. Some of the principles discussed may also be applicable to certain conditions within buildings (walls and floors) or to roofs when sealants may be required to increase the resistance of joints, particularly in large rigid units, to penetration by rainwater, fine snow or air.

Unlike the joints in roofs, the joints in external walls have, in general, been characterised by the fact that, in order to exclude rainwater and to some extent to meet other requirements, greater reliance has been placed on the use of sealants. In the case of brickwork, for example, the mortar in

*This classification is taken from practice in the United States of America and Canada; there does not appear to be any standard classification in this country. BRS Digest (2nd Series) No. 39, *Cellular plastics*, HMSO, October, 1963, includes the same classification at the foot of Table 2, p. 4.

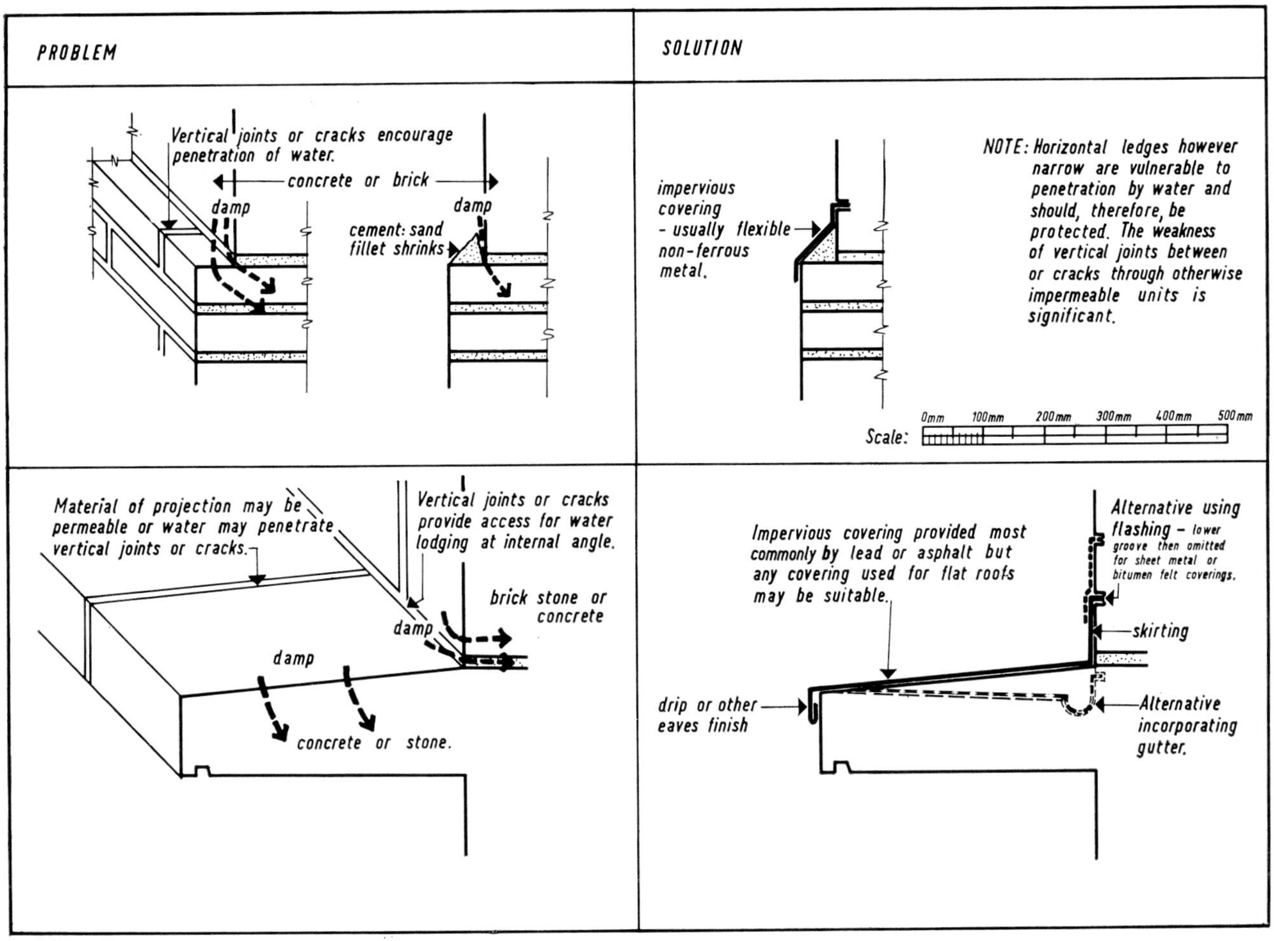


*D*.3.04/24
*Some examples of the application of weatherings*

the joints not only excludes rainwater, but is also necessary for structural reasons. However, the mortar, as already discussed under 'External walls' (see particularly '3. Solid walling'—pp. 98-103), should ideally have properties similar to and behave very much like the walling units themselves. Other types of traditional sealing materials which are themselves impervious to water include glazing putties or bituminous and other compounds used in pavement work.

It is possible in certain cases (in others it may be desirable though sometimes impracticable) to design suitable dry and open joints which exclude rainwater and which, together with other features, may also meet other requirements, as in the case of tile hanging (see pp. 99–100). Nevertheless, in this study it has been considered necessary, in the light of current building practice and experience, to deal with the design of joints primarily assuming the use of some form of sealant. The main emphasis is, therefore, placed on the use of sealants such as mastics and gaskets, with mortars also included. However, it should be noted, with due caution, that this emphasis is not intended to pre-suppose that sealants provide the only or, for that matter, the most appropriate method of excluding rainwater and meeting the general requirements of the joint. In fact, sealants, particularly mastics, may not necessarily provide the only means of excluding rainwater, while in some cases they may not be used at all or possibly only in a comparatively minor way. Consequently, the use of open or drained joints, which may or may not incorporate mastics, is also considered.

The need for joints at all in any form of construction is due to factors such as provision for movements, manufacturing techniques of the units or component parts and possible methods of site assembly. It is in the light of these and other factors that exclusion of rainwater must be seen. Although ideally it would seem better, in view of the problems and difficulties involved, to secure a weathertight joint, if the number of joints were limited. However, this implies *larger units* and consequently *greater movement* at the joint and *greater demands* on the sealant used. In addition, each joint will be subjected to greater quantities of water, with the quantities increasing the more impermeable the materials used on the exposed face. Height is, of course, also significant. (See *3.02 Exposure,* pp. 32–35).

There is a tendency nowadays towards the increased use of materials in larger units, many of which have significant movements particularly when associated with thermal insulants, and taller buildings. The effect of these developments has meant that special consideration must now be given to the problems and requirements of joint design. The latter are not new to building practice. In most traditional constructions, however, empirical methods proved adequate in their own terms. These methods have been found to be quite inadequate in the new forms of constructions, including the use of traditional materials in new ways. Despite the availability of some quantitative methods for assessment, joint design is still, on the whole, in its formative stages. The results of long-term field studies are still awaited, while improvements in the performance of sealants are continually being sought.

In order to cover as many aspects as possible associated with joint design, including the interrelationship (in some cases interaction) of the various factors involved which influence the techniques suitable to exclude rainwater, it has been considered convenient to use three basic headings. These are: (1) *General principles,* in

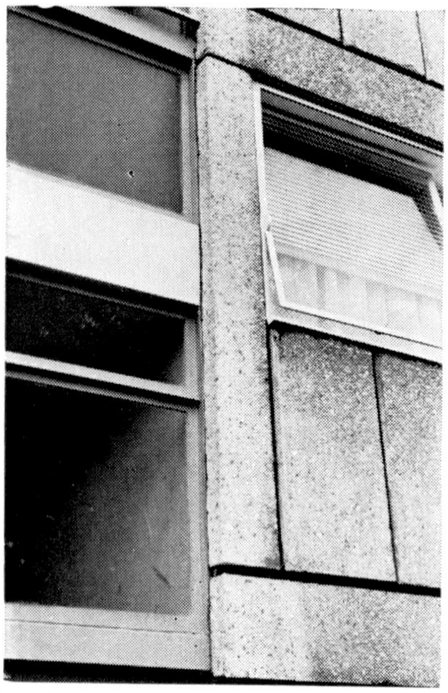

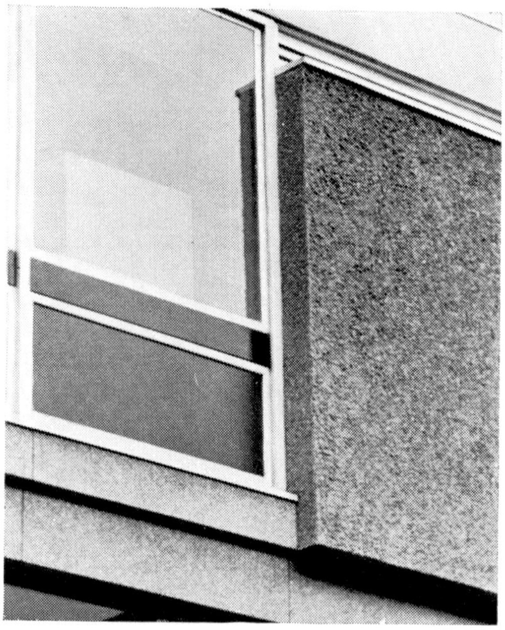

*'. . . the joints in external walls have, in general, been characterised by the fact that, in order to exclude rainwater and to some extent to meet other requirements, greater reliance has been placed on the use of sealants.'*

*Examples of joints between units of the same material, joints between units of different materials and joints between different elements*

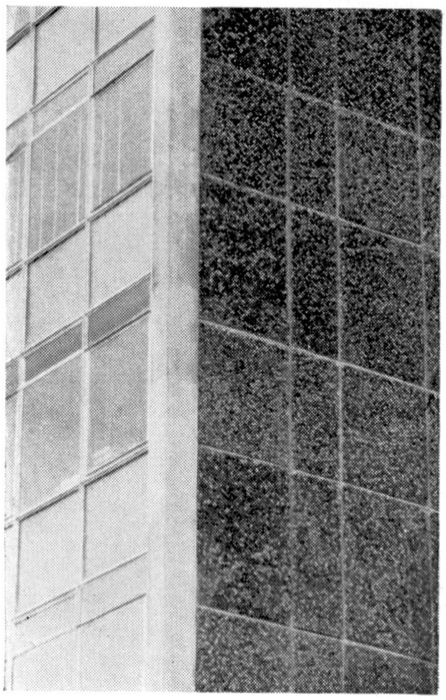

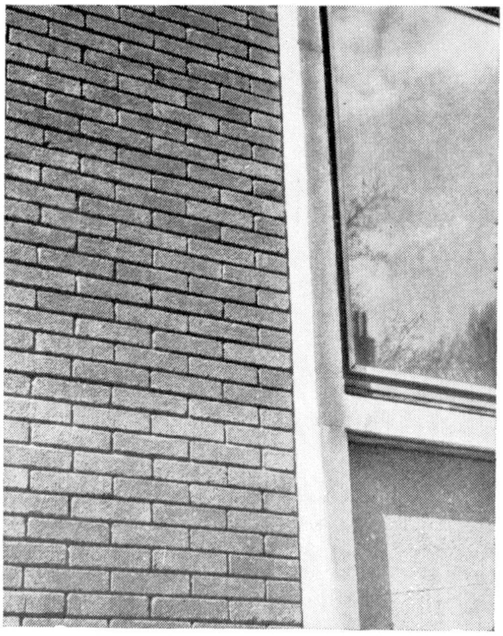

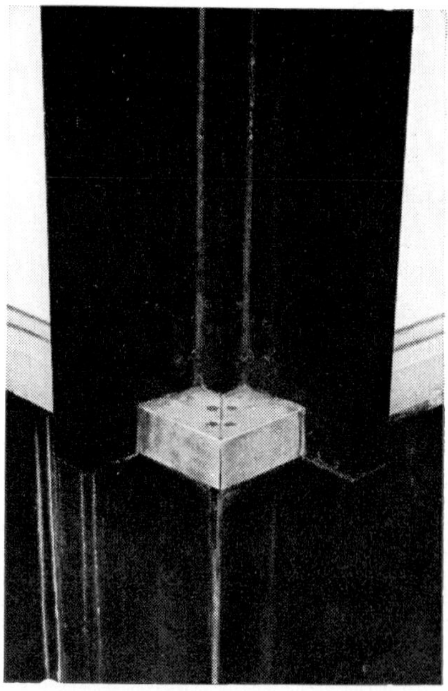

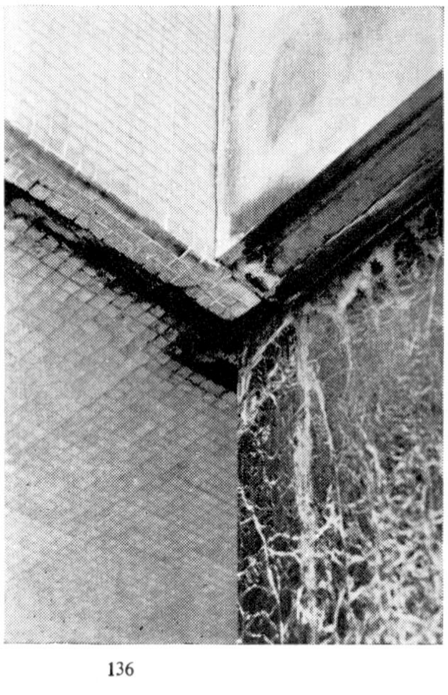

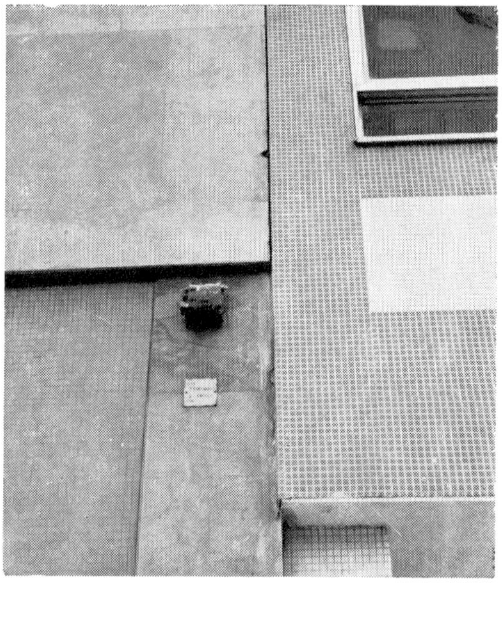

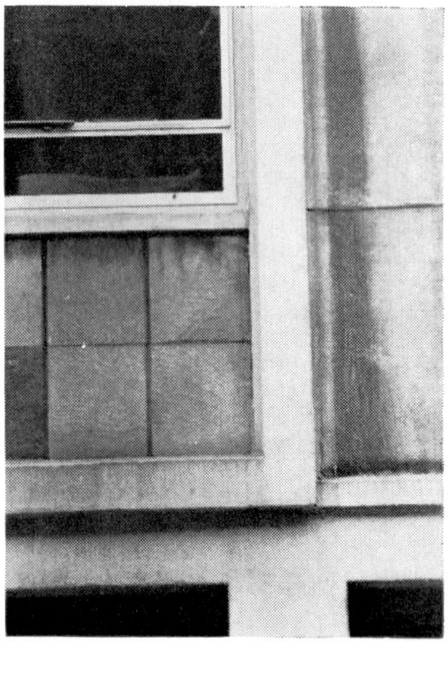

which the main factors are set out; (2) *Sealing materials,* which includes the general properties and behaviour of mortars, mastics and gaskets; and (3) *Specific applications,* which includes selected examples of joints for various parts of a construction or for specific materials.

## 1. General principles

Although principles may be established for the design of joints in general, the detailed application of these principles will be influenced by factors such as the properties of the materials used and related methods of fixing. The effects of these and other factors are illustrated in '3. Specific applications' later.

(a) *Requirements of the joint*

Mention has already been made of the fact that joints have to fulfil many requirements other than exclusion of rainwater. Ideally, joints should then be designed so that they meet the following requirements:

(i) *Exclusion of the weather,* namely rain, wind, air and snow.

(ii) *Allowance for thermal and moisture movements.* These are closely related to the properties of those sealants, such as mortars and mastics, which effect complete weathertightness by adhesion with the faces of the joint. The type of sealant must, therefore, be chosen according to the expected movements. The latter may be calculated from available information on the properties of materials and the range of environmental conditions* to be anticipated during fixing and the life of a building.

For design purposes it is, at present, advisable to assume that porous materials will undergo their full range of reversible moisture movements; those cast *in situ* will also undergo initial drying shrinkage. Any known sheltering effect would allow some relaxation in the values used.

Thermal and moisture movements often oppose one another and thus tend to have a cancelling effect. On the other hand, it is possible that they will work together when, for example, a joint is made when a unit is cold and dry or when it is warm and wet. For design purposes it is safer to assume, unless the conditions likely to prevail are more accurately known, that thermal and moisture movement will work together. The calculated movements must, therefore, be added together to give the maximum movement at the joint.

(iii) *Allowance for working loads.* It is important that the weight of units being fixed or the loads imposed on the units by wind do not distort the joint and particularly the sealant used.

The imposed loads, whether due to the weight of the unit or to wind, may cause the sealants which remain plastic to extrude. Plasticity may, however,

*Thermal movements and anticipated temperatures in buildings are included in *4.00 Heat and its effects.* Moisture movements are included in *3.03 Moisture content.*

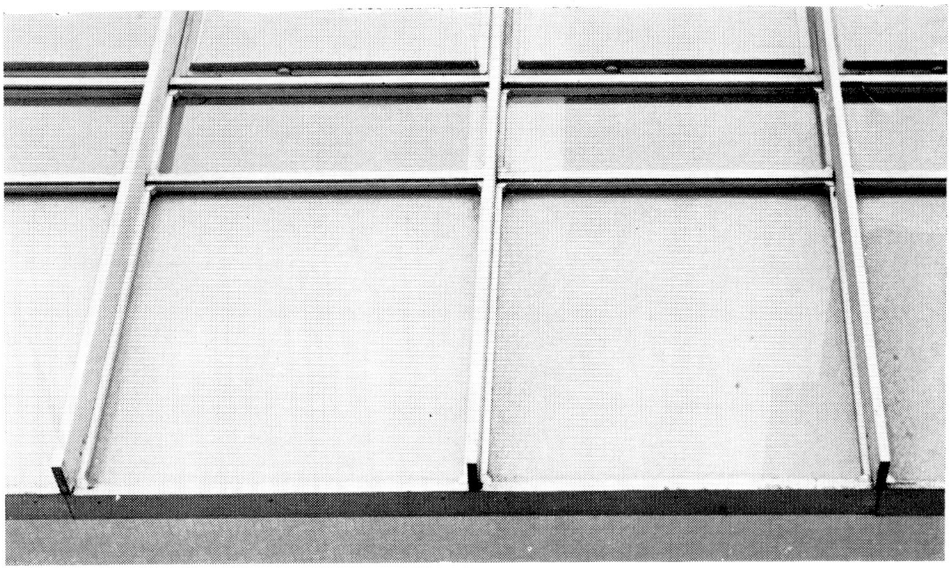

*Above, a continuation of the examples from p. 136*

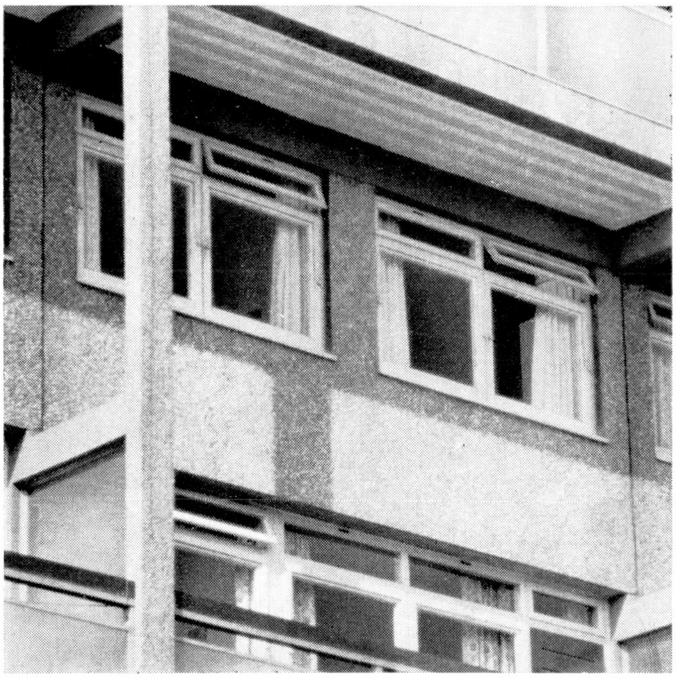

*Right, with the increased use of materials in larger units special consideration must be given to joint design. An example of a large precast concrete walling unit. Below, a comparative example of changes in both scale and type of joint between a 'traditional' wall of brick and stonework and precast concrete cladding. This example typifies the effects of the need to provide for movement and to take into account manufacturing techniques and methods of site assembly, particularly when large units are used*

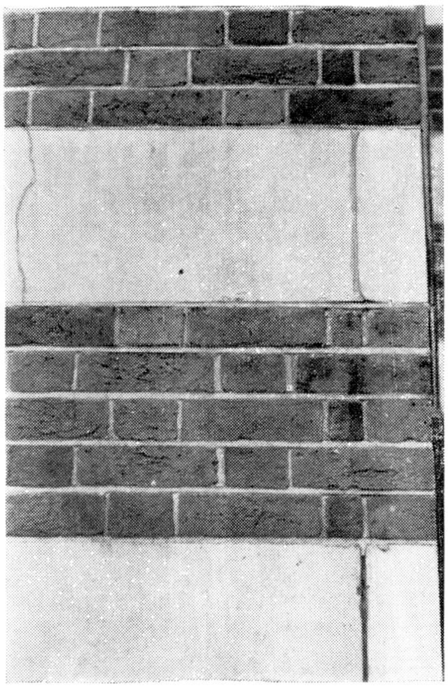

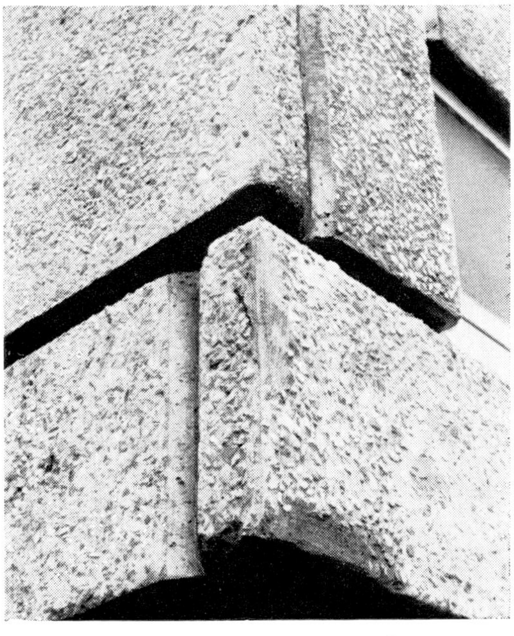

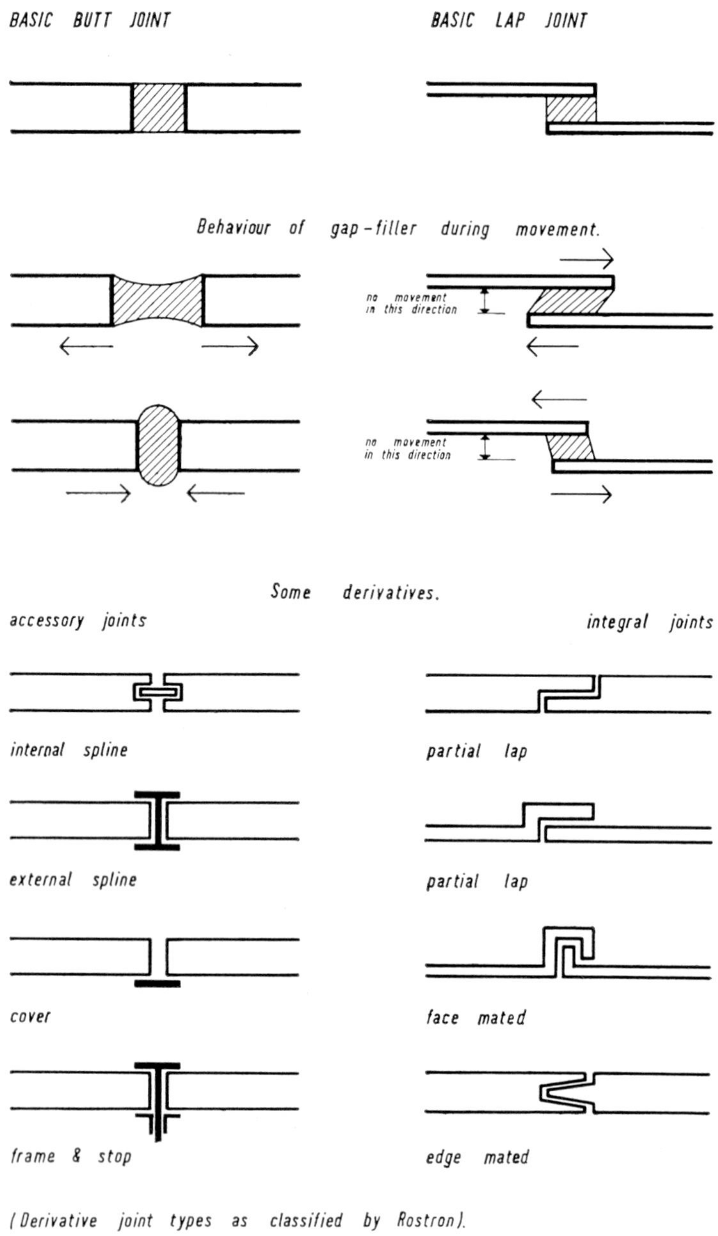


*D.3.04/25*
*Types of joint—see text*

only be temporary and required so as to be able to apply the sealant, as in the case of mortars and some mastics. In this the mastics are particularly significant as it is possible to suitably control the plasticity of mortars. It may, therefore, be necessary to ensure that the loads are carried mechanically by spacers (may include the use of mortar bed or pads), setting blocks or other devices (fixing devices on the structural frame as used with concrete slabs are notable).

(iv) *Durability*. Materials used to seal joints must themselves be durable. This also applies to the other components of the joint, but, in general, experience suggests that special consideration should be given to the sealant. Mastics, in particular, require special care. Compatibility, shielding from the deteriorating effects of the weather, but particularly sunlight, and adequate thickness of material are among other factors of primary importance.

The durability of the joint (only applicable to mortars and mastics) is also primarily dependent on the maintenance of good adhesion between the sealant and the faces of the joint. All the requirements for good adhesion (see 'Adhesion' in *Section 1.11*), should, therefore, be observed.

(v) *Ease of repair*. The extent to which joints should be easily repaired will depend on circumstances. The anticipated durability of a sealant (again mastics are significant) will be important. At present it would seem advisable to ensure that mastics are so used as to ensure that replacement is possible.

(vi) *Preservation of thermal and sound insulation*. Any continuous break in a construction is likely to reduce both thermal and sound insulation. The joint should, therefore, be designed to ensure that the insulation of the construction is preserved as much as possible.

(vii) *Ease of assembly*. It is important that the units and component parts are easily assembled. In this it is necessary to take dimensional and fixing tolerances into account.

(b) *Methods of approach*

There are three basic methods of approach which may be adopted to deal with the exclusion of rainwater. These are:

(i) *One line of defence*. In this method a sealant is used at or near the exposed surface. The success of the joint to exclude rainwater depends entirely on the durability of the sealant. As most sealants (mastics and gaskets) are themselves impervious, durability and good adhesion (mastics) or the maintenance of a compression seal (gaskets), are fundamental, as water must not be allowed to pass the surface. With porous sealants, such as mortar, the maintenance of good adhesion is still important, although the principle of controlled penetration of water may be used.

(ii) *Two lines of defence*. In this method, which has been used in this country for many years in patent glazing, the possibility of water penetration through the seal provided at or near the exposed surface or between cracks at the interface of the sealing material and joint is anticipated. Any water which may penetrate is then allowed to drain away to the outside by means of suitable channels or cavities incorporated in the construction behind the joint. The drainage channels or cavities form the second line of defence and are, in many ways, analogous to the traditional cavity wall. The first line of defence may be effected by the use of spring clips, cover strips, gaskets or mastic.

Obvious advantages are to be gained with this method. Although it may seem possible to dispense with the first line of defence and merely to allow for drainage, some form of sealing is usually required to ensure that there is no infiltration of air, particularly during high winds. Other factors which may make the use of the principle of drainage difficult, include the necessity of avoiding water being blown up the channel or cavity at the outlet points. On tall buildings this can present an extremely difficult problem.

(iii) *Joint geometry*. In this method the opposing faces of the joint are so profiled to include what may best be termed anti-capillary and pressure equalizing grooves or cavities. Rainwater is then allowed to penetrate the joint to a predetermined zone and subsequently to drain away to the outside. Drainage, it should be noted, takes place within the thickness of the joint. Water is, therefore, not allowed to penetrate and subsequently drain behind the joint as in the case of a second line of defence (see (ii) above). Accordingly, a prerequisite is sufficient thickness of the units or panels being joined. Concrete slabs may be made in thicknesses suitable for the incorporation of the necessary profile more conveniently than in other materials. It is, therefore, with concrete slabs that developments of joint geometry to exclude rainwater have taken place.

(c) *Types of joint* (diagram D.3.04/25)
There are basically two types of joint which may be used. These are: (1) *The butt joint* (sometimes also known as a push-pull joint) and (2) *The lap joint* (also known as a shear joint) as shown at the top of the diagram. The reasons for the alternative names of both joints may be appreciated by reference to the manner in which sealants filling the joints behave relative to expansion or contraction in the joint, as shown in the diagram.

From the two basic types of joint a number of permutations are possible in terms of detail. Some derivatives are included in the diagram. The 'accessory joints' are essentially butt joint types while the 'integral joints' lap joint types. In regard to the latter it should be noted that certain features, particularly a limitation on the extent of movement, are similar to the butt joint. This means care in the determination of the minimum width of the joint to avoid opposing faces meeting. Theoretically, the true lap joint does not restrict the movement of the opposing surfaces.

(d) *Direction of the joint*
In some cases the precise detail of any particular type of joint will depend on its direction, that is whether it runs vertically or horizontally. It is possible to consider vertical and horizontal joints separately. Their design relative to the exclusion of rainwater may be different, mainly because of the effects of driving rain and the related flow of water over the exposed surfaces and hence the demand at the joint itself.

However, before outlining the factors which may result in detailed differences between vertical or horizontal joints it is necessary to note that the junction of vertical and horizontal joints, whether different in detail or not, needs special consideration, so as to ensure complete weather-tightness. Separate two-dimensional drawings are often inadequate to understand or resolve the difficulties which may be involved. In some cases even three-dimensional drawings may not illustrate the implications clearly. Consequently, it may be advisable, at the design stage, to construct simple models of the joint itself. In the case of concrete panels, for example, balsa wood may be a convenient medium to use. It has been suggested that, where models are used, they should not be made less than half full-size.

With horizontal joints it is possible

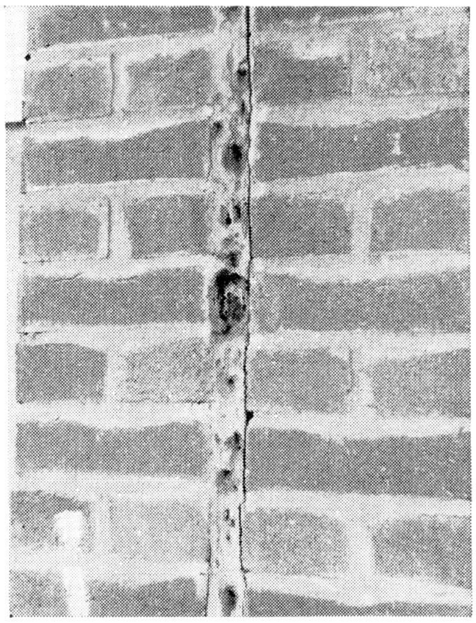

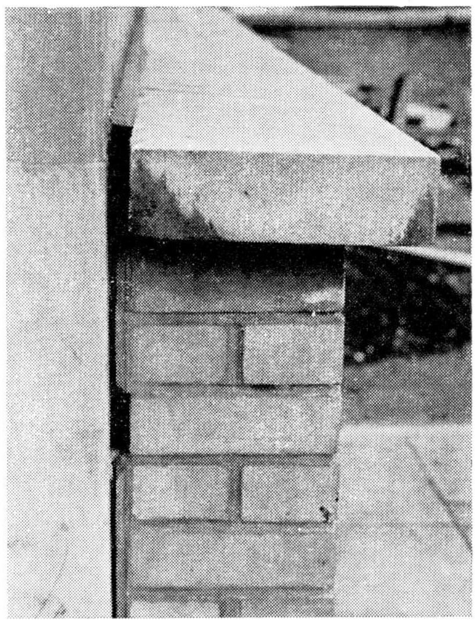

*Curiosity can lead to premature deterioration of a plastic mastic used within human reach as shown in the example above.* (*Building about four years old*). *The mastic has, however, also failed to maintain adhesion with the faces of the joint. An obvious example of incorrect choice of mastic aggravated by lack of maintenance. Right, two examples of the failure of sealants to accommodate movements. In the picture* (*top right*) *mortar has been used as a sealant and in the picture below it a mastic has been used. These examples underline the importance of the relationship between the properties of a sealant* (*particularly when complete watertightness is effected by adhesion*) *and the movements which it can accommodate*

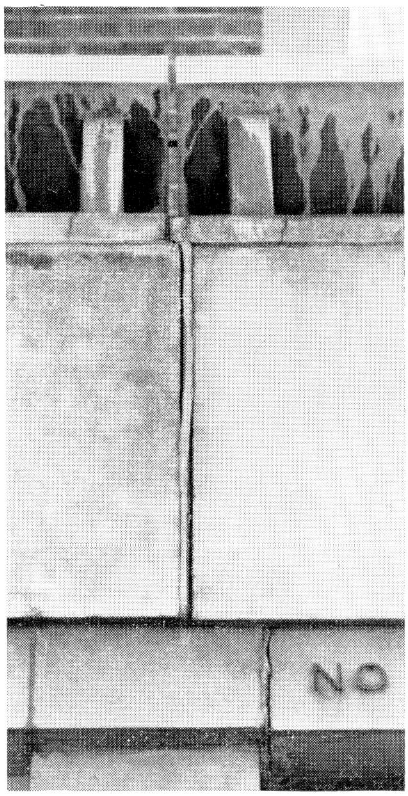


*The junction of vertical and horizontal joints always needs special consideration. An example of the use of staggered joints in precast concrete cladding to avoid the 'four corner clash' is given below*

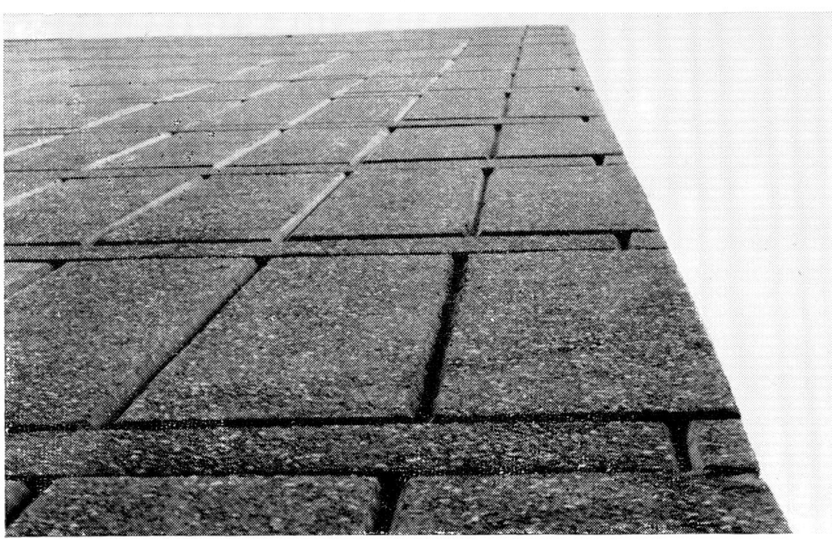

to solve the problem of exclusion of rainwater by simply using a form of lap joint, placing little reliance on a seal, although a seal may be desirable for other reasons. In the main it is safe to assume, except of course where exposure may result in the wind causing an upward flow of water, that the flow of water is essentially downwards. However, the flow of water down the surface may, when rain is accompanied by wind, take on a diagonal creep (similar to that discussed under 'Roofs' previously). This places an additional demand on the vertical joint and its detailed design will be influenced accordingly.

## 2. Sealing materials

All materials used to fill joints are required to maintain a weatherproof seal between the sides of a joint. The nature of the materials required for a particular circumstance is, to a large extent, dependent on the degree of movement which they can tolerate without failure. Looked at in another way, the choice of a sealant is primarily dictated by the movement expected to take place. However, the nature of the materials to be joined may influence the choice of material. In masonry, for example, the choice lies chiefly in a range of mortars.

Broadly speaking, sealing materials range between those which are rigid and those which are resilient. *Rigid sealants,* such as mortars and some of the traditional glazing putties, are characterised by the fact that they can only withstand *slight movements.* The *resilient sealing materials,* such as mastics and gaskets, on the other hand, have been specifically formulated to accommodate much *larger movements.* There is a considerable range of movements which can be accommodated by sealing materials as a whole. Among other things, it is always important to ascertain the extent of movement which a specific material can accommodate. The general properties and behaviour of mortars, mastics and gaskets are now dealt with separately.

### (a) *Mortars**

A mortar consists basically of a binding agent (various types of cement and/or lime) mixed together with water, is made *in situ* and may, in building practice, be used either as a jointing or as a surfacing material in all forms of masonry. Only jointing is considered here. The properties of the mortar may be altered by varying the proportions of the constituents, the type of constituents or by the inclusion of certain additives.

The basic differences between lime : sand and cement : sand mixes may be conveniently noted here. Traditional mortars were made of at least 1 part* lime to 3 parts sand. Such mixes are workable, i.e. good plasticity, but develop strength slowly, relying on absorption or evaporation of the water and subsequent reaction with carbon dioxide in the air. Slow strength development and low eventual strength make lime mortars unsuitable for most present-day needs. Cement mortars, on the other hand, develop strength rapidly and possess greater strength in the hardened mortar, but also undergo fairly large drying shrinkage (see 'Movement in cement-based products', *Section 3.03,* pp. 82–85). Strength cannot simply be varied by using lean mixes and 1 part of cement to 3 parts sand is the minimum requirement for reasonable workability. A 1 : 3 cement : sand mix is far too strong for most general uses. Cement and lime may, however, be combined so as to take advantage of the useful properties of each. Thus a range of strengths and degrees of plasticity may be obtained. Cement mortars may also be varied in strength and given better plasticity by the use of 'plasticisers' (air entraining agents) or by the sole use of masonry cement and sand.

When freshly made, a good mortar should hang on a trowel, spread easily, not lose water readily and stiffen in contact with absorptive walling units and remain plastic for long enough for the walling units to be easily adjusted to line and level. These properties are important to aid adhesion between the mortar and the walling units, thereby reducing the likelihood of cracking and consequently reducing the likelihood of penetration of rainwater through the wall. All these properties cannot necessarily be found in practice in any one mortar, although traditional lime : sand mixes possessed many of them. Consequently, a mortar mix must be designed to provide those which are most important in any particular circumstance. Other factors which influence good adhesion and cracking, such as strength and durability, must also be taken into account.

In general, one of the chief disadvantages of mortars is that, being rigid when set, they can only accommodate slight movements in the walling units or as the result of settlements, etc. As important, however, mortars are also susceptible, in varying degrees, to drying out shrinkage which may result in loss of adhesion and/or cracking. The extent to which a mortar is able to withstand the induced stresses, without loss of adhesion or cracking, is primarily dependent on the *strength* of the mortar, although this is closely related to the strength and movements of the walling units.

The guiding principle to be adopted in the selection of a suitable mortar is that it should not contain any more cement (important for strength but not for plasticity) than is necessary to give adequate strength in the units used. In general, there are two main reasons for *avoiding* the use of *rich mixes,* except for specific applications. These are: (1) Strong mortars are less able to accommodate movements caused by shrinkage, settlement, etc., and tend to concentrate the effects of differential movement in fewer and wider cracks. Weaker mortars, although they may still yield to the induced stresses in the form of cracking, tend to distribute fine hair cracks in the joints inconspicuously. This type of cracking is less likely to produce continuous capillary paths, thus reducing the likelihood of penetration by rainwater through the wall. In this it is to be remembered that cracking is more frequent when strong mortars are used with sand-lime or concrete bricks and lightweight concrete blocks, as all these units are unable to withstand the restraints imposed on their moisture movements by the strength of the mortar. The increased size, when compared to traditional bricks, of lightweight concrete blocks which have inherently large moisture movements (see comparative charts C.3.03/1 and C.3.03/10), is also significant. The magnitude of movement in large panels of precast concrete, together with the wide joints necessary, usually precludes the use of mortar as the sole means of sealing the joints between units (see '3. Specific applications' later). The same is not necessarily true of ashlar work (natural or precast stone) in which the units are adequately restrained by a background.

(2) The strength of the mortar does not make a significant contribution to the strength of the wall in which it is used. The strength of the units themselves is far more significant. Consequently the use of a mortar of a lower strength than the walling units may be justified.

The choice of a richer mix may, however, be justified, if not imperative, when there is a risk of frost action (see *3.08 Frost action,* for detailed consideration of the factors involved) either during construction or during the life of the building. Types of construction and time of construction are important. In order to resist deterioration due to frost action, durability of the mortar is necessary. The requisite durability may be provided by strong mortars, which, among other things, develop their durability fairly quickly after being laid, particularly in winter.

Another factor which does, in part, influence loss of adhesion and the extent of cracking which may occur in a mortar whatever its strength is the width of the joint. The wider the joint the greater the risk of loss of adhesion and/or cracking. In most brick and block masonry it is, however, difficult to reduce the width of the joint to less than a nominal 9·5mm. Except in special circumstances, the nominal width of joint

*References: (1) *Mortars for jointing,* BRS Digest (2nd Series) No. 58, HMSO, May, 1965. (2) *Principles of Modern Building,* Vol. I, 3rd Ed., pp. 112–7 and p. 245, HMSO, 1959.

*In the context of mortars, use of the terms 'part' or 'parts' implies part or parts *by volume,* i.e. the quantitative measurement of the constituents.

should not exceed 16·0mm. In ashlar work it is possible to reduce the joint width to as little as 3·2mm, although 4·5mm is common. (See diagram D.3.04/6, included under 'Solid walling', p. 103).

There is a fairly wide range of mortar mixes available to suit the requirements of any particular circumstance or condition. In making a selection account must be taken of the factors already discussed and their relationship to (1) the type of construction, (2) its exposure, and (3) the time of construction. It is, however, convenient to consider mortars suitable for bricks and blocks separately from stone masonry.

*Brick and block masonry.* In order to facilitate the selection of mortars for various uses, the Building Research Station has designated mortars 1–5 according to type of construction, conditions of exposure, early frost hazard and type of brick and block used. These are given in Table 3.04/4. A further choice has, however, also to be made of mortar mix in any one designation to satisfy other requirements. Table 3.04/5 classifies the mortar mixes in each designation and shows by indicating arrows how they compare as regards strength and resistance to frost and rain penetration. It should be noted that in Table 3.04/4 internal walls and partitions have been included. In many cases these may, during construction that is, be as exposed as external walls. Hence the inclusion of the risk of early frost hazard.

*Stone masonry.* In general the mixes quoted above are also suitable for stone masonry, either as jointing or pointing. However, account has also to be taken of other requirements, such as colour and texture, permeability relative to the stone and low soluble alkali content (to avoid staining).

Typical mixes* in general use which satisfactorily fulfil the requirements of stone masonry are:

(1) 16 parts fine crushed stone,
4 parts lime putty or hydrated lime,
1 part Portland cement.

Although the mix is a little lean, thus suffering in plasticity, it has made a good hard joint.

(2) 12 parts fine crushed stone,
3 parts lime putty or hydrated lime,
1 part Portland cement.

Stronger than the first and probably quite satisfactory.

(3) 7 parts fine crushed stone,
5 parts lime putty,
1 part Portland cement.

A mix recommended by a firm of stonemasons. Although highly plastic, it is rather stronger than either (1) or (2). In some cases shrinkage may prove troublesome.

*Reference: *Principles of Modern Building,* Vol. I, 3rd Ed., p. 245, HMSO, 1959.

**Table 3·04/4. Selection of mortar types**

| *Type of construction* | *Exposure conditions*[1] | *Early frost hazard* | *Type of bricks or blocks* | *Mortar designation* |
|---|---|---|---|---|
| *External walls:* Retaining walls | Any | Yes or no | Clay, concrete or calcium silicate | 1 |
| Parapet, free standing wall or below damp-proof course[3] | Any | Yes or no | Clay | **1, 2 or 3** |
| | | | Concrete or calcium silicate[2] | 3 |
| Between eaves and damp-proof course | Severe | Yes or no | Clay, concrete or calcium silicate | 3 |
| | Sheltered or moderate | Yes | Clay, concrete or calcium silicate | 3 |
| | | No | Clay | **3 or 4** |
| | | | Concrete or calcium silicate[2] | 4 |
| *Internal walls and partitions*[4] | — | Yes | Clay | 3 |
| | | | Concrete or calcium silicate | 4 |
| | | No | Clay, concrete or calcium silicate | **4 or 5** |

*Notes:* 1. Severe exposure conditions apply to external walls in districts with a driving-rain index of $7m^2/s$ or more, and to high walls in districts with an index of $6m^2/s$ or more. See *Section 3.02,* pp. 35–38.

2. When a 1:1:5–6 mix is used with calcium silicate or concrete bricks, the bricks should be Class A(i) quality or better (BS 187:1955 and 1180:1944).

3. Special attention should be paid to the quality of bricks used for these purposes; calcium silicate and concrete bricks should be special-purpose type (BS 187:1955 and 1180:1944) and clay products should have a low content of sulphate salts. Magnesium lime mortars should not be used below damp-proof course unless the lime has been fully hydrated.

4. For concrete partition blocks that have an appreciable drying shrinkage the mix with the lower cement content is preferable. For some types of partition blocks, e.g. gypsum or anhydrite plaster blocks, a mortar based on a gypsum or anhydrite plaster may be used.



*Reference: Mortars for jointing,* BRS Digest (2nd Series) No. 58, Table 1, p. 2, HMSO, May, 1965.

**Table 3·04/5. Equivalent mortar mixes[1] (proportions by volume)**

| | *Mortar designation (from Table 3.04/4)* | *Hydraulic –lime:sand* | *Cement: lime[2]: sand* | *Masonry –cement: sand* | *Cement: sand with plasticiser* |
|---|---|---|---|---|---|
| ↑ Increasing strength but decreasing ability to accommodate movements caused by settlement, shrinkage, etc. | 1 | — | $1:0–\frac{1}{4}:3$[3] | — | — |
| | 2 | — | $1:\frac{1}{2}:4–4\frac{1}{2}$ | — | — |
| | 3 | — | 1:1:5–6 | $1:4\frac{1}{2}$ | 1:5–6 |
| | 4 | 1:2–3 | 1:2:8–9 | 1:6 | 1:7–8 |
| | 5 | 1:3 | 1:3:10–12 | 1:7 | 1:8 |
| Direction of change in properties (within any one mortar designation) | ——→ Increasing resistance to ——→ damage by freezing. ←—— Improving bond and consequent ←—— resistance to rain penetration. | | | | |

*Notes:* 1. The different types of mortar that comprise any one designation in the above table are approximately equivalent in strength, and do not differ greatly in their other properties Such differences as do exist (indicated by the arrows at the bottom of the table) can be reduced by additives or special treatments. Thus the bond of aerated mortars to dry bricks can be considerably improved by water-retaining additives, e.g. cellulose ethers and aeration of cement–lime mortars will improve their resistance to early damage by freezing.

2. 'Lime' refers to non-hydraulic or semi-hydraulic lime. The proportions given are for lime putty. If the lime is measured as the dry hydrate, the amount can be increased by up to $1\frac{1}{2}$ volumes for each volume of lime putty; the hydrate should preferably be soaked at least overnight before use. Where a range of sand contents is given (e.g. 5–6, 8–9 or 10–12), the higher should be used for sand that is well graded, and the lower for coarse or uniformly fine sand.

3. The recommendation applies only when the maximum possible strength is needed. Otherwise, it is better to adopt the recommendations given for clay bricks generally.



*Reference: Mortars for jointing,* BRS Digest (2nd Series) No. 58, Table 2, p. 2, HMSO, May, 1965.

## (b) *Mastics**

Mastics, sometimes known as caulking compounds or sealants (the latter may include gaskets), include a wide range of compositions (see Table 3.04/6) to suit a wide range of joint filling or sealing conditions for exclusion of rainwater and air or infiltration of snow. Selection of a mastic suitable for a particular circumstance requires extreme care. Glazing putties are an early, if not traditional, form of mastic, which are readily formed into desired shapes but harden rapidly, need protection by paint and are only capable of accommodating slight

*References: (1) *Jointing with mastics and gaskets—1 and 2,* BRS Digests (2nd Series) Nos. 36 and 37, HMSO, July and August, 1963, respectively. (2) Baker, T. A., *Guide to choosing a mastic* (Materials Division, the BRS), article in Building Materials, pp. 12–17, August, 1965. (3) Rostron, R. Michael, *Light cladding of buildings* (Architectural Press), 1964, particularly chapter 15. (4) Trade literature, but particularly *Designing and sealing of joints in building,* by Bostik Ltd., 1965.

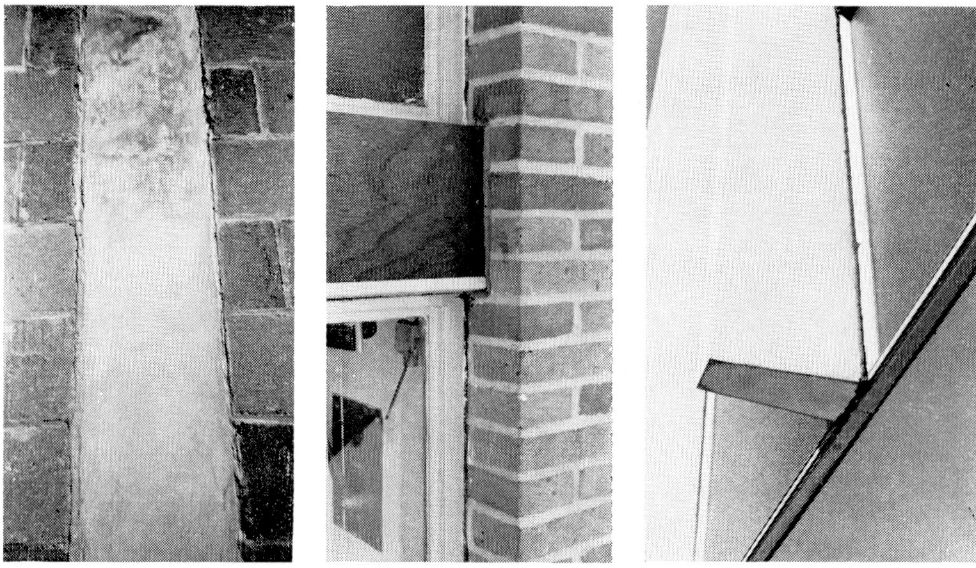

*The selection of a mastic suitable for a particular circumstance requires extreme care. A wide range of compositions are available to suit a wide range of joint filling or sealing conditions The photographs above illustrate messy applications of a mastic to an ill-considered joint. Those below show the incorrect choice of mastic for the particular circumstance (left) to a building after four years and (right) after six months*

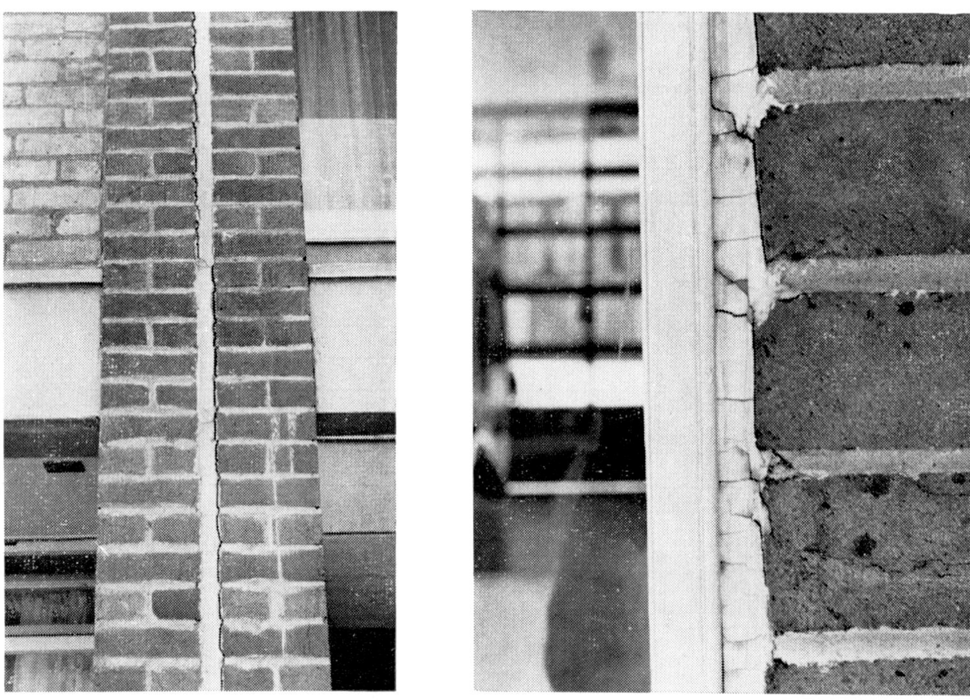

movements. Recent developments in mastics have, therefore, aimed to formulate materials which do not slump and retain plasticity or elasticity for long periods of time while accommodating fairly large movements. The performance of the newer mastics to meet the rigorous requirements imposed on them has varied considerably. In many cases failure to take those precautions which aid durability, including the actual design of the joint, have been significant.

At present, experience suggests that the life of a mastic cannot be expected to be the same as that of the building, short-life buildings apart. The need for replacement of the mastic and the manner in which this is to be accomplished should, therefore, be carefully considered in the design of all joints. The absence of comprehensive standards and codes means that manufacturers should be consulted, although reference to those standards and codes that are available together with the advice available from the Building Research Station, much of which (currently available, that is) is included here, should be of assistance in understanding the significance of some of the basic problems involved. It should be emphasised that although there may, from Table 3.04/6, appear to be a comparatively small number of mastics, there may, in fact, be a number of different materials available containing any one medium.* The precise composition and related properties of any particular mastic should, therefore, be checked. It has been considered convenient to outline first

***Standards and codes on mastics, including putties, available or pending*: the first three are particularly relevant to most of the mastics listed in Table 3.04/6. Tests included in British Standards may be useful in some cases. (1) US Federal Specification TT-C-598, *Compound caulking: Plastic (for masonry and other structures)*. (2) American Standards Association Specification A 116.1-1960, *Polysulfide-Base Sealing Compounds for the Building Trade*. (3) Draft Specification No. 1, *Two-part polysulphide based sealing compositions for the Building Industry*, The Sealant

*Continued on p. 143*

**Table 3.04/6. Composition of Mastics**

| Medium | Nature of mastic | Usual method of application | *Volume of mastic* | | | Life expectancy* (years) | Comments |
|---|---|---|---|---|---|---|---|
| | | | | *Width Max.* | *Depth Min.* | | |
| Drying and non-drying oils | Plastic | Gun, knife or trowel, tape | — | 16·0mm | 9·5mm (preferably 12·7mm or more) | 5–10 | Many harden after a few years. The best are probably the gun mastics which remain soft under a leathery skin for prolonged periods if used in adequate depth, preferably over 12·7mm. Should only be used if expected elongation is not more than 10%. Must be accessible for maintenance and renewal. Suitable for painting |
| Bitumen and rubber-bitumen | Mainly plastic, some partly elastic | Gun, knife or trowel, tape, poured | — | — | — | — | Cheap materials of good resistance to water, dilute acids and alkalies. Many harden in a few years if exposed. Softened by oil, grease and some solvents. Primer may be required. Difficult to paint |
| Butyl rubber | Mainly plastic, some partly elastic | Gun, knife or trowel, tape | Non-curing | 9·5mm | 6·4mm | 15–20 | Recent materials retain softness well. May lose adhesion to glass when sunlight gains access to glass/mastic interface. Subject to flow under pressure, particularly non-curing types. Exposed surfaces may collect dirt |
| | | | Curing | 1·6mm | 3·2–6·4mm | Unknown: 15–20 likely | |
| Polyisobutylene | Plastic | Tape, usually soft | — | — | — | — | Retains softness well. Adhesion to glass when sunlight gains access to the glass/mastic interface is relatively good |
| Polysulphide rubber ('Thiokol'†) | Elastic | Mostly two-part gun-applied or poured. Some one-part materials available | One-part | 12·7–25·4mm | 6·4mm | Unknown: 15–20 likely | Sets to a rubber in a day or so at temperatures above 7°C (two-part materials; one-part materials set more slowly). Not tolerant of grease on surfaces. Good durability, but loses adhesion to glass when sunlight gains access to glass/mastic interface. One-part materials may exude from joint before onset of cure. Some materials stain white marble. Smears may be hard to remove (two-part materials) |
| | | | Two-part | 50·8mm | 6·4mm | 20 minimum | |
| Urethane | Elastic | Two-part, gun-applied or poured | — | 50·8mm | 6·4mm | Unknown: 15–20 likely | Special mixers are required. Sets to rubber in a day or so at temperatures above 7°C. Good adhesion difficult to obtain; all surfaces require priming. Mainly recommended with primer for concrete. Sensitive to moisture until cured |
| 'Neoprene' | Elastic | Two-part, gun-applied | — | — | — | — | Good reports from America—little British experience |
| Silicone | Elastic | One-part, gun-applied | — | 0·8–25·4mm | 0·8–9·5mm | Unknown: 15–20 likely | Good reports from America—little British experience. Sets fairly quickly. Some loss of properties at high temperatures |
| Acrylic | Plastic | Gun-applied | — | 12·7mm | 6·4mm | Unknown: 15 likely | Relatively new. Behaviour expected similar to butyl mastics. Little known of their durability |

*Important:* * The values quoted in this column represent the minimum and maximum life that can reasonably be expected and assume good quality materials and, above all, joint design and workmanship which aid durability—see text.
† Registered trade name of Thiokol Chemical Corporation and refers to liquid polymer made by them.

*References:* (1) *Jointing with Mastic and Gaskets—1*, BRS Digest (2nd Series), No. 36, HMSO, July 1963.
(2) Rostron, R. M., *Light Cladding of Buildings*, (Architectural Press), 1964 (particularly for 'Volume of mastic' and 'Life expectancy').
(3) *Designing and Sealing of Joints in Buildings*, published by Bostik Limited, 1965 (particularly for information on 'Acrylic' mastic).

the application and basic characteristics of mastics and then to discuss under various headings the significance of those factors which influence durability, including adhesion.

*Application.* Mastics may be applied by gun, knife or trowel or by pouring, while some are available as tapes or strips. Those intended for pouring in horizontal surfaces are usually based on bitumen and require heating; mastics for cold pouring are based on 'Thiokol' or urethane. Although mastics are available ready for use (one-part mastics), others are supplied in two separate packs (two-part mastics) for mixing immediately prior to use, usually for gun application. All mastics require care in their application. Among other things, two-part mastics have a short pot life, from $\frac{1}{2}$ to 32 hr, depending on material and temperature.

*Basic characteristics.* Two broad groups may be identified each with its own characteristics: (1) *Plastic mastics,* which implies that the mastic is capable of plastic flow and not that it is based on plastics. This group includes most mastics based on oils, bitumen or polyisobutylene and some butyl mastics. Under continuing load they may be extruded, in which case spacers of a more rigid material should carry the load. They have the ability to flow slowly with the movement of the joint (dependent on speed rather than extent of the movement), thus reducing the demand on the adhesion and cohesion of the mastic. (2) *Elastic mastics* include those based on 'Thiokol', 'Neoprene', silicones or urethane and some butyl mastics. On curing (comparatively short-time) most of the compositions change from a plastic state to form a rubber-like mass, which is not extruded when subjected to load. The demands on adhesion are proportional to the extent of the movement and are not greatly affected by its rate. The rubber-like mastics are difficult to remove.

*Effect of joint type.* Both butt and lap joints may be sealed with mastics (diagram D.3.04/26). *Butt joints* are easy to fill and often easy to replace. Against this, when the mastic fails the widest part of the joint is only partly filled by the mastic and leakage may be severe. *Lap joints* are more difficult to fill and to replace. Against this, the surfaces being joined remain the same distance apart, although moving parallel to each other, i.e. the joint does not gape even if the adhesion fails and the mastic still fills the joint. For equal movement of the surfaces, the extension of the mastic in a lap joint is only about half that in a butt joint. This is important when choosing a mastic according to calculated movement (see Table 3.04/7 and 'Effect of joint dimensions' below). Another advantage is that the mastic in a lap joint is better protected from the weather, thus aiding durability.

*Effect of joint dimensions.* Both the width and depth of the joint are important. Taken together, they influence the volume of mastic used. Their inter-related dimensions may influence slumping of the mastic or may affect the extensibility of the mastic.

*The width* of the joint must be

*Continued from p. 142*

Conferences of the Federation of British Rubber and Allied Manufacturers. (4) BS 3712 : 1964, *Parts I and II, Methods of tests for building mastics.* Unifies test procedure and facilitates comparison. Further parts are to be published. (5) BS 3245 : 1960, *Jointing compounds for the use in liquified petroleum gas appliances and installations.* (6) BS 2499 : 1954, *Tests to assess the properties of hot applied joint sealing compounds for concrete pavements.* (7) BS 1737 : 1951, *Jointing materials and compounds for water, town gas and low-pressure steam installations.* (8) BS 544 : 1934 (including a number of amendments), *Linseed oil putty for use in wooden frames.* Being revised and may be followed by one for metal casement putty. (9) BS Code of Practice, CP 152 : 1960, Glazing and fixing of glass for buildings. Gives guidance on the choice of compounds for various glazing techniques, etc.

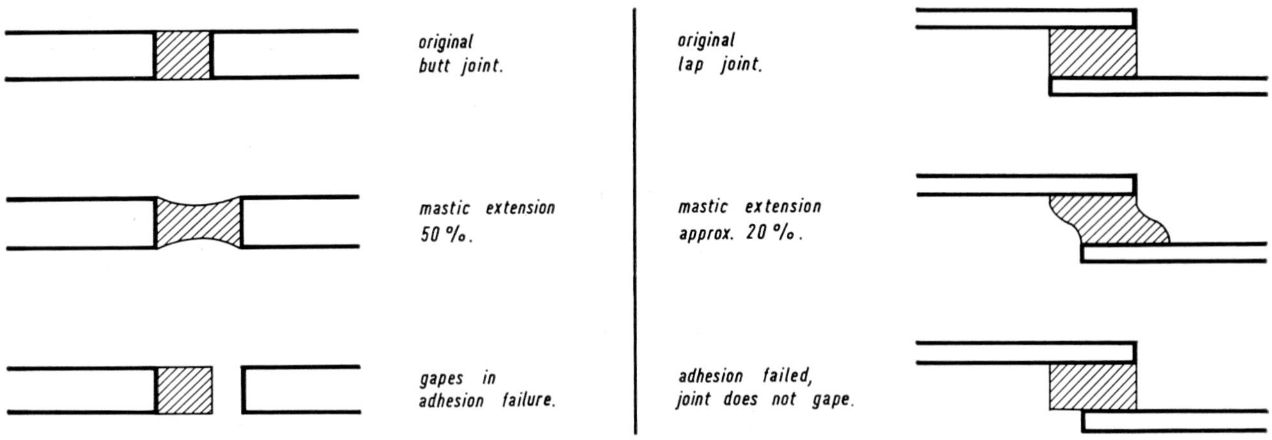


*D.3.04/26*
*Effect of joint type on mastic seal*

**Table 3.04/7. Choice of mastic according to calculated movement**

| *Movement as a percentage of minimum mastic width** | | *Mastics suggested* |
|---|---|---|
| Butt joint | Lap joint | |
| 1 | 5 | Putties are adequate, but must be painted |
| Under 10 | Under 40 | Any soft mastic or gasket. Oil or bitumen-based mastics are adequate if shielded or easily renewed |
| 10–25 | 40–75 | Plastic or elastic mastics or gaskets are suitable. Where movement is slow (less than 25mm/h) or if the joint is likely to spend long periods at full extension, a plastic mastic (e.g. butyl, polyisobutylene or oil-based gun mastic) is better. Where there is stick-slip movement or only short periods are spent at full extension, an elastic mastic should be used (e.g. 'Thiokol', urethane). The greater the movement, the softer the mastic should be |
| Over 25 | Over 75 | It is probably better to rely on gaskets in shear or on specially designed joints without mastics |


* The minimum mastic width in terms of dimensions can only be calculated once the maximum possible movement in the joint has been determined. For design purposes the movement in the joint is assumed to be the total for the two units separated by the joint. Thus the total movement, due either to thermal or moisture or both depending on the materials concerned, in each unit must be doubled. If, for example, the total movement in one unit = 1·27mm, then the maximum possible movement in the joint will be = 2·54mm. Assuming the latter represents the maximum joint movement of 25% or 75% which the best mastics can tolerate in butt or lap joints respectively given in the table, then the minimum mastic width will need to be as follows:

For the butt joint: $\frac{100}{25} \times 2{\cdot}54 = 10{\cdot}16$mm.

For the lap joint: $\frac{100}{75} \times 2{\cdot}54 = 3{\cdot}38$mm.

See text for other adjustments which must be made to determine the actual width.

*Reference: Jointing with mastics and gaskets*—2, BRS Digest (2nd Series) No. 37, Table 2, p. 3, HMSO, August, 1963.

sufficient to accommodate the expected movement and be appropriate to the movement properties of the mastic. The Building Research Station has prepared a table to aid the choice of mastic according to calculated movement. This is given in Table 3.04/7. In order to use this table it is first necessary to calculate* the maximum movement of a panel (thermal or combined thermal and moisture as relevant), taking any special circumstances such as conditions (temperature or moisture) to be expected at the time of erection, ease of replacement or inconsequence of joint failure (i.e. water penetration may not be important) and the degree of restraint. The maximum movement of the panel has to be doubled to give the maximum movement of the joint. From this the minimum mastic width (usually falls between 0·8mm and 25·4mm) can be calculated according to the movement properties of the mastic to be used. The minimum mastic width then forms the basis upon which the actual width, which will include tolerance, will be determined. This width is of importance if slumping is to be avoided. However, in order to ensure that no joint is less than the minimum mastic width a *design joint width* must be calculated on the basis of $W + 2T$, as shown in diagram D.3.04/27, which also illustrates that the actual joint may vary between $W$ and $W + 4T$.

*The depth* (usually measured perpendicular to the weathering or exposed surface) is primarily important for the durability of the mastic, which can be associated with the surface skin which forms during the curing of the mastic. In the case of the oil-based mastics, the rapid formation of a surface skin delays further drying out, and hence hardening, of the mastic. Greater depth (9·5mm or more) is, therefore, an advantage, if not imperative. In the case of one-part polysulphide mastics, the formation of the skin retards curing, and hence the formation of an elastic material. The depth has, therefore, to be restricted so as to avoid long-curing periods. The same consideration does not apply to the two-part polysulphide mastics as they cure by a chemical reaction, which is initiated as soon as the sealants are mixed. However, it should be noted that for optimum durability a minimum depth of 6·4mm is applicable to all polysulphide mastics.

*The ratio* of the width to the depth is important relative to the extensibility of the mastic. In the first place there must be sufficient depth to enable the particular mastic to accept deformation. For the oil-based mastics a depth of at least 9·5mm below the surface skin should be regarded as a minimum—12·7mm or more should preferably be used to compensate for workmanship and/or site difficulties. For polysulphide sealed joints the recommended* relationship between the width and the depth for both butt and lap joints is illustrated in diagram D.3.04/28.

*Effect of filling the joint.* In general the cost of mastics increases with performance; the higher the expected performance the higher the cost. On the other hand, excessively deep-filled mastic joints are not normally essential nor necessarily desirable. The bulk of the joint could, therefore, be filled with back-up materials, such as fibreboard, rope and expanded plastics, thus limiting the amount of sealant used (diagram D.3.04/29). The use of back-up materials can aid adhesion

*Calculations of this kind will be included in *7.00 Production and use generally*. Examples are, however, included in BRS Digest (2nd Series) No. 37—included in references 4 (1).

*Bostik Ltd. Different manufacturers, it should be noted, recommend different thicknesses.

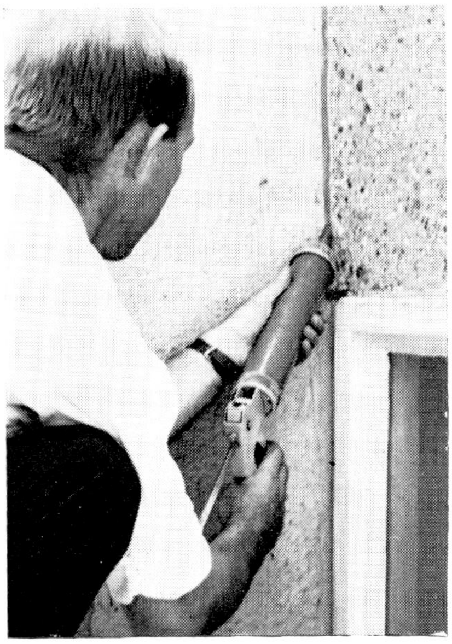

*Two examples of mastics applied with a gun. Above, oil bound mastic to a joint between concrete panels*

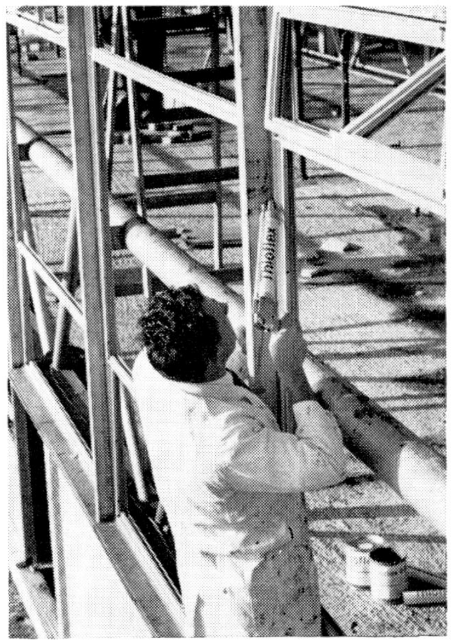

*A polysulphide mastic to a joint between window frames and mullion. Photographs are published by courtesy of Expandite Ltd.*

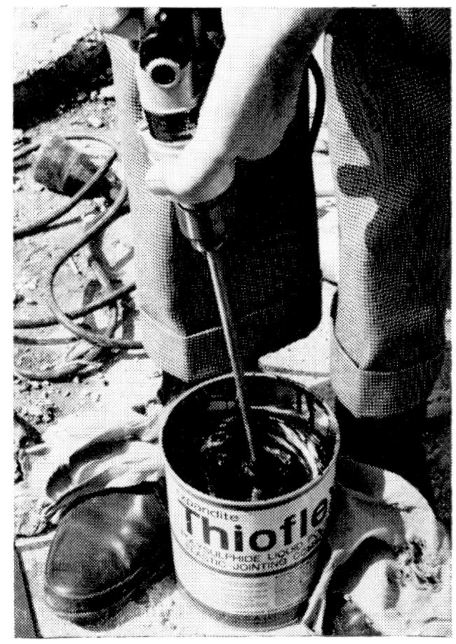


*Two-part mastics require careful and thorough mixing prior to use. The photograph above shows the mixing of a two-part polysulphide mastic*

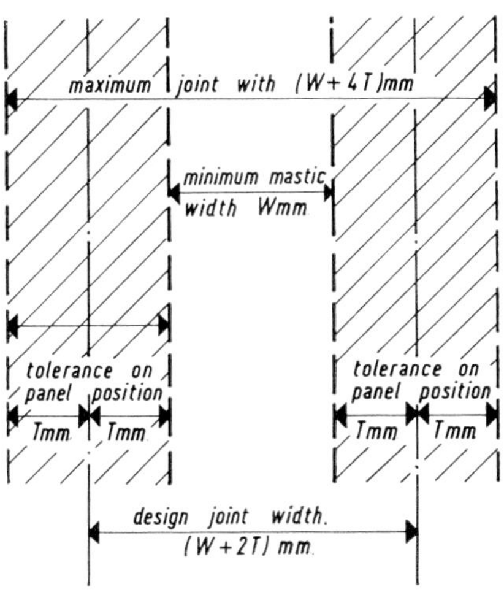


*D*.3.04/27
*To illustrate maximum and design joint width and maximum width*

*D*.3.04/28
*Width/depth ratios of polysulphide mastic seals for butt and lap joints.* (*Recommendation of Bostik Ltd.*)

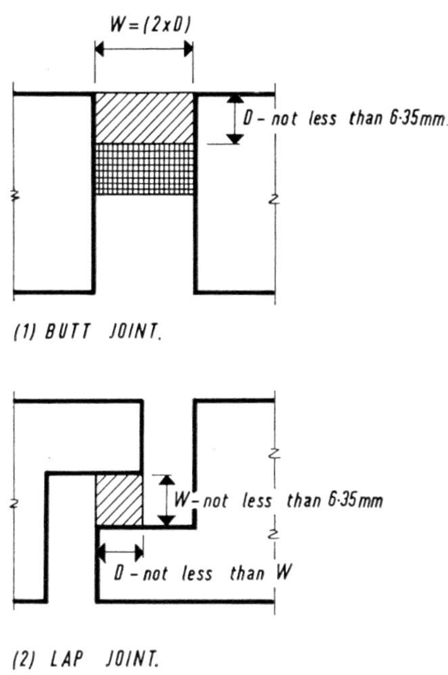


by providing a stop against which the sealant can be forced. It will then spread to the side of the joint, thus obtaining good contact with the joint faces. Back-up materials may also be required to avoid points or areas of high stress in the sealant.

The nature of the back-up material is not critical with most of the plastic mastics, particularly those which are oil-based. However, back-up material should not provide restraint to the elastic mastics and some of the plastic mastics. Consequently, the mastics should either not be allowed to adhere to the back-up material or the back-up material should have the same compression or extensibility as that of the mastic. Plastics-based sponges are often suitable.

*Effect of incompatibility*. As more than one mastic may be used in a particular condition it is important that those used must be compatible with one another. Furthermore, mastics must be compatible with other materials with which they come into contact. Incompatibility may reduce durability and/or the maintenance of good adhesion.

For good adhesion all surfaces must be properly prepared. Basically this includes cleanliness and dryness of the joints. Other precautions may, subject to the mastic being used (manufacturer's instructions need to be carefully followed), include (1) removal of paint or lacquer, or (2) priming or sealing to avoid loss of medium from the mastic, alkali attack by cement-based products, loss of adhesion to oily timbers or to improve the bond.

*Effect of exposure*. In general, the durability of mastics is effected by direct exposure to light, particularly sunlight, air, and in some cases the erosive effects of driving rain and/or wind (high buildings notable).



L

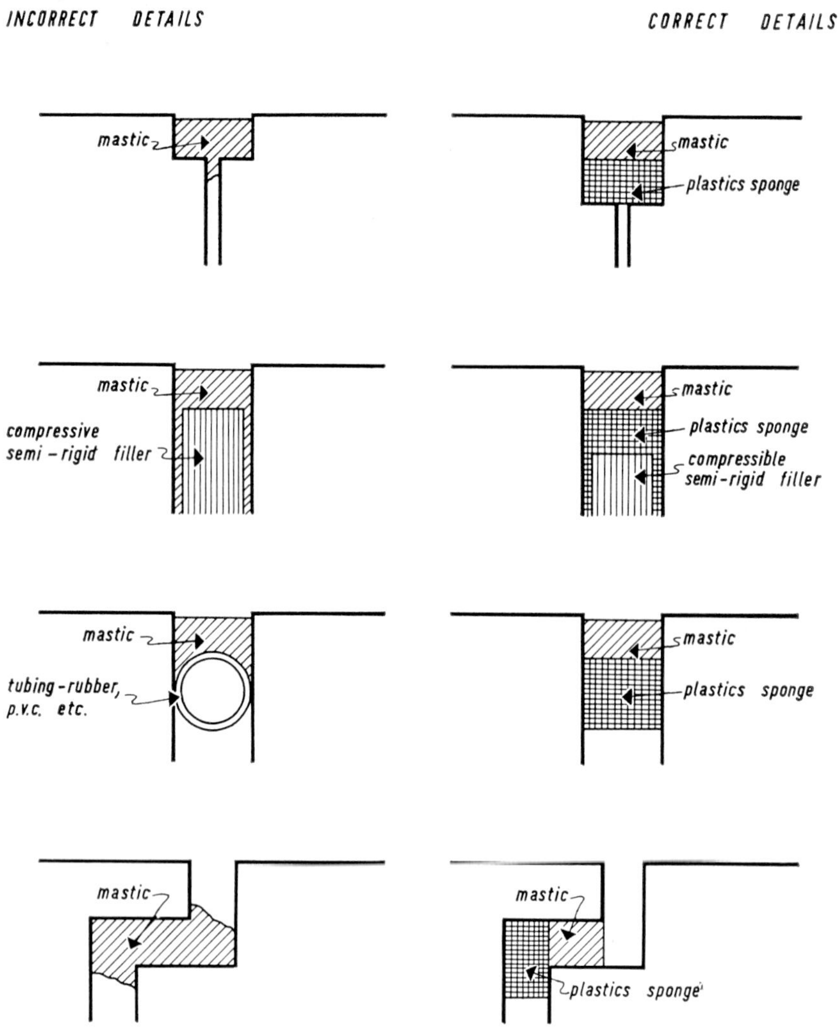


*D.3.04/29*
*The use of 'back-up' materials for deep joints to be filled with mastic. Back-up materials not only save mastic but also aid adhesion and help to avoid points or areas of high stress in the sealant. Properties of the back-up material may be critical for some types of sealant. (Based on information supplied by Bostik Ltd.)*

Mastics may, therefore, be assisted in retaining their original properties if they are suitably shielded—cover strips, overhangs, drips, etc., or drained and ventilated cavities. Some methods of affording protection are illustrated, in principle, in diagram D.3.04/30.

*Effect of size.* The extent of both thermal and moisture movements will be effected by size (superficial dimensions rather than thickness). It is always important to remember that, in general, the greater the size the greater the demands on the mastic. Other factors, such as the nature of the material, environmental conditions, etc., must, however, also be taken into account.

Designed panel and thus joint sizes should take manufacturing and assembly accuracy into account. Some materials can either be made or assembled more accurately than others. It is unfair to require the mastic to make up for excessive tolerances due to faulty design or bad workmanship.

Size as it affects weight of panels, including imposed wind loads, may be important relative to the ability of the mastic to resist extrusion. Setting blocks or distance pieces may be imperative to prevent extrusion (see diagram D.3.04/31).

*Effects of application techniques.* All mastics must be applied by the correct technique so as to ensure good adhesion and complete filling of the joint. In some cases it may be advisable to use specialist applicators.

Thorough mixing of two-part compounds in the right proportions and used within the stipulated pot-life are necessary to ensure a good quality material.

(c) *Gaskets*

Unlike mastics, gaskets rely for their efficiency on the maintenance of a compressive stress within the sealing material rather than on adhesion. Preformed strips are inserted in the joint in such a way that there is a continuing pressure on the sides of the joint. As they do not rely on adhesion, gaskets can tolerate large movements.

The function of gaskets* and hence the requirements needed in the joint, are essentially the same as those of mastics. Stiff tape mastics, oiled cords in patent glazing or bitumen felt on which concrete panels are bedded could be regarded, in many ways, as fulfilling the functions of a gasket.

It has now become common to regard preformed strips made of fully cured elastic compounds such as natural rubber, 'Neoprene' or PVC as the true gaskets. Notwithstanding this, it may be noted that spring clips, as commonly used in patent glazing and other forms of cover strips, if not used in exactly the same way as gaskets, do perform in much the same way. Forms of draughtstripping as applied to doors and windows or pile and plush tapes for sliding points are also forms of gasket, although not inserted into a joint. For comparison these are included in diagram D.3.04/32, although the remainder of the text deals only with true gaskets.

Gaskets are preferably placed in a recess in the joint under sufficient compression to ensure that they are not released by subsequent movements. Gaskets made of foamed material or those which contain pockets of air can be compressed more readily into the joint and can tolerate greater movement than solid ones.

As gaskets do not require hardening or curing they are fully functional as soon as they are installed. As protection during handling or transportation, gaskets may be attached to fragile materials like glass. Although cleaning of surfaces is advisable, this does not require the same rigid precautions as in the case of mastics which rely so much on good adhesion.

One disadvantage of gaskets is that they cannot, like mastics, accommodate rough or irregular surfaces. Consequently, on such surfaces it may be necessary to use mastics or adhesives with gaskets to fill any slight gaps. Another potential weakness is the mitre formed at corners. This can be overcome if special care is taken to ensure that a sound weld is made.

### 3. Specific applications

The purpose of this part is to include some additional examples of the application of mastics and gaskets under various headings. The examples, illustrated in the diagrams and described in the text, are not intended to be exhaustive. Particular emphasis

*References

(1) *Jointing with mastics and gaskets—1 and 2*, BRS Digests (2nd Series) Nos. 36 and 37, HMSO, July and August, 1963, respectively. (2) Rostron, R. Michael, *Light Cladding of Buildings* (Architectural Press), 1964. (3) Trade literature (mainly for diagrams).

is, however, placed on the joints in light cladding generally and between precast concrete panels. In most cases it is not possible to give precise information on the efficacy of the particular application due mainly to the lack of sufficient experience 'in the field'. However, where possible, an indication is given of potential advantages and disadvantages, together with other significant features.

(a) *Light cladding (diagrams* D.3.04/33–35)

The term 'light' used here is that previously defined in p. 96, namely the use of relatively thin materials which are light in terms of their normally usable thicknesses as claddings. For convenience, the use of glass in windows is included in the examples.

*Socket joints* (diagram D.3.04/33) are frequently used for fixing infill panels. Subject to detail, such a joint may have the features of both a butt and lap joint ((1) of the diagram) or be essentially of the lap type ((2) of the diagram). In (1) the mastic is substantially incompressible. If the infill panel expands relative to the frame either the mastic is extruded and becomes unsightly or, because of the forces exerted during expansion, the seal of a double glazed unit may be broken or a plastic panel may buckle. The use of an expansion space, preferably filled with a strip of close-cell foamed plastic, as shown in (2) can help to prevent these failures occurring.

Conflicting requirements often result in difficulties in selecting a mastic, particularly for glass in window frames. Diagram D.3.04/34 illustrates three commonly used applications. In (1) a polysulphide sealant is used at the bottom of the joint, with a butyl mastic above. In this position the glass/polysulphide interface is shielded from sunlight, but the butyl mastic may be damaged by window cleaners and children. To provide greater surface resistance, it is more usual to have a polysulphide mastic gunned in at the top of the joint on the outside, as in (2).

The use of two mastics can be avoided by the use of oval spacers incorporated in a joint using a plastic mastic (3). The spacers are necessary to carry wind loads, thus avoiding extrusion of the mastic. A feature also illustrated in the diagram is the external bead which has been faired off to 40 degrees to the horizontal. The advantages of a bead profiled in this way are that, at the bottom, rain is shed more easily, while at the top, the bead prevents a shadow being cast on the glass. This reduces the risk of the glass cracking when the cladding to the wall is most heated by the sun, namely when the sun is 40 degrees above the horizon.

*Gaskets*, for use with or as framing, are available in a number of sections. H-sections, V-sections and I-sections are common, but other more complex

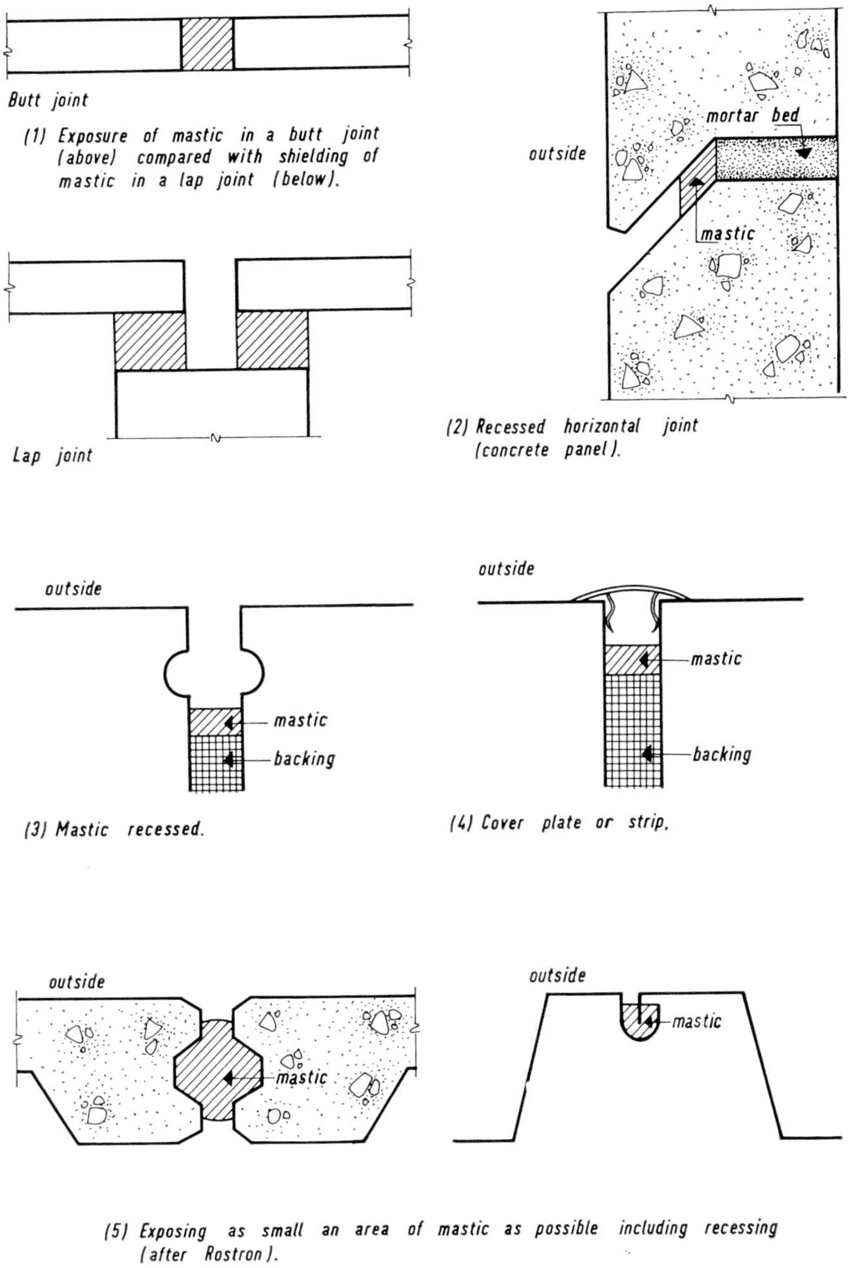


*D.3.04/30*
*Basic exposure of sealants in butt and lap joints and some methods of affording protection of the sealant*

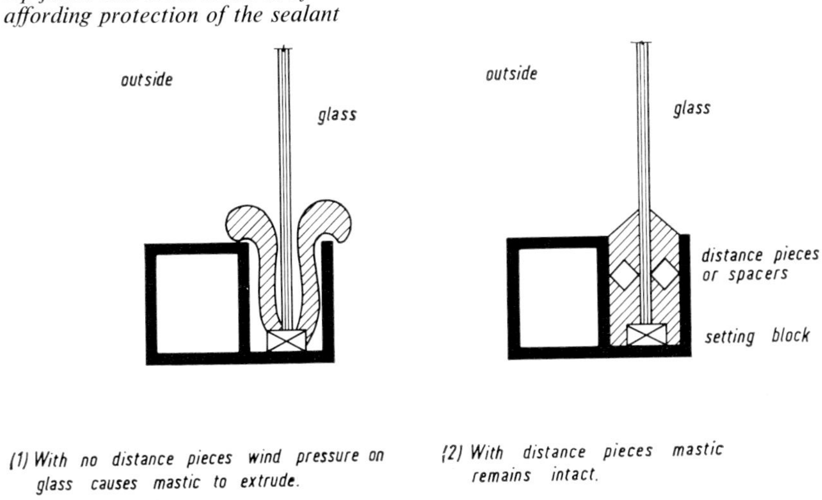


*D.3.04/31*
*Effects of wind pressure on mastic—air currents are not shown*

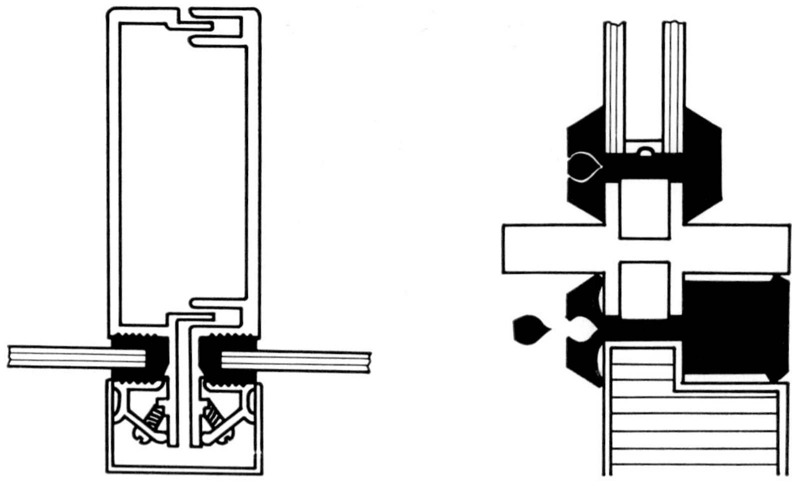

(1) TWO EXAMPLES OF TRUE GASKETS.

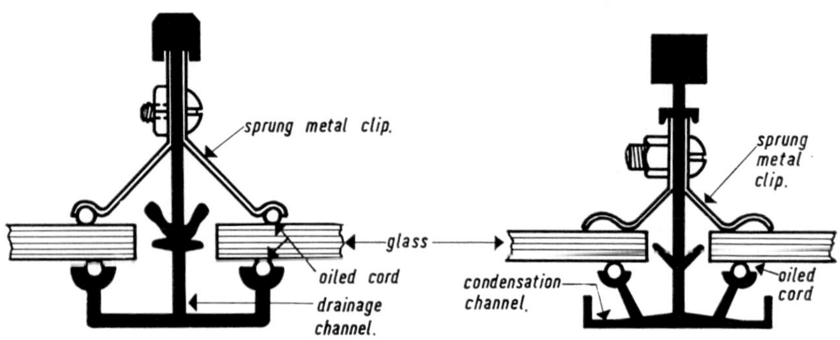


(2) GASKET TYPE USED IN PATENT GLAZING.

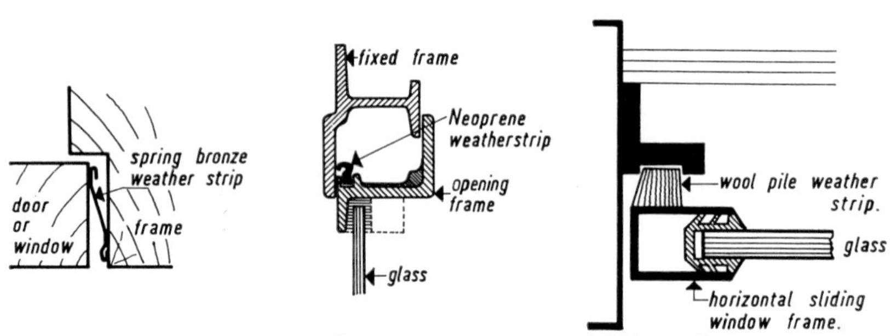


(a) Metal. (b) Neoprene. (c) Wool pile.

(3) GASKET TYPE USED AS WEATHER STRIPPING.

*D.3.04/32*
*Illustrations of some true gaskets and gasket types*

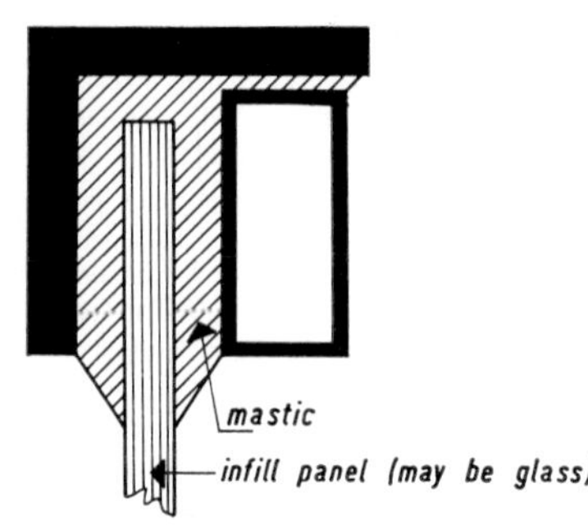


(1) No provision for expansion of panel relative to the frame.

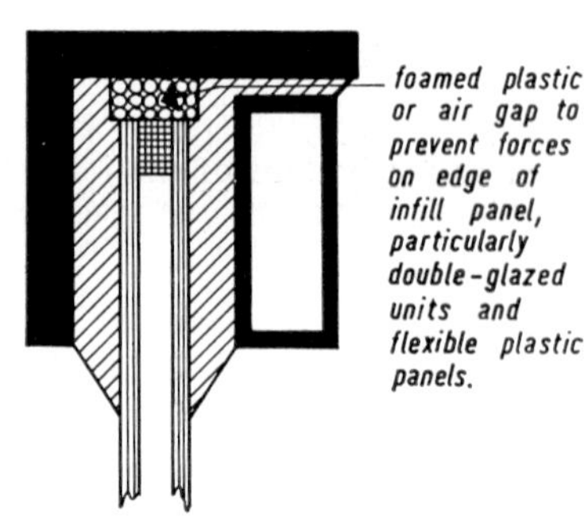


(2) Allowing an expansion space.

*D.3.04/33*
*Butt and lap joint features of a socket joint*

sections are also made. There are four basic methods by which the requisite pressure may be applied, as illustrated in diagram D.3.04/35. In (1), pressure is applied essentially by a movable metal pressure bead which forces the gasket into position while the screws are applied. (2) illustrates the self locking or zipper gasket, where compression is achieved by forcing an oversized strip (material the same as the gasket but harder) into a channel in the gasket. An example of compression of the gasket by distortion is illustrated in (3). Finally, (4) includes examples of evacuated gaskets. The hollow extrusion (plain tubing in its simplest form) is first evacuated, fitted into position and then punctured to allow air to enter so that the tube expands.

(b) *Gutters and sheets* (diagram D.3.04/36)

Although apparently a little out of context, the method of detailing a joint in a gutter using a loadbearing rope gasket and a soft bituminous mastic is also equally applicable for sheets. It is important to note that expansion is allowed for by ensuring that the top bolt hole is slightly enlarged. The mastic, well shielded, helps to maintain watertightness.

(c) *Openings* (diagram D.3.04/37)

The use of mastics for setting windows, doors, etc., openings is now widespread. The diagram illustrates in (1) the joint for setting a window with a timber sub-frame and metal frame in brickwork requiring mastic

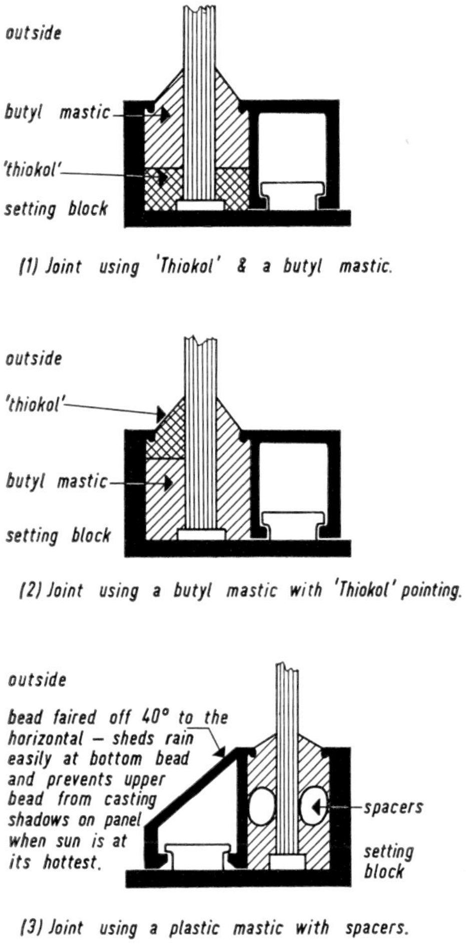


*D*.3.04/34
*Three common applications of mastics for glazing. Note: 'Thiokol' is not a product but refers to liquid polymer made by and the registered trade name of Thiokol Chemical Corporation*

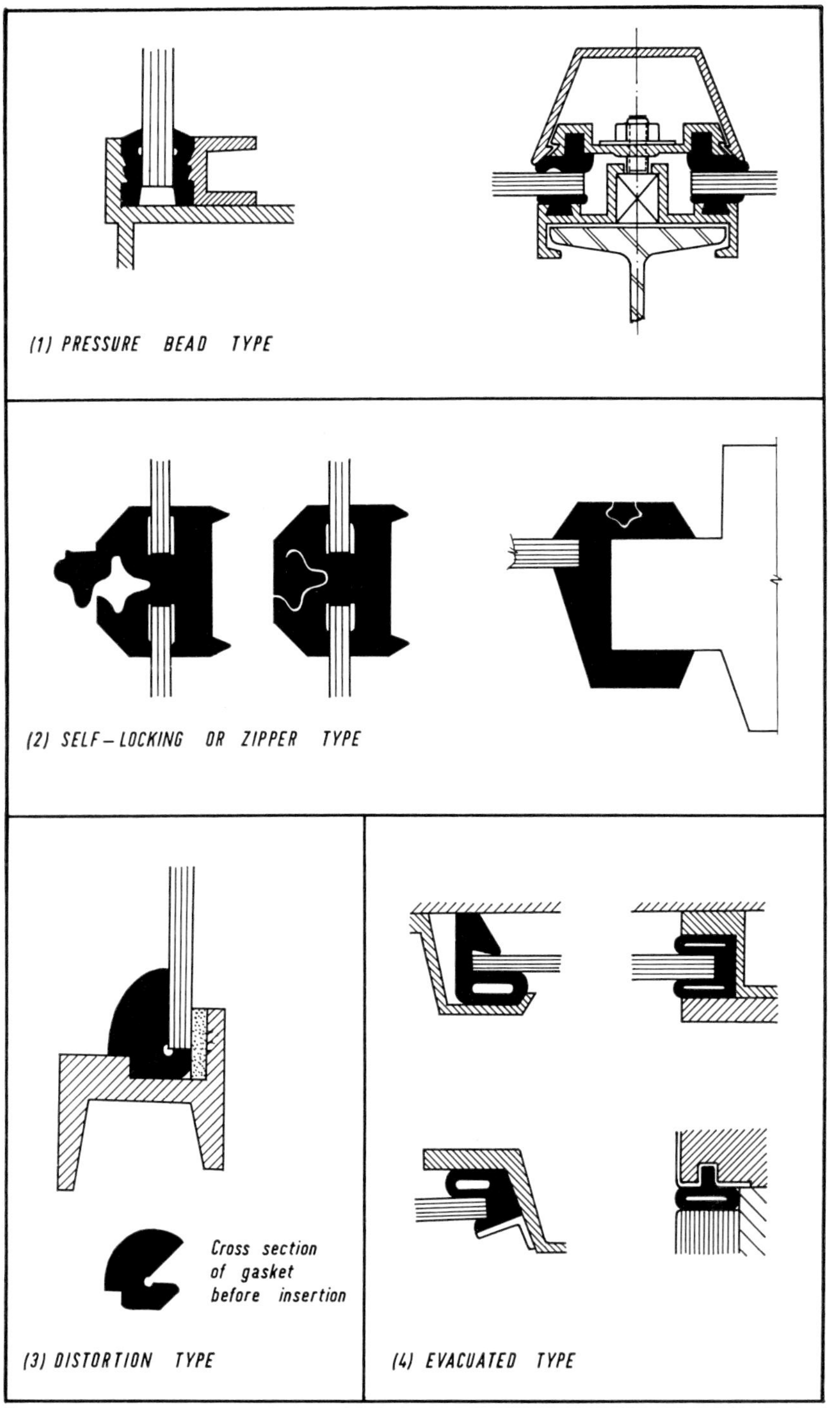


*D*.3.04/35
*Various types of gasket illustrating the four basic methods by which the requisite pressure may be applied.*

(*Based on information from Pilkington Bros. Ltd. and DuPont Co.* (*UK*) *Ltd.*)

pointing and bedding respectively, and (2) the joint for a metal window without a sub-frame, requiring mastic pointing.

It may be noted here that the use of a mastic as pointing follows very closely the use of other gap-filling materials (often mortar or putty) in traditional building methods. Although obviously superior to these in many respects, the mastics are sometimes required, often to their detriment, to fill rather large gaps which, in part, appear to result from a failure to appreciate the significance of tolerances, particularly when frames are not built-in as the wall proceeds. (Building-in of frames which results in smaller gaps to fill is a significant feature of much traditional work.) One notable departure (as described by Rostron) is to be seen in

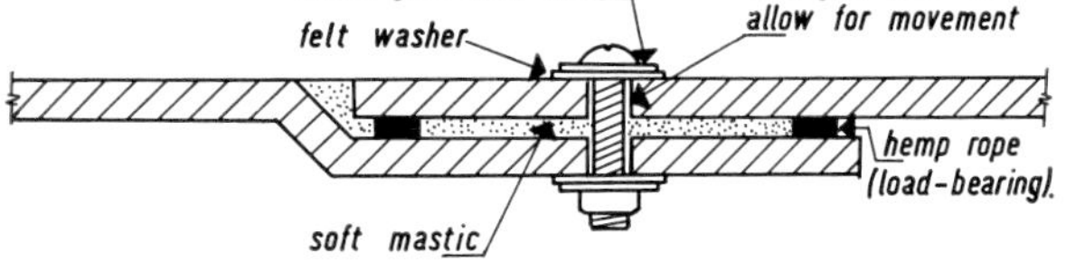


*D*.3.04/36
*Use of loadbearing rope and soft bituminous mastic for a joint in a gutter—also applicable to sheets. Note method of allowing for expansion*

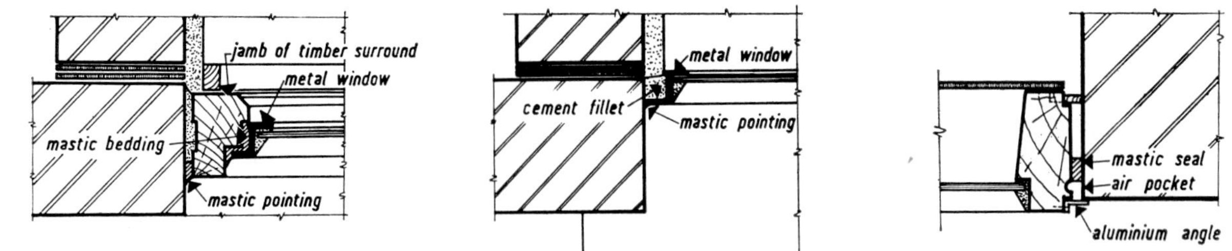


(1) Metal frame in timber sub-frame in brickwork – mastic bedding & pointing.

(2) Metal frame in brickwork – mastic pointing.

(3) Protection & accessibility of mastic seal – timber in brickwork.

*D*.3.04/37
*Use of mastic for setting frames in openings ((3) Courtesy: Powell and Moya, architects)*

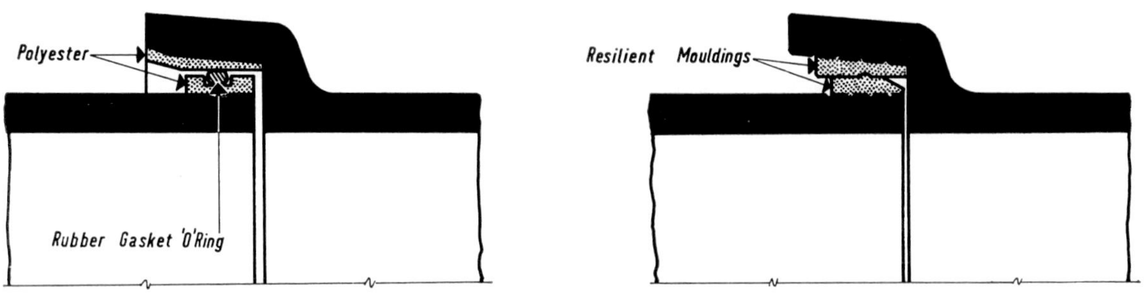


'O'RING JOINT.

JOINT WITH RESILIENT MOULDINGS.

*D*.3.04/38
*Two types of 'push-fit' joints for using gaskets for jointing in vitrified clay pipes. (Based on information from Clay Pipe Development Association Ltd.)*

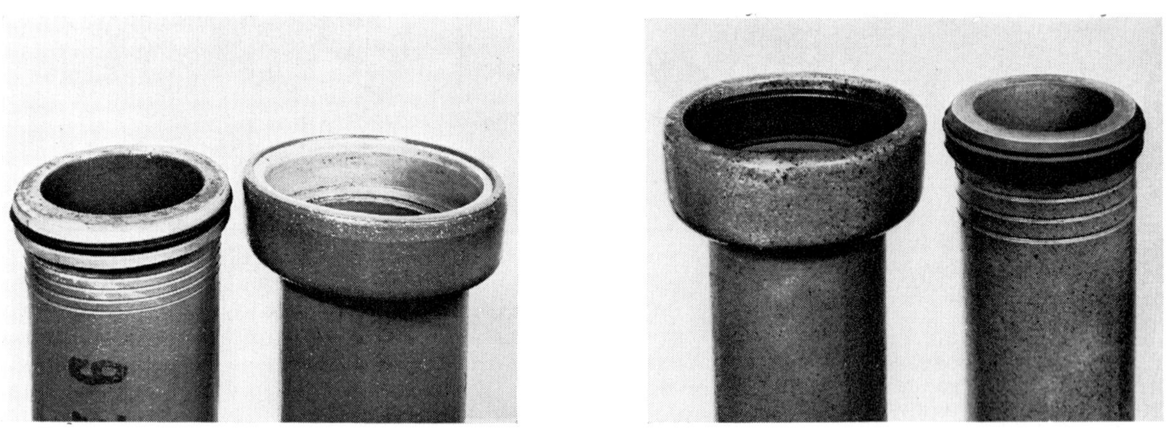

*Photographic examples of 'push-fit' joints shown in diagram* D.3.04/38. *That on the left is an 'O' ring joint and that on the right a joint with resilient mouldings*

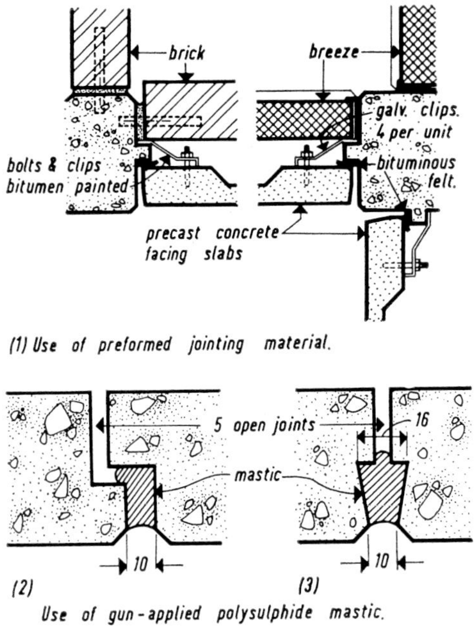


D.3.04/39
*Vertical joints for precast concrete cladding panels ((1) Courtesy: Johns, Slater and Haward architects, (2) and (3) after Gilchrist)—dimensions in mm*

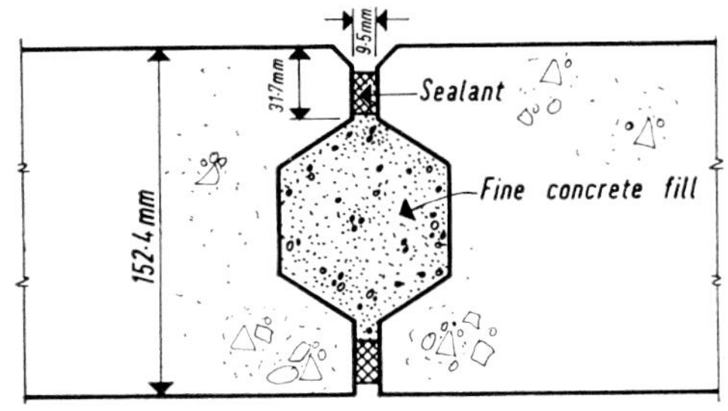


D.3.04/40
*Gap-filled joints (after Gilchrist)—dimensions in mm*

example (3), where the pointing as such has been omitted. Instead the mastic is used as a seal with an air pocket to discourage suction through the joint behind an aluminium angle, which, in addition to protecting the mastic, can also take up a certain amount of tolerance. A further point worth noting is that, despite being concealed, the mastic is still accessible.

(d) *Pipes* (diagram D.3.04/38)

Although not applicable to external walls, it has been considered convenient to include here two types of 'push-fit' joints using gaskets for jointing in vitrified clay pipes. (1) illustrates the use of the 'O' ring, while (2) resilient mouldings. The socket and spigot of each is shown in the accompanying photographs.

(e) *Precast concrete panels*

Because of the relative importance which precast concrete panels are now assuming (perhaps, better, have already assumed) in building practice, not only as cladding but also more significantly as the basic structure (i.e. without any backing, cavities or linings) fixed to floor and roof slabs, various types of joints are included here and covered in detail. For convenience, vertical and horizontal joints are considered separately.*

*Vertical joints* (diagrams D.3.04/39–50). When panels are used as cladding in light forms of construction, backing materials, cavities or separate internal linings help to reduce the rainwater load on the joint. Consequently satisfactory joints, left open or sealed, have been formed when the cladding has been pulled back at columns by clips or straps against a strip of preformed jointing material (diagram D.3.04/39 (1) ). Where this is not possible, alternative joints such as those shown in (2) and (3) can be used.

When the panels are used in heavy forms of construction to form the structure of the building, the joint assumes greater importance. Not only must it now resist the penetration of rainwater (still probably the most important factor in this country) but it must also prevent infiltration of air (exclusion of draughts is important) and provide sufficient thermal insulation (insulation equivalent to that of the panels themselves being ideal). From the various attempts which have been made to solve this problem, four classes of joints may be identified. These are:

(1) Gap-filled joints,
(2) Joints sealed by cover strips,
(3) Lapped joints with a preformed (usually elastic) jointing material encased in the joint, and
(4) Open-drained joints.

*Gap-filled joints* (diagram D.3.04/40). Whatever the section, the joint relies on a gap-filling material which does not crack or shrink from the components on either side of the joint. Complete filling of the joint is imperative.

For joints of comparatively small sections, mastics can be used; for joints of larger sections cement mortar or a fine concrete can be used.

The rigid requirements of mastics can usually only be met by the polysulphide compounds.

When mortar or fine concrete infill is used, the cross sectional area of the joint should be *at least* 13 000mm² so as (1) to fill the joint completely (narrow joints are difficult to fill), (2) to reduce shrinkage cracking and loss of adhesion, and (3) to reduce the strain due to movements of the panels. Because cracks between the panels and the fill are almost inevitable, it is advisable to seal the outer face with a gun applied mastic as shown.

*Joints sealed by cover strips* (diagram D.3.04/41). Cover strips provide a continuous mechanical barrier against the weather independent of any sealant (mastic or any other gap-filler). One advantage of cover strips is that they conceal the edges of the panel, while also providing large tolerances.

The zinc cover strip developed at the BRS is illustrated in (1), while a proprietary one, in aluminium, is illustrated in (2). The latter has been specially designed to deflect water away from the junction of the cover strip and panel. It may not provide a seal against infiltration of air, so an additional seal should be provided. In some cases, it may be advisable, as a precaution, to provide a mastic seal

*References: (1) This part was originally mostly based on an interim report of a Building Rereach Station study by D. Bishop published in *The Builder* (now *Building*) for January 5, 1962 (pp. 31–35) and entitled *Waterproof joints between precast concrete panels*. The station has been pursuing its study but it is understood that there is no reason for any fundamental changes in the principles originally proposed. Among details which appear to be important are the problems of tolerance and junctions of vertical and horizontal joints with the correct use and fixing of flashings when incorporated in the design. The information has now been brought up-to-date *in Joints between concrete wall panels: open drained joints*, BRS Digest (2nd Series) No. 85, HMSO, August, 1967, which has been used in this study. (2) Details have also been taken from *Concrete facing slabs*, by J. Gilchrist Wilson, published by The Cement and Concrete Association, 4th (revised) Ed., pp. 34–38, November, 1963. (It is understood that this publication is now out of print.)

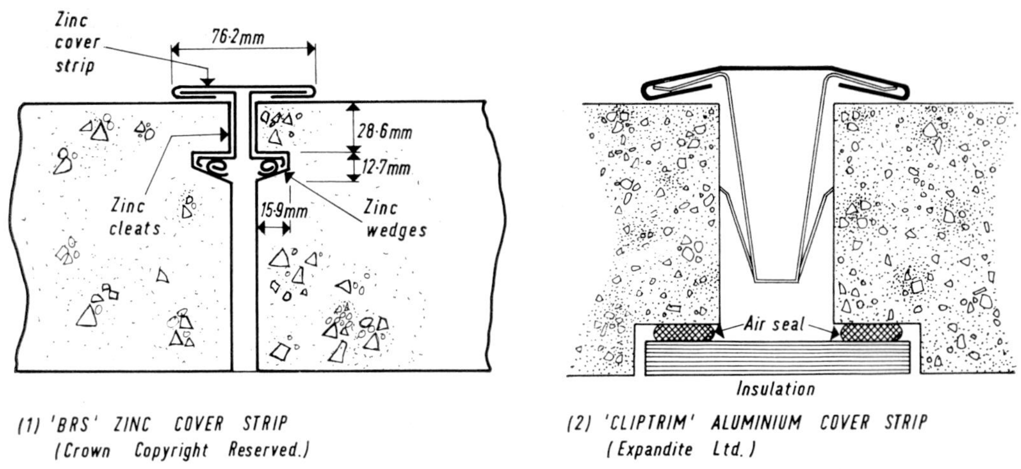


(1) 'BRS' ZINC COVER STRIP (Crown Copyright Reserved.)

(2) 'CLIPTRIM' ALUMINIUM COVER STRIP (Expandite Ltd.)

D.3.04/41
*Joints sealed by cover strips*

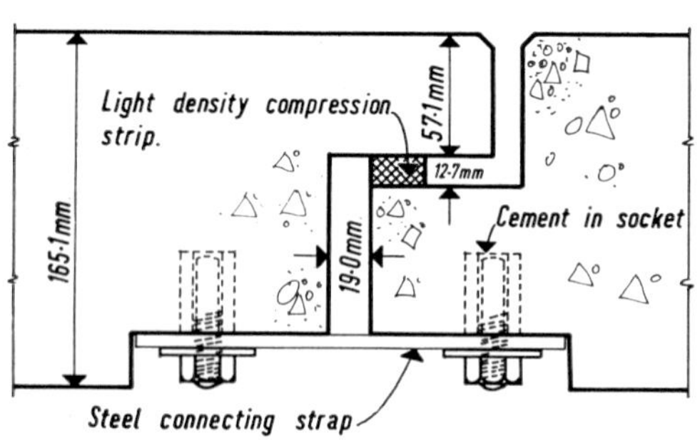


D.3.04/42
*Lapped joint (after Gilchrist)*

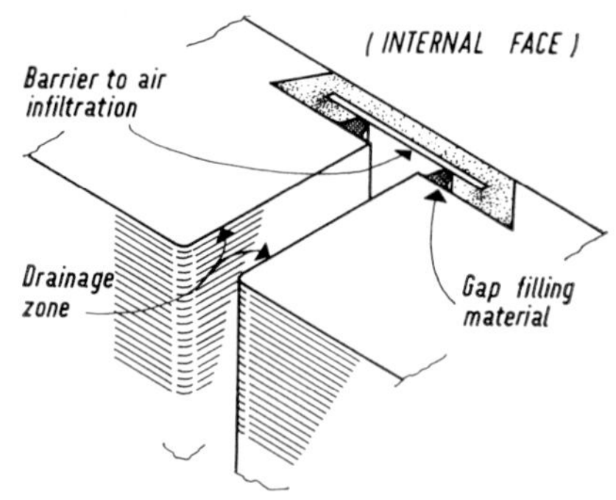


D.3.04/43
*Basic features of a vertical open drained joint. (Crown Copyright from BRS Digest (2nd Series), No. 85)*

at the back of the joint as a second line of defence.

*Lapped joints* (diagram D.3.04/42). A compressed sealing strip is used to form a channel in which water is trapped and drained. For success the jointing material must satisfy four requirements: (1) be capable of being compressed to two-thirds of its thickness by a pressure not exceeding 0·07N/mm²; (2) have a closed cell structure to prevent capillary action; (3) remain elastic; and (4) have a life equal to the estimated life of the building. 'Light' density (about 176kg/m³) preformed strips of Neoprene, polysulphide or butyl base, are likely to meet these requirements.

During erection the sealing strips are easily susceptible to damage, particularly in windy weather. Careful handling of the panels is, therefore, essential. The seal is, of course, inaccessible for inspection or repair.

*Open-drained joints* (diagrams D.3.04/43–51). Failure of the three types of joints already described may be caused by: (1) the limits of tolerance provided for in the design being exceeded; (2) insufficient care being exercised during erection of the panels; and (3) differential movement in the panels causing either fracture or loss of adhesion of the sealing material.

To avoid these difficulties, one method is to omit the material bridging the gap between the panels and to rely instead on (1) an *air-tight barrier* at the back of the joint to prevent air flow through it, and (2) the *geometry* of the joint to trap most of the rain in an outer zone. The principles of the design of such a joint are illustrated in diagram D.3.04/43. The vertical joint is normally divided into two zones, an inner and outer zone, by an intermediate baffle as shown in diagram D.3.04/44. Most of the water entering the outer zone is drained away and the little that does manage to penetrate past the baffle drains away in the inner zone. (The air pressure on either side of the baffle is more or less equal and this helps to prevent penetration of water past the baffle.) It is important to note that the joint is only effectively sealed at the back in which position the seal is least exposed to weathering action.

The features and dimensions important to the successful performance of the open-drained joint illustrated in diagram D.3.04/44 (developed by BRS) and likely to perform satisfactorily even in conditions of severe exposure are:

1. An air barrier is required at the back of both horizontal and vertical joints to prevent air infiltration.
2. Most of the water entering a vertical joint drains away within a zone 50mm deep measured from the face of the joint.
3. A baffle at a depth of 50mm, i.e. placed at the back edge of the drainage zone, in a vertical joint, arrests wind-driven rain.
4. Horizontal joints should be protected by a 50mm upstand on sheltered sites and a 100mm upstand on exposed sites. This upstand must be carried effectively across the intersection with the vertical joints.
5. The width of the joint should not be less than 10mm—smaller joints may become blocked with debris and lead to failure by capillarity.

The flashing at the intersection of vertical with horizontal joints, it is important to note, must ensure that the rainwater shed by the baffle, plus any that has penetrated to the air barrier, is brought to the front of the joint at each intersection. This precaution is necessary to overcome the effects of misalignment of vertical joints, and to ensure continuity of the upstand in the horizontal joints. The distance $x$ in diagram D.3.04/44 measured from the *foot* of the baffle is the *effective* upstand overlap at the joint intersection. The positioning of the baffle is important because if the lower ends of the baffles are dragged downwards into position during assembly they may subsequently creep back and so reduce the overlap. Similarly the top ends of the baffles should be carried well up under the flashings.

The idea of the open drained joint is not new. Early types of patent glazing used it, while in the 1950's it was applied to concrete cladding panels by Reema and in joint systems of Scandinavian origin as shown in diagram D.3.04/45. An early open drained joint developed by BRS and following tests on joints with various profiles is shown in diagram D.3.04/46. The two grooves, one in the outer zone and one in the inner zone, were incorporated to provide vertical discontinuities. These grooves have now been omitted in the latest version (diagram D.3.04/44). However, there seems to be some justification for the use of inclined washboard grooves on the faces of the joints. These grooves help to drain rainwater towards the front and so offer additional protection. Such protection may be sufficient to suggest the omission of intermediate baffles except in high or very exposed buildings and only if the fixing of the air barrier can be guaranteed.

From tests carried out by BRS open drained joints have three important features, namely (1) the drainage zone, (2) the baffle and the ventilated cavity, and (3) the air barrier. The joints illustrated in diagrams D.3.04/47–51 illustrate the importance of these features either separately or in combination and are discussed separately below:

1. *The drainage zone.* An intermediate baffle is not always necessary, as the drainage zone is sometimes sufficient to provide adequate protection to the air barrier. Additional protection is provided when the vertical edges of the zone prevent sideways flow of water or when inclined grooves lead water to the front of the joint. If, as illustrated in diagram D.3.04/47, the air barrier can be sealed from the back, there are no constructional problems. However, if panels are hung from a frame, joints are best sealed from outside the building in which case a slightly lapped joint, as shown in diagram D.3.04/48, will provide a stop against which the gap sealing material can be gunned into position.

2. *The baffle and the ventilated cavity.* The joint illustrated in diagram D.3.04/49 follows the fundamental principles of the open-drained joint exactly with two zones. The small quantities of water that penetrate past the barrier will drain away in the cavity rather than impinge on the barrier, especially if the faces of the joint are provided with inclined (washboard) grooves. For panels with joint faces parallel, that is edges of panels which are straight and square, the baffle can take the form of a neoprene tube or cruciform plastics strip.

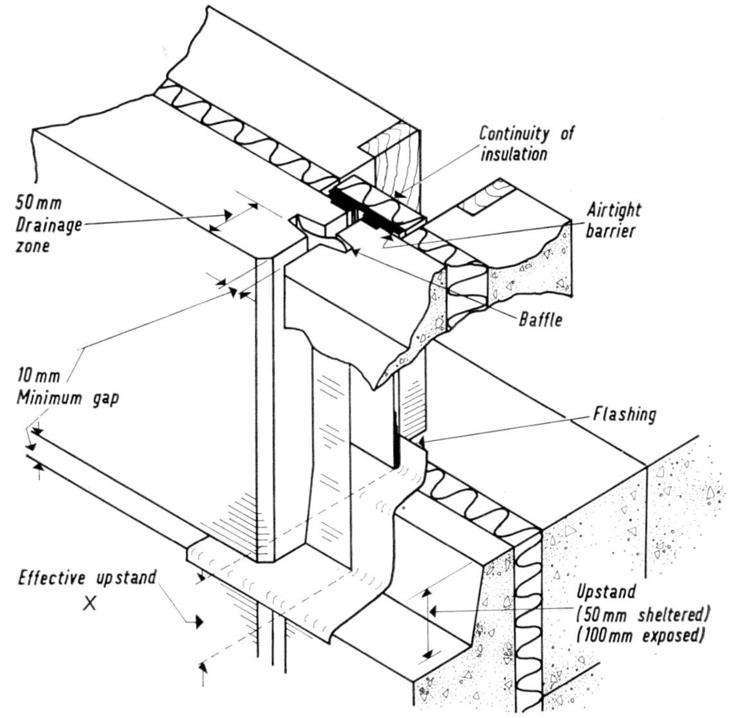


*D.3.04/44*
*Drained joints between façade panels. (Crown Copyright from: BRS Digest (2nd Series), No. 85)*

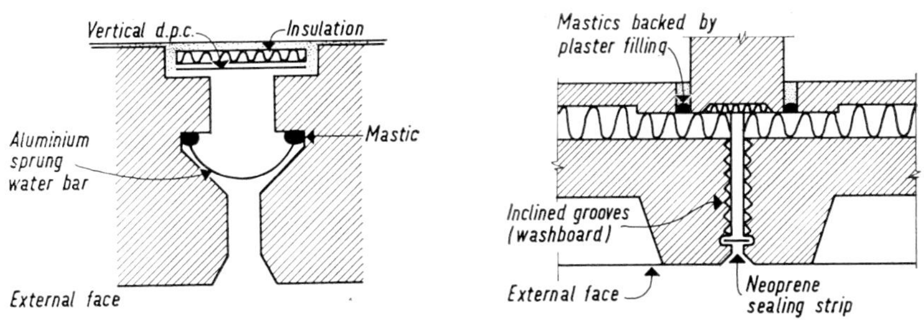


(1) VERTICAL DRAINED JOINT (REEMA)

(2) VERTICAL DRAINED JOINT (MALMSTROM)

*D.3.04/45*
*Two early examples of vertical open drained joints*

*D.3.04/46*
*Early BRS vertical open drained joint (Crown Copyright)*

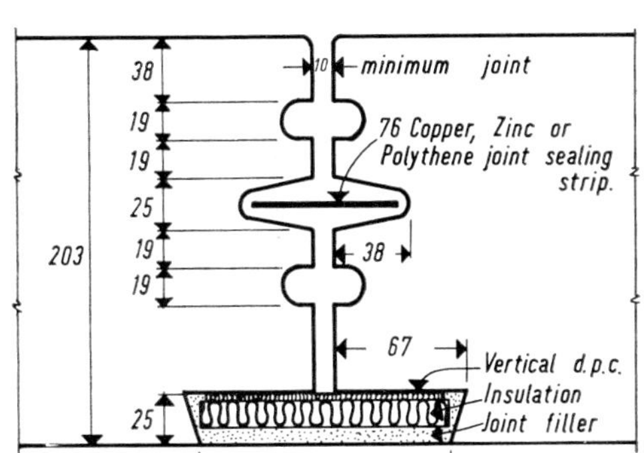


JOINT PROTECTED BY GROOVES
(Crown Copyright Reserved.)

NOTE: All dimensions are in millimetres.

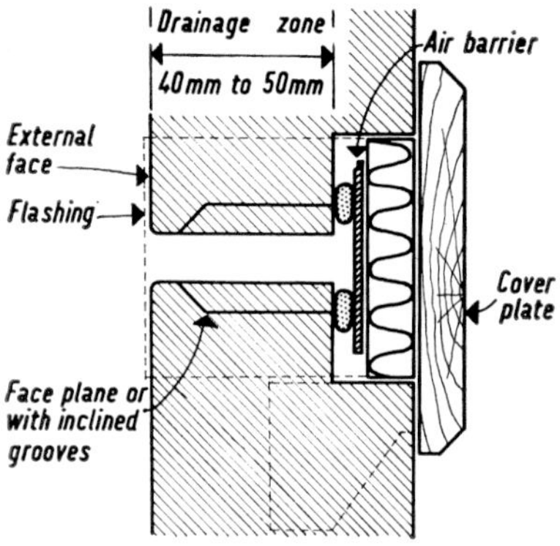


*D.3.04/47*
*Drained vertical joint without baffle and sealed from the back.* (*Crown Copyright from: BRS Digest* (*2nd Series*), *No. 85*)

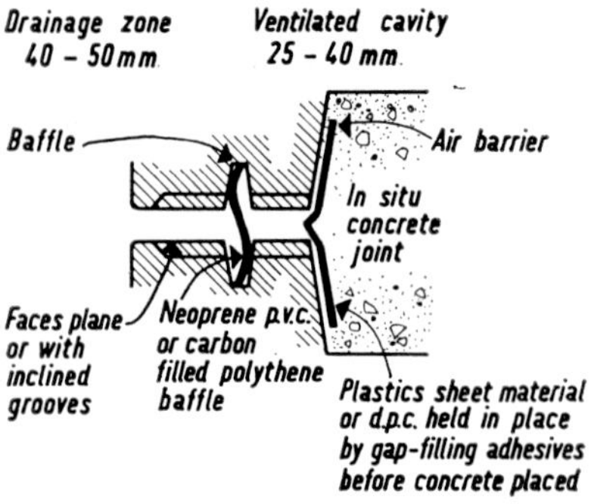


*D.3.04/49*
*Drained vertical joint with baffle and ventilated cavity.* (*Crown Copyright from: BRS Digest* (*2nd Series*), *No. 85*)

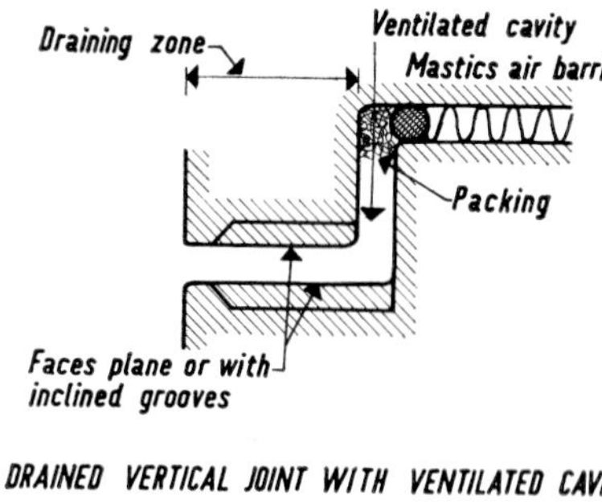


*D.3.04/51*
*Drained vertical joint with ventilated cavity.* (*Crown Copyright from: BRS Digest* (*2nd Series*), *No. 85*)

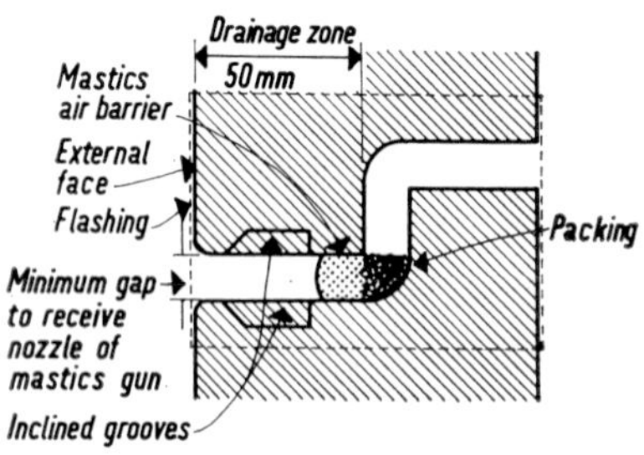


*D.3.04/48*
*Drained vertical joint without baffle and sealed from the front.* (*Crown Copyright from: BRS Digest* (*2nd Series*), *No. 85*)

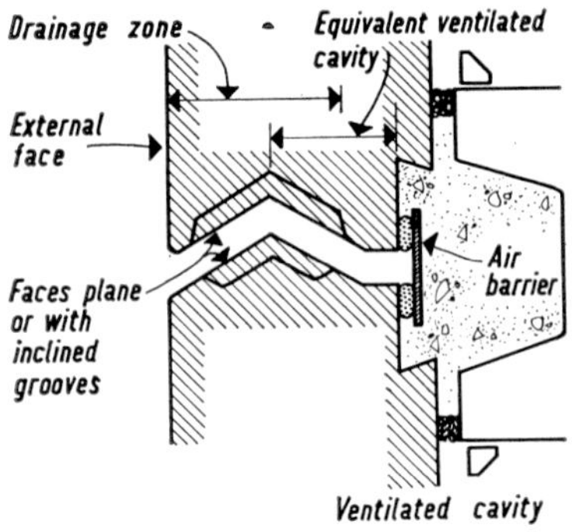


*D.3.04/50*
*Drained vertical joint with ventilated cavity equivalent.* (*Crown Copyright from: BRS Digest* (*2nd Series*), *No. 85*)

When the tolerances of joint sizes are not known or are suspect, a simple baffle of the kind illustrated in diagram D.3.04/48, held loosely in vertical grooves should be used. Furthermore the grooves should be designed to accommodate the tolerance range while baffles of several widths should be provided.

Diagram D.3.04/50 shows a joggled drainage zone, while diagram D.3.04/51 shows the return of the open section of the joint in the plane of the panel to form a ventilated cavity. The first example illustrates a labyrinth which is the equivalent of a baffle and ventilated cavity and so can be used as an alternative for the latter.

3. *The air barrier*. The air barrier is relieved of most of the waterload which it would otherwise receive when proper provision is made for the drainage zone, the baffle and the ventilated cavity. Ideally, sealants forming the air barrier should be in rolling shear, as shown in diagram D.3.04/47, rather than in tension, as shown in diagrams D.3.04/48 and 51. Very simple air barriers (perhaps of d.p.c. felt temporarily held in place with gap-filling bituminous adhesive, as shown in diagram D.3.04/44) have been found satisfactory when joints in low buildings are backed by *in situ* concrete. Care is needed to overcome difficulties in sticking the air seal across adjacent faces when these are not in line.

*Horizontal joints* (diagrams D.3.04/52–54). Among problems which may be associated with the joints between panels used as cladding in light forms of construction is support and extrusion of the mastic. There are a number of different methods in common use for supporting the panels from the main frame or structure of a building. Nevertheless, a feature common to a number of joints is the provision of a mortar bed. This acts as a support, in the loose sense, to prevent the mastic being extruded during erection and before the main method of support has been achieved. Furthermore, the mortar acts as a backing against which the mastic may be gunned.

Diagram D.3.04/52 illustrates some examples of joints applicable mainly to panels used as cladding in light forms of construction. Other methods commonly used for claddings and found sound and watertight are variations of the rebated joint which has been sealed off at the back to prevent rain being blown up between the slabs.

In heavy forms of construction, the open-drained joint, of the lap type shown in diagram D.3.04/53 (1) has been found to be successful. An important requirement for this type of joint is the minimum overlap of 50mm shown in the diagram. Furthermore, the width between the opposing faces of the panels must be sufficient to prevent capillary action, while free drainage must be maintained.

In the BRS study an attempt was made to develop the water-bar

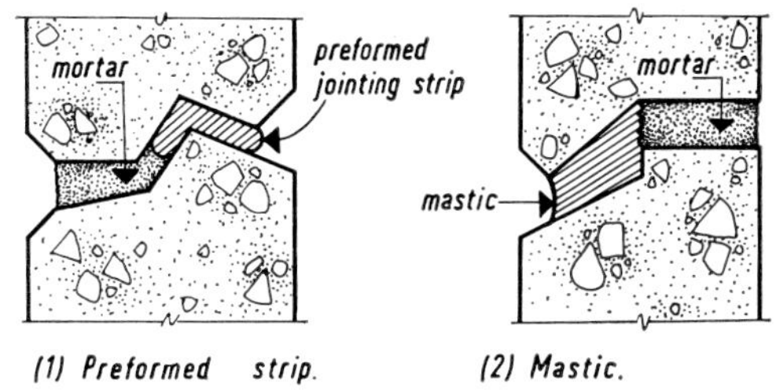


*D.3.04/52*
*Horizontal joints for precast concrete cladding panels (after Gilchrist)*

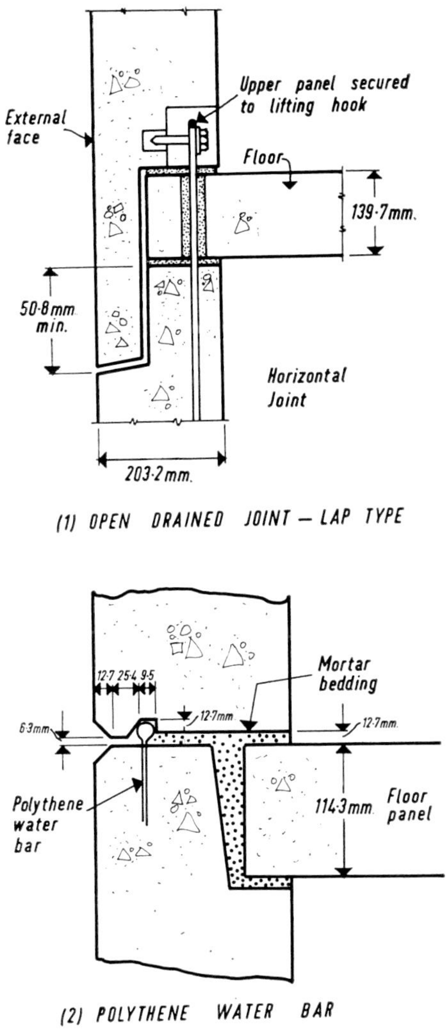


*D.3.04/53*
*Horizontal joints for heavy forms of precast concrete construction (Crown Copyright)*

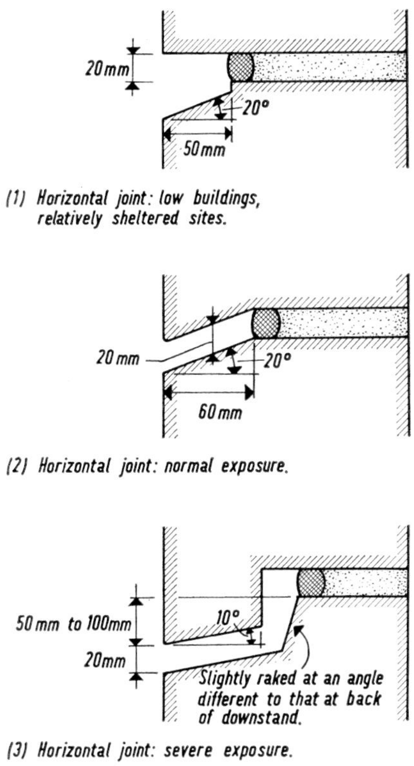


*D.3.04/54*
*Open drained horizontal joints for varying conditions of exposure. (Crown Copyright from: BRS Digest (2nd Series), No. 85)*

principle as shown in diagram D.3.04/53 (2). The panel tested did not, however, prove satisfactory. Rain penetration was evident at several places, mainly where the water bar did not take up the contour of the rebate in the upper panel. This problem, it was suggested, could probably be solved by a larger rebate, but this was considered to be impracticable. It was further noted that the advantage of low cost is outweighed by the disadvantages of the difficulty of forming the water bar and the possibility of damage during handling and erection.

The open-drained lap type joint illustrated in diagram D.3.04/53 (1) is successful because of the upstands and sloping sills which reduce water penetration. However, it has been shown that an effective air barrier is more important and the best weapon against water penetration. Such a barrier can be effected by sealing the backs of horizontal joints. Horizontal joints based on this principle and for various conditions of exposure are illustrated in diagram D.3.04/54. In (1) only the lower surface of the joint needs to be slightly weathered. However, in a more exposed site, both the upper and lower surfaces should be weathered as in (2), while with severe exposure weathering and an overlap are required as in (3). It would appear that little is to be gained by providing an upstand with an effective height greater than 50mm, unless the filling is likely to be ineffective or the exposure severe. In these circumstances up to 100mm may be necessary. These dimensions take no account of tolerances; these must be allowed for by additional overlap. It is safest, as suggested in connection with diagram D.3.04/44, to design for a 50–100mm upstand as appropriate for sheltered or exposed situations.

## Entrapped water*

### 1. Scope

Entrapped water (sometimes also known as 'Entrapped moisture') is a term now used to describe water which may be held, usually for a considerable length of time, in flat roof constructions. The entrapped water may eventually escape but only after a protracted drying-out period, involving years† rather than months after completion of a building or, as is also common, leak out of the construction as liquid by way of weak points such as cracks or other through routes provided, for example, by electrical conduits. The sources of water may be attributable *either* to water introduced during construction (mixing, cleaning or rainwater) *or,* as important, to water formed as a result of interstitial condensation. Both sources of water, it should be strongly emphasized, are important, and thus the problems associated with entrapped water are not only dynamic rather than static, but are also applicable to both wet (usually the most severe) and dry forms of construction. Failure to appreciate the significance of both sources of water can lead to a misunderstanding of the necessity of taking the correct precautions in particular circumstances.

The reasons for the water becoming entrapped are complex but, in the main, can be associated with difficulties created in the transmission of the entrapped water to the free surface of the construction so that evaporation and eventual drying out can take place. Although the transmission of water from the interior to the surface of the construction will be influenced by the structure of the materials making up the construction (see *Section 3.03,* 'Capillarity (a) The drying out of a porous body'—p. 68), thermal effects, particularly temperature gradients, are significant. Not only do they tend to reduce the rate of drying out by causing the migration of moisture within the construction, but they also tend to encourage condensation of the moisture *already* entrapped which results in the formation of liquid water. It is the latter which collects in pools and subsequently leaks out under gravity. Water may, of course, be added to the construction as a result of the condensation of water vapour from the interior of the building permeating through the construction towards the external surface. Such condensation which would normally occur during cold weather may also account for leakage of water.

From these general considerations it will be seen that thermal effects do play an important part in the occurrence of entrapped water which may, of course, also occur in external walls having an impervious covering. However, on the whole, entrapped water problems appear, in recent years, to have been more commonly associated with flat roofs, particularly those using *in situ* lightweight insulating screeds. This has been due, not only to the presence of mixing water* which has not been allowed to dry out prior to the application of the waterproof covering, but also to the susceptibility of unprotected horizontal surfaces to accumulate large quantities of water during rain. The latter may also not have had sufficient time 'to escape' before the waterproof covering is laid. Other factors which are equally important derive from the nature of the construction of the whole roof deck, which usually presents difficulties of providing, below the waterproof covering, either the requisite drainage or ventilation which would allow the moisture to escape.

In the case of walls such problems as have occurred can be or, better, have been associated with interstitial condensation rather than water introduced into construction. Methods of providing drainage and ventilation are also not as difficult as in the case of roofs. Thus it has been considered more convenient to deal, in this section, with the problems of entrapped water due to water introduced during construction and from interstitial condensation in flat roofs only, but with particular emphasis on those constructions using *in situ* lightweight screeds. Walls are included in *4.00 Heat and its effects,* in which details of the mechanisms of and factors affecting condensation, together with possible methods of prevention, are covered.

### 2. Precedent

It is perhaps ironic that all problems associated with entrapped water result from the substantial increase in the thermal insulation of the envelope of buildings. The problems are, therefore, comparatively new to building practice. Although the principles involved are clear, many details, particularly those related to actual practice, are somewhat obscure. There is at the present time a lack of any quantitative method of assessing the severity of conditions and thus the particular solutions which should be adopted. A great deal of work has been done, in theory and in practice, in Scandinavia, where climatic conditions are, on the whole, somewhat more severe than those normally encountered in the British Isles. Despite this, Scandinavian practice provides a useful basis.*

### 3. Effects

Entrapped water implies dampness. Consequently it should not be allowed to remain as moisture within a construction or, alternatively, be allowed to condense into liquid form, if decay and deterioration is to be prevented. In the case of roofs, entrapped water, in either state, may result in staining of ceilings (leaching of bitumen from the waterproof covering by alkalis derived from the cement in screeds is significant); rotting of organic matter; frost damage or blistering and subsequent tearing of the roof covering. Dripping water may not only cause inconvenience, but also damage to the interior of a building. Finally, and by no means least, high moisture contents lead to a loss, sometimes substantial, of thermal insulation. In this connection it is useful to note that, on occasions, it may be more practical to accept reduced thermal efficiency of the roof during the initial life of a new building, provided adequate precautions have been taken to ensure that the entrapped water can escape to the outside air over a comparatively short period of time.

### 4. Quantity of water

Whether or not entrapped water in roofs is likely to cause decay or deterioration, including loss of thermal insulation, will, in the first instance, be dependent on the quantity of water entrapped at any time beneath the waterproof covering. At the same time the quantity of water involved will also determine the precise nature of precautions which should be taken to allow the water to escape, particularly once the roof covering has been laid. In general terms the greater the quantities of water involved, the more elaborate the precautions necessary to ensure that the entrapped water can, in fact, escape. Other related factors, such as the area of the roof, are, however, also important.

It may not be possible to evaluate precisely the quantities of water which may be involved. In the case of interstitial condensation, for example, the ability to predict the likelihood of the risk of condensation occurring is, at present, of greater value than a prediction of the actual quantity which may be formed. Nevertheless, it is possible to form some basis for assessment of the necessity of incorporating any particular type of precaution by taking

*References: (1) *Developments in Roofing*, BRS Digest (2nd Series), No. 51, October, 1964, revised 1968. (2) *Principles of Modern Building—Vol. II,* Chapter 7, HMSO, 1961. (3) Tolhurst, A. J. M., *Trapped Moisture in Roofs,* Articles in the Journal of the Mastic Asphalte Advisory Council, pp. 31–33, January, 1963, and pp. 33–37, July, 1963. (4) Billington, N. S., *Thermal Properties of Building* (Clever-Hume Press Ltd.), Chapter 5, pp. 136–138, 1952. (5) *Roof Waterproofing Problems,* translation from the German by H. W. McInnes, article in *The Builder,* pp. 1081–1082, November 22, 1963.

†In bad cases it has been calculated by one authority that periods up to 20 years would be necessary for complete drying out.

*In general, lightweight insulating screeds require the use of greater quantities of mixing water than in the case of 'traditional' dense screeds.

*Cognisance is also taken of the useful work which has been carried out in America, and in other parts of Europe, such as Germany. Much of this, it would appear, stems from the work originally carried out in Scandinavia. Furthermore, it should be noted that at the present time opinions vary (in some cases quite violently) as to the 'best' solution which should be used. Building practice being what it is, this only supports the justifiable contention that there is no panacea for all problems and so each situation must be considered 'on its own merits'.

into account the nature of the sources of water. Subject to circumstances these must, in turn, be related to the drying-out process which may take place prior to the laying of the roof covering. The two chief sources of water, namely that introduced during construction and that formed as a result of interstitial condensation, i.e. after construction, are not strictly interrelated. However, water formed as a result of interstitial condensation may, subject to the amount involved, subsequently behave in the same way as water introduced during construction. Thus it would appear more realistic, and perhaps less confusing, to deal with their basic nature separately.

(a) *During construction*

The quantities of water which may be contained in the roof deck at the time the waterproof covering is being laid, and which will subsequently become entrapped, will be dependent on:

(i) The amount of water which is necessary for mixing of *in situ* screeds. In the case of lightweight screeds considerable quantities of water (up to 10·87 litres/m$^2$—see Table 3.02/2, p. 46) are normally required.

(ii) The amount of water which is allowed to evaporate from the screed (in some cases the structural background too) before the waterproof covering is laid.

(iii) The amount of water which is allowed to be absorbed by the roof deck during rain before the waterproof covering is laid. From the example given previously in *Section 3.02* (p. 46) it will be seen that it is possible for a dry screed to absorb nearly as much rainwater as that used initially for mixing. The quantity of mixing water required for a 76·2mm aerated cement screed is between 5·44 and 10·87 litres/m$^2$, while approximately 8·16 litres/m$^2$ may be picked up by the screed having a fall of 1 : 60 during four days of rain.

It is important to note here that both *in situ* screeds and other dry forms of background (often used specifically to try to overcome entrapped water associated with wet screeds) upon which the roof covering will be subsequently laid are also susceptible to absorbing rainwater, unless suitably protected.

(iv) The amount of absorbed rainwater which is allowed to evaporate before the waterproof covering is laid.

(b) *After construction*

The quantity of water already contained in the roof deck after the waterproof covering has been laid may be increased as a result of interstitial condensation. Looked at in another way, a relatively dry roof may become damp at any time as a result of the formation of interstitial condensation. The risk of such condensation occurring is dependent on the following interrelated factors:

(i) The relative humidity of the air in the space below the roof. Generally, the higher the quantity of water in the internal atmosphere, the greater the risk of interstitial condensation occurring.

(ii) The temperature gradient through the roof in which dew point is important. Generally there is a greater risk of interstitial condensation occurring when there is an appreciable difference in temperature between the internal and external air, particularly when high internal temperatures are accompanied by high relative humidities. Thus the condensation usually takes place during the winter, although the fact that it has taken place may not manifest itself until the spring or summer.*

(iii) The vapour diffusing characteristics of the materials making up the roof deck. Thus water vapour barriers may be used (usually on the warm side —winter condition) to control the permeation of vapour through the construction and so prevent the formation of condensation.

It may be noted here that the use of vapour barriers is more strongly favoured in North America than it is in Scandinavia, where greater reliance is placed on drainage and/or ventilation of the roof deck. One of the arguments against the use of vapour barriers is that although they may prevent the formation of interstitial condensation, entrapped water from other sources may still leak out at the joints or at the edges of the barrier.

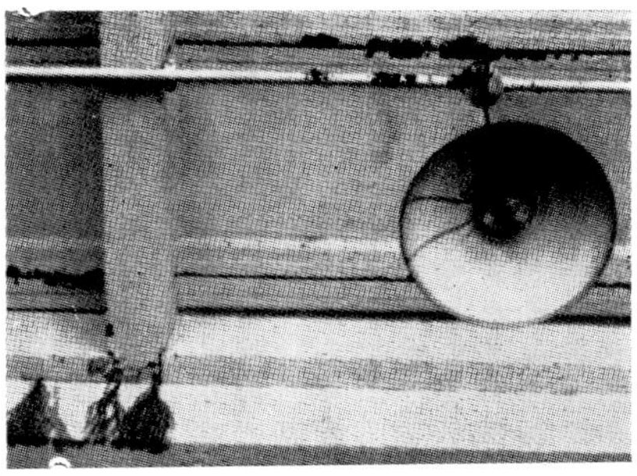

*Leaching of bitumen from the roof covering due to the action of alkalis derived from the cement and staining ceilings above and, below, walls (Top and centre photographs, Courtesy: Parovents Ltd.)*

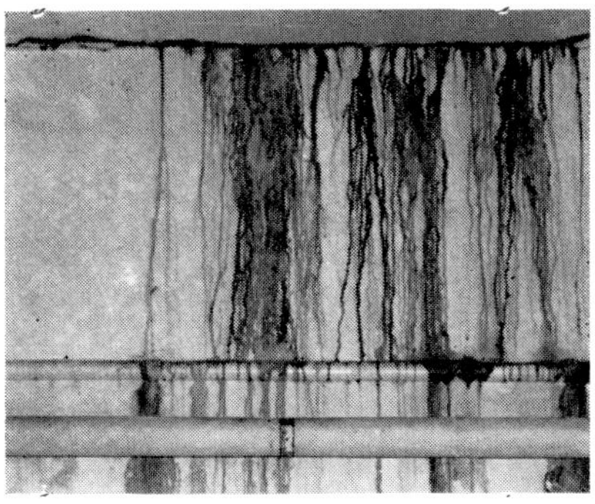

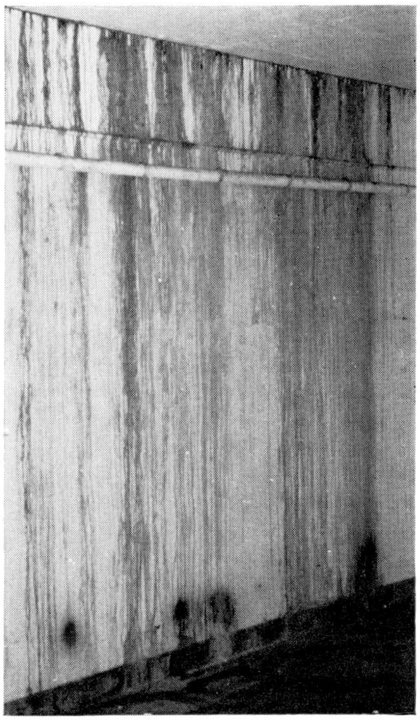

**5. Moisture transmission**

Water trapped in a screed or structure will at first be generally evenly distributed, thus creating, in a sense, a condition of equilibrium. However, this equilibrium is later broken and the water then moves and subsequently settles in ponds or hollows of the roof slab itself or at the bottom of falls, sometimes near rainwater outlets, for example.

Temperature gradients also account for further movement of water. There is a tendency for the water to 'migrate' from warmer to cooler zones (see diagram D.3.04/21 earlier). Thus, in summer water will tend to be 'pushed' towards the internal face of a construction or to any other area that may be shaded, particularly when the sun is shining. In winter, on the other hand, the water will be 'pushed' in the opposite direction, that is towards the external face of the construction and underneath the waterproof covering. In general terms the effect of seasonal variations in temperature is to cause the lower part of a construction to be wetter than the upper part in summer, with the converse occurring during the winter. For this reason the positioning of organic materials within the roof deck so as to avoid their decay will be important, if no provision has been made for the entrapped water to escape.

During winter water vapour from the interior of a building which is allowed to permeate through the roof construction will normally condense on the underside of the roof covering. The condensed water may, subject to pore structure, be able to find its

*The fact that interstitial condensation may not manifest itself until there has been a change in the thermal gradient in the roof structure is indicative of the difficulty of distinguishing whether failures due to entrapped water have been due to water introduced during construction or as a result of interstitial condensation. This is particularly true in the early life of new buildings.

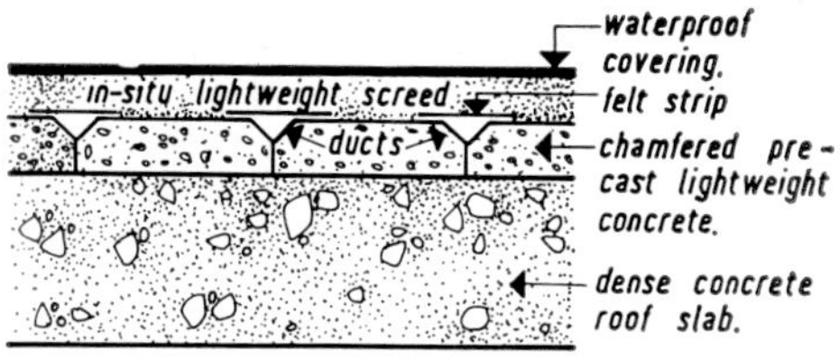


(1) Using chamfered precast blocks - face up.

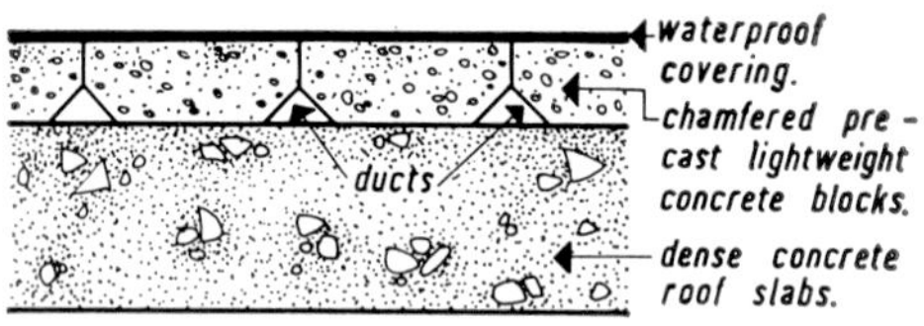


(2) Using chamfered precast blocks - face down.

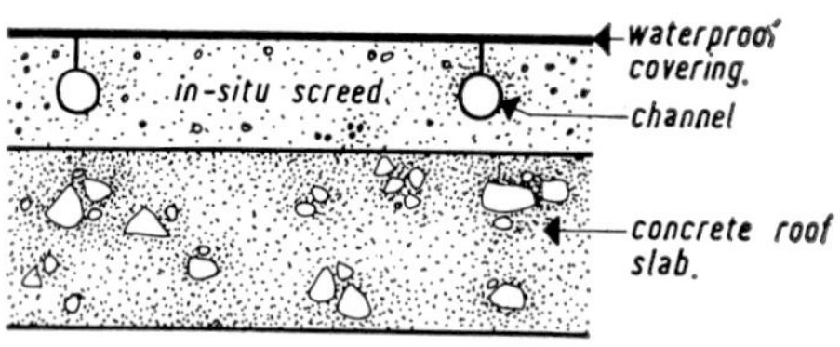


(3) Channels within in-situ screed.

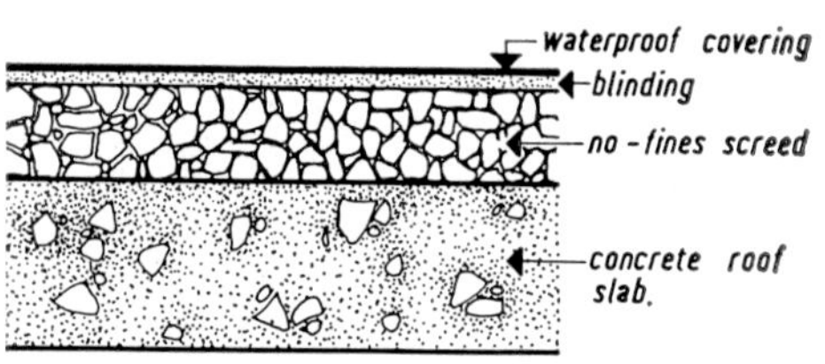


(4) Using no-fines screed.

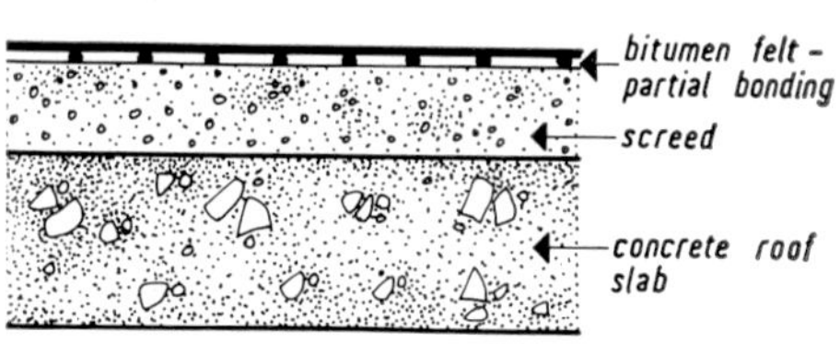


(5) Partial bonding of bitumen felt.

*D.3.04/55*
*Alternative methods of providing ventilation ducts under a waterproof covering of asphalt or bitumen felt to a flat roof (plastics-based sheets are also available)*

way back to the soffit from which, subject to environmental conditions, it may evaporate. However, this condition of equilibrium in which there is a transmission of water vapour in one direction and liquid water in the opposite direction, may be upset by cracks, in which case the water will drain at localised points instead of being evenly distributed. This may then result in dripping.

Finally, there is one other thermal effect which leads to blistering and eventual tearing of the roof covering (particularly bitumen felt and asphalt) which should be considered. During the summer, solar radiation on the roof will cause the moisture entrapped within the construction to vaporise, with the result that considerable pressure is exerted on the underside of the waterproof covering. At best, the pressure will tend to weaken adhesion (the adhesive is in any case weakened by heat) in the case of felt roofs or, at worst, cause small areas to blister in the case of either asphalt or bitumen. Once formed, the blisters help to reduce the vapour pressure. In extreme cases the pressure may be sufficient to actually tear the covering. However, tearing may still take place even when there is no longer any pressure acting on the underside of the covering, as the blister will remain behind and is thus capable of being damaged by other causes. Such blisters may, under certain circumstances, become filled with water which in turn may, during extreme winter conditions, freeze and tear the covering. Tearing may also occur during maintenance.

## 6. Drying out

In general, drying out of the entrapped water in a screed (the principles outlined here are with some slight modification also applicable to other materials used instead of the screed) is severely restricted because free ventilation at the surface is not possible. Solutions designed to allow the entrapped water to evaporate (preferably to the outside air) aim, therefore, to provide a means by which through ventilation can take place somewhere between the top of the structural deck and the underside of the roof covering.

In order to allow the ventilation to take place, ducts of some description are required and, as important, these must have adequate access to the outside air. This means that the duct system must be an open rather than a closed system with at least two outlets, reasonably well spaced apart, to the outside air. Although the rate of natural ventilation will be influenced by environmental conditions, particularly air movement, and the size and distribution of the ducts and outlets, it is nevertheless important that the latter should be distributed so as to reduce as much as possible the distance which the entrapped water will have to diffuse. The longer the distance the slower the evaporation and thus the slower the drying out. Where the ducts and/or outlets are limited, they may only assist in reducing pressure build-up.

(a) *Ducts* (Diagram D.3.04/55)

In Scandinavia it is not uncommon to find that fairly elaborate ducting systems are used with lightweight screeds on dense concrete slabs. Some of the systems are in some ways miniature versions of the herring-bone ground water drainage adopted in this country to drain heavy clay soils or sports fields. Diagram D.3.04/55 (1) illustrates a system in which chamfered blocks are abutted to form a groove, which is covered with felt before the screed is laid. In (2) chamfered insulating slabs are abutted so as to form a groove above the dense slab. An alternative (3) would be to form channels within the screed which should be protected from cracking in the zone of the channel while bonding of the roof covering in this zone should be avoided. On the whole, ducts may be more easily formed in precast insulation slabs. To remove the surplus water present initially and also to prevent the accumulation of interstitial condensation it is recommended that the cross sectional area of the ducts should be 1/1 000 of the roof area. Some authorities feel that a ratio of this order would not be necessary in this country where thermal conditions are not as severe as in Scandinavia. At present, no alternative reduced ratio has been recommended.

A multiplicity or complete network of small ducts throughout the whole volume of the screed can be obtained by the use of blinded no-fines aggregate (4). Any type of aggregate may be used, although care must sometimes be exercised to avoid breakage, particularly with vermiculite. The honeycomb may then be linked to outlets.

It is possible to provide ventilation of the surface of the screed (or other insulant) by the use of heavily gritted first felts or special channelled underlays and, to a lesser extent, by partial bonding (5). With these systems it is important to ensure that ducting formed under the felt is not blocked or otherwise damaged, either during laying or later during maintenance.

(b) *Outlets* (Diagram D.3.04/56)

Outlets, sometimes also referred to as ventilators, may be provided in two basic positions, namely (i) at the edges of the roof (eaves or parapet) or (ii) through the roof covering itself.

Edge ventilation may form an integral part of the built-up felt roof, as shown diagrammatically in diagram D.3.04/56 (1). At parapets care must be taken to ensure that rainwater does not find its way behind the covering. Where a honeycomb screed is used the vents at eaves should have, the BRS suggest, an area of 1 065–4 258mm²/metre run.

Roof-top ventilators all require proper sealing where they pierce the roof covering and must be designed accordingly. They must also be designed to prevent the entry of rainwater through the opening they form. Three types of ventilators have been developed (diagram D.3.04/56 (2–4) ). These are:

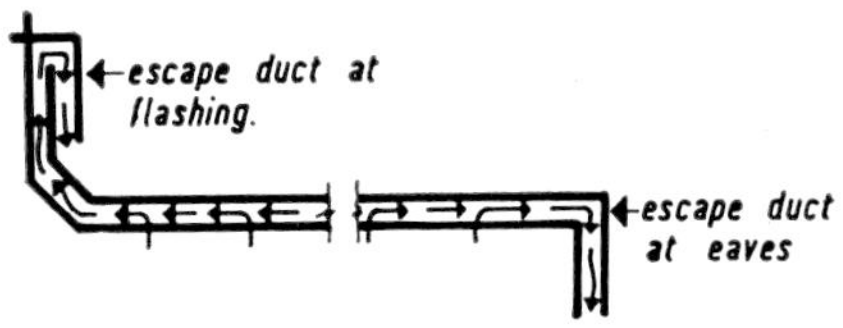


(1) Outlets for bitumen felt partially bonded (diagrammatic only).

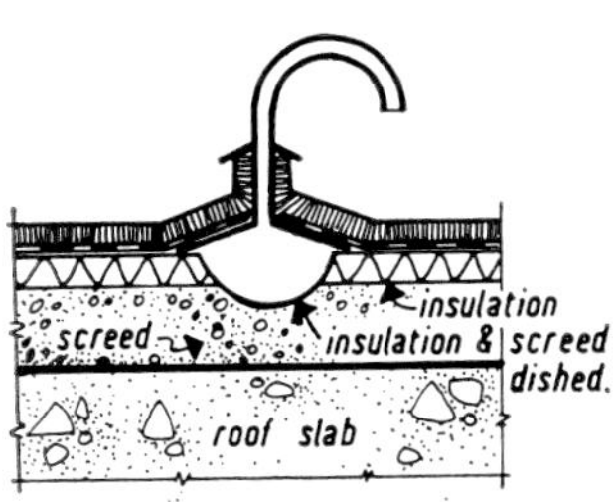


(2) Bent copper tubes as Parovent

Note: For comparison diagrams 2–4 have been drawn to approximately the same scale, viz. 1:12

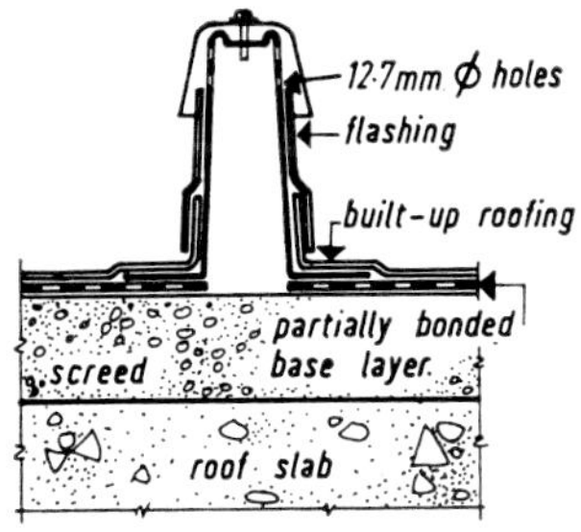


(3) Mushroom Vent as Breather Vent (D. Anderson Ltd.)

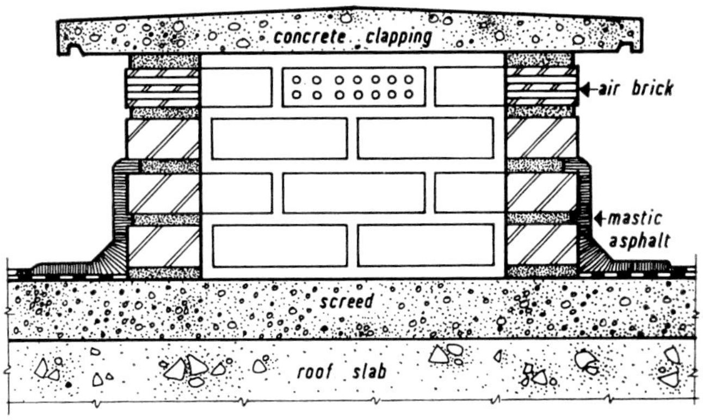


(4) Brick box ventilator. (Mastic Asphalte Advisory Council).

*D*.3.04/56

*Alternative methods of providing ventilation outlets for the release of entrapped water*

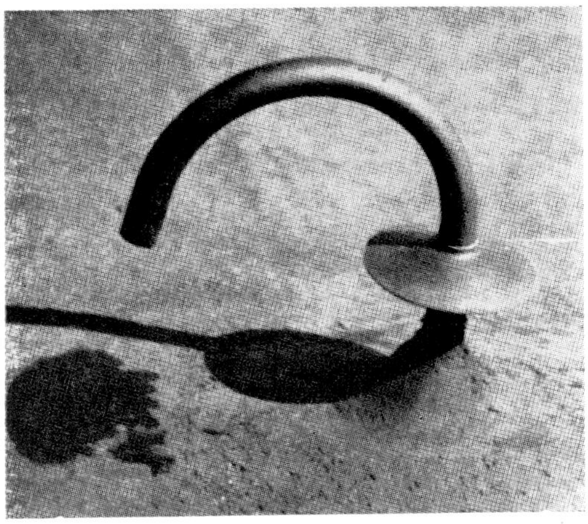

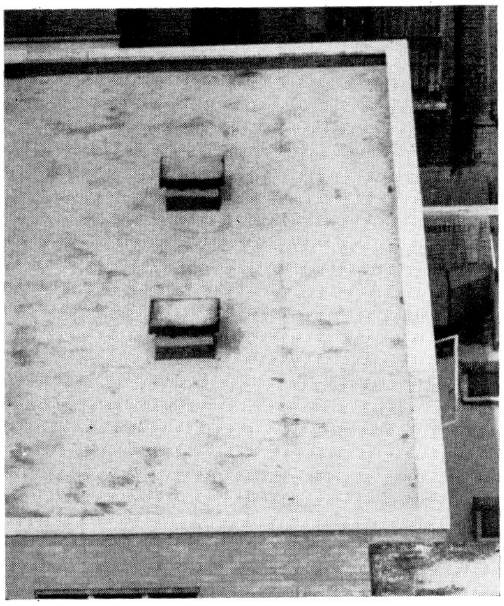

*Examples of two of the ventilators illustrated in diagram D.3.04/56. Above, 'Parovent' bent copper tube ( (2) in diagram)—note water line on the left which is the result of the dripping of condensed water from the roof deck during drying out. Right, brick box ventilators ( (4) in the diagram) (Courtesy: Parovents Ltd.)*

(i) Bent copper tubes which are easy to install but through which ventilation is limited and thus are more useful for releasing pressure than drying out.

(ii) Mushroom vents of metal or plastics which are also easy to install. The extent of drying depends very much on design and the ease of the passage of air over or through the screed. The spacing of vents should be at approximately 6·0m centres.*

(iii) Brick box ventilators, as developed by The Mastic Asphalte Advisory Council, are constructed *in situ* on the screed. The boxes have an internal area of just over 0·09m² (459mm by 229mm internal dimensions) with 229mm by 76mm air bricks on all four sides. The council recommends that there should be one box per 56m² of roof area with a minimum of two.

In all cases the ventilators should preferably be placed over low points to which water can drain and over high points to which water may be driven by warmth. It is also important that the screed or insulant should not be omitted* or taken up inside the area of a ventilator.

*Forced ventilation.* Whatever system of ducting and ventilators is adopted, it is unlikely whether under natural conditions, including warmth from the building, screeds will dry out much before one year has elapsed. The whole process may be speeded up if, where ducting has been incorporated, a conventional roof ventilator with a slow-speed fan is installed instead of a brick box ventilator. The speed of drying out would have to be carefully controlled in order to avoid damage to the screed (moisture movement and cracking) and the covering.

*Maintenance of ventilation.* Ventilation, whether natural or forced,

*As recommended by D. Anderson & Son Ltd. for their 'Breather Vents'.

*Some manufacturers of vents advise 'dishing' of the insulant, presumably in an attempt to increase the free area from which ventilation can take place.

# Index

# Index

# Index

# Index

# Index

# Index

# Index

www.ingramcontent.com/pod-product-compliance
Lightning Source LLC
LaVergne TN
LVHW010933061026
849535LV00007B/2373
* 9 7 8 2 3 4 3 1 0 4 5 2 2 *

Achevé d'imprimer par Corlet Numérique - 14110 Condé-sur-Noireau
N° d'Imprimeur : 133065 - Dépôt légal : octobre 2016 - *Imprimé en France*

**L'HARMATTAN ITALIA**
Via Degli Artisti 15; 10124 Torino
harmattan.italia@gmail.com

**L'HARMATTAN HONGRIE**
Könyvesbolt ; Kossuth L. u. 14-16
1053 Budapest

**L'HARMATTAN KINSHASA**
185, avenue Nyangwe
Commune de Lingwala
Kinshasa, R.D. Congo
(00243) 998697603 ou (00243) 999229662

**L'HARMATTAN CONGO**
67, av. E. P. Lumumba
Bât. – Congo Pharmacie (Bib. Nat.)
BP2874 Brazzaville
harmattan.congo@yahoo.fr

**L'HARMATTAN GUINÉE**
Almamya Rue KA 028, en face
du restaurant Le Cèdre
OKB agency BP 3470 Conakry
(00224) 657 20 85 08 / 664 28 91 96
harmattanguinee@yahoo.fr

**L'HARMATTAN MALI**
Rue 73, Porte 536, Niamakoro,
Cité Unicef, Bamako
Tél. 00 (223) 20205724 / +(223) 76378082
poudiougopaul@yahoo.fr
pp.harmattan@gmail.com

**L'HARMATTAN CAMEROUN**
BP 11486
Face à la SNI, immeuble Don Bosco
Yaoundé
(00237) 99 76 61 66
harmattancam@yahoo.fr

**L'HARMATTAN CÔTE D'IVOIRE**
Résidence Karl / cité des arts
Abidjan-Cocody 03 BP 1588 Abidjan 03
(00225) 05 77 87 31
etien_nda@yahoo.fr

**L'HARMATTAN BURKINA**
Penou Achille Some
Ouagadougou
(+226) 70 26 88 27

**L'HARMATTAN SÉNÉGAL**
10 VDN en face Mermoz, après le pont de Fann
BP 45034 Dakar Fann
33 825 98 58 / 33 860 9858
senharmattan@gmail.com / senlibraire@gmail.com
www.harmattansenegal.com

**L'HARMATTAN BÉNIN**
ISOR-BENIN
01 BP 359 COTONOU-RP
Quartier Gbèdjromèdé,
Rue Agbélenco, Lot 1247 I
Tél : 00 229 21 32 53 79
christian_dablaka123@yahoo.fr

à vivre avec ce diabète, cette « sale bête » qui l'accompagne désormais. Dans son imaginaire d'enfant, Léa devient Super Léa, une super-héroïne du quotidien, une dompteuse... La « sale bête » n'a qu'à bien se tenir ! «Écrite par deux mères d'enfants qui souffrent de ce mal, la pièce a des accents de vérité d'autant plus convaincants que le rôle de la fillette est endossé par Rébecca Stella, l'une des mamans qui est de surcroît une comédienne d'une subtile envergure.» (Pariscope). «Un joli spectacle.» (www.froggydelight.com)
*(15.00 euros) ISBN : 978-2-336-2-97408*

**SE LIBÉRER D'UNE ADDICTION SANS DROGUE**
**Baclofène et boulimie : une expérience**
*Goffart Claude*
Ce livre retrace l'itinéraire d'une «toxico de la bouffe», aidée dans son combat par l'usage du baclofène, molécule ancienne redécouverte par un professeur alcoolique. Elle s'avère efficace pour supprimer l'envie irrésistible qui mène à la bouteille mais semble aussi apte à aider les boulimiques. Décrit dans ces pages, ce traitement demande surtout de la ténacité et un travail sur soi attentif mené avec un thérapeute et en lien avec une association dédiée aux utilisateurs de ce traitement.
*(20.50 euros, 198 p.)*
*ISBN : 978-2-343-06233-4, ISBN EBOOK : 978-2-336-38817-5*

**AUTISME**
**Le sacrifice invisible**
**Trajectoires des familles et regards croisés des professionnels**
*Jean-Bart Christiane*
Malgré des évolutions positives dans l'accompagnement des enfants autistes, l'auteure sort de l'institution et va à la rencontre des familles. Retracer leurs trajectoires lui semble indispensable à la compréhension de l'environnement de l'enfant autiste. Il s'agit d'avoir une vision globale de l'enfant autiste, de prendre en compte tout ce qui influe sur lui dans des cadres comme l'institution qui le prend en charge, sa famille, l'école, son voisinage...
*(Coll. Réseau Tessitures, 25.00 euros, 256 p.)*
*ISBN : 978-2-343-06565-6, ISBN EBOOK : 978-2-336-38662-1*

**FRAGMENTS POUR UNE HISTOIRE DE LA GÉRONTOLOGIE (Volume 1)**
*OAREIL*
Ce livre raconte avec force anecdotes la naissance de l'action gérontologique : les errements, les oppositions et les luttes des acteurs qui ont ouvert cette voie nouvelle. Ce tome rassemble les entretiens individuels de ces femmes et hommes, pionniers chacun dans leur domaine. Ils narrent leurs parcours, leurs rencontres, la manière dont ils s'y sont pris pour construire pas à pas des actions, des services, des organisations sur des terrains en friche.
*(Coll. La gérontologie en actes, 23.50 euros, 220 p.)*
*ISBN : 978-2-343-06908-1, ISBN EBOOK : 978-2-336-38920-2*

se métamorphoser au fil des ans, avant de questionner la problématique de la classification. Passant ensuite en revue les facteurs, corrélats et autres théories, il lève un bout de voile sur la complexité de ce trouble de l'humeur, tout en faisant un détour dans ses spécificités africaines.
*(26.50 euros, 270 p.)*
*ISBN : 978-2-343-06235-8, ISBN EBOOK : 978-2-336-39178-6*

**SCIENCE ET HUILES ESSENTIELLES**
*Baumann Alexandre*
Les huiles essentielles sont fortes là où les médicaments sont faibles : maux de dos, maladies cardiovasculaires, infections chroniques, anxiété « ordinaire »... Cela est étayé par de nombreuses études scientifiques. Pourtant elles continuent à être vues comme de simples substances agréablement odorantes. Ce livre combat cette injustice en détaillant une centaine d'études scientifiques démontrant de réels effets thérapeutiques.
*(17.50 euros, 172 p.)*
*ISBN : 978-2-343-07469-6, ISBN EBOOK : 978-2-336-39322-3*

**LA MALTRAITANCE DES PERSONNES ÂGÉES**
**L'envers du décor**
*Sauveur Yannick - Postface de Pascal Lardellier*
Ce livre interroge les causes de la maltraitance des personnes âgées. L'auteur cible les responsabilités de l'État et la faiblesse des moyens mis au service des personnes âgées. Il offre ainsi une réflexion sur le jeunisme, l'âgisme et la société marchande. Fort de son expérience du milieu médicosocial, l'auteur apporte un éclairage original sur l'envers du décor, les personnels maltraités. De nombreux témoignages illustrent son propos.
*(Coll. Des Hauts et Débats, 19.00 euros, 186 p.)*
*ISBN : 978-2-343-07283-8, ISBN EBOOK : 978-2-336-39357-5*

**ACCOMPAGNER LA VIE JUSQUE-LÀ**
*Feroumont Bernadette - Préface de Gabriel Ringlet*
Ouvrir ce livre, c'est plonger dans l'univers de l'accompagnement de la fin de vie et comprendre combien des attitudes simples et spontanées peuvent compter pour le patient, l'entourage ou l'équipe soignante. Les récits parlent de tendresse et de moments heureux, mais aussi de tristesses, de colères, d'injustices. Ouvrir ce livre, c'est aussi découvrir que le temps nous rappelle l'urgence de savourer la vie : il nous invite à porter sur nos rencontres et nos gestes un regard intérieur qui leur donnera du sens.
*(Coll. Encres de vie, 16.50 euros, 162 p.)*
*ISBN : 978-2-336-30839-5, ISBN EBOOK : 978-2-336-39254-7*

**LES ÎLES DÉSERTES**
*Avela Guilloux, Rébecca Stella*
Léa a 9 ans. Un jour, elle découvre qu'elle est diabétique. À partir de ce moment-là, sa vie change, devient compliquée. Elle doit faire face à sa colère, ses propres peurs, à un traitement difficile, à des contraintes auxquelles elle ne s'attendait pas, aux réflexions pas toujours délicates de son entourage. Léa va devoir apprendre

et future. La bioéthique questionne finalement la nature même de l'être humain et offre la perspective d'un nouvel avenir.
*(Coll. Cultures et Médecines, 17.00 euros, 154 p.)*
*ISBN : 978-2-343-07225-8, ISBN EBOOK : 978-2-336-39901-0*

## TRANSGRESSIONS DES FRONTIÈRES DU CORPS
**La chirurgie esthétique**
*Mitz Vladimir*
Les frontières de la chirurgie esthétique délimitent, avec difficulté, une spécialité chirurgicale qui est expansive. Cette chirurgie transgressive dérange les concepts philosophiques du «accepte-toi tel que tu es», elle bénéficie d'innovations tumultueuses telles les homogreffes du visage ou des membres, elle est constamment soumise à l'œil éveillé des médias. Cet ouvrage se propose d'en exposer les facettes en explorant ses mythes, ses bases conscientes et inconscientes et ses limites.
*(Coll. Eidos série Retina, 16.50 euros, 156 p.)*
*ISBN : 978-2-343-07729-1, ISBN EBOOK : 978-2-336-39759-7*

## VERS LA CÉCITÉ
**Un étrange parcours – Récit**
*Abbadie-Douce Paulette*
Dans son précédent ouvrage « Voyage vers la cécité », l'auteur se penchait sur le choc éprouvé à l'annonce du verdict de cette maladie des yeux qui l'affecte : la « DMLA ». Dans ce nouvel ouvrage, elle nous dévoile d'étranges phénomènes qui l'assaillent et la troublent. À la suite de recherches, elle découvre avec stupéfaction que ces phénomènes sont une conséquence prévisible de la maladie des yeux qui l'affecte. Alors pourquoi ce silence autour de ces phénomènes reconnus par les spécialistes ?
*(8.00 euros, 50 p.)*
*ISBN : 978-2-343-07608-9, ISBN EBOOK : 978-2-336-39792-4*

## MÉDECINE À TRAVERS LES SIÈCLES
**Entre rencontres et découverte**
Sous la direction de Xavier Riaud
Si la médecine et ses acteurs ont contribué incontestablement au bien-être de l'humanité, les dérives de quelques-uns ou les zones d'ombre amènent inévitablement à une discussion à propos de l'éthique qui doit la régir. Forts de ce postulat, les auteurs de cette collection ont souhaité décrire les avancées et les évolutions des sciences médicales.
*(Coll. Médecine à travers les siècles, 19.00 euros, 182 p., Illustré en couleur)*
*ISBN : 978-2-343-07425-2, ISBN EBOOK : 978-2-336-39465-7*

## LA DÉPRESSION
**Une pathologie à visage multiple**
*Lamessi Alain - Préfaces du docteur Thierry Malassiné et du professeur Michel Dieudonné Vohito*
Le présent ouvrage tente de présenter les multiples visages de la dépression. Pour cela, Alain Lamessi retrace la longue histoire de cette maladie qui n'a cessé de

# Recours aux soins
# et couverture médicale au Liban

# Logiques sociales

*Collection dirigée par Bruno Péquignot*

En réunissant des chercheurs, des praticiens et des essayistes, même si la dominante reste universitaire, la collection « Logiques Sociales » entend favoriser les liens entre la recherche non finalisée et l'action sociale.

En laissant toute liberté théorique aux auteurs, elle cherche à promouvoir les recherches qui partent d'un terrain, d'une enquête ou d'une expérience qui augmentent la connaissance empirique des phénomènes sociaux ou qui proposent une innovation méthodologique ou théorique, voire une réévaluation de méthodes ou de systèmes conceptuels classiques.

## Dernières parutions

Anja HESS, *Les habitants des chambres de bonne à Paris. Étude filmique des usages de l'espace quotidien*, 2016.

Christophe CAMUS, *Mais que fait vraiment l'architecte ?, Enquête sur les pratiques et modes d'existence de l'architecture*, 2016.

Roland GUILLON, *Mes années 1950 et 1960 ou l'éveil d'une sensibilité,* 2016.

Louis DURRIVE, *Compétence et activité de travail*, 2016.

Laurent AUCHER, *Le Tribunal des ouvriers, Enquête aux prud'hommes de Vierzon*, 2016.

Benoît SOUROU, *Stratégies identitaires chez les migrants turcs en France*, 2016.

Michel BOURDINOT, *Vers de nouvelles fonctions pour le permanent UD CFDT ?,* 2016.

Isabelle PAPIEAU, *Il y avait des fois,* La Belle et la Bête. *Réalités et magie à l'italienne*, 2016.

Yvon CORAIN, *L'expérience dans tous ses états, Une approche méthodologique*, 2016.

Cécile NOESSER, La résistible ascension du cinéma d'animation. *Socio-genèse d'un cinéma-bis en France (1950-2010),* 2016.

Aurélien CINTRACT, *La mort inégale. Du recul de la mort à l'analyse socio-historique de la mortalité différentielle*, 2016.

Éric LE BRETON, *Mobilité et société dispersée, Une approche sociologique*, 2016.

Christiane Saliba Sfeir

# Recours aux soins et couverture médicale au Liban

L'Harmattan

5-7, rue de l'Ecole-Polytechnique, 75005 Paris

www.harmattan.com
diffusion.harmattan@wanadoo.fr

ISBN : 978-2-343-10452-2
EAN : 9782343104522

# Remerciements

Tous mes remerciements vont à l'Université libanaise représentée par :

Son président professeur Adnan El Sayyed Hussein,

La doyenne de la faculté de Santé publique professeure Nina Saadallah-Zeidan,

Le directeur de la faculté de Santé publique-section 2 professeur Joseph Bechara,

Pour le soutien financier et la confiance académique qui m'ont été accordés pour ce projet de recherche financé par l'Université.

Je voudrais remercier également les professeures et chercheures Pascale Salameh et Marie-Thérèse Sabbagh pour leurs précieux conseils et lectures qui n'ont fait que rajouter à la valeur scientifique de ce rapport.

Tous mes remerciements vont à la direction générale de la Caisse nationale de Sécurité sociale en la personne de son directeur général Dr Mohammad Karaki et au directeur du centre du Kesrouan Dr Jean-Pierre Boutros pour leur confiance et leur encouragement pour cette recherche.

Mes remerciements vont également aux représentants du ministère de la Santé publique pour avoir répondu aux innombrables questions ainsi qu'à toutes les directions des structures sanitaires, dispensaires et hôpitaux, pour leur accueil et leur coopération à cette recherche.

Je tiens également à remercier mes étudiantes en master de Santé publique option Education et Promotion de la santé, Carla Njeim, Hanane Chaybane et Joëlle Touma qui

ont contribué à l’étude qualitative de cette recherche ainsi qu’à tous les employés de la CNSS qui ont assuré toute la coopération possible pour le déroulement de l’enquête quantitative.

Toute ma gratitude va aussi aux 53 personnes interviewées lors de cette recherche pour le partage de leur vécu.

# Résumé

L'expression recours aux soins désigne dans cette recherche une composante de l'« accès aux soins ». L'accès aux soins est un élément essentiel du droit fondamental à la santé. Il présente un double objectif de réflexion en sociologie de santé. Il s'agit bien de la possibilité ou de l'accessibilité aux soins en termes, de droits sociaux autant que l'usage ou le recours qui en est fait ou pas. Les inégalités d'accès aux soins de santé sont présentes partout dans le monde. Elles touchent particulièrement les groupes vulnérables et conduisent à un phénomène du non-recours ou du recours tardif aux soins, susceptible d'avoir des conséquences catastrophiques tant pour la santé individuelle que publique.

L'aspect abordé dans cette étude vise à identifier les facteurs déterminants les comportements du recours ou du non-recours aux soins des Libanais face aux épisodes de maladies et d'explorer l'influence d'une couverture maladie et du coût socio-économique des soins sur l'état et la fréquence du recours. La démarche méthodologique se base sur une étude qualitative et sur une enquête quantitative. L'étude qualitative repose sur une observation directe du terrain et des entretiens semi-directifs menés auprès de cinquante-trois Libanais, rencontrés dans huit établissements sanitaires localisés dans les cazas du Kesrouan, Metn et Beyrouth. L'enquête quantitative se base sur des données de 102 dossiers de la CNSS du caza du Kesrouan allant de début janvier 2012 à fin juin 2015.

Les principaux résultats de cette étude révèlent que les barrières financières et géographiques réduisent l'accès

aux soins. En parallèle, les déterminants socio-culturels et les croyances héritées influencent directement la décision du recours aux services de santé. La perception de la santé, de la gravité de la maladie et des établissements sanitaires sont des facteurs motivant ou entravant ce recours. La relation établie avec l'équipe soignante, ainsi que l'influence des expériences vécues par la famille et l'entourage apparaissent comme des facteurs de renforcement à adopter ou à abandonner un comportement en santé. Les résultats quantitatifs ont renforcé ces résultats en montrant qu'une couverture médicale favorise les recours aux soins, le lien continu avec les professionnels de santé et un accès régulier aux services de santé prescrits. Elle contribue à un meilleur contrôle sur la santé, mais le coût restant à la charge des ménages constitue un recours sélectif selon l'âge et la gravité de la maladie de la personne couverte.

La conclusion de ce travail ouvre des perspectives vers une nouvelle stratégie de promotion de la santé au Liban qui favorisera une couverture plus généralisée et un recours aux soins plus structuré et plus accessible à l'ensemble de la population.

**Mots clefs :** accès aux soins, recours aux soins, renoncement aux soins, inégalités en santé, perception de la santé, croyances en santé, comportement en santé, déterminants sociaux en santé, accessibilité financière, accessibilité géographique, couverture médicale, fréquence du recours, politiques sociales, protection sociale.

# Liste des sigles et des abréviations

MSP : Ministère de Santé publique.

OMS : Organisation mondiale de la santé.

ONG : Organisation non gouvernementale.

MAS : Ministère des Affaires sociales.

CNSS : Caisse nationale de Sécurité sociale.

PRECEDE : Predisposing, Reinforcing and Enabling Constructs in Educational/Environment Diagnosis and Evaluation.

PROCEED : Policy, Regulatory and Organizational Constructs in Educational and Environmental Development.

# Liste des figures

# Liste des tableaux

# Liste des annexes

# Introduction

Ce travail de recherche s'intitule *Recours aux soins et couverture médicale au Liban* en considérant le Recours aux soins comme une composante de l'accès aux soins. Le recours aux soins en santé résulte à la fois des caractéristiques du système de soins en santé et des caractéristiques de la population (Aday et Andersen, 1974). Il s'agit de l'accès multidimensionnel aux soins, du rapport entre les besoins en soins de la population libanaise et l'utilisation du système de soins, l'offre de soins et le recours aux soins (Perchansky, Thomas, 1981), mais également des différentes représentations de santé pouvant définir des barrières à cet accès aux soins. Il s'agit bien de la possibilité ou de l'accessibilité aux soins en termes de droits sociaux autant que de l'usage ou le recours qui est fait ou pas (Lombrail et Pascal, 2005).

Le ministère de la Santé publique au Liban révèle dans ses rapports des inégalités sociales en matière de santé dues essentiellement à des déterminants sociaux (pauvreté, chômage, analphabétisme, logement) et environnementaux (système de soins, assainissement de l'eau...) de santé. Le nombre effectif des bénéficiaires est estimé à 240 000 composés de patients ayant recours à des opérations coûteuses et un nombre d'ayant droit estimé à 2 millions (Ammar, 2012). Ce rapport-ci montre également qu'un taux de mortalité infantile assez élevé (16,1/1000 naissances en 2004 ; en France c'est 3,1/1 000 en 2004 selon l'Ined), un taux de mortalité maternelle encore élevé (23/100 000 naissances en 2008 ; en France c'est 9,6/100 000 naissances selon l'InVS, bilan 2001-2006). Le

bulletin statistique 2013 du ministère montre une mortalité infantile qui passe à 9/1 000 en 2009 pour 3,33% en France en 2009 (Ined). La mortalité maternelle montre une amélioration allant de 25/100 000 naissances en 2011 pour passer à 18/100 000 en 2013 (Statistical Bulletin MOPH, 2013). Le rapport de l'Inserm (2013) montre une mortalité maternelle en France entre 2007 et 2009 de 10,3/100 000 naissances.

De plus, certains hôpitaux refusent d'admettre des patients avec une prise en charge du ministère de la Santé publique et que les dépenses de santé incombent de 60% à la seule charge des familles (Ammar, 2012). Il s'agit donc d'un concept de recours aux soins peu exploré et d'un manque de stratégies définies et planifiées au niveau du système de santé libanais.

La problématique de ce projet de recherche tourne autour du questionnement suivant : quels seraient les facteurs d'influence possible sur le recours aux soins chez les Libanais ? Serait-il un problème de perception de la santé ou de répercussion d'une situation socio-économique lourde faute de moyens assurés par un système libanais de protection sociale ?

Ce projet vise à analyser les dimensions de ces inégalités dans l'expérience quotidienne des citoyens Libanais couverts soient-ils ou non par un régime officiel de protection sociale et d'explorer à travers une sociologie qualitative les représentations de santé et les caractéristiques psychosociologiques contribuant à un accès ou à un renoncement aux soins.

En effet, celui-ci étant considéré comme un comportement à adopter vis-à-vis du risque santé (Dourgnon et Sermet, 2002), un recours conceptuel au modèle psychosocial de prédiction des comportements de Fishbein et Ajzen (1975 in Godin 1991) sera effectué dans

un cadre plus général de planification santé inspiré du modèle Precede de Green et Kreuter (2005).

Un travail d'évaluation sur dossier de personnes couvertes par la Caisse nationale de Sécurité sociale est réalisé pour évaluer l'impact de l'existence d'une couverture médicale sur la fréquence du recours aux soins d'une part et le coût socio-économique laissé à la charge des familles d'autre part. C'est une étude sur certaines caractéristiques actuelles de ce système de protection sociale.

Selon l'Organisation mondiale de la santé, il est important de considérer la santé comme un bien-être complet physique, social et mental et ne consiste pas seulement en une absence de maladie ou d'infirmité (OMS, 1946). Or depuis la conférence d'Alma Ata en 1978 qui a préconisé l'accès de tous les individus aux services de santé, celui-ci reste déterminé par ces choix et des contraintes qui dépendent aussi bien des croyances, des arbitrages individuels et collectifs que de l'environnement physique et psychosocial.

Les objectifs de ce projet de recherche se résument dans les points suivants :

- Déterminer les différentes composantes du recours aux soins en fonction de la perception de la santé comme bien-être physique, social et mental.
- Faire ressortir les comportements psychosociaux dans un contexte d'après-guerre pour analyser la motivation de la population concernant sa propre santé, l'attitude vis-à-vis du risque de santé et leur influence dans le choix d'une couverture médicale.
- Analyser les déterminants sociaux en santé spécifiques à la population libanaise dans le cadre référentiel d'une société patriarcale confessionnelle qui développe un ensemble de discriminations liées au genre masculin et féminin.

- Faire ressortir les représentations sociales en santé des citoyens concernant le système de santé, le rôle de l'Etat libanais, l'offre perçue en santé.
- Inciter par cette étude exploratoire à développer des études épidémiologiques et à construire une base commune de données nationales permettant une meilleure analyse des déterminants sociaux de la santé sachant que le terme de « déterminants sociaux de santé » renvoie à un objet commun à diverses disciplines scientifiques.

Cette recherche est composée de huit chapitres :
- Les trois premiers chapitres présentent la revue de littérature, les concepts d'accès et de recours aux soins, d'inégalités sociales en santé, les systèmes de santé et le cadre conceptuel adopté.
- Le chapitre quatre, celui de la méthodologie de la recherche, définit le choix de la méthode de l'étude empirique qualitative et quantitative de cette recherche.
- Les chapitres cinq, six et sept sont les résultats de l'observation ; des entretiens semi-directifs et de l'enquête quantitative.
- Le chapitre huit est celui de la discussion des résultats de la recherche.
- La Conclusion traite d'une ouverture vers une stratégie de promotion de la santé à travers des recommandations basées sur les axes de la charte d'Ottawa.

# Chapitre I
# Définitions des concepts de santé

L'OMS (1946) considère actuellement la santé « comme un état de complet bien-être physique, mental et social et non simplement comme l'absence de maladie et d'infirmité ». Il s'agit d'une définition idéaliste qui a néanmoins le mérite de clarifier la distinction essentielle entre maladie et santé. Dans ce contexte, la maladie est un concept relativement étroit qui peut faire référence à des processus pathologiques, compromettant l'intégrité anatomique ou physiologique du corps. La santé fait référence à quelque chose de plus large. Elle concerne l'expérience subjective qu'ont les individus de leurs corps et d'eux-mêmes et les conséquences sur leur vie quotidienne. Tandis que la maladie appartient au domaine de la biologie, la santé appartient au domaine de la sociologie et de la psychologie, englobant comme lui les sentiments, les comportements et, in fine, la qualité de la vie (Pouëzat, 2002).

Une bonne santé est une ressource capitale pour le développement social, économique et personnel. Certains facteurs politiques, économiques, sociaux, culturels, environnementaux, comportementaux et biologiques peuvent améliorer la santé ou au contraire lui nuire. On parle alors de déterminants sociaux qui interagissent entre eux pour devenir des générateurs d'inégalités sociales en santé (Lombrail et Pascal, 2005).

Améliorer l'état de santé de la population dans son ensemble et de chacun en particulier, quelle que soit son

origine ou son appartenance sociale, est un objectif largement partagé et par ailleurs inscrit dans les textes fondamentaux nationaux et internationaux. La conférence internationale sur les soins de santé primaires réunie à Alma Ata en 1978, affirme que la santé est un droit fondamental de l'être humain et que les inégalités flagrantes dans la situation sanitaire des peuples, aussi bien entre pays développés et pays en développement qu'à l'intérieur même des pays sont politiquement, socialement et économiquement inacceptables. Les participants à la conférence considèrent que les soins de santé primaires sont des soins de santé essentiels et qu'ils doivent être rendus universellement accessibles à tous les individus et à toutes les familles de la communauté (OMS, 1978). Durant cette conférence, l'OMS lance son grand mot « la santé pour tous en l'an 2000 » qui préconise en fait l'accès de tous aux soins préventifs et curatifs. Le Liban avait signé cette convention et a développé une stratégie pour mettre en place les soins de santé primaire. Cet objectif trop ambitieux de « santé pour tous » dans la majorité des pays du monde ne sera jamais réalisé étant donné les ressources humaines et financières disponibles (Potvin, Moquet, Jones, 2010, p. 74). Dès lors, une définition du concept d'accès aux soins devient nécessaire.

## 1.1. Concept d'accès aux soins de santé

Le recours aux soins est une composante de l'accès aux soins. L'accès est une préoccupation majeure dans la politique de santé, il est également l'un des mots les plus fréquemment utilisés dans les discussions du système de soins de santé, mais il est souvent non défini ou utilisé précisément. Pour certains, l'accès se réfère à l'entrée ou l'utilisation du système des services de santé, tandis que pour d'autres, il caractérise les facteurs qui influencent l'entrée ou l'utilisation (Clark, Coffee, 2011).

Depuis les années soixante, de nombreux chercheurs, essentiellement en sociologie médicale, puis aussi en santé publique, ont cherché à définir le concept d'accès aux soins pour améliorer la performance de tout système de santé. Pour L.A. Aday et R.M. Anderson, le concept d'accès se définit comme le rapport entre les besoins en soins d'une population (caractéristiques sociodémographiques) et l'utilisation du système de soins (prise en charge effective des patients). Définie comme l'analyse spatiale de l'offre des soins et du recours aux soins, la géographie des soins de santé repose sur le concept d'accès ou d'accessibilité, deux termes non équivalents pour certains auteurs, mais synonymes pour d'autres (Aday, Andersen, 1974). Penchansky et Thomas (1981), prolongent cette réflexion, en décomposant le concept d'accès en cinq dimensions bien définies : la disponibilité, l'accessibilité, la commodité, la capacité financière et l'acceptabilité.

### 1.1.1. Disponibilité

Elle est définie comme la relation entre, d'une part, le volume et le type des services existants et, d'autre part, le volume et le type de besoins des patients. Face à un besoin en santé, une offre de services de santé doit exister. La disponibilité des services de santé comporte au moins trois composantes essentielles qui sont : la présence physique, la disponibilité temporelle et la fourniture de prestations adaptées en volume et en nature aux besoins des personnes.

Par disponibilité, il ne faudrait pas entendre la simple présence physique d'une infrastructure sanitaire, mais sa capacité réelle à produire un service. Dans les pays en développement, il est primordial de vérifier d'une part, l'existence effective d'une infrastructure de santé et d'autre part, l'existence de personnel adéquat avant de

considérer le volume et la qualité des prestations fournies ou même le niveau de l'équipement médical.

### 1.1.2. Accessibilité

L'accessibilité est la relation entre la localisation des services et celle des patients, prenant en compte la mobilité des patients, la durée, la distance et le coût du trajet, c'est une mesure de proximité (Penchansky et Thomas, 1981).

Il s'agit de quantifier la fraction de la distance qui devrait diminuer progressivement l'interaction entre les services de santé et leurs patients potentiels et au fur et à mesure que croît la distance les séparant. Cet effet de dissolution par la distance existe toujours. Mais son intensité est fort variable en fonction d'autres facteurs comme le niveau hiérarchique du service de santé, l'âge et le sexe du malade, la disponibilité du véhicule ou le type de problème de santé.

L'accessibilité peut être considérée comme équitable lorsque des variables non « contrôlables » comme l'âge, le sexe, ou la nature de la maladie peuvent expliquer l'utilisation des services. Par contre elle ne l'est pas si cette dernière est liée à des variables comme l'éducation, le revenu ou l'absence de ressources.

Différentes mesures de la distance séparant les services de la santé de leurs utilisateurs potentiels sont communément utilisées pour décrire l'accessibilité. Certaines d'entre elles sont fortement influencées par la densité et la qualité des voies de communication, ainsi que par le mode de transport utilisé.

La capacité à être atteint par une clientèle, un message et un service, dépend de l'état des moyens de transport et représente un coût : le monde entier est accessible en tous ses points, mais le coût d'accès peut être très élevé. L'accès aux services entre dans la qualité de la vie, le prix

du logement, les stratégies de l'habitation. L'accessibilité peut se définir selon divers critères (aller et retour dans la journée, dans la demi-journée, aller et retour permettant une journée complète de travail, tout ceci supposé à des tarifs acceptables).

### *1.1.2.1. Accessibilité de point de vue géographique*

Selon Picheral (2001), l'accessibilité reflète la capacité matérielle d'accéder aux ressources sanitaires et aux services de santé, elle présente au moins deux dimensions : matérielle et sociale. Elle traduit la possibilité de recourir aux prestataires de soins, c'est une condition de l'accès aux soins, mais ne détermine pas à elle seule le recours aux soins effectif (c'est-à-dire l'utilisation effective du système). L'accessibilité géographique est reliée à la notion de distance entre offre et demande : distance géométrique, distance longueur des trajets-routes, distance temps donc de la proximité ou de l'éloignement du cabinet médical, de l'établissement de soins et de la longueur du trajet à effectuer.

C'est un indicateur social qui traduit les inégalités sociales existantes et de plus c'est un indicateur de santé fréquemment utilisé.

### *1.1.2.2. Accessibilité en économie de santé*

L'accessibilité économique est la possibilité financière de recourir à des services de santé ou à une pratique, technique ou équipement médical assurés par une couverture ou une assurance sociale.

Pour Lambert (1985), les conditions d'accessibilité aux équipements collectifs sont toujours contrastées dans les grandes nations où persistent des inégalités régionales et des régions de peuplement dispersé (zones de montagne, régions sous-peuplées ou dépeuplées). Des enquêtes d'économie de la santé permettent d'identifier, sur l'espace sanitaire, les principaux déséquilibres entre offre

et demande de soins. La progression du taux d'utilisation des services existants (consultation, hospitalisation) accompagne la diminution des barrières d'accès aux soins (fréquence et commodité des transports, prise en charge des dépenses par les assurances).

Les mesures de l'accessibilité potentielle des divers types de services de santé sont indispensables d'ailleurs pour planifier et localiser de nouveaux services de santé. La plus grande accessibilité est donc un des objectifs premiers de tout système de santé dans sa dimension sociale et qu'est l'équité (IRDES, 2013).

### 1.1.3. Commodité

La commodité est la relation entre la manière dont les ressources sanitaires sont organisées pour accueillir le patient et la capacité de celui-ci à s'adapter à cette offre. La notion de commodité renvoie à la possibilité d'un contact pratique et facile (ou non) entre le patient et le système de santé. Les aspects temporels sont ici souvent prépondérants : jours et heures d'ouverture des services de santé, présence régulière d'un agent de santé, temps d'attente. Toutefois, cela n'est pas exclusif, il faudra y ajouter le système de paiement, la prise en charge des urgences, la consultation téléphonique, le système de référence... Par exemple, en milieu rural, les heures d'ouverture des services de santé sont souvent peu adaptées au rythme de travail des paysans. En contrepartie, dans les sociétés peu monétarisées, l'impossibilité de payer en nature les praticiens de la médecine moderne en limité fortement l'accès (Bonnet, 2002).

### 1.1.4. Capacité financière

La capacité financière peut se définir comme la relation entre le prix des prestations et la capacité du patient ou de

sa famille, ou de son assurance à payer ou à emprunter ou encore à recevoir une aide de son entourage.

Dans les pays en développement, très rares sont les personnes couvertes par une assurance-maladie. De plus, les bénéficiaires d'une telle prestation sociale comme les fonctionnaires et les employés du secteur public ne se recrutent généralement pas dans les couches les plus démunies de la population ni dans les plus à risque.

Dans ces pays en développement, la capacité financière de la population constitue souvent une des principales raisons de l'inaction thérapeutique face à la maladie ou du choix d'un recours particulier. L'introduction d'un paiement ou d'une rapide augmentation des tarifs se répercutent généralement fortement sur le choix thérapeutique, surtout si elles ne sont pas accompagnées d'une amélioration de la qualité des soins (Bonnet, 2002).

### 1.1.5. Acceptabilité

L'acceptabilité est définie selon Penchansky et Thomas (1981) comme la relation entre les caractéristiques (âge, sexe, ethnie, langue, religion, localisation…) et les attitudes des patients et celles du personnel et des structures de santé. Elle fait essentiellement référence à la capacité du prestataire du service et du patient, de surmonter des barrières sociales et culturelles qui empêchent ou altèrent le contact entre eux.

Au regard du problème de santé qui se pose, tous les recours thérapeutiques ne sont pas équivalents. Un hôpital peut être plus acceptable qu'un autre en raison de son affiliation religieuse, de la présence de proches parmi les employés, gage d'un meilleur accueil, ou de parents à proximité ce qui facilite l'hébergement et la pension des accompagnateurs.

Ces dimensions sont étroitement liées et constituent autant de difficultés potentielles pour le patient qui

souhaite obtenir une consultation. Il s'y ajoute l'existence des inégalités sociales de santé liées à des situations sociales et étatiques différentes telles que le chômage, la pauvreté et l'éducation…

## 1.2. Inégalités sociales de santé

La notion des inégalités sociales de santé (ISS) est définie comme étant l'existence de différences d'état de santé entre des individus de situations sociales différentes : revenu, éducation, catégorie sociale (Jusot, 2010).

Selon Cantoreggi (2010), les déterminants sociaux interagissent sur l'état de santé et renvoient à des conditions de vie, de travail et des déterminants collectifs matériels, psychosociaux ou socio-environnementaux générateurs d'inégalités sociales.

Jusot (2010), quant à lui, identifie quatre grands types de causes sociales dans la littérature scientifique :

- Les conditions matérielles de vie (logement, nutrition, travail dangereux…) qui constituent le gradient social de santé. Partout dans le monde, plus on est pauvre, moins on est en bonne santé. À l'intérieur des pays, les données montrent qu'en général, plus un individu occupe une position socio-économique défavorable, plus il est en mauvaise santé : ce gradient social concerne toute l'échelle socio-économique, de haut en bas. Il s'agit d'un phénomène mondial, que l'on constate dans les pays à revenu faible ou intermédiaire comme dans ceux à revenu élevé.
- L'effet inverse de l'état de santé sur le statut économique et social.
- Les comportements à risque (tabac, alcool, obésité) qui possèdent des conséquences différentes selon les groupes sociaux.

- Les déterminants psycho-sociaux comme la susceptibilité aux maladies et la capacité de les combattre qui dépendent du soutien social reçu, de la place dans la hiérarchie et des événements survenus depuis l'enfance.

Fassin (2004) définit les inégalités sociales de santé comme l'aboutissement des disparités structurelles (ressources, logement, alimentation, emploi et travail, école et formation) qui caractérisent l'état de la justice sociale dans un pays ou dans un territoire à un moment de son histoire et de son développement économique.

### 1.2.1. Egalité et inégalités dans l'accès aux soins

L'égalité en matière de soins peut se définir comme l'égalité d'accès aux soins disponibles pour des besoins équivalents, l'égalité d'utilisation des soins disponibles pour des besoins équivalents et l'égalité de qualité des soins. L'égalité d'accès aux soins implique que chacun ait un droit égal à utiliser les services disponibles, que ces derniers soient répartis équitablement dans tout le pays en fonction des besoins et qu'ils soient facilement accessibles. L'inégalité d'utilisation des soins disponibles est remarquée lorsque des conditions économiques ou sociales défavorables limitent l'utilisation des services. Quant à la notion d'égalité de qualité de soins, elle revient à ce que chacun puisse être traité en fonction de ses besoins et non pas en fonction de sa position sociale. Elle implique aussi que les dispensateurs de soins soignent avec le même dévouement tous les groupes de la société (Braveman, Gruskin, 2003).

Les inégalités d'accès aux soins se produisent à différentes étapes qui vont du « contact » avec le système de soins (professionnel/institution), jusqu'à la délivrance du soin nécessaire (provision), en passant par l'identification du besoin de soin (recognition). Cette inégalité peut s'analyser alors, selon deux volets celui de

la possibilité de se faire soigner donc l'accès potentiel et celui de l'utilisation qui est faite de cette potentialité donc l'accès effectif. L'utilisation est habituellement considérée sous le seul angle de l'accès primaire, mais une particulière attention mérite d'être portée à l'accès secondaire (Lombrail, Pascal, 2005).

### 1.2.2. Accès primaire et accès secondaire

Les soins de santé primaires renvoient aux soins de premier niveau. C'est la porte d'entrée dans le système de soins, qui offre des soins généralistes, globaux, continus, intégrés, accessibles à toute la population, et qui coordonne et intègre des services nécessaires à d'autres niveaux de soins (Bourgueil, Marek, Mousques, 2009). Les inégalités d'accès aux soins primaires peuvent être le fait d'un refus de soins par les professionnels, d'un non-recours aux soins par les personnes qui ressentent un besoin ou de la méconnaissance du besoin ou tout simplement la non-disponibilité de ces soins (Benattar, 2010).

L'accès secondaire correspond à la manière structurellement déterminée dont se déroulent les soins après un premier contact. Le renoncement aux soins se produit après la phase de contact avec le système de soins et va de l'identification du besoin jusqu'à la délivrance du soin nécessaire. Les obstacles qui grèvent l'accès primaire continuent d'opérer. D'autres s'y ajoutent, liés aux acteurs et au système (Lombrail, Pascal, 2005).

Donc, certaines inégalités d'accès aux soins relèvent du système de soins sous les aspects des déterminants géographiques, du financement des soins et des modes de prise en charge, d'autres relèvent de facteurs individuels comme le capital santé, le niveau d'éducation, l'information sur le système de santé... L'ensemble de ces

facteurs contribue au non-recours ou au renoncement aux soins de la part des patients.

### 1.2.3. Inégalités de recours aux soins

Une variante des inégalités sociales de santé est celle des inégalités sociales de recours aux soins. Les études ont démontré que ces différences sont d'autant plus fortes pour les recours aux soins de spécialistes et le recours aux soins préventifs.

Le travail d'identification des facteurs liés à l'accès et à l'utilisation des services de santé, les organise et les regroupe dans des modèles. L'un des modèles le plus ancien et le plus utilisé revient à Andersen et Aday. Dans ce modèle, les mesures d'accès ont été très proches des mesures d'inégalité de recours aux soins. Les obstacles aux soins concernent les non assurés, qui doivent payer l'intégralité des soins au moment de la consommation, et les ruraux ou les résidents de zones défavorisées, qui font face à une rareté relative de l'offre.

Selon Anderson et Aday, le recours aux services de santé résulte à la fois des caractéristiques du système de soins de santé et des caractéristiques de la population. Dans ces modèles, le comportement humain individuel est considéré comme influencé par les faits sociaux, il est donc possible de le modifier en agissant sur le groupe en particulier pour la modification des comportements à risque ou l'orientation vers une offre de soins. Depuis le modèle d'Anderson, la plupart des modèles regroupe les caractéristiques de la population pouvant influencer l'accès et l'utilisation des soins en trois catégories : facteurs prédisposants (variables démographiques, structure sociale, valeurs et croyances en santé, connaissances), facteurs de capacité ou de réalisation (indicateurs communautaires, disponibilité de ressources) et facteurs déclenchants (besoins perçus face à la maladie,

symptômes, diagnostics et conséquences) (Aday, Andersen, 1974).

Le modèle de Green et Kreuter adopté comme cadre conceptuel de cette étude (voir chapitre 3) comporte ces trois catégories dans une approche écologique plus globale avec des appellations de facteurs prédisposants, facteurs facilitants où sont inclus les facteurs déclenchants et facteurs de renforcement où sont inclus les facteurs de capacité ou de réalisation de Aday et Andersen.

En effet, la perception d'un besoin de santé constitue le moteur du processus pouvant conduire à l'utilisation d'un service de santé. Pour qu'il y ait passage à l'acte, d'autres facteurs doivent être présents chez le malade et son entourage. Tout d'abord les facteurs prédisposants qui incitent à l'utilisation puis les facteurs de réalisation qui permettent l'utilisation. Ces facteurs sont reliés plus spécifiquement à l'accessibilité géographique et économique. De plus, les facteurs déclenchants selon Grignon et Naudin (2002) réunissent les besoins perçus et exprimés face à la maladie à l'évaluation experte des symptômes, des diagnostics et des conséquences établis par des experts.

Les trois facteurs prédisposants, de capacité et déclenchants réunis ensemble doivent rencontrer une offre adéquate dépendante des spécialistes en santé, du volume du service de santé, du nombre de lits d'hospitalisation… disponible pour une population vivant dans un espace donné.

## 1.3. Justice sociale et équité

L'espérance de vie a augmenté dans le monde au cours de la seconde moitié du XXe siècle, mais de fortes inégalités face à la mort, à la maladie, au handicap et à l'accès aux soins sont toujours présentes. Les causes des inégalités sont multiples et traversent l'ensemble du corps

social. Ainsi pouvoir bénéficier d'un logement décent, avoir accès à un emploi satisfaisant et suffisamment rémunéré, vivre dans un environnement de qualité, profiter d'une meilleure éducation sont des facteurs déterminants d'une bonne santé au côté de la qualité des soins offerts et de l'obtention d'une réelle égalité d'accès aux soins.

Certaines disparités en santé pourront être attendues, légitimes comme une plus grande consommation de soins pour les personnes âgées ou un meilleur état de santé des plus jeunes. A l'inverse, certaines disparités telles qu'un moindre accès aux soins en zone rurale ou un renoncement aux soins pour des motifs économiques ou pour une disparité de l'offre de soins sont jugées inacceptables (Rochaix, Tubeuf, 2009). Ces quelques exemples montrent que le problème des inégalités de santé ne peut s'envisager que si deux questions sont posées au préalable. Sont-elles évitables ? Sont-elles tolérables ? Ces questions font basculer la réflexion du champ des inégalités à celui de l'équité et de la justice sociale.

### 1.3.1. Justice sociale

La justice sociale peut se définir de manière négative, et donc est injuste ce qui n'est pas acceptable socialement. C'est aussi une notion qui évolue dans le temps, ce qui est juste socialement peut devenir injuste si le contexte change. C'est essentiellement une projection vers une société plus juste, ce n'est pas réellement une fin en soi, il y a toujours des injustices. Elle peut être perçue soit comme une utopie, soit comme une démarche progressive (Braveman, Gruskin, 2003). Les actions ayant pour objectif la justice sociale visent à donner à chacun les mêmes chances de réussite, d'où il s'agit du principe d'« égalité des chances ». Les corrections nécessaires peuvent être sociales, financières ou culturelles. John Rawls en 1971, considère qu'une société est juste si elle

respecte trois principes dans l'ordre, la garantie des libertés de base pour tous, l'égalité « équitable » des chances et le maintien des seules inégalités qui profitent aux plus défavorisés (IRDES, 2014).

### 1.3.2. Equité verticale et équité horizontale

L'équité se mesure en effet en considérant un jugement de valeur selon lequel une inégalité sera qualifiée de juste ou d'injuste. L'OMS définit l'équité comme « l'absence de différences systématiques et potentiellement évitables pour un ou plusieurs aspects de la santé de sous-groupes de populations définis socialement, économiquement, démographiquement ou géographiquement ». Dans le champ des systèmes de santé, les modalités concrètes de financement et de l'accès aux soins reflètent l'importance attachée au principe d'équité. Les systèmes de santé partagent certes des objectifs à caractère égalitariste, mais ils les mettent en œuvre sous des formes diverses soit un égalitariste de type bismarckien ou un égalitariste de type bévéridgien, définis dans le chapitre suivant. En conséquence, les règles de financement d'une part, et d'accès aux soins d'autre part sont déconnectées, chacune pouvant jouer un rôle dans la recherche d'une plus grande équité. Cette déconnexion est appliquée par les concepts d'équité verticale et d'équité horizontale définis par Aristote (Rochaix, Tubeuf, 2009).

L'équité verticale requiert que les inégaux soient traités inégalement. Si les individus diffèrent selon leur propension à payer, le respect de l'équité verticale suggère que les plus riches contribuent davantage que les plus pauvres. De manière générale, si les individus diffèrent au titre de toute autre caractéristique individuelle jugée pertinente dans l'allocation des soins de santé, un système de santé « verticalement équitable » veillera alors à ce que les individus soient traités différemment au titre de cette

caractéristique. En France, la couverture maladie universelle illustre un objectif d'équité verticale dans la propension à payer en favorisant l'accès et le recours aux soins d'une classe de la population ayant de plus faibles moyens financiers (Benattar, 2012).

L'équité horizontale correspond au principe de justice distributive selon lequel des individus égaux doivent être traités également. Ce principe stipule donc en matière de santé que des individus qui présentent des caractéristiques similaires en termes d'état de santé ou de pathologies reçoivent des prestations de soins similaires et que toute discrimination en fonction d'une autre caractéristique individuelle, quelle qu'elle soit, ne peut être tolérée (Benattar, 2012).

Le terme équitable a alors une dimension éthique. Il désigne les inégalités qui sont à la fois évitables et injustes. Par conséquent, avant d'affirmer qu'une situation est inéquitable, il faut étudier la cause et déterminer qu'elle est injuste par rapport à la situation dans le reste de la société (Braveman, Gruskin, 2003).

# Chapitre 2
# Systèmes de santé et recours aux soins

## 2.1. Systèmes de santé dans le monde

Depuis des décennies, la crise des systèmes de santé fait l'objet de débats dans tous les pays. Tout le monde convient que les systèmes de santé sont en crise, à des degrés divers certes. Ils sont classés en fonction de leur organisation suivant une inspiration libérale bévéridgienne, ou bismarckienne.

En effet, aucun système n'est parfaitement libéral ou planifié. Un système de santé libéral serait caractérisé par des consommateurs assurés auprès de compagnies d'assurance privées en versant des primes en fonction des risques, des biens et services médicaux vendus sur des marchés concurrentiels, des prix formés librement, et des offreurs guidés par la recherche du profit. Ce système reste loin de la justice sociale et de l'égalité devant la maladie et se caractérise par un niveau élevé des prix. Le système de santé américain est l'un des plus libéraux au monde (Azar, 2000).

A l'opposé, un système de santé centralisé serait caractérisé par des consommateurs délégant les décisions à l'État. Celui-ci gère et planifie l'offre, détermine les capacités de production et assure le financement par l'impôt (Azar, 2000).

Le système bévéridgien est celui des pays du nord et du sud de l'Europe. Il repose sur le principe d'un accès universel au système de soins sans lien avec la notion de

travail. C’est donc la puissance publique qui assure le financement de ce système par voie fiscale et non par des cotisations sociales. C’est un système de solidarité nationale ayant pour principes l’universalité, l’unité et l’uniformité.

Le système bismarckien est le système d’assurance sociale du centre de l’Europe où les droits sociaux sont liés à l’activité professionnelle, et géré à parité par les partenaires sociaux responsables. Les usagers de ce système bénéficient d’une quadruple liberté : liberté du choix du producteur de soins, liberté de s’adresser à des spécialistes ou généralistes sans que la demande ne doive être médiatisée par un offreur primaire spécifique, liberté de s’adresser à plusieurs producteurs, et liberté de choix de l’établissement de soins (Vie publique, 2014).

## 2.2. Système de santé au Liban

La santé au Liban fait partie de l’éventail de services auxquels le citoyen devrait normalement avoir droit, mais ne peut y accéder compte tenu des structures du système. La gestion de la maladie au Liban reste principalement du ressort de l’individu et du secteur privé, aussi bien pour la prestation des services de santé que pour leur financement. Certes, l’État intervient dans ce domaine, mais son action directe a toujours été insuffisante et liée aux besoins des personnes défavorisées. Elle s’est d’ailleurs profondément transformée au cours des années de crise (Melki, 2000).

Après l'indépendance en 1943, le Liban construit une disposition de la santé publique, sous la rubrique des programmes nationaux de développement social. L'État a construit un réseau de district et des hôpitaux ruraux qui opérait au sein d'un système de référence, mais axé sur le service des défavorisés. Les patients ont été tenus de prouver des difficultés pour l’accès aux soins.

La guerre au Liban de 1975 à 1990 a consolidé la fourniture de l'aide sociale par des groupes sectaires et a permis la croissance illimitée de services de santé privés. Durant cette période, le pourcentage de lits d'hôpitaux publics a chuté de 26% à 10% et plus de 50% de la capacité en lits de l'hôpital privé a été concentrée dans les coûts élevés des soins curatifs. Après la guerre, le secteur public a continué à jouer un rôle minime dans la prestation directe de services de santé. Actuellement, le système de santé est décrit par de nombreux auteurs comme étant très fragmenté et pluraliste. Le secteur public a été longtemps absent en raison de la guerre au Liban. Depuis, le MSP a effectué de nombreuses réalisations. En 1998, les dépenses directes des ménages, représentant 60% des dépenses de santé totales, constituaient un obstacle important pour les personnes à faible revenu. Dès lors, une série de réformes a été mise en place par le ministère afin d'améliorer l'équité et l'efficience (Chen, Cammett, 2012).

Les composantes clés de cette réforme ont été : la réorganisation du réseau des soins primaires du secteur public, l'amélioration de la qualité des hôpitaux publics et de l'utilisation rationnelle des technologies médicales et des médicaments. Ce dernier point comprenait l'augmentation de l'utilisation de médicaments génériques de qualité assurée. Le MSP a aussi cherché à renforcer son leadership et ses fonctions de gouvernance. L'amélioration de la qualité des services dans le secteur public a donné lieu à une augmentation de l'utilisation, en particulier chez les pauvres. Le ministère de Santé publique (MSP) en 2013 a pris à sa charge 1 600 000 Libanais. Le budget total payé était de 420 milliards livres libanaises distribuées entre les hospitalisations du secteur privé, celles du secteur public, les médicaments et d'autres

dépenses[1]. Aujourd'hui, les deux secteurs publics et privés sont les acteurs clés au sein du système de santé libanais, mais leurs efforts non coordonnés fragmentent les services de ce système. Tandis que le secteur privé a une prédominance significative, les deux secteurs financent et fournissent des services de santé en l'absence d'une stratégie nationale en santé (Zakia, 2008).

## 2.3. Impact de la guerre en Syrie sur les services de soins libanais

Ajoutons aux difficultés et obstacles envahissant le système de santé au Liban, l'arrivée des réfugiés syriens qui perturbe davantage le secteur des services sociaux et sanitaires publics déjà fragilisé, alors même que les tensions sociales s'intensifient entre réfugiés et Libanais. La hausse de la demande de services de santé générée par le conflit syrien grève le système de santé libanais. Les retombées du conflit syrien sur le système de santé libanais se manifestent par une demande accrue des services de santé, une accumulation des impayés du ministère de Santé publique auprès des hôpitaux sous contrat, un déficit de professionnels de la santé comme les médecins spécialistes et les infirmiers, une flambée des maladies transmissibles et l'apparition de nouvelles maladies.

Ainsi, la demande des services de santé s'est intensifiée. Cette forte demande de soins hospitaliers crée des encombrements dans les hôpitaux et entrave l'accès aux soins, avec pour conséquences une pression financière sur le secteur hospitalier, le renchérissement des coûts et des pénuries de médicaments (World Bank, 2013).

---

[1] Données obtenues par l'entretien avec Dr. Joseph Hanna El Helou, directeur des soins médicaux au MSP, réalisé le 3/11/2014).

D'ailleurs le bulletin statistique 2013 du ministère détaille les chiffres correspondant aux deux populations bénéficiaires des soins au Liban : libanaise et syrienne par caza.

## 2.4. Financement du système de santé libanais

Le financement du système de santé libanais se présente selon trois modalités principales : publique ou fiscalisée, privée et parapublique ou socialisé (Azar, 2000). Les dépenses publiques en matière de santé c'est-à-dire celles relevant du budget de l'État émanent de plusieurs ministères et organismes autonomes : les ministères, de la Santé, de la Défense, de l'Intérieur et des Affaires sociales et la Mutuelle des fonctionnaires. L'État participe aussi au financement des prestations maladie et maternité de la CNSS.

Le financement privé des dépenses de santé se fait soit directement par les ménages, soit indirectement par l'intermédiaire de contrats avec des compagnies d'assurance privées, considérées être en 2010 au nombre de cinquante-deux compagnies. Ses primes souscrites sur le marché libanais sont estimées à 1,2 milliard de dollars. Le financement parapublic se fait essentiellement à travers la CNSS (Université Saint-Joseph [USJ], OMS, MSP, 2012). Cette modalité de couverture sociale sera développée dans ce qui suivra.

## 2.5. Protection sociale au Liban

Dans les pays en développement, le modèle de protection sociale est mis en place pendant les périodes de gouvernance coloniale. Le système de protection sociale au Liban est effectivement mis en place pendant la période du mandat français. Les contours de la politique familiale se sont dessinés au début des années 1940 et n'ont pas

connu de changements majeurs depuis à l'exception de l'introduction de mesures fiscales en 1959 (Azar, 2015). Historiquement, pour la plupart des mesures, le système de protection sociale couvre exclusivement les salariés. Son étendue reste assez limitée en ignorant une grande partie de la population notamment les travailleurs Libanais, les chômeurs et les personnes non actives.

### 2.5.1. Formes de protection sociale

Deux formes de protection sociale sont assurées aujourd'hui au Liban. L'une est institutionnelle, réservée principalement aux salariés pour une partie de leurs besoins sociaux, l'autre informelle et revêt essentiellement un caractère d'assistance, souple et précaire. Ces deux formes s'appuient sur plusieurs piliers. Les uns sont publics d'autres sont privés, et à l'intérieur de chaque catégorie plusieurs distinctions peuvent être effectuées. Ainsi pour les couvertures institutionnalisées, l'État est présent à côté d'organismes impliquant le secteur privé. L'action publique n'est pas concentrée dans une seule institution et plusieurs formules de protection existent. Même constat pour l'assistance informelle où l'on retrouve plusieurs organismes et structures publiques qui s'occupent de l'aide sociale, à côté d'une multitude de sources privées, les unes religieuses, les autres familiales, sans oublier les élans de générosité externes ou patronaux (Melki, 2000).

### 2.5.2. Caisse nationale de Sécurité sociale au Liban

Parmi les institutions de protection sociale formelle, figure le premier régime de protection sociale au Liban, institué en 1963, par la création de la Caisse nationale de Sécurité sociale (CNSS) couvrant les salariés du secteur privé, puis la mutuelle des fonctionnaires trois mois plus tard. Le contexte politique et social était alors

propice entre expansion économique avec de fortes inégalités sociales d'une part et le Chéhabisme, doté d'une doctrine sociale relativement progressiste d'autre part.

### *2.5.2.1. Système patriarcal et discrimination genrée*

C'est un régime imprégné par les valeurs du système patriarcal, marquant une sorte de discrimination genrée positive et négative reflétant le « modèle pro-traditionnel » et encourageant celui du « monsieur gagne-pain » à la différence près, avec certains pays occidentaux où ce modèle existe tel que l'Allemagne (Gautier, 1998 in Azar 2015), l'égalité homme/femme est loin d'être atteinte au niveau du droit familial rattaché au régime confessionnel libanais.

Le statut personnel relève des compétences des diverses juridictions religieuses que l'Etat s'engage à respecter : mariage, divorce, héritage... Le principe de l'égalité des femmes et des hommes est assez flou sinon inexistant chez certaines communautés à plusieurs niveaux : héritage par exemple chez les sunnites du Liban : 2/3 pour le garçon et 1/3 pour la fille (« Dieu vous recommande concernant vos enfants, le fils hérite comme deux filles » [sôurat An-Niçâ'/11], c'est toujours l'autorité paternelle et non parentale partagée qui est de mise malgré les avancées de ces derniers temps (Legal agenda, 2015).

Les références patriarcales déterminent les rapports de genre homme/femme au Liban à ce jour. Une inégalité dans les normes d'usage pour les uns et dans les normes juridiques pour les autres. Par exemple, dans certaines communautés, la femme est considérée comme mineure ayant besoin d'une protection permanente de l'homme.

Ces principes se traduisent dans le système de protection sociale en une sorte de discrimination positive envers les femmes au niveau de la couverture médicale telle que l'épouse au foyer, assimilée à un enfant à charge ainsi que la fille célibataire de moins de 25 ans étudiante

ou pas, sont couvertes alors que le garçon de plus de 18 ans et de moins de 25 ans ne pourra être couvert qu'en étant étudiant.

Néanmoins, dans les conditions requises pour une couverture médicale, une femme ne peut couvrir son mari à la CNSS s'il a moins de 60 ans que s'il a un handicap de plus de 50%. De plus, une discrimination négative envers les femmes travailleuses et les facilités qui leur permettent de concilier une vie familiale et une vie professionnelle en découlent également. Certains chiffres démontrent la sortie définitive du marché de l'emploi durant la période de maternité : le taux d'occupation professionnelle des femmes reflète le poids des contraintes familiales sur la vie professionnelle des femmes. Selon l'administration centrale de la statistique (2010), en 2009, il atteint sa valeur la plus élevée chez les femmes de 25 à 29 ans (47%) pour diminuer progressivement avec l'âge entre 30 et 34 ans (27%) et atteindre 23% entre 40 et 44 ans. Ce même taux est de 94% chez les hommes de la première tranche d'âge, 97% pour la deuxième et 97% pour la troisième. Parmi les femmes actives, 57% sont célibataires (contre 35% pour les hommes) (Azar, 2016).

#### *2.5.2.2. Couverture de la CNSS*

La couverture de la CNSS assure en 2012 environ 30% de la population libanaise soit 1 322 749 Libanais (cnss.gov.lb). Elle demeure la source d'assurance la plus importante au Liban (Kronfol, 2003). Elle touche les ouvriers et les salariés et leurs ayants droit du secteur privé, les ouvriers, les salariés et les retraités des institutions publiques et des offices autonomes non soumis au régime des fonctionnaires, les enseignants des écoles privées, les chauffeurs et les propriétaires de taxi, les employés et les employeurs du secteur de la boulangerie, les vendeurs de journaux, les médecins et les étudiants universitaires.

En effet, les protections offertes ne concernent que la couverture maladie/maternité (hospitalisation, médecine ambulatoire, médicaments, indemnité-décès), les allocations familiales et les indemnités de fin de service. Sont exclus le chômage, l'invalidité et même les accidents de travail qui sont à la charge de l'employeur, les prises en charge de plusieurs services notamment, les soins dentaires et l'ophtalmologie.

De plus, les salariés sont exclus de la couverture sanitaire dès qu'ils atteignent l'âge de la retraite, c'est-à-dire au moment où ils en ont le plus besoin. Par ailleurs, les tarifs appliqués par la CNSS sont souvent insuffisants et les salariés sont obligés de compenser eux-mêmes la différence.

Pour les indemnités de fin de service, le système se base uniquement sur une indemnité de capitalisation de fin de service et ne prévoit aucune autre forme de retraite par redistribution (Chamseddine, 2012). Un changement d'employeur en cours de carrière pourrait être pénalisant pour le calcul des droits du salarié en influençant le calcul de ses indemnités. En effet, le dernier salaire chez chaque employeur est pris en considération indépendamment s'il est inférieur ou supérieur à ce qui a précédé et une moyenne du tout devient la base du calcul.

Le financement de la CNSS, est assuré par des sources diverses : les cotisations supportées essentiellement par l'employeur, les revenus des fonds employés et les subventions exceptionnelles de l'État accordées en cas de catastrophe nationale entraînant un déficit de la caisse. La CNSS suppose une gestion paritaire à égalité entre État, employeurs et employés, mais dans les faits, les décisions sont totalement politisées et l'État reste le principal décideur (Kronfol, 2003).

Un travail sur dossiers des bénéficiaires sera fait dans cette recherche afin d'évaluer l'impact positif sur le

recours aux soins des bénéficiaires ainsi que sur le coût socio-économique restant à la charge des familles affiliées à la CNSS. Dans le cadre de cette enquête quantitative, la recherche visera uniquement la couverture maladie/maternité.

#### *2.5.2.3. Conditions pour bénéficier de la couverture maladie/maternité*

L'adhérent principal à la CNSS est appelé bénéficiaire. Chaque bénéficiaire peut avoir des ayants droit à sa charge. Le nombre total des bénéficiaires au 30 septembre 2014 est de 620 656 et le nombre des ayants droit est 787 429 personnes (CNSS, 2014).

L'affiliation des bénéficiaires s'effectue par le travail rémunéré. Ceux-ci peuvent faire partie de plusieurs catégories de métiers (voir tableau 2.1).

Au niveau de la CNSS au Liban, les ayants droit vivant sous le même toit du bénéficiaire et sont à sa charge peuvent être de trois catégories.

- L'épouse du bénéficiaire (masculin) à la CNSS si elle ne travaille pas. Le système de couverture est plutôt « Monsieur gagne-pain » (Azar, 2015), donc le nombre d'hommes bénéficiaires est dominant par rapport à celui des femmes. Quand il s'agit de plusieurs épouses, la CNSS couvre totalement la première épouse et couvre uniquement la deuxième au niveau maladie/maternité.

Concernant l'époux de la bénéficiaire femme, il faut qu'il ait atteint 60 ans et prouver qu'il ne travaille. S'il a moins de 60 ans, il doit prouver qu'il a un handicap physique ou mental l'empêchant d'assumer sa vie.

- Les enfants du bénéficiaire : pour les moins de 18 ans ; pour les filles de moins de 25 ans ; pour les garçons entre 18 et 25 ans s'ils sont uniquement des étudiants. La CNSS peut couvrir un maximum de 5 pour

les allocations familiales et tous les enfants en couverture médicale (maladie/maternité).

- Les parents du bénéficiaire : quand ils ont 60 ans et plus. S'ils ont moins de 60 ans, il faudra prouver sur expertise médicale qu'ils souffrent d'un handicap physique ou mental qui les empêche d'assumer leur vie. Une enquête sociale validera les conditions requises (CNSS, 2010).

***A ces conditions d'adhésion, s'ajoute le fait de :***

- Consulter des médecins ou institutions agréés auprès de la CNSS.
- Se procurer une ordonnance pour médicaments ou pour chaque acte médical à effectuer et les accords au préalable pour certains services : radiologie, échographie, imagerie par résonnance magnétique (IRM), scanner, examens de laboratoire et autres.
- Fournir une attestation de travail tous les trois mois.
- Présenter les factures dans un délai de six mois maximum de la date du recours aux soins.

***Institutions et professionnels de santé contractuels avec la CNSS***

Le nombre des institutions sanitaires et de spécialistes contractuels avec la CNSS au niveau national est de 17 146 au 30 septembre 2014 dont 148 hôpitaux, 11 345 médecins, 3 020 pharmaciens, 461 laboratoires d'analyses médicales, 248 centres de radiologie, etc. (voir Annexe 1).

Cette liste ne comporte pas la profession de psychologues, de nutritionnistes, d'orthophonistes alors que ce sont des métiers paramédicaux exercés en clinique privée ou dans des centres de consultations médicales en plus des institutions de santé. Par ailleurs, les soins à domicile ne sont pas couverts par la CNSS, ce qui oblige certains à prolonger leur séjour hospitalier pour couvrir les frais d'un traitement, de soins spécifiques qui peuvent être

réalisés par des soignants à domicile (pansement, injection, soins des plaies et escarres, gestion d'une thérapie…)

***Taux de remboursement maladie/maternité CNSS***

En se basant sur la tarification de la CNSS concernant les services maladie/maternité à rembourser, les taux de remboursement du recours aux soins sont les suivants :

- 80% pour les actes médicaux hors hospitalisation ;
- 90% des frais hospitaliers ;
- 95% du prix des médicaments du cancer dans/à l'extérieur de l'hôpital ;
- 100% du prix de la dialyse intra hôpital ;
- 100% des frais de l'accouchement effectué par un médecin ou une sage-femme.

Citons les statistiques disponibles au niveau national qui permettent de définir les catégories de bénéficiaires couverts, leurs ayants droit et leurs nombres correspondants.

**Tableau 2.1. Statistiques nationales bénéficiaires/type de travail au 30 septembre 2014**

| **Bénéficiaire** | **Nombre** |
|---|---|
| Employé | 459 048 |
| Chauffeur taxi propriétaire | 36 452 |
| Etudiant | 55 448 |
| Enseignant | 33 145 |
| Facultatif | 11 771 |
| Contractuels Etat | 10 447 |
| Médecin | 7 610 |
| Chauffeur employé | 3 661 |
| Maire | 2 069 |
| Boulangerie | 878 |
| Secteur maritime | 87 |
| Vendeur de journaux | 40 |
| **Total** | **620 656** |

**Tableau 2.2. Statistiques nationales des CNSS au 30 septembre 2014**

| Type de travail | Epoux/ épouse | Enfants | Père/Mère | Total |
|---|---|---|---|---|
| Employé | 165 004 | 375 748 | 93 336 | 64 088 |
| Chauffeur propriétaire | 31 156 | 52 693 | 10 022 | 93 871 |
| Enseignant | 2 654 | 16 250 | 5 954 | 24 858 |
| Facultatif | 6 978 | 4 650 | 1 397 | 13 025 |
| Médecin | 2 828 | 4 845 | 2 137 | 9 810 |
| Chauffeur employé | 1 850 | 4 282 | 208 | 6 340 |
| Maire | 1 543 | 1 800 | 447 | 3 790 |
| Boulangerie | 340 | 736 | 248 | 1 324 |
| Secteur maritime | 62 | 124 | 10 | 196 |
| Vendeur de journaux | 32 | 57 | 6 | 95 |
| Etudiant | 12 | 13 | 7 | 32 |
| **Total** | **212 459** | **461 198** | **113 772** | **787 429** |

**Source :** CNSS. 2014
https://www.cnss.gov.lb/index.php/statisctics/cnssstatprod

## 2.6. Infrastructures sanitaires au Liban

Les infrastructures sanitaires au Liban assurant les soins de santé primaires sont de deux types.

- **Les services ambulatoires** qui comptent 950 dispensaires et centres de santé primaires. Les dispensaires fonctionnent généralement avec des capacités humaines et physiques limitées et offrent des services restreints. Les centres de santé primaires offrent plus de services et s'impliquent dans des programmes de prévention, de planning familial et de soins prénataux. Cependant, le nombre de personnes fréquentant ces centres reste limité et

ne dépasse pas 20% de la population libanaise. Ces centres appartiennent soit à des organismes non gouvernementaux (ONG), soit au ministère de Santé publique (MSP), au ministère des Affaires sociales (MAS), ou aux municipalités. Quelques centres ont une gestion commune (Université Saint-Joseph [USJ], OMS, MSP, 2012).

- **Les institutions hospitalières** qui comprennent 150 institutions publiques et privées réparties sur l'ensemble du territoire libanais. Les hôpitaux publics sont aujourd'hui au nombre de 31, représentant un total de 2 550 lits. Ceci équivaut à 16,6% de la capacité totale des lits privés et publics fonctionnels. L'hôpital public fonctionne comme une institution semi-autonome responsable vis-à-vis d'un conseil d'administration nommé par le Conseil des ministres. Le secteur privé, comprenant 119 institutions, est le pilier du système de soins libanais. Il compte 12 148 lits. Ils sont majoritairement des hôpitaux généraux multidisciplinaires (Université Saint-Joseph [USJ], OMS, MSP, 2012).

L'acceptabilité des soins fait partie des facteurs entravant ou facilitant le recours aux soins des Libanais. Ceci amène obligatoirement à l'exploration des attitudes des patients et à l'étude des perceptions de la population et de leurs significations, comme des facteurs déterminant le comportement de recours aux soins. Cette étude est faite dans le cadre conceptuel adopté et détaillé dans le prochain chapitre.

# Chapitre 3
# Perception de la santé et cadre conceptuel

Dans cette étude, l'intérêt sera de comprendre les comportements des acteurs qui rentrent en jeu dans la problématique du recours aux soins dans un cadre conceptuel qui permet une vision de ce comportement en santé dans une optique de diagnostic, de planification et de promotion de la santé.

La perception ou l'autoévaluation de la santé constitue un indicateur important de l'état de santé de la population. Elle reflète l'appréciation globale que l'individu fait de son propre état de santé en intégrant ses connaissances et son expérience de la santé ou de la maladie (Levasseur, 1995). Parmi les éléments susceptibles d'expliquer le décalage entre état et perception de santé, divers processus de comparaison jouent un rôle décisif. En matière de santé comme dans d'autres domaines, l'individu définit moins sa situation dans l'absolu qu'en fonction de certains repères. Il peut notamment se comparer avec une autre personne se trouvant dans des circonstances analogues comme il peut également mettre en regard sa situation actuelle avec son sort à un autre moment de son parcours de vie (Henchoz, Cavalli, Girardin, 2008).

Levasseur (1995) mentionne plusieurs études montrant que la perception de l'état de santé est associée non seulement à la morbidité déclarée, sous forme de symptômes ou de maladies aiguës ou chroniques, mais également à la morbidité diagnostiquée. La perception de

l'état de santé a aussi été reliée aux mesures d'incapacité fonctionnelle et de limitation des activités. Au surplus, elle est reconnue comme étant un bon prédicteur de la mortalité (Levasseur, 1995).

## 3.1. Déterminants de l'autoévaluation de la santé

Outre les caractéristiques démographiques et socio-économiques, les comportements individuels, de même que le milieu social, l'utilisation des services de santé et la consommation de médicaments sont aussi associés à la perception de l'état de santé.

### 3.1.1. Âge, genre et milieu de vie

Etant donné que les problèmes physiques et la survenance des maladies ont tendance à augmenter avec l'âge, les perceptions moins positives de la santé sont attendues à un âge avancé. Cependant, lorsque l'état physique, les variables socio-économiques, les variables de comportement de santé et psychosociaux sont pris en considération, l'association entre l'état de santé perçue et l'âge disparaît. Ainsi, l'association entre l'âge et la perception de la santé ne serait pas directement attribuable à l'âge, mais à d'autres facteurs tels que le départ à la retraite et la solitude (Shields et Shooshtari, 2001).

Les femmes, malgré leur espérance de vie supérieure à celle des hommes, ont plus tendance que ceux-ci, à porter un jugement négatif sur leur santé. Les travaux de Shields et Shoostari (2001) et de Alexopoulos et Geitona (2009) montrent que les hommes se déclarent plus en bonne santé que les femmes. Cette mauvaise perception de l'état de santé par les femmes se révèle en lien avec le rôle joué par celles-ci dans la société, par lequel elles ressentent plus facilement la douleur et l'inconfort du fait de leur forte exposition aux services de santé par rapport aux hommes.

Concernant le milieu de vie, des résultats d'étude montrent que les individus vivant en milieu rural ont une meilleure santé perçue que ceux vivant en milieu urbain bien qu'en milieu rural la mortalité soit plus élevée (Grigorieve et Grigorieva, 2011).

### 3.1.2. Soutien social perçu, éducation, niveau socio-économique et mode de vie

La perception de la santé varie aussi selon le niveau de soutien social perçu. Les personnes se classant au niveau faible de l'indice de soutien social jugent plus négativement leur état de santé que les personnes qui se classent au niveau élevé (Guyon, 1988).

En effet, l'éducation contribue à améliorer l'état de santé en développant chez l'individu les habilités à rechercher le savoir, à comprendre les informations et à résoudre ses problèmes. L'éducation influence les styles de vie et les comportements de santé, grâce aux connaissances acquises, à la capacité à en acquérir d'autres et à travers les revenus élevés qu'elle permet d'acquérir (Guyon, 1988).

Plus le revenu est élevé, plus les gens déclarent avoir une excellente ou une très bonne santé. En revanche, les personnes qui font partie d'un ménage pauvre ou très pauvre sont beaucoup plus susceptibles de qualifier leur état de santé de moyen ou mauvais que les personnes provenant de ménages dont le revenu se classe au niveau moyen ou supérieur (Levasseur, 1995).

Le mode de vie au quotidien représente un facteur lié à la perception de l'état de santé des individus. Cependant, les contraintes économiques et sociales influencent les comportements en santé et imposent un ensemble de choix possibles. Les individus doivent alors choisir soit d'adopter des modes de vie favorables à la santé ou plutôt

des modes de vie défavorables à la santé (pratique du sport, consommation d'alcool…).

La perception de l'état de santé varie effectivement en fonction des comportements individuels tels que la pratique d'activités physiques durant les loisirs. C'est parmi les personnes dont la pratique de l'activité physique durant les loisirs est la plus fréquente (au moins trois fois par semaine) que se trouve la plus forte proportion d'individus qui déclarent avoir une excellente santé. Les moins actifs, c'est-à-dire ceux qui pratiquent des activités physiques une fois par mois ou moins, sont environ deux fois plus nombreux à qualifier leur santé de moyenne ou de mauvaise que les individus dont la pratique est plus fréquente (Guyon, 1988).

### 3.1.3. Evaluation de santé et promotion de la santé

L'évaluation de l'état de santé qui diffère d'un individu à un autre rappelle une fois de plus, l'existence d'inégalités en matière de santé. Si celles qui sont reliées à l'âge ne sont pas totalement évitables, d'autres le sont, du moins elles peuvent être atténuées par des actions qui relèvent principalement de la promotion de la santé.

L'autoévaluation de l'état de santé constitue un indicateur appréciable de l'état de santé de la population. Facile d'application, l'indicateur peut être utilisé autant au niveau national que régional et local comme instrument de surveillance de l'état général de santé des populations. Tout en permettant d'identifier les groupes de la population qui nécessitent une attention particulière, cet indicateur devient alors utile pour les interventions en santé publique et, en particulier, pour celles qui visent à mieux gérer l'utilisation et l'allocation des ressources.

Après avoir défini les concepts et présenté les facteurs influençant l'accès aux soins, il s'agit maintenant d'exposer le cadre de référence choisi pour guider la

construction de l'outil, analyser les données et élaborer une stratégie de promotion en santé.

## 3.2. Déterminants conceptuels

La problématique d'accès aux soins est composée de plusieurs facettes qu'il faudrait prendre en considération pour que cette étude ait un impact réel sur la santé et la qualité de vie des personnes concernées. Dans cette perspective, fut choisie la théorie du comportement planifié intégrée dans le modèle « PRECEDE/PROCEED », élaboré par Green et Kreuter comme cadre conceptuel de cette recherche afin de comprendre clairement la question du recours aux soins de santé chez la population libanaise ainsi que les facteurs influençant ce recours.

### 3.2.1. Modèle de Green et Kreuter

Le modèle « PRECEDE- PROCEED » est un modèle socio-écologique de planification de programmes de promotion de la santé. L'approche écologique propose une vision interactionniste, multifactorielle et socio-environnementale des problèmes psychosociaux. D'une part, elle porte son attention sur la relation réciproque entre l'individu et son environnement et, d'autre part, elle tient compte des interactions qui s'établissent entre les différents niveaux systémiques, ces dernières pouvant avoir une influence directe et indirecte sur la conduite de l'individu. Elle propose également d'intervenir simultanément sur plusieurs niveaux systémiques à la fois.

Le modèle de Green et Kreuter est basé sur les disciplines de l'épidémiologie, des sciences sociales, comportementales et de l'éducation. Les principes fondamentaux qui sont à l'origine de la construction de cette approche proviennent de la nature multifactorielle de toute problématique. Ce modèle aide à diagnostiquer,

planifier et évaluer toute action de promotion de la santé. Son but est alors d'expliquer les comportements vis-à-vis de la santé, et de concevoir et d'évaluer les interventions mises en œuvre pour influencer à la fois le comportement et les conditions de vie. L'acronyme « PRECEDE » signifie « Predisposing, Reinforcing and Enabling Constructs in Educational/Environment Diagnosis and Evaluation » - « facteurs prédisposants, facilitants et de renforcement identifiés par le diagnostic éducationnel et environnemental et évaluation de ce diagnostic » (Institut national de prévention et d'éducation pour la santé [inpes], 2014). L'acronyme « PROCEED » signifie « Policy, Regulatory and Organizational Contructs in Educational and Environmental Development » - « Politiques, réglementations et organisations dans le développement éducationnel et environnemental ». Ce modèle comprend neuf étapes divisées en deux parties. Les cinq premières étapes du modèle (PRECEDE) servent à faire un diagnostic de la situation afin de mieux saisir les facteurs qui déterminent l'état de santé ou ceux qui aboutissent aux problèmes de santé qui doivent être modifiés. Les quatre dernières étapes (PROCEED) servent à guider l'implantation et l'évaluation des programmes ou des politiques (Beaudry, Hamelin, 2006). Ce modèle permet de mettre en lumière la relation qui peut prévaloir entre les facteurs environnementaux et les comportements individuels (Green & Kreuter, 2005).

De ce modèle, sera retenu le diagnostic éducationnel et d'environnement, qui identifie les facteurs qui doivent être modifiés pour qu'un changement comportemental soit établi et maintenu. Ces facteurs seront classés en trois catégories : les facteurs prédisposants, les facteurs de renforcement et les facteurs facilitants.

### 3.2.2. Théorie du comportement planifié

Une théorie est une explication générale du comment les gens agissent ou non pour maintenir et promouvoir leur santé, celle de leurs familles et communauté. C'est un ensemble de concepts, définitions et propositions qui présente une vue systématique des situations en spécifiant les relations entre les variables pour expliquer ou prédire les évènements.

Le changement d'un comportement d'un individu, surtout en promotion de la santé, est caractérisé par la modification d'une action et d'une façon de se comporter. Lorsqu'un individu décide de changer son comportement, il suit une démarche de modification d'actions pour arriver à son but, celui de passer d'un comportement actuel non désiré au comportement souhaité.

Un certain nombre de théories issues de la psychologie sociale ont été élaborées et ont fait preuve d'efficacité concernant l'analyse des comportements sociaux. Elles expliquent pourquoi les individus adoptent ou non un comportement donné. La théorie du comportement planifié en fait partie.

En effet, la théorie de l'action raisonnée vise à prédire et par le fait même, à comprendre les comportements sociaux. La prédiction doit se faire par rapport à un comportement spécifique et volitif et dans une situation bien définie. Le déterminant immédiat d'un acte comportemental est l'intention de la personne de poser ou de ne pas poser l'action donnée. Ainsi l'intention d'une personne à adopter ou ne pas adopter un comportement est déterminée par son attitude à l'égard du comportement, et l'importance qu'elle accorde à l'opinion des gens qui lui sont proches, ceux-ci croient-ils qu'elle devrait ou ne devrait pas adopter le comportement en question.

Il a été déterminé que la théorie de l'action raisonnée est surtout valable pour les comportements qui sont sous le

contrôle volontaire. Il y a contrôle total lorsqu'il n'existe aucune contrainte à l'adoption d'un comportement, mais à l'inverse, il y aura un manque de contrôle si l'adoption de ce dernier nécessite opportunités, ressources et habiletés (Godin, 1991). D'où la théorie du comportement planifié proposée par Ajzen qui découle des précédents travaux qu'il a réalisés avec Fishben lors de l'élaboration de la théorie de l'action raisonnée. Ainsi cette théorie conserve les éléments de la théorie raisonnée tout en incluant le contrôle comportemental perçu par le sujet comme antécédent des intentions comportementales. Le modèle d'Ajzen part donc du principe que trois variables (l'attitude, les normes subjectives et la perception du contrôle) influencent directement les intentions d'effectuer un comportement. Cette intention influence à son tour le comportement (Godin, 1991).

A partir de cette classification, la théorie du comportement planifié sera combinée au modèle de PRECEDE/PROCEED dans un schéma afin de mieux comprendre et de pouvoir entamer un projet de promotion de santé dans le but d'améliorer l'état de santé et d'obtenir une meilleure qualité de vie.

## 3.3. Justification du choix du modèle du comportement planifié

Le choix de la théorie du comportement planifié pour comprendre les facteurs influençant le comportement est justifié par le fait que :

- l'intention de changer un comportement est influencée par l'entourage et par l'intention de la personne à agir selon cette influence ;
- l'adoption d'un comportement nécessite un degré de contrôle sur la situation. Le contexte de la recherche montre que plusieurs facteurs influencent ce contrôle tels

que les facteurs économiques : manque de moyen et absence de couverture ;

- le niveau de connaissance concernant l'utilité d'un recours aux soins joue un rôle dans la perception négative ou positive de ce recours.

## 3.4. Composantes du modèle de planification de Green et Kreuter

### 3.4.1. Facteurs prédisposants

Ils sont antérieurs au comportement, correspondent aux facteurs qui nourrissent le rationnel ou la motivation du comportement (Renaud & Zanurdi, 1998). Ils font référence aux connaissances individuelles et collectives, aux attitudes, aux croyances, aux valeurs, aux habiletés perçues et aux perceptions qui aident ou font obstacle à la motivation de changer un comportement (Green et Kreuter, 2005). L'utilisation des modèles psychosociaux de prédiction des comportements sont utiles pour la mesure de ces facteurs et celui du comportement planifié trouvera sa pertinence dans la dimension de la perception du contrôle.

Les facteurs prédisposants sont une combinaison de facteurs qui définissent la prédisposition à agir d'une certaine façon (Beaudry, Hamelin, 2006). Ces facteurs peuvent influencer le comportement de recours aux soins chez la population. D'où une présentation de ces facteurs (valeurs, connaissance, croyance) s'impose.

***Les valeurs*** correspondent aux principes qui orientent l'action d'un individu, d'un groupe ou d'une organisation en société. Les valeurs sont plus ancrées que les attitudes et les croyances. Elles sont aussi plus difficiles à changer surtout à court terme. Les attitudes sont souvent fondées sur des valeurs, mais aussi influencées par les croyances.

Cependant les croyances sont plus facilement modifiables que les valeurs.

***Une connaissance*** correspond à l'information factuelle et interprétative qui mène à la compréhension qui est utile pour entamer une action sur une base informée. C'est une condition nécessaire, mais habituellement insuffisante pour mener un changement de comportement individuel ou collectif.

La connaissance ou l'apprentissage cognitif peut découler de l'expérience, menant ainsi à des croyances qui, à la longue, se combinent et produisent des valeurs. Ajoutées aux influences sociales, elles mènent à leur tour à des attitudes.

***Une croyance*** est une conviction que quelque chose est vraie ou réelle. Diverses croyances définissent notre attitude envers le comportement en question. Elles reflètent aussi comment nous percevons autour de nous la norme sociale associée à ce comportement (il est plus ou moins acceptable dans notre environnement significatif) ou encore notre habileté (capacité) ou notre efficacité personnelle (ou perception du contrôle) à effectuer le comportement.

***Une attitude*** peut être définie comme un jugement, une évaluation envers une certaine catégorie d'objets, de personnes ou de situations. Elle peut prendre une forme « cognitive » ou « affective ».

La structure de l'attitude inclut toujours un élément d'évaluation (bon-mauvais, favorable-défavorable). Cette évaluation dépend des croyances qui la sous-tendent. L'attitude reste souvent une combinaison constante entre croyances, valeurs et intention.

L'attitude vis-à-vis du comportement est déterminée par la croyance qu'un résultat désiré est atteignable si un comportement particulier est maintenu et que ce résultat est bénéfique à sa santé (Zitouni, Ezzina, 2007). Il s'agit

en fait du jugement subjectif par rapport à un comportement et à ses conséquences ou résultats possibles, multiplié par l'évaluation que fait la personne de ces conséquences (Godin, 1991). En résumé, l'attitude d'une personne est le produit de

**« Croyance x Evaluation »** (Zitouni, Ezzina, 2007).

***Les normes subjectives*** sont reliées aux croyances de l'individu face à ce que les autres pensent qu'il/elle devrait faire (croyances normatives) et sa motivation de plaire à autrui (Zitouni, Ezzina, 2007). Dans la formation de la norme subjective, chaque croyance normative est pondérée par la motivation correspondante à s'y conformer. Le produit **« Croyances normatives x Motivation à se conformer »** représente la norme subjective de l'individu (Godin, 1991).

***Les habiletés*** existantes et les capacités auxquelles nous avons accès peuvent aussi prédisposer à adopter le comportement ou à le faciliter. Elles augmentent le sentiment d'auto-efficacité (perception du contrôle), et vice-versa. Plus la perception du contrôle ou le sentiment d'auto-efficacité d'une personne est positif face à un comportement à adopter, plus elle sera prédisposée à l'adopter.

**Le contrôle comportemental perçu** correspond à la facilité ou la difficulté perçue pour réaliser un comportement (Azjen, 1991). Il renvoie également à la perception qu'une personne de sa capacité à effectuer ou non le comportement en question. C'est le produit : **« Croyance de contrôle x facilitations perçues ».**

### 3.4.2. Facteurs facilitants

Ce sont des facteurs également antérieurs au comportement. Ils facilitent la réalisation d'une action motivée (Renaud, Zarnudio, 1998). Ils correspondent aux habiletés, aux ressources, aux barrières qui aident ou

nuisent aux changements comportementaux ou environnementaux.

Les facteurs facilitants incluent l'ensemble des facteurs qui rendent possible le changement de comportement ou de l'environnement. Ces facteurs incluent la disponibilité et l'accessibilité tant physique que financière des ressources personnelles et communautaires nécessaires à l'individu pour qu'il adopte le comportement visé. Ils font partie de l'environnement physique. Dans certaines communautés, une décision d'agir d'emblée sur l'environnement et donc directement sur les facteurs « facilitants » est prise après avoir examiné les motivations au comportement à adopter. C'est le cas lorsque le contrôle est objectivement hors de la portée des individus (Beaudry, Hamelin, 2006).

### 3.4.3. Facteurs de renforcement

Ces facteurs sont subséquents et postérieurs aux comportements. Ils sont la récompense ou l'incitatif à l'adoption du comportement et contribuent à son maintien, à sa répétition ou à son élimination (Renaud et Zarnurdio, 1998). Ils sont constitués des renforcements positifs ou négatifs provenant de l'entourage de la personne qui adopte le comportement. Ils peuvent l'encourager ou le décourager (Green et Kreuter, 1991). Le renforcement devra donc venir de personnes significatives ou considérées comme étant importantes à leurs yeux (Beaudry, Hamelin, 2006).

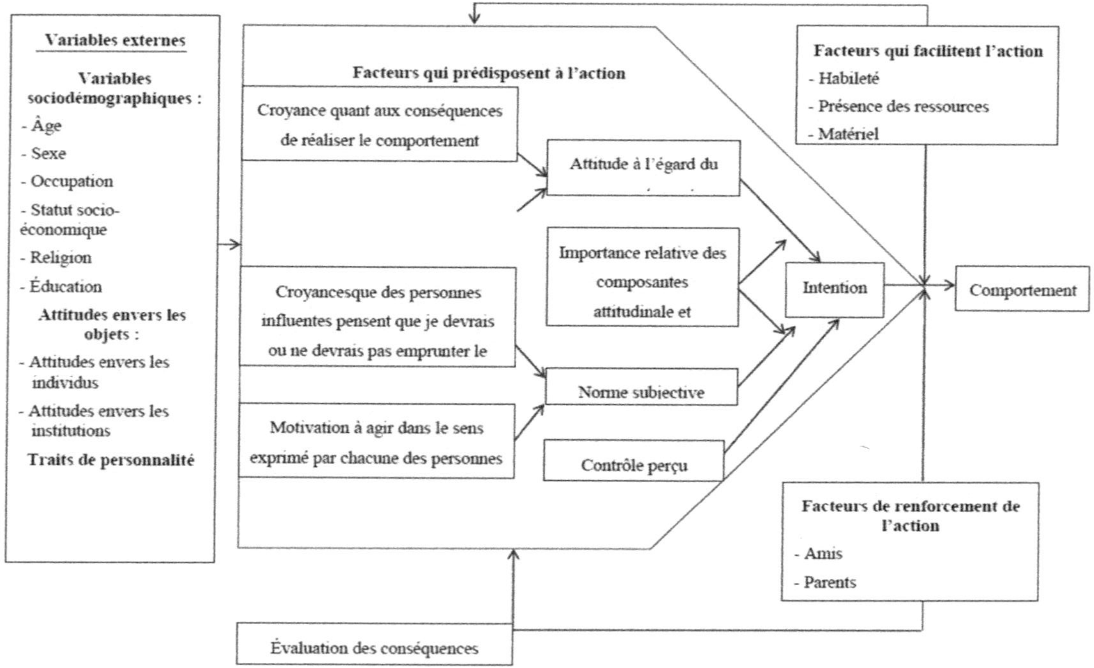


**Schéma du modèle de la théorie du comportement planifié et démarche de planification**

# Chapitre 4
# Méthodologie de la recherche

La méthodologie de cette recherche s'appuie sur une diversité d'approches essentiellement compréhensives de l'objet de recherche (Bourdieu, 1993). Elle comprendra une approche qualitative de type socioethnologique composée d'une observation de la réalité du recours aux soins et une exploration du comportement de ce recours chez la population libanaise. Elle a également recours à une approche quantitative à travers l'étude des dossiers des adhérents de la Caisse nationale de Sécurité sociale (CNSS) libanaise.

C'est l'étape d'exploration d'une recherche-action dans la mesure où elle permet l'étude d'une situation donnée et débouche sur des recommandations et des stratégies d'actions concrètes en Promotion de la santé. Il s'agit de mettre à l'épreuve une conception particulière du processus de connaissance et son objet est défini en fonction d'une expérience, d'un problème concret vécu par des acteurs notamment le recours aux soins au Liban. Le rôle du chercheur sera de favoriser la prise de conscience de ce problème et d'aider les individus et les groupes à le solutionner par une action collective (Mayer et al., 2000).

Cette démarche méthodologique est adoptée en fonction du choix et des objectifs du sujet de la recherche « Recours aux soins et couverture médicale ».

Trois étudiantes en master 2 de Santé publique option Education et promotion de la santé ont contribué avec le

chercheur principal à l'étude qualitative dans toutes ses étapes. L'une des étudiantes est assistante de service social et les deux autres sont infirmières. Elle s'est déroulée sur le terrain du mois de mars 2014 à décembre 2014.

## 4.1. Choix du sujet

Il n'existe pas d'études spécifiques autour de la question de l'accès aux soins au Liban en général. Des études épidémiologiques sont retrouvées sur la question de l'obésité ou du tabagisme (Salameh et Barbour, 2007, 2011), mais il n'existe pas à ce jour au Liban, à l'instar d'autres pays, des données de base obtenues par observation systématique des inégalités en santé.

Néanmoins, des études épidémiologiques similaires sont menées depuis les années quatre-vingts dans des pays développés tels que la France où des enquêtes nationales de l'Institut de recherche et de documentation en économie de la santé (IRDES) telles que l'Enquête santé protection sociale (ESPS) et l'Echantillon permanent d'assurés sociaux (EPAS) actualisent régulièrement ces données afin que les chercheurs puissent analyser la causalité et les composantes des inégalités sociales en santé (Bazin et al., 2006). Des études en épidémiologie et en économie de santé sont également financées en priorité par les Etats pour entretenir des bases de données permanentes.

L'accès et le recours aux soins sont cruciaux pour un bon état de santé et des conditions sanitaires équitables. Viser à produire des données qualitatives et quantitatives pertinentes permet d'explorer les déterminants sociaux de la santé au Liban.

Cette exploration pourrait servir à faire ressortir les indicateurs conceptuels nécessaires à faire valoir la mise en place des études épidémiologiques, socio-économiques, sociologiques, psychosociologiques et environnementales

à un niveau national et étatique afin de produire des données de base spécifiques sur les inégalités en santé. Elle cherche à se placer dans la mouvance internationale de la commission des déterminants sociaux des inégalités sanitaires de l'OMS qui préconise dans son rapport de 2009 de promouvoir des études de ce genre afin de favoriser la dynamique de l'action de recherche et de promotion de l'équité en santé.

La problématique des inégalités du recours aux soins interpelle tous les acteurs de santé publique indépendamment de leur formation, de leur discipline ou de leur champ d'expertise. Une prise de conscience de l'ampleur des disparités qui existent entre les groupes sociaux au Liban s'impose sachant que 45,6% de la population libanaise ne bénéficient d'aucune couverture sociale (Kronfol, 2003).

Le choix du sujet comporte aussi une dimension citoyenne chère au cœur de tout agent de santé et cela ne doit pas être minimisé. Pour ces raisons, le choix fut d'entreprendre une première étude des mécanismes en cause dans la construction des inégalités du recours aux soins chez la population libanaise, analyser les stratégies, réfléchir aux rôles de chacun dans la réduction de ces inégalités afin de permettre aux Libanais d'accéder au niveau de santé le plus élevé étant affirmé comme droit fondamental de tout être humain par la déclaration d'Alma Ata en 1978 (OMS, 1978). En effet, cette perspective se situe dans les recommandations internationales sur les soins en santé primaire et la stratégie de « santé pour tous » de cette déclaration, de la promotion de la santé dans la charte d'Ottawa (1986) ainsi que dans toutes celles visant la réflexion sur la place et la priorité de la santé dans la vie.

## 4.2. Objectifs de l'étude

### 4.2.1. Objectif général

Cette étude vise à définir les facteurs déterminant le comportement de recours ou de non-recours aux soins des individus au Liban face aux épisodes de maladies.

### 4 .2.2. Objectifs spécifiques

Les objectifs spécifiques se résument comme suit.

- Identifier la pratique et les connaissances des individus à avoir recours aux soins et l'utilisation des services de santé.
- Identifier l'impact de l'accessibilité géographique et de l'accessibilité économique sur l'utilisation des services de santé et le recours aux soins.
- Identifier la perception d'un besoin en santé et les facteurs socio-culturels qui peuvent déterminer le comportement d'un recours aux soins.
- Identifier l'influence des valeurs et des croyances concernant la santé et la perception du public des maladies sur les attitudes et les comportements en santé.
- Etudier l'impact du recours aux soins quand il y a une couverture médicale chez les adhérents de la CNSS : fréquence des recours observés, normes de couverture existantes en lien avec les valeurs et les références sociétales patriarcales, coût socio-économique pour les ménages…

## 4.3. Délimitation du champ de l'étude qualitative

Le thème du recours aux soins chez la population libanaise implique une étude des facteurs déterminant l'accès et le recours aux soins de cette population, question étendue sur tout le territoire libanais, donc il a fallu délimiter le champ de cette étude. Il s'agit

d'identifier les perceptions, les attitudes et les facteurs d'influence du recours aux soins. Cette étude est du type ethnographique donc l'observation et les autres sources de données jouent un rôle important et aident les chercheurs à comprendre une culture (Loiselle et Profetto-McGrath, 2007).

La recherche est donc menée dans des institutions de santé des Casas (districts) du Kesrouan, du Metn et de Beyrouth. A la suite de la première phase exploratoire, détaillée ultérieurement, la décision est prise d'élargir le champ de cette étude et d'intégrer de nouveaux établissements sanitaires. L'observation s'est alors déroulée dans un hôpital public, un hôpital privé et deux dispensaires au Kesrouan ; un hôpital privé et deux dispensaires au Metn ; un hôpital public à Beyrouth.

## 4.4. Critères d'inclusion de la population cible

### 4.4.1. Population participante à l'étude qualitative

L'échantillon de cette étude est non probabiliste et accidentel. Il repose toutefois sur un échantillonnage par critères d'admissibilité correspondant le mieux aux besoins en matière d'information (Loiselle et Profetto-McGrath, 2007).

La procédure de sélection de la population participante à l'étude qualitative s'est basée sur des critères d'inclusion et d'exclusion. Les **critères d'inclusion** de cette population, rencontrée et interviewée au sein des dispensaires et des hôpitaux publics et privés sont :

- ayant la nationalité libanaise ;
- âgés de plus de 18 ans ;
- bénéficiant d'une assurance privée, de la CNSS ou ne bénéficiant d'aucune couverture ;

- conscients, non atteints de maladies psychiques, de maladies graves ou en phase terminale, non admis à l'hôpital pour un accident ;
- disponibles pour la réalisation de l'entretien le jour même de leur venue, avant ou après la consultation médicale pour les interviewés dans les dispensaires et après leur admission hospitalière pour les interviewés dans les hôpitaux.

Un seul critère **d'exclusion** était établi et il concernait les bénéficiaires non civils de la protection sociale.

### 4.4.2. Population cible de l'enquête quantitative

Le travail d'enquête sur dossier au niveau de la Caisse nationale de Sécurité sociale a nécessité un accord au préalable au niveau de la direction supérieure de la Caisse par rapport à l'objectif de l'enquête et les engagements éthiques et scientifiques du chercheur.

Le terrain choisi de l'enquête est le centre du casa du Kesrouan, un casa qui compte 168 460 Libanais en 2013 et 6 321 réfugiés syriens. Il y a eu 1 330 naissances en 2013 et l'espérance de vie pour les Libanais en 2013 se situe autour de 81 ans.

Les tranches d'âge de la population dans Kesrouan sont de 11 624 enfants de 0-4 ans, 29 817 de 5-14 ans, 32 934 de 15-24 ans, 21 782 de 35-44 ans, 12 634 de 55-64 ans et 16 341 de plus de 65 ans (Statistical Bulletin MOPH, 2013).

Le directeur général de la CNSS donne un accord enthousiaste pour cette étude et pour le site demandé dans le Kesrouan. Il y a eu de la réserve émise de la part du comité médical qui a été rassuré par l'engagement académique du chercheur autour de l'anonymat et de la confidentialité des informations.

Les dossiers des adhérents sont informatisés depuis 2009. Le logiciel permet de saisir les actes médicaux et ne

donne qu'une notion floue des accords pour hospitalisation. Tout ce qui concerne les hospitalisations est inaccessible au niveau des dossiers. Les dossiers correspondants sont encore sur papier et sont stockés dans les archives.

Au départ de cette recherche, on avait projeté d'avoir recours à l'étude de 50 dossiers d'adhérents de la CNSS d'une part ; de constituer un carnet de santé et de le distribuer sur une cinquantaine de ménages d'autre part. Ceux-ci auront à remplir sur ce carnet chaque acte médical au cours d'une année pour pouvoir évaluer sur l'année les circonstances du recours aux soins et de la consommation médicale.

Le projet du carnet de santé était difficile à mettre en place à tous les niveaux. Il fallait suivre de près le remplissage des ménages or les possibilités du chercheur ne permettaient pas de le faire étant donné les ajouts en cours de travail de techniques par nécessité de pertinence et de fiabilité de la recherche entreprise (plusieurs sites d'observation, entretiens…).

Cependant, un travail d'évaluation des parcours sur la base de carnets de santé remplis par les ménages à court et moyen terme mériterait une étude spécifique pour obtenir des résultats fiables et valides.

Suite à cela, une décision de faire passer le nombre de travail sur dossiers des adhérents de la CNSS de 50 à 100 dossiers est prise pour permettre une meilleure visibilité de la fréquence du recours de personnes couvertes ainsi que du coût socio-économique de la santé laissé à la charge des ménages. Donc les hypothèses posées pour ce travail d'exploration sont les suivantes :

- une couverture médicale réduit les barrières du recours aux soins ;
- une couverture médicale motive un meilleur contrôle sur sa santé en consultant un professionnel de santé ;

- le recours aux soins est fréquent chez les bénéficiaires CNSS ;
- une priorité est donnée par âge et par type de maladie malgré le coût socio-économique correspondant ;
- le coût des soins laissé à la charge des familles est lourd pour le budget moyen des familles adhérentes.

***Travail exploratoire des dossiers***

Le travail exploratoire des dossiers et des possibilités de l'enquête dans le temps imparti a permis de définir des critères d'inclusion de la population cible de l'enquête.

En effet, le délai de traitement des dossiers entre dépôt et remboursement est de trois mois. Pas de sélection automatique possible au niveau du logiciel donc l'aide des employés de la CNSS est sollicitée afin de mettre en place une liste accidentelle avec critères de période de soins allant de 2012 à fin juin 2015. Donc l'échantillon accidentel se basait sur des ***critères retenus***.

- Nombre pris = 102 dossiers.
- Période de recours aux soins remboursés : de janvier 2012 jusqu'à fin juin 2015.
- Pas de critères de genre, car le nombre de bénéficiaires principaux est à majorité d'hommes.
- Un codage est fait et un code est attribué à chaque dossier dans un souci de confidentialité et d'anonymat.

En parallèle, le chercheur a tenu un cahier de notes pour les remarques importantes concernant les dossiers, les pratiques, les procédures et les décisions prises…

## 4.5. Techniques d'enquête

Il s'agit d'une exploration du domaine de l'étude et du choix des techniques d'enquête utilisées pour approfondir cette recherche. Elle comporte les méthodes adoptées :

Recherche documentaire, observation et entretiens semi-directifs, Enquête par questionnaire CNSS.

### 4.5.1. Recherche documentaire

Au début de cette étude, puis tout au long du travail effectué, une recherche documentaire est effectué sur plusieurs bases de données que celles-ci soient médicales, issues de sciences sociales ou générales. Les ouvrages abordant cette thématique ne sont pas faciles à trouver. Cependant, quelques-uns, retrouvés à « la Bibliothèque nationale de François Mitterrand » et la bibliothèque des Sciences Sociales en France, à la bibliothèque de plusieurs universités privées (Balamand, Usek) et de l'Université libanaise (Faculté de Droit – Faculté de Santé publique – Institut de Sciences sociales) ont été utilisés comme moyens de réflexion. Une recherche dans les bases de données électroniques et à partir des portails électroniques des revues scientifiques (CINAHL – EBSCO ; cairn.info ; persee.fr…) a été également possible au sein des bibliothèques citées ; les articles et ouvrages pertinents ont été retenus. En parallèle deux entretiens exploratoires ont été menés l'un auprès d'une assistante médico-sociale employée à la CNSS du Kesrouan, l'autre auprès du directeur des soins médicaux au MSP, pour combler le manque en informations.

### 4.5.2. Méthodes de recueil de données et déroulement de la collecte des données de l'étude qualitative

L'enquête de terrain s'est déroulée sur environ trois mois, entre juin et août 2014, réalisée sur la base d'observations et d'entretiens semi-directifs. Deux méthodes de recueil de données ont été utilisées : une observation directe et une enquête terrain basée sur la méthode de l'entretien semi-directif.

Une observation des interactions était rendue possible grâce à des observations directes de type ethnologique effectuées dans les salles d'urgence des hôpitaux et les salles d'attente des dispensaires. Des notes étaient prises, des discussions étaient entamées avec les patients. La transcription du journal de bord se faisait le jour même. En parallèle, les entretiens ont été effectués.

### *4.5.2.1. Observation directe*

Il s'agit d'une observation de type ethnologique qui s'est déroulée dans les cazas du Kesrouan et du Metn comme champ géographique de la recherche. Il était important de démarrer une observation sur place parmi les personnes bénéficiaires des services de soins, de s'adapter au milieu et d'observer le déroulement ordinaire des événements.

L'observation s'est réalisée en plusieurs étapes. Dans un premier temps, une collecte de données est faite dans un hôpital public, un hôpital privé et un dispensaire de chaque caza implantés dans des zones rurales et urbaines, afin de rencontrer des personnes de différentes catégories sociodémographiques et culturelles. Les informations concernant l'étude étaient communiquées aux directions des centres par écrit et une présentation orale a été faite durant un rendez-vous fixé par appel téléphonique.

Malgré un accord de principe, un hôpital public à Metn a refusé de collaborer, donc le choix s'est imposé de l'hôpital public le plus proche du caza, localisé à Beyrouth. De même, le dispensaire contacté dans la région du Kesrouan a refusé l'accueil des chercheures le premier jour de l'observation en disant : "غيرت رأيي ما بدّي وجعة راس". Alors, un autre dispensaire à proximité a été choisi.

La phase d'observation s'est accompagnée par la tenue d'un journal de bord. Le choix d'un hôpital et d'un dispensaire dans la zone rurale du Kesrouan était

nécessaire pour compléter l'échantillon de personnes participantes.

De plus, presque la majorité de la population rencontrée dans les différents établissements appartiennent à une même religion (religion chrétienne), donc le choix d'un autre dispensaire du Metn était fait pour découvrir différentes attitudes, croyances et connaissances d'une population de religion musulmane concernant le sujet de la recherche.

La phase observation s'est déroulée du 1er juin au 31 août 2014 étalée sur environ 50 heures. En parallèle, des entretiens semi-directifs ont été effectués pour enrichir l'étude exploratoire.

### *4.5.2.2. Entretiens semi-directifs*

Des entretiens semi-directifs sont menés auprès de cinquante-trois personnes libanaises, se présentant aux institutions sanitaires pour bénéficier des soins primaires. Les entretiens sont basés sur un guide élaboré suite à la recherche documentaire et la première phase d'exploration (Annexe 2 et 3). Comme le mentionnent Blanchet et Gotman (1992), la formalisation du guide est fonction de l'objet de l'étude (multidimensionalité), de l'usage de l'enquête et du type d'analyse que l'on projette d'en faire.

Il s'agit d'identifier les perceptions, les attitudes et les facteurs d'influence du recours à la santé. L'analyse du sens que les acteurs interviewés donnent à leur réalité, leurs pratiques en santé et aux événements auxquels ils sont confrontés permettra de faire ressortir les représentations sociales, leurs systèmes de valeurs, leurs repères normatifs, leurs lectures de leurs propres expériences (Quivy et Campenhoudt, 2006) et facilitera l'analyse des déterminants sociaux de santé qui influencent leur comportement vis-à-vis d'un recours ou d'un renoncement aux soins.

La reconstitution du processus social de la démarche des soins permettra de comprendre les facteurs individuels et psychosociaux déterminant l'adoption du comportement par la personne interviewée.

Le guide a été testé auprès de six personnes rencontrées dans un hôpital public, un hôpital privé et un dispensaire durant la phase d'observation. Plusieurs questions ont été rectifiées et d'autres y ont été ajoutées.

Dans la première partie, une grande attention a été accordée aux déterminants sociodémographiques et économiques dans l'objectif d'élaborer la relation entre ces différents déterminants, la prise en charge de la santé et le recours aux soins.

La deuxième partie de ce guide était formée de 12 questions ouvertes, divisées en cinq grandes thématiques.

- La connaissance des individus des lieux de soins dans leur milieu géographique, du système de santé et de leur propre santé.
- Leurs perceptions sur la santé, les maladies et les traitements.
- Leur comportement individuel et familial face à la maladie.
- La priorité donnée à la santé.
-L'influence économique sur la prise en charge de leur santé.

Chaque entretien était d'une durée de 30 à 45 minutes. Ces entretiens ont été réalisés dans les 8 établissements sanitaires du tableau qui suit.

**Tableau 4.1. Présentation des établissements sanitaires**

| Établissement/Code | Adresse | Secteur | Types de services offerts |
|---|---|---|---|
| Dispensaire 1 | Metn | Public MAS | Médicaux, paramédicaux, sociaux |
| Dispensaire 2 | Metn | Public MAS | Médicaux, paramédicaux |
| Dispensaire 3 | Kesrouan | Privé municipalité | Médicaux, paramédicaux |
| Dispensaire 4 | Kesrouan | Public MSP | Médicaux, paramédicaux |
| Hôpital 1 | Kesrouan | Public | Gynécologie, médecine, chirurgie |
| Hôpital 2 | Beyrouth | Public | Médecine, chirurgie |
| Hôpital 3 | Metn | Privé | Tous les services médicaux |
| Hôpital 4 | Kesrouan | Privé | Tous les services médicaux |

### 4.5.3. Elaboration du questionnaire quantitatif CNSS

Une analyse exploratoire approfondie de cinq dossiers a permis d'établir un questionnaire papier composé de variables à étudier selon le contenu des dossiers. Une liste de numéros de dossiers est établie par les employés de la CNSS en ne prenant comme critère que la période de soins allant de 2012 à fin juin 2015.

Le questionnaire comporte alors cinq parties (voir Annexe 8).

- Emploi du bénéficiaire.
- Période totale de couverture à la CNSS.

- Caractéristiques sociodémographiques et couverture des ayants droit.
- Nombre de demandes cumulées de remboursement de soins.
- Détails des recours par demande de remboursement déposée : Composants de chaque recours, nature du recours selon le classement CNSS (consultations, médicaments, radiologie, laboratoire), coût réel du recours, coût remboursé…).

Au sein de chaque partie, plusieurs items sont à remplir à partir des dossiers des bénéficiaires.

Un groupe de cinq employés de l'agence CNSS a contribué au remplissage du questionnaire ; une condition obligatoire pour respecter le secret médical.

La période de cette collecte s'étalait de mai 2015 (obtention de l'accord) à fin novembre 2015.

## 4.6. Méthodes d'analyse

### 4.6.1. Etude qualitative

Une analyse thématique de contenu des données issues des entretiens et des observations a été réalisée. Des catégories significatives ont été dégagées permettant l'évaluation des discours et une analyse des déterminants du recours aux soins (Quivy et Campenhoudt, 2006).

Dans un premier temps, les entretiens ont été tous retranscrits intégralement par écrit, suivis d'une première lecture flottante pour se familiariser avec les supports. Un découpage des entretiens, un codage et un classement en différentes catégories de réponses similaires sont faits. Le codage est central dans le processus de l'analyse, car il pose le problème du sens (Ghiglione et Matalon, 1995) et dans cette étude il est effectué dans un modèle ouvert dans lequel les catégories sont induites des discours analysés. Il

s'agit donc d'une opération intellectuelle qui consiste à transformer des données brutes (faits observés, paroles recueillies…) en une première formulation signifiante.

Les catégories ont été désignées donc par induction d'après les questions abordées suivant le guide d'entretien. La technique d'analyse de contenu est donc appliquée en s'intéressant au poids relatif de chaque thème composé de plusieurs catégories. Une analyse descriptive de ces résultats présentés en thèmes est appuyée par une restitution des verbatims des interviewés dans un souci de transparence des traitements des données.

Enfin, une mise en perspective des contenus des différents thèmes, afin de faire une analyse transversale et de comparer les données des différents entretiens entre elles et avec les données des observations également. Par la suite, une confrontation avec le modèle conceptuel et les données recueillies dans la littérature ont permis de produire une pertinence scientifique recherchée.

### 4.6.2. Analyse des données quantitatives

Une saisie des questionnaires est faite sur le logiciel Microsoft Access (2010). Le recours à ce logiciel est adopté, car il convenait à la mise en relation des variables qui correspondait aux objectifs de l'enquête :

Une table des bénéficiaires est liée à la table des transactions à travers « une à plusieurs » relations. La clef première de la saisie était le code donné à chaque bénéficiaire principal de la CNSS.

Après la saisie complète des données, celles-ci étaient exportées sur la base de données SQL (2008) (Structured Query Langage) pour l'analyse.

La base de données SQL a été utilisée pour l'analyse en raison de ses capacités d'agrégation. Agrégations de valeurs ont été effectuées pour le coût et le nombre de

transactions par famille, par bénéficiaire et par intervalles de dates.

Un cahier de notes est tenu au cours de l'enquête pour les détails pertinents en lien avec les objectifs de la recherche (procédure, pratiques des employés, du médecin contrôleur...). Ces notes ont également aidé à éclaircir des points importants concernant certaines décisions prises ou certains remboursements non effectués.

## 4.7. Considérations éthiques

La collecte de données dans les deux approches qualitatives et quantitatives a respecté les conditions éthiques d'une recherche scientifique.

- Le respect des règlements des institutions contactées : leur accord est donné suite à des demandes faites par lettre écrite définissant les objectifs de la recherche et ses conditions.
- L'anonymat et la confidentialité des données recueillies sont pris comme engagement de la part du chercheur. Cet engagement est également exprimé auprès des personnes à interviewer et un consentement libre de participer aux entretiens était proposé tout en expliquant à chaque participant les objectifs de la recherche.
- Tous les enregistrements d'entretiens sont faits avec le consentement de l'interviewé.
- Ces considérations éthiques sont également présentes dans la rédaction du rapport de recherche en évitant de mentionner des informations menant à l'identification des personnes et des structures.

## 4.8. Difficultés et limites de la recherche

### 4.8.1. Durant l'étude qualitative

Durant la réalisation de la recherche, plusieurs difficultés se présentaient :

- renoncement de deux établissements sanitaires à participer malgré l'obtention d'un accord oral ;
- manque d'ouvrages et d'articles traitant le sujet du recours aux soins au Liban ;
- nombre limité des Libanais rencontrés dans quelques centres sanitaires à cause du nombre élevé des syriens présents dans ces centres ;
- la grève, qui a eu lieu à un hôpital public de Beyrouth, a retardé l'enquête de plusieurs semaines ;
- le nombre élevé des personnes accidentées qui se sont présentées aux urgences ;
- la direction d'un centre qui a limité la possibilité d'effectuer l'étude à quatre jours et n'a pas accepté de la renouveler malgré le besoin de rencontrer plus de personnes.

Les difficultés étaient à relativiser en évaluant les facilités décelées :

- la collaboration de la plupart des équipes de travail de différentes institutions sanitaires a facilité la communication des interviewers avec la population ;
- le statut d'étudiants des interviewers et la caution académique qui s'y rattache ont favorisé l'obtention du consentement des interviewés ;
- la cohésion de l'équipe de travail a facilité l'atteinte du but visé grâce à l'existence d'une interdisciplinarité, d'un partage des tâches, d'une collaboration et d'un soutien mutuel.

Les limites de cette étude se situent dans le fait qu'elle est loin d'être exhaustive. Elle répond toutefois à l'objet

de l'étude donc elle pourrait être utilisée pour une extrapolation.

### 4.8.2. Durant l'enquête quantitative

L'enquête quantitative s'est déroulée du 1er mai 2015 au 30 novembre 2015.

Beaucoup de difficultés de remplissage ont surgi du fait des horaires et du logiciel de la base de données spécifique à la Caisse Nationale de Sécurité sociale. En effet, cela se traduisait par une réduction de la marge dédiée au remplissage possible des questionnaires :

- les horaires d'ouverture des bureaux du centre CNSS sont de 7h30 du matin jusqu'à 14h30 de l'après-midi. Ces horaires étaient réduits au cours de cette enquête à cause du mois du Ramadan et le centre fermait les samedis pendant les vacances d'été. Ces aménagements augmentaient la charge de travail des employés en réduisant les marges d'accueil et de traitement de dossiers ;
- au niveau de tout le centre, il n'y avait pas de poste d'ordinateur libre pour le mettre à la disposition de la recherche, car le nombre des postes correspond à celui des employés. Donc il fallait attendre qu'un poste se libère (celui des remboursements) à l'arrêt de l'accueil ouvert au public ne laissant qu'une marge de deux heures de travail possible avant la fermeture du centre et l'arrêt du système informatique. Aucune possibilité d'avoir accès aux dossiers informatiques en dehors des horaires ;
- le recours aux soins hospitaliers prévu au départ dans le cadre de l'étude des dossiers n'était pas accessible, car l'essentiel de ce recours est encore sur papier et dans les archives. Le temps imparti à l'enquête ne permettait pas d'y accéder. Il faudrait une étude spécifique sur cette question-là ;

- aucune étude visant les mêmes objectifs n'a été effectuée à ce jour au niveau de la CNSS.

Les facilités de cette enquête étaient l'accueil et la coopération de l'équipe du centre de la CNSS. Ils ont tout mis en œuvre pour faciliter les conditions de l'enquête malgré toutes les difficultés déjà citées.

## 4.9. Validité de l'étude

### 4.9.1. Validité interne

L'analyse qualitative répond aux critères de validité interne pour les raisons ci-dessous.

- Elle est crédible en fonction des méthodes scientifiques utilisées dans la collecte des données basée sur une observation et des entretiens semi-directifs enregistrés.
- Elle est plausible par rapport à d'autres informations et connaissances retrouvées dans la revue de la littérature montrant les trois facteurs qui influencent le recours aux soins : facteurs prédisposants, facilitants et de renforcement.
- Elle est fiable, car les dires des personnes interviewées qui ont été retranscrits soigneusement et vérifiés auprès d'une partie d'eux par la suite.
- L'analyse des observations et des entretiens menés a révélé une certaine similitude avec la littérature.
- Une triangulation des données entre chercheurs est faite pour la validation des résultats de la recherche (chercheur principal, étudiants en master et deux autres professeurs universitaires.
- La triangulation des données basée sur la comparaison des interprétations issues de différents échantillons (population hétérogène ayant différentes caractéristiques sociodémographiques et culturelles), de méthodes de collecte des informations diverses (entretiens

semi-directifs et observation directe de type ethnologique) et un cadre théorique qui revient à la théorie du comportement planifié qui sera étudié au sein du cadre développé par Green et Kreuter, notamment le modèle PRECEDE/PROCEED.

- Le questionnaire quantitatif a montré dans son aspect exploratoire l'influence de la couverture médicale sur la fréquence du recours aux soins. Les résultats statistiques concertés et travaillés bénéficient d'une validité interne liée à la fiabilité des sources des données et des techniques de traitement statistique Access et SQL d'une part et à la validation des hypothèses posées d'autre part.

### 4.9.2. Validité externe

La validité externe concerne la transférabilité de l'étude qualitative et la généralisation des résultats quantitatifs à d'autres contextes. L'échantillon choisi est représentatif de la problématique vu la pluralité des niveaux socio-culturels et économiques des interviewés, rencontrés dans différents types d'institutions sanitaires localisées dans plusieurs régions. De plus, une saturation des données est atteinte pour décrire le plus exactement possible la population étudiée. Enfin, les données recueillies sont superposables à celles exposées dans la revue de la littérature.

De ce fait, l'échantillon qualitatif choisi décrit correctement la population étudiée. Pourtant cette étude pourra par la suite être complétée par une étude quantitative ou même une étude qualitative au sein d'autres régions libanaises vers une démarche plus globale.

Le questionnaire quantitatif n'est nullement exhaustif, mais les résultats statistiques obtenus et les hypothèses ont une validité externe, car ils correspondent aux éléments de la littérature concernant les recours aux soins analysés.

# Chapitre 5
# Description des résultats de l'observation

Le terrain décrit dans les chapitres cinq et six est réalisé dans huit institutions sanitaires, par observation et par entretiens menés auprès de cinquante-trois citoyens fréquentant les établissements de santé choisis pour cette étude.

Dans ce qui suivra, sera abordée, en premier lieu, la description de l'observation menée et dans le chapitre suivant l'analyse des entretiens effectués.

La phase d'observation s'est réalisée dans huit établissements sanitaires pour une durée de 50 heures environ, réparties sur 22 heures aux dispensaires, 15 heures dans les hôpitaux privés et 13 heures dans les hôpitaux publics.

## 5.1. Observation dans les dispensaires

Dans les salles d'attente des dispensaires, la présence de plusieurs pancartes et brochures informatives sur plusieurs thèmes médicaux et des campagnes de prévention concernant surtout la poliomyélite et le cancer du sein est notée. De plus, l'horaire des visites des médecins est affiché dans trois dispensaires ainsi que les services rendus.

Les bénéficiaires de trois dispensaires se trouvaient séparés en deux groupes ; d'un côté les Libanais et de l'autre les syriens.

***Dispensaire 1***

Financé par le ministère des Affaires sociales, il assure des services médico-sociaux. Le centre est formé de trois étages. Dans le premier se déroulent les consultations médicales. L'accessibilité pour les personnes âgées et les personnes handicapées est presque impossible ou difficile vu l'absence d'ascenseur.

Durant l'observation dans ce centre, plusieurs évènements ont été remarqués :

Trois femmes sont venues pour se procurer du traitement, mais en vain ;

" ما بقى عمنلاقي الدوا هون، عمنتعذّب بالدوا";

quatre femmes sont venues pour déjeuner au centre ;"نحنا منتروّق ومنتغدّا بالمؤسسات وبالعطلة الله بدبرنا",

et elles disent que leur priorité n'est pas la santé et leur souci est d'assurer les besoins les plus élémentaires ;

" مين بالو بالصحّة خلّينا نشوف قبل كيف بدنا ندبّر الأكل والشرب."

Une dame, n'ayant aucune couverture sociale, est venue consulter le gynécologue. Elle souffre d'un saignement depuis un certain temps. Elle a bénéficié d'examens médicaux divers et il s'est avéré qu'elle a besoin d'une opération. L'objectif de sa consultation aujourd'hui est de convaincre le médecin de reporter la date de l'opération pour des raisons financières.

Une autre dame aussi ne bénéficiant d'aucune couverture sociale raconte aux chercheures qu'une fois elle a été heurtée par une voiture et que le conducteur s'est enfui. Elle fut obligée d'aller aux urgences et pour pouvoir payer les frais élevés des soins, elle a dû s'endetter.

De même, un monsieur se présente avec son fils pour consulter le pédiatre. L'enfant présente une hyperthermie depuis 24 heures, mais les parents ont attendu la consultation du pédiatre du dispensaire par manque de moyens financiers.

De ces faits, on constate que les conditions économiques de cette population constituent un obstacle majeur pour l'accès aux soins.

***Dispensaire 2***

Financé et supporté par le ministère des Affaires sociales, il assure des services médico-sociaux. Ce centre est composé de trois étages et les salles de consultation se trouvent au troisième étage, ce qui rend l'accès aux personnes âgées ou atteintes de handicap très difficile.

Durant cette observation, un nombre élevé d'étrangers présents dans le centre est remarqué et une totalité des bénéficiaires du sexe féminin est constatée. Une majorité des femmes viennent au centre pour la consultation du gynécologue et un grand souci face aux maladies génitales est ressenti.

Une femme de vingt ans est rencontrée, sans couverture sociale, nouvellement mariée, très anxieuse, en train de fumer malgré tous les signes d'interdiction de fumer. Elle présente depuis quatre mois un saignement vaginal et ne s'est adressée à aucun gynécologue par peur du diagnostic et de la consultation. Aujourd'hui, son amie l'a convaincue que la sage-femme peut l'examiner et qu'elle est très compétente.

Quant aux femmes qui attendent le pédiatre avec leurs enfants, la majorité raconte qu'elle vienne au dispensaire pour la vaccination vu le prix et que le suivi médical se fait dans les cliniques privées ;

"الطعم نفسو، ليش لادفع حقّو كتير برّا، منجي منعملو هون بس المتابعة عند حكيمن"

Au cours de la présence des chercheures effectuant l'observation, les étrangers se dirigent vers elles pour demander si elles représentaient les Nations unies et apparaissent déçus face à leur réponse négative.

***Dispensaire 3***

Nouvellement fondé et équipé, il est financé par la municipalité de la région. Il fournit des services médicaux et paramédicaux. L'accès est facile pour toutes les personnes. La salle d'attente est vaste et contient des jouets pour les enfants.

Durant les heures passées dans la salle d'attente, les bénéficiaires étaient assez satisfaits des services rendus et exprimaient leur reconnaissance à toute l'équipe soignante et surtout à l'infirmière responsable ;

" عسلامتها، تركنا غير مستوصف وجينا لهون لأنّا شاطرة وخدومة" ، "الحكما يلّي بيجوا لهون كتير شاطرين، بحكّموا بأهمّا مستشفيات".

Une constatation est donc faite que les bénéficiaires de ce centre cherchent des soins de qualité, car l'équipe de travail est assez compétente et les matériaux sont nouveaux. Les personnes visitant ce centre représentent toutes les classes socio-économiques.

Durant les conversations, tout le monde signale qu'il ne peut plus consulter les centres de la région à cause de la prédominance syrienne ;

"ما بقى يطلع دور للبناني منروح مننطر ساعات، عجقة وضجّة."

***Dispensaire 4***

Situé à une altitude de 1 400 mètres de la surface de la mer, c'est le centre de soins de santé primaire le plus récent de la région. Il offre des soins médicaux et paramédicaux. Il est financé par le MAS et le MSP.

Le nombre le plus élevé des bénéficiaires revient à la population syrienne. La responsable du centre exprime qu'ils essaient de convaincre même les Libanais de venir au dispensaire qui y renoncent à cause de la population syrienne ;

" عمنبرم على أهالي الضيعة تنقنعن يجوا عالمستوصف".

Les Libanais fréquentant le centre, se sentent à l'aise, car ils se connaissent. Eux aussi ont exprimé leur insatisfaction envers la présence élevée des syriens. Par contre, ils sont fiers d'avoir ce centre de santé dans leur région surtout que le centre le plus proche est à un minimum de vingt minutes du village en voiture.

Une femme qui boitait est rencontrée. Elle a demandé si son médecin viendra ce jour. Après trente minutes d'attente, l'infirmière lui signale que le médecin sera absent à cause d'une urgence. Elle tombe en colère et se plaint du service offert par le dispensaire ;

" يلّي ما معو مصاري بيتبهدل، يعني إذا واحد بيجي على المستوصف بيستلشقو في لأنّو ببلاش."

Une jeune femme vivant en France, est venue avec sa fille au centre pour une consultation pédiatrique. De son point de vue, les Libanais ont honte de venir aux dispensaires et sous-estiment la qualité offerte. Ceci pourrait montrer que les européens ont une différente perception des Libanais concernant le centre médico-social.

## 5.2. Observations dans les hôpitaux

***Hôpital 1***

Il s'agit d'un hôpital contenant 100 lits dont seulement 30 sont fonctionnels. Il dispose des services de gynécologie, de médecine et de chirurgie et d'une salle d'accueil remplaçant la salle d'urgence.

Durant la lecture des dossiers médicaux, il a été remarqué que les patients sont admis non seulement à la charge du ministère, mais aussi à la charge de la CNSS, de la protection sociale des secteurs non civils et à leur propre charge (étrangers).

Dans cet hôpital, trois patients rencontrés se sont plaints du manque de places vacantes et qu'à plusieurs reprises ils ont été transférés vers d'autres hôpitaux publics loin de la région ;

"مش دايماً هون بيكون في محلّات، كزا مرّة ودّوني عغير محل، مع إنّو هون أقربلي".

Un homme âgé de soixante-cinq ans, ne bénéficiant d'aucune couverture sociale se lamente de son hospitalisation en décrivant l'hôpital comme un « garage » ;

" زتّوني بهالكاراج"

De même, un homme libanais vivant à l'étranger, passant les vacances au Liban, a retardé son hospitalisation par manque de confiance dans les structures sanitaires.

Par contre, une femme âgée de quatre-vingt-quatre ans était ravie de son hospitalisation et comparait la prise en charge avec d'autres centres qu'elle a déjà visités.

La direction de l'hôpital a reporté les opérations de deux patients en attendant que ces derniers assurent les frais. Le cas observé d'une femme admise pour une fracture du fémur montre qu'elle s'est adressée en premier lieu à un hôpital privé, mais le coût de l'opération était trop élevé, elle s'est donc décidé de venir à l'hôpital public s'attendant à une prise en charge gratuite. Elle a été désappointée lorsqu'ils lui ont suspendu l'opération pour des raisons financières.

***Hôpital 2***

Il comporte un seul service de médecine-chirurgie, un bloc opératoire et une petite salle d'urgence contenant deux lits pour accueillir les patients avant 14 heures.

C'est un ancien bâtiment dont les chambres sont trop sombres et les lits à mobilisation manuelle. L'absence

d'équipement et de matériel affecte aussi l'hygiène hospitalière.

Il n'y avait pas de possibilité de se laver les mains, car il n'y avait pas de savon antiseptique ni d'essuie-mains. L'infirmière responsable, qui porte les mêmes gants durant sa visite aux patients, a raconté que c'était leur situation depuis un an.

Les personnes observées et avec lesquelles les chercheures ont pu parler, signalent qu'elles pouvaient prévenir leur état aggravé, si elles avaient les moyens économiques et elles préfèrent être prises en charge ou hospitalisées dans un autre établissement sanitaire de qualité.

Une femme qui avait une assurance privée auparavant est également rencontrée, mais puisque son fils unique s'occupe d'elle, et ne peut plus payer les frais, elle a dû l'annuler. Aujourd'hui, elle est admise aux frais du MSP.

"كل شي بتقدمو الدولة منو على قد المستوى. كنت assurance ومريحة راسي، بس الوضع خلانا ننذلّ وندق ابواب الوزارة" (*en souriant d'une façon sarcastique)*

Il est constaté que les bénéficiaires de cet hôpital regrettent leur hospitalisation et leur prise en charge dans ce centre, mais n'ont pas d'autre choix.

***Hôpital 3***

Il accueille des patients ayant différentes couvertures sociales, sauf ceux couverts par la protection sociale des secteurs non civils. Il est divisé en deux bâtiments, un pour le séjour hospitalier, l'autre renferme les services d'exploration, le bloc opératoire, les salles de soins intensifs et le service d'urgence qui peut recevoir onze patients. Le nombre de lits s'élève à 150 tous fonctionnels.

Durant l'observation aux urgences, plusieurs accidentés de la voie publique se sont présentés. Une femme est arrivée avec son mari pour une sensation de vertige. Elle a

raconté que son frère est tombé de l'arbre suite à un vertige et qu'il est décédé. Elle est venue par peur de mourir de la même manière. Ceci pousse à réfléchir sur l'éventuelle influence de l'expérience familiale sur la décision du recours aux soins.

Une jeune fille couverte par une assurance privée, a été admise aux urgences pour un malaise suite à une exposition au soleil. Elle a avoué à la compagnie d'assurance et à l'équipe soignante qu'elle a feint l'évanouissement pour pouvoir être admise.

Un infirmier bénéficiaire d'une assurance privée en plus de la CNSS s'est présenté pour une sensation de reflux. Il s'est adressé aux urgences, car, selon lui, il sera « *mieux examiné* » et ne paiera pas le coût de la consultation.

Une femme ayant une couverture médicale d'une assurance privée, arrive aux urgences suite à une chute et un trauma de la cheville. Elle demande au médecin résident de lui faire une radiographie de la cheville, du dos et de la hanche. N'ayant pas de réponse convaincante concernant l'utilité de ces examens, il explique qu'il répondait aux demandes exigées par la dame ;

"هيك بدّا، شفتيا قدّي عم بتنق، امرأة كبيرة وحكيما بالمستشفى وهي عندا تغطية".

Une femme de cinquante-deux ans, hémiplégique et aphasique, n'ayant aucune couverture sociale, se présente aux urgences pour vomissements depuis trois jours, mais vu l'état économique, elle n'est pas venue auparavant. L'équipe soignante l'a prise en charge et lui a administré le traitement nécessaire. Elle a été transférée à domicile, car elle n'a pas les moyens de payer l'hospitalisation. L'hôpital a pris à sa charge le coût des premiers soins.

Un homme âgé de cinquante-quatre ans, couvert par une assurance privée, se présente pour une dyspnée. Après

deux heures d'attente, la compagnie d'assurance a refusé sa prise en charge. Son médecin a insisté pour lui faire passer un examen spécifique même si le patient allait payer les charges. L'examen a montré une embolie pulmonaire donc l'urgence d'être hospitalisé. Ceci pousse à se dire que parfois les opérations administratives retardent la prise en charge des personnes et affectent leur état de santé.

Enfin, plusieurs personnes sont arrivées pour des cas urgents comme une colique néphrétique, des accidents de la voie publique, mais puisque les compagnies d'assurance ne les ont pas couvertes, ces personnes ont dû quitter l'établissement sans être prises en charge.

***Hôpital 4***

Il offre des soins médicaux et paramédicaux : hospitalisation, services d'exploration, bloc opératoire, soins intensifs et service d'urgence. Le nombre de lits s'élève à 150 tous fonctionnels. Tous les patients sont admis dans cet hôpital sans distinction de couverture sociale.

Plusieurs heures d'observation sont passées dans les salles d'urgence de ce centre, et durant tous les moments de la journée. La plupart des gens qui se présentaient aux urgences, étaient des étrangers accueillis pour des accidents ou des chutes.

Une minorité de Libanais était rencontrée. Parmi eux, une femme, couverte par la CNSS qui arrive avec une douleur au bras. Elle raconte qu'elle a eu un accident de travail. La secrétaire lui conseille de dire qu'elle est tombée à domicile pour pouvoir effectuer les examens aux frais de la CNSS car celle-ci ne couvre pas les accidents de travail.

Une autre dame arrive avec sa fille âgée de seize ans, couverte par la CNSS et une assurance privée, ayant une

douleur à la main après une chute. A l'examen clinique, le médecin n'a trouvé aucun signe de fracture ou d'entorse, mais la mère insiste qu'il lui fasse une radiographie. Et malgré que l'examen effectué s'avère négatif, elle presse le médecin à lui faire un bandage ;

"بدّي طمّن بالي هيك هيك في ضمان و تأمين"

Cela explique, que parfois le professionnel de santé se soumet à la volonté du patient et de sa famille pour calmer leur angoisse.

# Chapitre 6
# Description et analyse des résultats des entretiens semi-directifs

L'entretien semi-directif est un échange de perceptions, d'expériences et de connaissances. Dans ce chapitre, il s'agit d'exposer les données retenues des entretiens effectués dans les différents centres sanitaires.

## 6.1. Phase d'exécution des entretiens

Dans les dispensaires, les entretiens se déroulaient dans une salle de consultation disponible au moment de l'entretien, un peu à l'écart afin d'assurer un cadre favorisant la parole et le climat de confiance chez l'interviewé, après s'être présenté en tant qu'intervieweur et avoir obtenu le consentement des interviewés.

Dans les hôpitaux, la population cible était les patients arrivant aux urgences. Les entretiens étaient effectués dans leurs chambres d'hospitalisation après leur admission à cause de leur état de santé parfois critique aux urgences qui ne permettait pas de discuter avec eux. L'accord et le consentement des patients concernés étaient pris avant d'accéder à leurs chambres.

Tous les entretiens effectués dans les dispensaires ont été réalisés avec l'interviewé seul, rencontré le jour de sa venue au centre soit en attendant la consultation si le temps le permettait, soit immédiatement après celle-ci. La décision est prise de ne pas donner de rendez-vous aux

patients après avoir fait face à la faible probabilité que ceux-ci s'y tiennent.

Quant aux hôpitaux, les dossiers des patients étaient consultés avant l'entretien et la demande était formulée au patient de le rencontrer seul, excepté quatre entretiens où un membre de la famille était présent à la demande de l'interviewé sans pour autant intervenir. L'entretien était présenté comme une étude universitaire ayant pour but d'étudier les inégalités dans l'accès aux soins.

La durée de chaque entretien s'étendait de 30 à 45 minutes, avec la confirmation d'une garantie d'anonymat. Les intervieweurs étaient habillés en blouse blanche suite à la demande de la direction des centres afin de faire croire aux patients qu'ils faisaient partie de l'équipe du centre.

Tous les entretiens étaient enregistrés après avoir pris l'accord des interviewés. L'enregistrement d'un des entretiens a été malencontreusement effacé, mais heureusement des notes ont été prises afin de garder les éléments essentiels de l'entretien.

Comme cette étude ne porte pas sur l'expérimentation du corps humain et n'entre pas dans le champ d'application de la loi sur la recherche biomédicale, seul le consentement oral des patients a été demandé.

Huit personnes ont été exclues, deux n'ayant pas pris l'entretien au sérieux, deux étaient interrompues par l'arrivée du médecin, deux n'avaient pas la possibilité de continuer l'entretien faute de temps, une interviewée interrompue à cause de l'arrivée des visiteurs et une à cause de l'aggravation de sa douleur.

La confidentialité des données a été possible grâce à une attribution d'un code à chaque entretien réalisé, rendant ainsi les entretiens anonymes.

Les tableaux représentant les caractéristiques sociodémographiques des 53 interviewés sont placés dans la partie des annexes (Annexe 4, 5 et 6).

## 6.2. Analyse par thème des entretiens semi-directifs

La collecte des données auprès de la population cible représente une phase primordiale pour tout travail de recherche. En effet, cette étape consiste à extraire du discours recueilli auprès des interviewés les facteurs déterminant l'accès aux services de soins. Dans cette partie, le traitement des informations sera abordé suivant des catégories composant des thèmes qui seront traités selon la pertinence des discours analysés.

### 6.2.1. Choix du centre visité et attentes des bénéficiaires

Au cours des entretiens, des tentatives sont faites pour comprendre le contexte et les raisons qui ont poussé les interviewés à visiter les lieux de soins et les relations qu'ils ont pu établir au niveau des dispensaires, hôpitaux publics et hôpitaux privés.

*a - Accessibilité financière*

**Au niveau des dispensaires,** le coût des consultations, moins cher que celui des cliniques privées, est un élément marquant dans le choix (E7, 8, 12, 17, 23, 24, 25, 26,27).

" رفيقتي دلّتني عهون قالتلي الفحصيّة بس ب ٧٠٠٠ ل.ل. هون أرخص بكتير من العيادة." (E24)

Même les bénéficiaires de la CNSS se dirigent vers les dispensaires, car en privé le coût de la consultation est plus élevé et ils doivent attendre plusieurs mois pour récupérer l'argent à cause des longues procédures.

Sept personnes s'adressent aux dentistes de ces centres, signalant que les frais des soins dentaires sont chers au

Liban et ne sont couverts que par la protection sociale des secteurs non civils (E5, 6, 10, 11, 12, 13, 18).

"أنا بجي لهون كرمال الأسنان. بالمستوصف أرخص والضمان ما بيغطيون." (E13)

Trois personnes se trouvent obligées à venir au dispensaire par manque de moyens financiers (E 5, 6,14).

" بصراحة أنا ما كتير حابّة إجي عالمستوصف بس مجبورة ما في مصاري." (E5)

**Au niveau des hôpitaux publics,** le critère qui pousse les individus à s'y adresser s'avère être l'état économique des patients et l'absence de couverture sociale. En effet, douze des quatorze interviewés ne bénéficient d'aucune couverture médicale. Cette situation les oblige à fréquenter les établissements publics. En traitant ce sujet, il est remarquable qu'ils aient beaucoup utilisé les verbes *« falloir et devoir »*, comme si la question du recours à ce secteur est incontournable (E 28, 29, 31, 32, 33, 35, 36, 37, 38, 39, 40, 41).

" ما في حل ثاني غير إنّو نجي لهون، هيك ومش عارفين كيف بدنا نغطّي الفرق" (E36)

**Au niveau des hôpitaux privés,** les patients rencontrés jouissent tous d'une couverture médicale, ce qui constitue le premier facteur dans le choix de ce secteur pour la prise en charge médicale.

***b - Accessibilité géographique***

**Au niveau des dispensaires**, la facilité de l'accès géographique est un facteur influençant le choix de consulter un dispensaire. Sept personnes réclament qu'elles s'y dirigent, car il se situe à proximité de leur milieu de résidence (E4, 6, 8, 12,16, 21, 22).

**Au niveau des hôpitaux publics,** l'accès géographique ne s'avère pas être un facteur facilitant la consultation

d'un hôpital public, vue la disparité dans la répartition de ces établissements sur le territoire libanais. A noter qu'une personne seulement s'est dirigée vers un hôpital public, car il se trouve à proximité (E34).

**Au niveau des hôpitaux privés,** deux interviewés fréquentant l'hôpital 4 mentionnent que l'accès géographique est pour eux une cause fondamentale dans le choix du centre (E43, 44).

"جيت لهون بحالة طارئة، لأنن قراب عليي." (E43)

## *c - Offre de soins*

**Au niveau des dispensaires,** pour certains interviewés, l'objectif de la visite du centre est la consultation des spécialistes surtout gynécologue (E9, 15, 21, 23, 24, 25,27), pédiatre (E8, 21), dentiste (E5, 6, 10, 11, 12, 13, 18) et cardiologue (E2, 20). D'autres demandent des services paramédicaux ou sociaux (E1, 7, 10, 19, 21, 22, 26).

" أنا بجي لهون مرتين بالجمعة كل اثنين وأربعاء لأنو بأمنولنا وجبات الغدا." (E1)

"أنا بجي لعند حكيم القلب، كتير شاطر وصار بيعرفلي." (E2)

Trois personnes signalent leur insatisfaction de consulter un dispensaire. Elles considèrent que la consultation en clinique privée est meilleure (E5, 6,14).

" المستوصفات بتقدّم خدمات، بس ما في متل الحكيم في نطرة كتير وعجقة." (E6)

Deux autres personnes se plaignent de la durée d'attente (E6, 17). Une personne note que l'horaire d'ouverture des dispensaires n'est pas adapté pour les personnes qui travaillent (E22).

**Au niveau des hôpitaux publics,** deux personnes non satisfaites du retard dans la prise en charge, montrent un

manque de confiance envers l'équipe soignante et regrettent leur consultation du centre (E28, 30).

"أنا جايي لهون بس ما عندي غير حلّ. ما بوثق بحكمتن وبخاف منّا." (E30)

En parallèle et malgré le sentiment d'obligation d'être hospitalisées dans le secteur public, deux personnes expriment leur satisfaction de la prise en charge offerte, de la qualité des soins et de l'hygiène à l'hôpital (E33, 35).

"والله ما في منن بالمستشفى هون. العناية والإهتمام top حتّى شوفو هون أنظف من أهمّ مستشفى ببيروت." (E33)

**Au niveau des hôpitaux privés**, il s'est avéré important pour les individus rencontrés, d'avoir un dossier complet à l'hôpital dans lequel sont notés tous leurs antécédents. Cette condition les amène à s'adresser à ces établissements (E43, 45, 47, 48, 49, 50, 51, 53).

" أنا جيت لهون لأنّو حكيمي بحكّم بهالمستشفى وملفّي فيا. صاروا بيعرفوا كل شي عنّي." (E49)

Ils trouvent que dans ces hôpitaux, leur santé est correctement prise en charge, avec sérieux et compétence. Ils sont attachés à ces services de qualité et par suite n'envisagent pas d'aller ailleurs (E42, 43, 46, 52, 53).

" المستشفى هون معروفة والحكمة فيا بتجنن أصلاً أحسن الحكما بحكموا هون." (E42)

*d - Aspect relationnel*

**Au niveau des dispensaires,** la relation avec l'équipe soignante, l'accueil chaleureux et le respect dont faisait preuve le personnel, la bonne réputation et la compétence des médecins sont des facteurs renforçant le recours aux soins (E 1,3, 4, 6, 8, 12, 15, 16, 19,20, 23, 24, 25).

" أنا بجي لهون لأنّو المستوصف كتير معروف بالضيعة والحكما شاطرين." (E12)

**Au niveau des hôpitaux privés,** le lien établi avec le médecin traitant qui connaît bien l'histoire médicale et qui prend en charge la personne depuis longtemps est une composante essentielle du choix du soin (E 45, 46, 49, 50).

"أنا ما بروح غير مطرح لأنّي بوثق بس بالحكيم هون." (E46)

*e - Limites d'accès socioculturel*

**Au niveau des dispensaires**, la majorité des femmes fréquentent le dispensaire 2 pour un suivi gynécologique par la sage-femme (E21, 23, 24, 25,27). Ceci est relié aux valeurs culturelles et religieuses de cette population, sachant que toutes les femmes rencontrées sont voilées et préfèrent que l'examen soit fait par un médecin du même sexe.

*f - Rapport à l'étranger*

**Au niveau des dispensaires,** trois interviewés paraissent gênés par la présence des syriens dans les dispensaires de leur région. Selon eux, la qualité des services offerts en souffre et le prix des services rendus a augmenté et ce sont les raisons qui les ont poussés à consulter ailleurs, dans des dispensaires hors de leur région (E18, 26, 27).

" بالمستوصف يلّي حدّ بيتنا في عجقة كتير، ملان سوريّة." (E18)

" بالمستوصف يلّي بمنطقتنا كانت المعاينة ب ٧٠٠٠ ل.ل قبل ما يجو السوريّة. هلّق صارت ب ٢٠،٠٠٠ ل.ل غلّو الأسعار عاللبناني ورخّصو للسوري." (E26)

*g - Abus du système*

**Au niveau des hôpitaux publics,** deux des interviewés avouent qu'ils viennent régulièrement à l'hôpital pour des bilans périodiques de santé en prétendant toujours des maux. Ils considèrent que les services semi-gratuits offerts

par l'Etat sont un droit acquis. Il s'agit d'un composant de l'abus du système de soins (E35, 37).

" بجي لهون تيعملولي فحوصات هيك هيك ما بدفع شي. أنا أصلاً كل شهرين بفوت عصحّة السلامة. شو بدّي أحلا من هيك خدمة وإهتمام وببلاش." (E35)

### 6.2.2. Connaissance des structures sanitaires hors du centre consulté et les représentations qu'en ont les personnes rencontrées

Durant les entretiens, une analyse du rapport des interviewés aux structures sanitaires en dehors du centre visité est faite, pour déceler leur ressenti, leurs représentations et leurs connaissances de cet « ailleurs ».

#### *a - Connaissances des structures de soins dans le milieu environnant*

**Au niveau des dispensaires,** vingt-cinq des interviewés aux dispensaires ont pu nommer au moins quatre centres sanitaires entre dispensaires, hôpitaux publics et hôpitaux privés.

Les interviewés au dispensaire 1 sont majoritairement inscrits dans un réseau régional et associatif. Ils sont dans une situation précaire et bénéficient d'aides apportées variées allant de l'aide alimentaire au suivi médical.

**Au niveau des hôpitaux publics,** les personnes rencontrées semblent avoir des connaissances diverses des centres sanitaires installés dans leurs régions (E29, 31, 34, 35, 36, 37). Elles sont aussi capables de nommer des hôpitaux publics localisés dans des régions lointaines consultés auparavant (E29, 33, 41).

**Au niveau des hôpitaux privés,** les interviewés dans les hôpitaux privés, citent facilement, en parlant du réseau sanitaire de leur région, d'autres hôpitaux du même secteur et mentionnent quelques dispensaires. Seulement

deux nomment un hôpital rattaché au secteur public (E45, 49).

***b- Représentations des structures de soins environnantes***

**Au niveau des dispensaires,** les représentations qu'ont les personnes rencontrées dans le caza du Kesrouan des institutions hospitalières de leur région sont surprenantes. Les unes relèvent de leur manque de confiance envers les hôpitaux privés (E8, 9, 10, 11, 12, 13, 18, 19), les autres considèrent que les professionnels de santé y travaillant sont incompétents (E8, 9, 10, 11, 14, 16, 19, 20). Cette perception est le résultat de diverses expériences vécues personnellement ou dans son entourage dans ces structures.

" نحن ما منسترجي نتحكّم بولا مستشفى بالمنطقة حتّى لو حالة طارئة. أصلاً كلّ ولاد المنطقة بيقولو إنّو يلّي فايت على هالمستشفيات مفقود ويلّي ضاهر مولود." (E19)

" مرّة جوزي فات بحالة طارئة على مستشفى X، منيح يلّي طلع عايش من بين إيدين الحكما. ما حدا عرف حكّمو إلّا تنزّلني على مستشفى ببيروت." (E10)

De ce fait, cette population préfère être hospitalisée dans les hôpitaux universitaires de Beyrouth (E8, 9, 10, 11, 19, 20).

" إذا بدنا نفوت عمستشفى، ما منوثق بحدا بهيدي المنطقة. منفضّل نروح عمستشفى ببيروت." (E11)

**Au niveau des hôpitaux publics,** les représentations, qu'ont les personnes interviewées dans les dispensaires, sont majoritairement négatives. Les unes se sont plaintes de la nature des services offerts, les autres de la qualité de ces services. Elles considèrent que les prestations fournies ne répondent pas à leurs besoins (E31, 33, 36, 37, 41).

" المستوصف يلّي عنّا بالمنطقة أنجأ في كم حكيم بيجوا عليه وهيدي هيي. لا في إدوية ولا فحوصات ولا حملات." (E36)

Quant aux hôpitaux privés, les interviewés montrent une appréhension à aller consulter dans ces établissements. Ils trouvent que leur situation économique ne leur permet même pas d'y penser. Pour eux, être admis dans un hôpital privé est à la fois un luxe et un privilège qui ne leur sont pas attribués (E31, 34, 35, 38, 40, 41).

" بس بالإسم منعرفن حتّى زيارة ما منسترجي نروح علين. هنّي كتير بعاد عنّا وعن الوزارة." (E41)

**Au niveau des hôpitaux privés,** la population, rencontrée dans les hôpitaux 3 et 4, conçoit le secteur public comme moins compétent et moins capable que le privé. Bénéficiant d'une couverture médicale, elle trouve que l'hôpital public ne la concerne pas et que les services fournis sont destinés aux plus pauvres (E42, 43, 45, 49, 52, 53).

" بمنطقتنا في مستشفى حكومي بس أنا ما بروح عليه، منّي معوّدي بحس إنّو منّو إلنا هوأكتر معمول للعالم يلّي ما معا مصاري وما في مين يدفع عنّا الحكمة." (E45)

Concernant les représentations des dispensaires, deux se plaignent des services offerts (E46, 47). Par contre, un des interviewés paraît fier de la présence d'un dispensaire bien équipé dans sa région (E49). En parallèle, une personne signale que l'horaire de travail des dispensaires n'est pas compatible avec celui des employés en général.

" المستوصف عنّا بالمنطقة كتير مجهّز وبلبّي عدد من حاجات السكان." (E49)

### 6.2.3. Perception de la santé

Comme la perception de la santé chez les individus influence leur recours aux soins, une définition de la santé est demandée aux interviewés.

***a - Registre symbolique***

La santé, pour huit interviewés **des différents établissements visités**, représente un signe de vie conforme à la volonté de Dieu. C'est *« un don »* que Lui seul peut fournir. Tandis que l'échec de la guérison, et/ou la souffrance quelle qu'elle soit, sont censés être dus *« à une malédiction ou à une désobéissance »* de la part de la personne souffrante envers Dieu et que la maladie est provoquée par *« la sanction de Dieu »* (E1, 7, 14, 15, 20, 32, 41).

" الله بجازي بالصحّة، وهو العاطي الصحّة." (E7)

" الصحّة نعمة من عند الله، يلّي ربنا غضبان علي بيضربو بصحتو." (E14)

Sept autres considèrent que la santé *« c'est la vie »*. Pour eux, la vraie richesse de l'être humain est d'être en bonne santé (E4, 6, 17, 18, 19, 22, 24, 28, 30, 36, 37).

" الصحّة هي الأساس، هي الدنيي. ما تاخدي شي من هالدنيي خدي بس صحّة." (E6)

A noter qu'un des interviewés de confession musulmane précise que le déterminant de la bonne santé se constitue de ne pas manger de la viande du porc et de ne pas consommer de l'alcool (E21).

***b - Résultat d'un équilibre psychologique, physique et spirituel***

**Au niveau des dispensaires,** cinq des interviewés perçoivent la bonne santé comme le résultat d'un bon équilibre psychologique. Ils affirment que le stress et la dépression sont deux facteurs renforçant l'apparition de la maladie (E2, 8, 13, 26, 27).

" الواحد بس تكون نفسيتو مرتاحة يعني صحتو منيحة وبيعيش."(E26)

Une autre personne trouve que la santé est égale à l'absence de maladie (E3). Deux autres y ajoutent le bon état physique et psychologique (E 10, 12).

" الصحّة يعني ما في مرض. يعني تكون نفسّياً وجسديّاً منيح." (E12)

**Au niveau des hôpitaux privés,** la définition de la santé donnée par la population rencontrée est particulière. Ces personnes ont attribué à la santé de nouvelles caractéristiques. Pour elles, c'est un mode de vie sain englobant une bonne alimentation et une pratique régulière d'activités physiques (E43, 47, 48, 51, 53).

" أهمّا الشي بالصحّة إنّك تعملي sport ويكون عندك نظام غذائي جيّد، يعني تشربي كتير ماي و تاكلي أكل صحّي." (E48)

C'est la prévention et le dépistage précoce de la maladie (E42). C'est un bon état physique, psychique et spirituel (E49). C'est la capacité de vivre heureux, sans douleur et sans peine (E44, 45).

" الصحّة كتير مهمّة. أهمّا شي فيا إنّوتتوقّي المرض و تكتشفي عبكّير." (E42)

### *c - Résultat d'un équilibre professionnel et financier*

Cinq personnes conçoivent la santé comme la capacité de mener une vie normale et d'être une personne rentable pouvant réaliser un travail fructueux. Elles estiment qu'être en bonne santé permet aux individus de mener leurs activités professionnelles et d'assurer ainsi les besoins quotidiens de leurs familles. Ainsi, elles craignent la maladie, car celle-ci influence leur rendement économique (E 9, 23, 29, 31, 46, 50, 52).

" إذا الواحد صحتو منيحة، بيقدر يعيش كيف ما بدّو. يعني إذا كان صاخن كيف بدّو يشتغل ويأمّن مصاري لعيلتو." (E9)

En parallèle, une personne pense que la bonne situation économique entraîne la bonne santé. Pour elle, il faut avoir de l'argent pour se traiter et être en bonne santé (E 25).

" أهمّا شي بالصحّة تكون أحوالو المادّية للواحد منيحة. هيك إذا مرض بيتعالج، وهيدا أصعب شي هالإيّام." (E25)

*d - Se sentir « désabusé »*

**Au niveau des hôpitaux publics,** en abordant le sujet de la santé et en demandant aux individus de donner une définition de ce concept, une majorité de personnes en pleine souffrance encombrées de douleurs ont été trahies par leurs larmes et dénoncées par les essoufflements en y répondant.

Pour eux, la santé n'existe plus. Envahie par la maladie, elle est perdue depuis longtemps. L'âge avancé ou l'atteinte d'une maladie grave comme la sclérose en plaques sont l'assise de cette perception négative de la santé (E33, 34, 35, 38, 39, 40).

" عن أيّا صحّة عمتحكيني بهالعمر، خلص بلّش هلّق العدّ العكسي، كلّو عميرجع لورا." (E33)

*e - Priorité dans la vie*

**Au niveau des dispensaires,** sont retrouvés des personnes qui perçoivent la santé comme une priorité qui ne doit pas être négligée quelle que soit la raison (E 12, 14, 23, 24).

### 6.2.4. Perception des couvertures médicales et de leur efficacité

En abordant le sujet des couvertures médicales, force était de constater que les connaissances et les représentations que possèdent les interviewés dépendent majoritairement de leurs expériences vécues.

*a - Choix de la meilleure couverture médicale*

Pour les personnes rencontrées **aux dispensaires,** les avis concernant le choix de la meilleure couverture médicale étaient variés. La plupart mentionne que la CNSS permet l'accès aux consultations médicales, au traitement et à l'hospitalisation (E3, 6, 8, 9, 11, 13, 17, 19, 22, 26, 27).

" لو ما بيّي عندو ضمان ما كنّا قدرنا حكّمنا." (E19)

Certains considèrent que l'assurance est *« la crème des couvertures »,* car l'hospitalisation est payée à 100%, les soins en urgence sont couverts et l'admission à l'hôpital est plus facile (E6, 8, 9, 16, 20, 24).

"أحسن شي الواحد يكون عندو تأمين، بالقليلة ما بتدفعي ولا ليرة فرق بس تفوتي على مستشفى." (E24)

Une minorité a pu relever d'autres types de couvertures médicales telles la protection sociale des non-civils (armée libanaise, forces de l'intérieur et de la gendarmerie), la combinaison entre la CNSS et l'assurance, et pour une personne, payer ses propres frais de soins semble être le meilleur moyen de couverture (E5, 10, 15, 19).

Neuf des personnes rencontrées dans **les hôpitaux publics** optent pour la CNSS comme meilleure couverture sociale. Ces personnes signalent que la CNSS leur donne le droit de choisir l'établissement sanitaire qui peut leur procurer les meilleurs soins. L'accessibilité géographique est garantie ainsi qu'un sentiment de sécurité interne de pouvoir accéder aux soins. Elle assure hospitalisation et traitement médical. Elle permet à l'individu d'avoir une variété dans le choix de l'institution sanitaire (E28, 29, 31, 33, 35, 37, 38, 40, 41).

" يا ريت في ضمان والله كنّا منرتاح نفسيّاً. بس تكوني مضمونة ما بتوفري عحالك لا حكمة ولا دوا." (E37)

Deux personnes disent que l'important c'est de jouir de n'importe quelle couverture médicale. Ceci leur permet d'être moins anxieux face à la maladie (E32, 36).

"يا ريت عنّا حيالّا تغطية ما كانت بنتي نجبرت تترك علمها تتحكمني." (E32)

L'argent est la meilleure couverture sociale pour un des interviewés (E39).

Il est important de noter que personne n'a mentionné l'assurance privée comme moyen de couverture médicale chez les interviewés à l'hôpital public.

Quatre des assurés rencontrés **dans les hôpitaux privés** attribuent à l'assurance la qualité de la meilleure couverture médicale, surtout pour les admis en 1ère classe. Les procédures sont faciles et la prise en charge est excellente malgré que, pour l'un d'eux l'assurance refuse de couvrir quelques actes médicaux, problème qui n'a pas d'importance vu que cette personne se permet de payer les frais de tout acte non couvert (E42, 44, 51, 52).

"أنا assurance درجة أولى ما بتصوّر في أحسن. كل شي مأمنلنا من إهتمام، خدمة وعناية." (E44)

Trois personnes jouissant de la CNSS la trouvent la meilleure, car tout est couvert (E 45, 47, 50).

Deux personnes préfèrent être couvertes par l'assurance à cause des procédures fastidieuses de la CNSS (E43, 46). Deux virent leurs choix vers les protections sociales des non-civiles qui paient même les frais de soins dentaires (E48, 53). Une personne signale que l'important c'est d'être couvert pour se protéger (E49).

### *b - Influence des couvertures médicales sur la qualité de la prise en charge*

La majorité des personnes interviewées dans **les dispensaires** n'a qu'une connaissance partielle de l'influence de la couverture médicale sur la prise en charge.

Cinq personnes ne trouvent pas de relation entre les deux et considèrent que l'équipe médicale est tenue à prendre soin de tout patient quelle que soit sa couverture (E3, 4, 14, 16, 17).

" ما في فرق بالمتابعة الطبّية، المريض بالنسبة للحكيم مريض مين ما كان عم يدفع عنّو." (E16)

Par contre deux trouvent que les soignants montrent une nonchalance à l'égard des patients admis aux frais du MSP (E20, 22).

" أكيد إذا فايتي على حساب الوزارة بدن يستلشقو فيكي. أنا جرّبتا وبعرف." (E20)

Une personne, elle-même professionnelle de santé, exprime que les hôpitaux abusent des soins en cas d'accueil des personnes assurées (E10).

"إذا الواحد فايت Assurance بينطلبلو فحوصات أكتر من غيرو، ومرّات كتير ما إلن لزوم." (E10)

Cinq des personnes dans **les hôpitaux publics** trouvent une grande différence entre l'hôpital public et l'hôpital privé. Elles pensent qu'au privé la prise en charge est plus rapide, l'admission est plus facile et l'équipe soignante est plus compétente (E30, 31, 38, 39, 40).

"وقت جيت عالمستشفى نطّروني شي ٧ ساعات قبل ما يفوتوني عأساس أنا بوضعي خرج أنطر. لو أنا بمستشفى خاص ومش عحساب الوزارة أكيد ما كنت نطرت هلقد." (E38)

Face à ces personnes, cinq autres perçoivent que les médecins sont les mêmes dans les deux secteurs. Elles disent que la qualité de soins et de prise en charge offerte est excellente et affirment que l'équipe médicale est tenue à prendre soin de tous les patients de la même manière (E28, 29, 33, 34, 35).

Les personnes rencontrées dans **les hôpitaux privés** ne trouvent dans la couverture aucune influence sur la prise

en charge (E42, 43, 44, 45, 46, 47, 49, 51, 52, 53). Deux seulement parlent de différence dans l'accueil. Elles trouvent que l'hôpital et l'équipe rattachée à cette structure accordent plus d'attention aux malades accueillis en *« première classe »* (E44, 48).

" أوّل سؤال بيسألوا بالمستشفى ضمان أو assuranceبحس إنّو بتأثّر كتير إذا كنت مضمون أو assuré على الإهتمام وخصوصي إذا كان الواحد درجة أولى أو ثانية." (E48)

***c - Problèmes des couvertures***

Pour les personnes rencontrées **dans les dispensaires,** les difficultés relevées concernant la CNSS étaient surtout d'ordre administratif : présentation des boîtes de médicaments vides pour preuve de consommation, longues files d'attente aux caisses, insuffisance d'informatisation technologique des centres de gestion, recours aux « pistons de passe-droits » et aux trafics d'influence ainsi que les problèmes rencontrés à l'admission à l'hôpital. Les personnes témoignent aussi une angoisse concernant l'avenir surtout à l'âge de la retraite, âge d'arrêt de la CNSS (E4, 10, 12, 18, 22).

"نحنا مضمونين وعمندفع الأدوية وعمنتأخّر كتير لنقبضن. المعاملات كمان صعبة. في نطرة وبهدلة" (E10)

Pour l'assurance, le problème majeur était le coût élevé des frais d'assurance et l'arrêt de la prise en charge au cas où une maladie chronique se déclenche (E8, 10, 15).

"أضرب شي ال Assurance بس تعوزيون بوقفو." (E15)

Pour les personnes rencontrées dans **les hôpitaux publics,** le sujet des couvertures sociales chez une population, majoritairement hospitalisée au compte du MSP, était douloureux. Ils regrettent l'arrêt de leur couverture CNSS et leurs expériences vécues avec la CNSS ou dans les établissements sanitaires marquaient

leurs réponses. En effet, trois des interviewés ont été couverts auparavant par la CNSS mais l'arrêt de la couverture à l'âge de la retraite (E33, 35) ou suite à l'arrêt du travail après avoir été atteints d'une maladie chronique grave (E31) est considéré par eux comme une injustice et un point faible non acceptable dans le fonctionnement de cette couverture. Ils signalent qu'après l'arrêt de la CNSS, la prise en charge de leur santé s'est complètement modifiée.

" وقت كنت مضمون كانت نفسيتي مرتاحة. كنت إقدر أمّن علاجاتي كلّا وإقدر روح على المستشفى يلّي بدّي. والله مش مقبول نظام الضمان عنّا وقت الواحد يعوزو بكبّو برّا." (E31)

Les expériences vécues par les interviewés des **hôpitaux privés,** les expériences ne montrent aucun problème vis-à-vis des couvertures médicales.

### 6.2.5. Facteurs du choix du recours et du renoncement aux soins

A la fois phénomène médical, social et économique, la notion du recours ou du renoncement aux soins couvre de multiples dimensions. En fait un comportement en santé renferme une dimension individuelle et une autre collective et sociale.

Dans l'objectif d'analyser ces comportements, la question du recours ou du renoncement aux soins en cas de maladies, ainsi que les types de remèdes utilisés sont abordés dans les entretiens.

Le choix diffère selon des variables socio-culturelles, économiques, familiales et psychologiques.

#### *a - L'âge*

L'âge constitue l'un des principaux déterminants des comportements du recours aux soins. Douze des interviewés trouvent que les enfants en bas âge sont

vulnérables et que la consultation d'un médecin est primordiale (E3, 6, 8, 9, 13, 14, 16, 20, 21, 22, 23, 26).

" لمّا بتشوفي ولدك مريض، ما بتعودي تسألي عن الدنيي كلّا، بتركضي في عند الحكيم." (E6)

" الولاد بعدن صغار ما بسترجي، دغري باخدن عند الحكيم،حرام هول طفالا." (E16)

Un interviewé considère que ses parents, âgés, ont besoin d'une prise en charge médicale immédiate devant toute symptomatologie (E11).

De manière remarquable, malgré que les frais de santé constituent un fardeau lourd pour la majorité des interviewés, ces derniers mobilisent des fonds personnels et des ressources de l'environnement pour assurer le traitement et la prise en charge médicale nécessaire aux enfants et aux personnes âgées atteintes de maladies graves. Face à ces besoins, les adultes renoncent aux soins et essaie par tous les moyens de trouver de l'argent pour les soins nécessaires. (E3, 6, 7, 9, 15, 16, 19, 21, 25).

" نحن ما وقّفنا علاج البابا ولا نهار مع إنّو علاج ال cancer مكلف كتير. العايلة ما تركتنا وبعنا شقفة أرض سيسرتنا شوي." (E19)

### *b - Situation économique*

**Au niveau des dispensaires,** trois personnes adoptent un comportement différent face à la maladie de l'enfant. La première prodigue des pratiques d'automédication (E10). La deuxième s'oriente vers le pharmacien en un premier temps (E22). La troisième résoud le problème par appel téléphonique. Tout cela pour économiser les frais des consultations (E5).

Concernant les adultes, par manque de moyens, ces derniers ne se permettent pas l'achat de leurs médicaments ou l'exécution des examens et des opérations demandées. Certains d'entre eux renoncent complètement aux soins

(E1, 5, 20, 22) d'autres reportent la prise en charge (E13, 18).

"إذا بتدقريني بإيدي بصرخ، بس ما في مادّيات. أنجأ قادرة آكل وإشرب." (E1)

**Au niveau des hôpitaux publics,** les conditions économiques constituent par excellence pour dix des interviewés le facteur majeur influençant les comportements du recours ou du renoncement aux soins. Ces personnes consultent les médecins lorsque la chance de guérison par les soins délivrés à domicile devient impossible. Leur premier choix du recours vire vers l'automédication, vers un coup de fil au médecin et vers les soins de type traditionnel. Ils supportent la douleur et cherchent à dépasser la maladie sans payer de l'argent. Ils peuvent se priver parfois des soins fondamentaux (E28, 29, 30, 31, 32, 37, 38, 39, 40, 41).

"هالمرّة لو حسّيت قادر عالج حالي ما كنت جيت عالمستشفى بس شفت حالتي بالويل خلص إجري رايحة." (E28)

" عندي مكنة oxygène بالبيت بدفع خمسين $ أجار بالشهر. الشهر يلّي بحسّ في حالي منيح بردّا توفّر شوي." (E31)

Une personne souffrant d'une maladie handicapante, se retrouve incapable d'avoir un recours adapté aux soins, en raison d'une solitude doublée d'une situation économique défavorisée. Par conséquent, elle ne peut même pas aller chercher son traitement du MSP ni se déplacer pour consulter un médecin ni solliciter une aide professionnelle qualifiée (E38).

" أنا مقطوعة من شجرة جيراني جابوني لهون. الحكيم بدّو يجددلي الإستشفا بس ما عندي حدا يعمل المعاملات. حتّى دوا ال sclérose ما في مين يأمنلي ياه." (E38)

**Au niveau des hôpitaux privés,** seulement une personne a évoqué le problème financier comme obstacle du recours, mais elle a bien précisé que la phase d'attente

avant de consulter un médecin est de deux jours seulement (E50).

" مننطر يومين بس قبل ما نروح عند الحكيم لأنّوما عمنلحّق دفع." (E50)

*c - Croyances et remèdes traditionnels*

La pratique en santé des adultes diffère selon les croyances et les valeurs personnelles. Deux grandes filières se distinguent dans le discours des interviewés : d'une part, celle faisant appel à des soins de types biomédicaux pratiqués au sein des institutions sanitaires et d'autre part, celle reposant sur des savoirs dits traditionnels.

Pour dix-huit interviewés **aux dispensaires,** l'autogestion de la maladie devance la consultation d'un spécialiste. Il s'agit soit d'une automédication ou d'usage de méthodes usuelles et traditionnelles, comme l'application sur le corps d'un linge humide visant à faire diminuer la fièvre ou aliments spéciaux, bouillis de plantes, massage d'huile…

Ces soins sont fortement inscrits dans une logique de transmission familiale ou appliqués à partir de recettes traditionnelles retirées des livres disponibles dans les maisons ou même recherchées sur internet. La gestion personnelle des maux à domicile se fait en tout début de maladie (E1, 2, 3, 5, 7, 8, 9, 10, 13, 15, 16, 18, 20, 24, 26, 27, 33, 34).

" عندي كتاب طبّ عربي، مرّة كان عندي زنّار نار، غليت بصل وزيت وشلت الزيت ودهنتو عبطني وتركتن على ٣ إيّام." (E13)

" رحت على محّل أعشاب، جبت من عندو حبوب بيوطّو الضغط، معن عمباخد حبق لأنّو الحبق كمان بيقشّط الضغط. أصلاً هلأ بوجود الinternet بيقدر الواحد يلاقي مليون وصفة." (E20)

Ces pratiques ont aussi été mentionnées par la population rencontrée dans **les hôpitaux publics.** Face à l'échec de la médecine conventionnelle, trois personnes se sont adressées aux médecins traditionnels pour traiter la

hernie discale et l'ostéoporose (E33, 35, 38) et une a visité un « *médecin voyant* » dans l'espoir de guérison (E36).

" إمّي كان عندا وجع ظهر شافت كتير حكما وما صحّت. قررنا ناخدا عند حكيم بيقرا بالكف ما صحّت رجعنا أخدناها عند حكيم عربي بصيدا." (E36)

**Au niveau des hôpitaux privés,** aucune personne n'a mentionné son recours aux pratiques traditionnelles et déclare ne pas croire à ses « *conneries* ».

" شو هالكلام الفارغ الما إلو معنى. حدا بصدّق هالأخبار وبآمن فيا." (E36)

*d - Expérience familiale*

L'expérience familiale de la maladie a provoqué le changement de comportement en santé chez trois interviewés. Ce vécu (négligence, accompagnement de malade) marquant leur histoire les pousse aujourd'hui vers la consultation médicale au moindre symptôme (E6, 17,19).

" أنا تعلّمت من تجربتي مع جوزي، توفّى من ورا الإهمال وقلّة المصاري. كنت متلو إسترخص على حالي بس اليوم إذا دقّتني شوكة بروح عند الحكيم." (E6)

" نمّلو أصابيعي جيت دغري عند حكيم المستوصف وعملت فحص دم. من بعد مرض بيّي كلّ شغلة بتقعّدني عأعصابي." (E19)

*e - Peur*

La peur prend différentes facettes dans le choix du recours ou du renoncement aux soins. Trois personnes ont recours à l'automédication comme premier comportement face à la maladie par peur de l'hospitalisation (E43, 46, 51).

"أنا بخاف من المستشفيات كتير من هيك إذا بتنزبّط بالبيت بلا روحة حكيم أحسن." (E43)

Trois autres n'osent pas s'adresser aux médecins par peur de l'annonce d'un mauvais diagnostic (E2, 4, 8)

"أنا بخاف روح أعمل فحوصات تما يبيّن شي معي بضل خايفة من النتيجة من بعد كل يلّي عمبسمعو عن الأمراض." (E8)

Pour une personne, elle se traduit par la prise de produits chimiques. Celle-ci préfère ne pas prendre des médicaments et renoncer au suivi médical (E 39). Cinq personnes ne renoncent à aucun traitement et insistent à assurer une prise en charge complète par peur d'aggravation de leur état sanitaire (E33, 34, 37, 40, 41). Deux autres suivent les traitements et les prescriptions minutieusement par peur des maladies (E42, 43).

### *f - Genre*

Une forte prévalence d'absence au recours aux soins est constatée dans le discours des hommes. Ils se considèrent plus capables de supporter la maladie et de reporter la prise en charge surtout ceux habitant la zone rurale (E 9, 11, 20).

" أنا رجّال بعالج حالي إذا صخنت.و لو في شي رجّال عكل آخ بروح عند الحكيم. بعدين نحن ولاد جبل." (E11)

### *g - Suivi thérapeutique*

Le renoncement aux soins est relié chez cinq personnes à l'amélioration de leur état de santé, lorsqu'elles se sentent mieux elles arrêtent le traitement et ne reconsultent plus le médecin (E45, 46, 47, 48, 52).

Deux autres ne donnent pas d'importance au suivi médical et disent qu'elles ont d'autres priorités. Quand elles tombent malades, elles prennent des médicaments déjà prescrits auparavant par les médecins et arrêtent leur traitement suite à une décision personnelle (E51, 53).

*h - Consultations et bilans périodiques*

**Ces pratiques de prévention ont été mentionnées uniquement par 8 personnes rencontrées dans les hôpitaux privés.** Ces interviewés font un suivi régulier chez un médecin de famille, un spécialiste et ont même avancé l'idée de l'importance de la prévention médicale (E42, 44, 45, 47, 48, 49, 52, 53).

"نحن بالبيت عنّا حكيم للعايلة، كل ما حدا صار معو شي منروح لعندو." (E45)

# Chapitre 7
# Résultats du questionnaire CNSS

Les résultats de l'enquête quantitative seront abordés dans ce chapitre sur la base du questionnaire CNSS rempli à partir des dossiers des adhérents.

## 7.1. Centre CNSS de l'enquête

### 7.1.1. Choix et description du centre

La CNSS se répartit sur 31 centres sur l'ensemble du territoire libanais. Une proximité géographique des services est assurée pour les bénéficiaires et le rattachement se fait normalement selon le siège social de la société affiliée. Un changement de centre d'affiliation est possible à effectuer par le bénéficiaire pour se rapprocher davantage de son domicile.

Cette enquête a comme objectifs d'évaluer la fréquence du recours aux soins et l'impact socio-économique laissé à la charge des familles.

Rappelons les hypothèses posées :

1 - Une couverture médicale réduit les barrières du recours aux soins.

2 - Une couverture médicale motive un meilleur contrôle sur sa santé en consultant un professionnel de santé.

3 - Le recours aux soins est fréquent chez les bénéficiaires CNSS.

4 - Une priorité est donnée par âge et par type de maladie malgré le coût socio-économique correspondant.

5 - Le coût des soins laissé à la charge des familles est lourd pour le budget moyen des familles adhérentes.

Le choix de faire l'étude de dossiers dans un centre du Kesrouan est fait pour faciliter au chercheur la collecte de données. Ce choix n'altère en rien la pertinence de l'étude étant donné que c'est le même logiciel dans tous les centres de la CNSS.

L'enquête s'est déroulée du 1er mai 2015 au 30 novembre 2015. Le centre du Kesrouan est composé de trois étages où la direction et les différents départements de la caisse se répartissent l'espace sur deux bâtiments. Il se situe en plein centre-ville de la capitale de la région, accessible par des autoroutes et par différents itinéraires des multiples villes et villages du caza.

Nombre total des employés du centre de l'enquête est de 41 employés dont 6 contractuels à l'heure et 35 contractuels permanents reçus sur concours de la fonction publique.

Nombre total des adhérents au centre de l'enquête est de 44 045 en 2015 selon le rapport d'activité du centre en question de ladite année dont 31 548 employés, 1 427 en facultatif, 83 du secteur de la boulangerie, 157 chauffeurs employés, 2 458 chauffeurs propriétaires, 5 705 étudiants, 377 médecins, 85 maires, 2 199 professeurs d'écoles, 2 du secteur maritime.

### 7.1.2. Estimation de la production du centre du Kesrouan

Au niveau de **la production du travail** de la CNSS au Liban tous centres confondus en 2011, 4234.088 demandes de remboursement de soins sont déposées et 2 939 174 demandes de soins finalisées. Au centre du Kesrouan, pour la même année, 300 000 demandes de

remboursement sont déposées et 150 000 demandes finalisées.

Une efficacité dans le rendement de travail du centre du Kesrouan est observée au cours de cette enquête à ce niveau, confirmée par les statistiques relevées en 2012 : Au cours des deux premiers semestres 2012, le centre du Kesrouan a reçu 160 000 demandes de remboursement et a pu finaliser 150 000 tandis qu'au niveau du centre de Beyrouth 340 000 demandes sont reçues à la même période et 150 000 sont finalisées (CNSS, 2014).

Une organisation du travail du centre s'est forcément améliorée et par conséquent le traitement des dossiers s'est accéléré. Le témoignage de certains adhérents d'autres centres recueillis ont confirmé l'efficacité actuelle de ce centre vis-à-vis de certains autres.

Le rapport d'activité de 2015 du centre de l'enquête montre une continuité dans cette dynamique : il y a eu 316 660 demandes de remboursement déposées et 258 218 demandes finalisées.

Dans le travail de dépouillement des questionnaires, la question 3.6 relative à la durée de la prise en charge des parents du bénéficiaire n'était pas pertinente à exploiter étant donné l'observation des changements dans les procédures concernant la couverture des parents. Une remise en priorité de la nécessité de couvrir les parents des adhérents se traduit depuis 2013 à travers des exigences réduites et une sorte de prolongation automatique suite à l'enquête à effectuer tous les cinq ans. C'est la prise de conscience par la CNSS de l'absence d'une assurance vieillesse au Liban et son souci de faire évoluer la conception de la protection sociale au Liban.

Il faut signaler que le remboursement de la CNSS a été valorisé en 2013 pour les tarifs reconnus par la caisse. Par exemple la consultation du généraliste est passée de 20 000 à

33 000 L.L. et celle d'un médecin spécialiste de 30 000 à 50 000 L.L.

### 7.1.3 Bénéficiaires et ayants droit

Rappelons que l'échantillon est accidentel et non probabiliste au sein de la population des bénéficiaires d'un centre de la région du Kesrouan. Le bénéficiaire est l'adhérent principal qui est spécifié dans certains tableaux et figures par « soi-même » pour marquer la différence avec le reste de la population décrite dans les tableaux.

### 7.1.4. Moyenne d'âge des bénéficiaires et des ayants droit

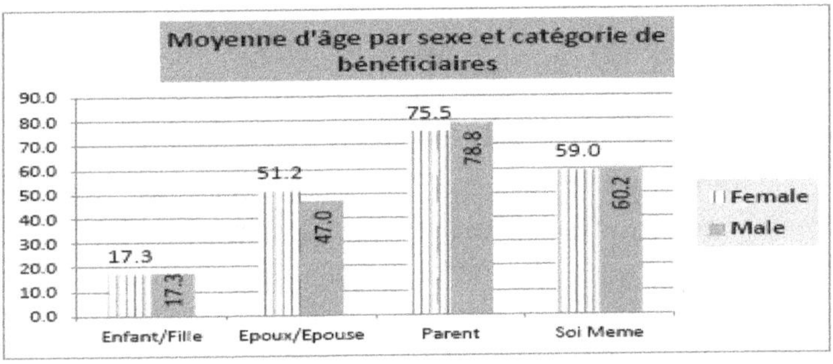


**Figure 7.1. Répartition par moyenne d'âge/ catégorie d'assurés**

**Source :** Croisement des réponses aux questions 3.1 et 3.2 du questionnaire.

La moyenne d'âge des enfants est de moins de 18 ans pour garçons et filles. Celle des épouses est de plus de 50 ans sachant qu'il n'y a qu'un seul époux parmi l'échantillon qui a 47 ans.

Tous les bénéficiaires et leurs époux/épouses ont plus de 25 ans.

### 7.1.5. Répartition par sexe

**Tableau 7.1. Bénéficiaires/type de travail**

| **Type de travail** | **N** | **%** |
|---|---|---|
| Employé | 72 | 70,6% |
| Chauffeur | 19 | 18,6% |
| Facultatif | 5 | 4,9% |
| Autres | 4 | 3,9% |
| Médecin | 2 | 2,0% |
| **Total** | **102** | **100%** |

**Source :** Réponses à la question 1 du questionnaire

**Tableau 7.2. Répartition par sexe**

| **Répartition par sexe** | | |
|---|---|---|
| Sexe | N | % |
| Femme | 203 | 57,3% |
| Homme | 151 | 42,7% |
| **Total** | **354** | **100,0%** |

**Source :** Réponses à la question 3.2 du questionnaire

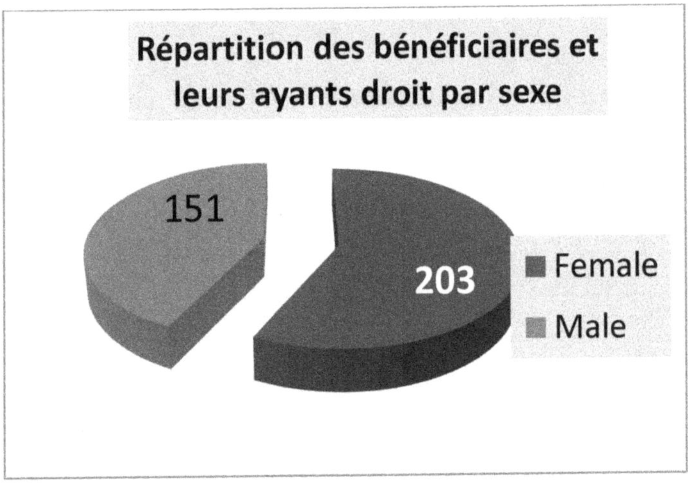


**Figure 7.2. Répartition des bénéficiaires et leurs ayants droit par sexe**

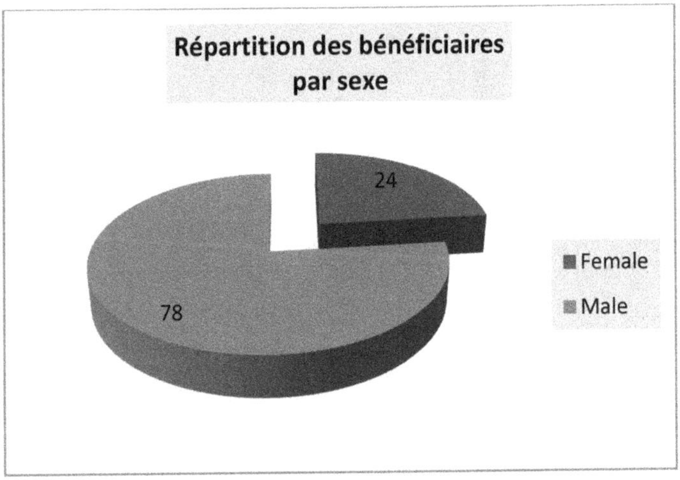


**Figure 7.3. Répartition bénéficiaires par sexe**

**Sources 7.2 et 7.3 :** Réponses à la question 3.2 du questionnaire.

La répartition par sexe (78 hommes et 24 femmes) montre que la prédominance du modèle « Monsieur gagne-pain » est présente par une majorité masculine des adhérents principaux à la CNSS.

### 7.1.6. Lien de parenté entre les bénéficiaires et les ayants droit

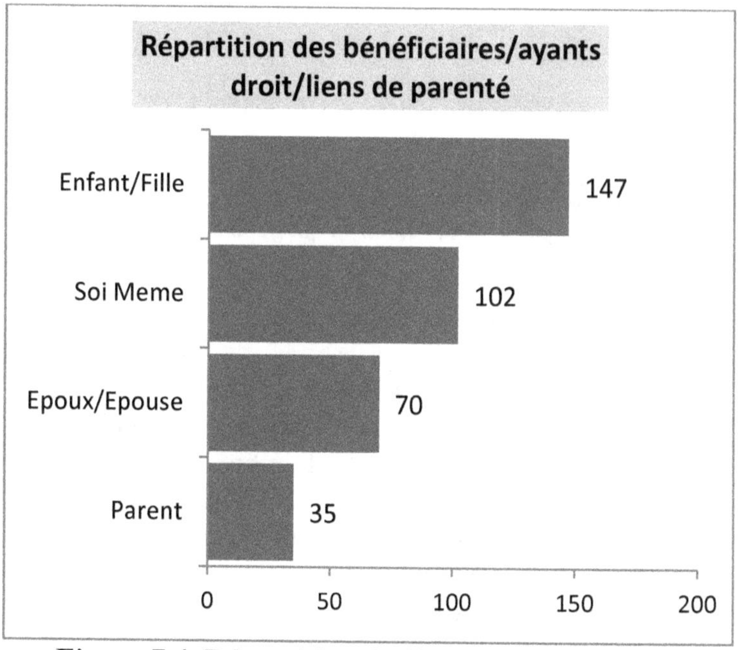


**Figure 7.4. Répartition du lien de parenté entre bénéficiaires et ayants droit**

Source : Réponses à la question 3.1 du questionnaire

**Tableau 7.3. Liens de parenté/genre.**

| **Relation** | **N** | **%** |
|---|---|---|
| Soi-même | 102 | 28,8% |
| Fille | 86 | 24,3% |
| Epouse | 69 | 19,5% |
| Enfant (garçon) | 61 | 17,2% |
| Mère | 24 | 6,8% |
| Père | 11 | 3,1% |
| Mari | 1 | 0,3% |
| **Total** | **354** | **100,0%** |

Source : Réponses des résultats des croisements entre variables des questions 3.1 et 3.2 du questionnaire.

Le nombre d'époux hommes est de 1 et celui d'épouses est de 69/70. En plus le nombre de mères couvertes est de 24/32.

Celui des filles est de 86 pour un nombre de 61 pour garçons. Pour les mères des personnes couvertes, ceci pourrait être en lien avec le nombre de femmes ne bénéficiant d'aucune ressource et d'aucune couverture médicale possible dues à l'absence d'un parcours de travail des générations précédentes de mères assignées au modèle traditionnel de femmes au foyer et d'absence d'assurance vieillesse au Liban.

## 7.2. Couverture CNSS

Les normes de couverture sont déjà décrites. Dans l'échantillon de l'enquête, elles sont réparties par sexe et par raison.

**Tableau 7.4. Couverture selon le sexe.**

| | Femme | | Homme | | Femme et Homme | |
|---|---|---|---|---|---|---|
| **Couverture** | **N** | **%** | **N** | **%** | **N** | **%** |
| Oui | 176 | 86,7% | 137 | 90,7% | 313 | 88,4% |
| Non | 27 | 13,3% | 14 | 9,3% | 41 | 11,6% |
| **Grand Total** | **203** | **100,0%** | **151** | **100,0%** | **354** | **100,0%** |

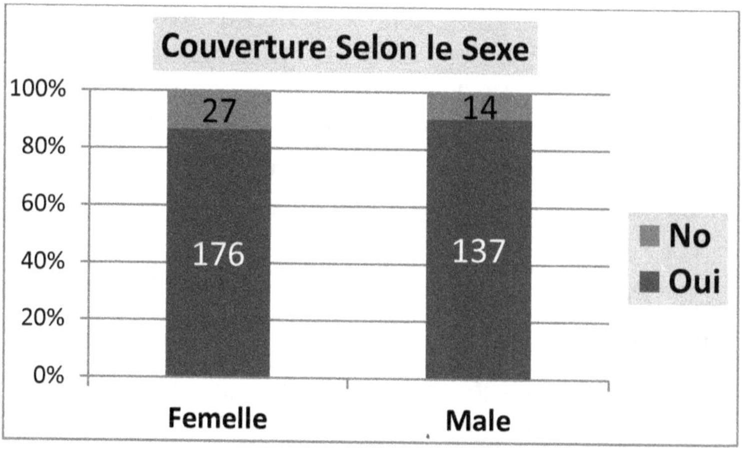


**Figure 7.5. Couverture selon le sexe.**

**Source :** Croisement des variables des questions 3.2 et 3.4.

Les personnes couvertes de l'échantillon sont 176 femmes et 137 hommes. Les 14 personnes de sexe masculin font partie de la catégorie enfants/garçons et ils ne répondent plus aux conditions requises donc ayant plus de 18 et n'effectuant pas des études ou ayant plus de 25 ans.

Pour les femmes, 27 femmes ne sont pas couvertes. Le tableau 7.5 informe sur les raisons de cette couverture et aide à déduire les raisons de la non-couverture.

**Tableau 7.5. Raison de couverture des ayants droit**

| Raison de couverture (autre que le bénéficiaire soi-même) | | |
|---|---|---|
| **Relation avec le bénéficiaire** | **N** | **%** |
| **Enfant/Fille** | | |
| < 18 ans | 85 | 41,1% |
| < 25 ans, étudiant | 28 | 13,5% |
| **Total (Enfant/Fille)** | **113** | **54,6%** |
| **Epoux/Epouse (Ne travaille pas)** | **63** | **30,4%** |
| **Parent (> 60 ans)** | **31** | **15,0%** |
| **Grand Total** | **207** | **100,0%** |

Source : Réponses à la question 3.5 du questionnaire.

Parmi la catégorie féminine non couverte, il y a 21 filles et 6 épouses. Six sur soixante-neuf épouses travaillent donc et bénéficient d'une autre couverture sociale. Vingt et une filles doivent avoir plus de 25 ans ou bien avoir moins de 25 ans, mais être travailleuses rémunérées ou mariées.

## 7.3. Période totale de couverture CNSS des bénéficiaires

Il s'agit dans cette variable du total de la période d'affiliation du bénéficiaire sur le long de sa vie à ce jour. Elle regroupe les différentes affiliations chez les mêmes employeurs ou différents employeurs même entrecoupées.

La durée de couverture est une condition pour l'obtention des indemnités de fin de service. Selon le guide de l'assuré (2010), il faudra valider un total de minimum de 20 ans cumulés pour avoir droit à un calcul d'indemnités de fin de service.

Les conditions pour l'obtention de ces indemnités permettent une sorte de protection sociale pour les bénéficiaires en cas d'incapacité… Elles se résument dans l'une des conditions suivantes :

- durée de travail minimum de 20 ans ;
- être atteint d'une invalidité de 50% minimum validée suite à une expertise médicale qui l'empêche de continuer à travailler ;
- la femme mariée peut en bénéficier si elle a quitté son travail au cours des douze mois suivant la date de son mariage ;
- avoir atteint l'âge légal (60-64 ans) ;
- en cas de décès de l'employé assuré, les ayants droit pourront bénéficier de ces indemnités citées.

**Tableau 7.6. Période de couverture des bénéficiaires**

| **Période de couverture (le bénéficiaire soi-même)** | | |
|---|---|---|
| **Période de couverture** | **N** | **%** |
| < 5 ans | 3 | 2,9% |
| 5- 10 ans | 24 | 23,5% |
| 11- 15 ans | 23 | 22,5% |
| 16- 20 ans | 15 | 14,7% |
| 21- 25 ans | 9 | 8,8% |
| > 25 ans | 22 | 21,6% |
| Missing Data | 6 | 5,9% |
| **Grand Total** | **102** | **100,0%** |

**Source :** Réponses à la question 2 du questionnaire.

**Tableau 7.7. Couverture par catégorie d'ayants droit par âge**

| Couverture par catégorie de bénéficiaire | Femme | Homme | Grand Total |
|---|---|---|---|
| **Couvert** | **176** | **137** | **313** |
| **Enfant/Fille** | **64** | **49** | **113** |
| < 25 | 63 | 40 | 103 |
| 25 + | 1 | 9 | 10 |
| **Epoux/Epouse** | **65** | | **65** |
| 25 + | 65 | | 65 |
| **Parent** | **23** | **10** | **33** |
| 25 + | 23 | 10 | 33 |
| **Soi-même** | **24** | **78** | **102** |
| 25 + | 24 | 78 | 102 |
| **Pas couvert** | **27** | **14** | **41** |
| **Enfant/Fille** | **22** | **12** | **34** |
| < 25 | 5 | | 5 |
| 25 + | 17 | 12 | 29 |
| **Epoux/Epouse** | **4** | **1** | **5** |
| 25 + | 4 | 1 | 5 |
| **Parent** | **1** | **1** | **2** |
| 25 + | 1 | 1 | 2 |
| **Grand Total** | **203** | **151** | **354** |

Source : Croisement des réponses aux questions 3.1., 3.2 et 3.3 du questionnaire.

Les résultats de la couverture en fonction de l'âge montrent :

- que tous les bénéficiaires en titre ont plus de 25 ans dans l'échantillon ;
- la continuité des couvertures des filles de moins de 25 ans sans condition de continuité des études comme pour les garçons ;
- le nombre de filles de moins de 25 ans non couvertes est de 5 sur 63. Elles ne sont plus à la charge du bénéficiaire (activité professionnelle rémunérée, mariage…).

## 7.4. Services utilisés

Au niveau du questionnaire, les détails des recours sont établis par type de bénéficiaire ou ayants droit, date du recours, type de service utilisé et coût de cette utilisation.

Cela est réparti sur la question 5 qui est divisée en plusieurs variables spécifiques en fonction des services assurés selon les conditions imposées par la CNSS.

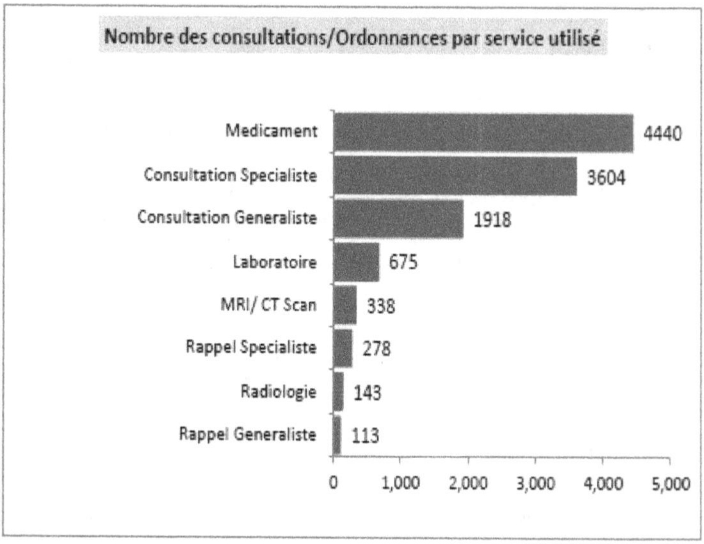


**Figure 7.6. Type de services de Recours demandés par les assurés.**

**Source :** Réponses à la question 5 du questionnaire.

**Tableau 7.8. Nombre total des transactions et pourcentage par type de service utilisé**

| | | |
|---|---|---|
| **Consultation generalist** | 1 918 | 32,3% |
| **Rappel generalist** | 113 | 1,9% |
| **Consultation specialist** | 3 604 | 60,6% |
| **Rappel specialist** | 278 | 4,7% |
| **Médicament** | 4 440 | 74,7% |
| **Laboratoire** | 675 | 11,4% |
| **Radiologie** | 143 | 2,4% |
| **IRM/CT Scan** | 338 | 5,7% |

**Source :** Réponses à la question 5 du questionnaire

N.B. Les nombres dans le tableau 7.8 sont pris des 5943 transactions traitées. On peut ajouter plusieurs transactions par assuré, car il peut avoir recours à plus d'un seul service par transaction. Pour cette raison, le total des pourcentages peut aller au-delà de 100%.

Le nombre de recours le plus fréquent est celui de la consommation de médicaments. Ce sont des médicaments délivrés sur ordonnance par un médecin agrée par la CNSS.

Le centre est dans la région du Kesrouan. Tous les médecins traitants et délivrant les ordonnances sont connus par le service médical et le médecin de la caisse se met en contact direct avec eux selon le besoin.

Une sorte de contrôle s'exerce dans l'estimation des remboursements de certaines consultations lorsqu'un abus est suspecté.

L'observation effectuée au sein du centre a montré l'exercice de ce contrôle qui est approuvé par les employés qui ont également le souci de réduire les abus. Ce contrôle pourrait dans certaines situations amener à une annulation des frais de consultations, mais pas à celle du remboursement du coût de médicaments. Cela explique

entre autres le nombre élevé de médicaments remboursés en comparaison avec celui des consultations.

Les rappels des consultations des généralistes et des spécialistes donc les questions 5.4 et 5.6 doivent être à un minimum de deux semaines pour qu'ils soient remboursés à moitié sinon aucun remboursement des frais n'est possible.

Les IRM/Scan doivent être faits après accord préalable de la caisse.

Les consultations des spécialistes sont nombreuses, mais constituent l'ensemble des spécialistes décrits dans le tableau 7.9. Au Liban il n'y a pas d'obligation de médecins traitants pour chaque famille comme en France par exemple. Le patient peut s'orienter directement vers un spécialiste sans passer par un généraliste.

## Tableau 7.9. Répartition consultation par catégorie d'assuré par spécialité de médecin

| | Enfant/Fille | | Epoux/Epouse | | Parent | | Soi-même | | Total | |
|---|---|---|---|---|---|---|---|---|---|---|
| Spécialité | N | % | N | % | N | % | N | % | N | % |
| Généraliste | 225 | 27,0% | 514 | 36,3% | 446 | 35,2% | 870 | 35,8% | 2055 | 34,6% |
| Cardiologie | 6 | 0,7% | 94 | 6,6% | 93 | 7,3% | 328 | 13,5% | 521 | 8,8% |
| Médecine interne | 15 | 1,8% | 72 | 5,1% | 174 | 13,7% | 123 | 5,1% | 384 | 6,5% |
| Pédiatrie | 347 | 41,7% | 8 | 0,6% | 1 | 0,1% | 7 | 0,3% | 363 | 6,1% |
| Gynécologie/Obstétrie | 14 | 1,7% | 191 | 13,5% | 6 | 0,5% | 84 | 3,5% | 295 | 5,0% |
| Urologie | 5 | 0,6% | 8 | 0,6% | 105 | 8,3% | 108 | 4,4% | 226 | 3,8% |
| Endocrinologie | 3 | 0,4% | 34 | 2,4% | 24 | 1,9% | 160 | 6,6% | 221 | 3,7% |
| Chirurgie générale | 24 | 2,9% | 51 | 3,6% | 47 | 3,7% | 86 | 3,5% | 208 | 3,5% |
| Chirurgie orthopédie | 5 | 0,6% | 40 | 2,8% | 71 | 5,6% | 70 | 2,9% | 186 | 3,1% |
| Oncologie | 24 | 2,9% | 118 | 8,3% | 23 | 1,8% | 17 | 0,7% | 182 | 3,1% |
| Maladies infectieuses | 5 | 0,6% | 67 | 4,7% | 41 | 3,2% | 46 | 1,9% | 159 | 2,7% |
| Néphrologie | 2 | 0,2% | 5 | 0,4% | 92 | 7,3% | 43 | 1,8% | 142 | 2,4% |
| Médecine de la famille | 4 | 0,5% | 32 | 2,3% | 11 | 0,9% | 81 | 3,3% | 128 | 2,2% |
| Otorhino | 31 | 3,7% | 29 | 2,0% | 9 | 0,7% | 57 | 2,3% | 126 | 2,1% |
| Pathologie clinique | | 0,0% | 29 | 2,0% | | 0,0% | 80 | 3,3% | 109 | 1,8% |
| Gastroentérologie | 16 | 1,9% | 19 | 1,3% | 6 | 0,5% | 67 | 2,8% | 108 | 1,8% |
| Ophtalmologie | 25 | 3,0% | 12 | 0,8% | 45 | 3,6% | 20 | 0,8% | 102 | 1,7% |
| Rhumatologie | 2 | 0,2% | 5 | 0,4% | 20 | 1,6% | 73 | 3,0% | 100 | 1,7% |
| Pneumonologie | 13 | 1,6% | 19 | 1,3% | 29 | 2,3% | 38 | 1,6% | 99 | 1,7% |
| Psychiatrie | 33 | 4,0% | 38 | 2,7% | 2 | 0,2% | 18 | 0,7% | 91 | 1,5% |
| Dermatologie | 26 | 3,1% | 14 | 1,0% | 2 | 0,2% | 8 | 0,3% | 50 | 0,8% |
| (blank) | 3 | 0,4% | 9 | 0,6% | 7 | 0,6% | 18 | 0,7% | 37 | 0,6% |
| Neurologie | | 0,0% | | 0,0% | 3 | 0,2% | 9 | 0,4% | 12 | 0,2% |
| Chirurgie cardiovasculaire | | 0,0% | 2 | 0,1% | 2 | 0,2% | 5 | 0,2% | 9 | 0,2% |
| Chirurgie esthétique | 1 | 0,1% | 2 | 0,1% | 3 | 0,2% | 2 | 0,1% | 8 | 0,1% |
| Spécialité non définie | 1 | 0,1% | 1 | 0,1% | 2 | 0,2% | 4 | 0,2% | 8 | 0,1% |
| Ansethésie réanimation | | 0,0% | 1 | 0,1% | | 0,0% | 5 | 0,2% | 6 | 0,1% |
| Médecine d'urgence | 2 | 0,2% | 1 | 0,1% | 1 | 0,1% | 1 | 0,0% | 5 | 0,1% |
| Allergologie | | 0,0% | 1 | 0,1% | | 0,0% | | 0,0% | 1 | 0,0% |
| Dentiste | | 0,0% | | 0,0% | | 0,0% | 1 | 0,0% | 1 | 0,0% |
| Chirurgie vasculaire | | 0,0% | | 0,0% | 1 | 0,1% | | 0,0% | 1 | 0,0% |
| Grand Total | 832 | 100,0% | 1416 | 100,0% | 1266 | 100,0% | 2429 | 100,0% | 5943 | 100,0% |

**Source :** Réponses aux questions 5.1 et 5.16 du questionnaire.

## Tableau 7.10. Consultations généralistes par Catégorie d'assuré

| | Enfant/Fille | | Epoux/Epouse | | Parent | | Soi-même | | Toutes catégories | |
|---|---|---|---|---|---|---|---|---|---|---|
| Catégorie d'utilisation | N | % | N | % | N | % | N | % | N | % |
| Utilisé | 220 | 26% | 471 | 33% | 412 | 33% | 815 | 34% | 1918 | 32% |
| Non utilize | 612 | 74% | 945 | 67% | 854 | 67% | 1614 | 66% | 4025 | 68% |
| Grand Total | 832 | 100% | 1416 | 100% | 1266 | 100% | 2429 | 100% | 5943 | 100% |

**Source :** Réponses aux questions 5.1 et 5.16 du questionnaire.

Les résultats obtenus au tableau 7.10 montrent une fréquentation importante de la totalité des assurés chez le généraliste. Les normes d'usage chez les personnes couvertes de l'échantillon consistent à consulter un généraliste en premier ou selon la situation du malade. Ces résultats montrent que le généraliste est le référent médical des ménages de l'échantillon de l'enquête.

## Tableau 7.11. Consultation généraliste par tranche d'âge

| | < 60 | | 60 et plus | | Toutes Catégories | |
|---|---|---|---|---|---|---|
| **Catégorie d'utilisation** | **N** | **%** | **N** | **%** | **N** | **%** |
| Utilisé | 948 | 32% | 970 | 33% | 1918 | 32% |
| Non Utilisé | 2045 | 68% | 1943 | 67% | 3988 | 68% |
| **Grand Total** | **2993** | **100%** | **2913** | **100%** | **5906** | **100%** |

**Source :** Réponses aux questions 5.2 et 5.16 du questionnaire.

La différence entre les moins et les plus de 60 ans n'est pas significative dans le recours à un généraliste ce qui confirme le recours premier des ménages à ses services. Le coût inférieur de la consultation du généraliste pourrait contribuer à favoriser ce facteur.

**Tableau 7.12. Consultations des spécialistes les plus utilisées par catégorie d'assuré.**

| **Les premiers trois services des médecins spécialistes les plus utilisés selon la catégorie de l'assuré** | | | |
|---|---|---|---|
| Catégorie | Spécialité | N | % |
| Soi-même | Cardiologie | 301 | 21,3% |
| | Endocrinologie | 142 | 10,0% |
| | Médecine Interne | 118 | 8,4% |
| Parent | Médecine Interne | 170 | 21,7% |
| | Urologie | 100 | 12,7% |
| | Néphrologie | 91 | 11,6% |
| Epoux/Epouse | Gynécologie Obstétrie | 178 | 21,1% |
| | Oncologie | 110 | 13,0% |
| | Cardiologie | 87 | 10,3% |
| Enfant/Fille | Pédiatrie | 304 | 54,1% |
| | Otorhino | 30 | 5,3% |
| | Psychiatrie | 29 | 5,2% |

**Source :** Réponses aux questions 5.1 et 5.16 du questionnaire.

Les résultats du tableau 7.12 montrent un taux de consultations par catégorie souvent liée aux exigences de l'âge et le sexe de l'assuré notamment en ce qui concerne la gynécologie/obstétrie pour les épouses en âge de procréer ; les pédiatres pour les enfants dont la moyenne d'âge est de moins de 17 ans et les cardiologues pour les bénéficiaires composés d'une majorité d'hommes avec une moyenne d'âge au-dessus de 40 ans.

La catégorie du Parent présente des recours ayant attrait aux maladies chroniques avec 170 consultations de médecine interne, 100 en urologie et 91 en néphrologie tout en présentant un recours régulier auprès des généralistes dans le tableau 7.11.

## 7.5. Fréquence des recours par famille

La fréquence des recours pourrait se constater par le nombre de recours aux services par famille par an.

**Tableau 7.13. Fréquence consultation généraliste par famille par mois**

| Année | Minimum | Maximum | Moyenne | Nombre total des consultations |
|---|---|---|---|---|
| 2012 | 1 | 7 | 1,6 | 605 |
| 2013 | 1 | 6 | 1,5 | 515 |
| 2014 | 1 | 6 | 1,5 | 551 |
| 2015 | 1 | 5 | 1,6 | 236 |
| Grand Total | 1 | 7 | 1,5 | 1907 |

**Source :** Réponses aux questions 5.1, 5.2, 5.3 et 5.4.

Un minimum d'une consultation de généraliste par mois est présent sur toutes les années. Le maximum de visite se situe de 5 à 7 consultations par mois. La moyenne est à peu près **d'une consultation et demie par mois par famille.**

Ce sont des moyennes stables qui marquent une régularité chez les familles enquêtées dans le recours à la consultation d'un généraliste.

**Tableau 7.14. Fréquence consultation spécialiste par famille par mois**

| Date | Minimum | Maximum | Moyenne | Nombre Total Des Consultations |
|---|---|---|---|---|
| 2012 | 1 | 10 | 2,0 | 1003 |
| 2013 | 1 | 11 | 2,0 | 1098 |
| 2014 | 1 | 11 | 1,9 | 1082 |
| 2015 | 1 | 7 | 1,9 | 412 |
| Grand Total | 1 | 11 | 2,0 | 3595 |

**Source :** Réponses aux questions 5.1, 5.2, 5.5, 5.6.

Un minimum autour de 1 et un maximum autour de 10 consultations par mois par famille. La moyenne varie autour de deux visites par mois par famille. En consultant le tableau des consultations des spécialistes 7.12, il est constaté que c'est lié à la priorité par âge et par pathologie : pédiatrie, oncologie et endocrinologie (pour le cancer), cardiologie, gynécologie obstétrie…

**Tableau 7.15. Fréquence du recours aux médicaments par famille par mois**

| Moyenne des ordonnances médicaments par famille par mois | | | | |
|---|---|---|---|---|
| Date | Minimum | Maximum | Moyenne | Ordonnances au Total |
| 2012 | 1 | 8 | 1,9 | 1290 |
| 2013 | 1 | 8 | 1,9 | 1275 |
| 2014 | 1 | 7 | 1,9 | 1329 |
| 2015 | 1 | 7 | 1,8 | 532 |
| Grand Total | 1 | 8 | 1,9 | 4426 |

**Source :** Réponses aux questions 5.1, 5.2 et 5.7.

La moyenne des ordonnances tourne autour de deux par mois et par famille. Le nombre total revient autour des mêmes valeurs tous les ans. Il n'y a pas de pics significatifs entre les différents mois dans les résultats obtenus ce qui montre une régularité dans l'achat des médicaments sur ordonnance pour obtenir le remboursement. Une légère hausse de 2013 à 2014 est observée. Elle pourrait être en lien avec les délais plus courts de traitement des dossiers et la revalorisation du seuil de remboursement également.

### 7.6. Coûts socio-économiques

Les coûts socio-économiques restant à la charge des familles se basent sur un calcul de la différence entre le prix réel payé par famille pour les services utilisés (consultations, médicaments et autres services…) d'une part et le remboursement à 80% ou à 90% du tarif fixé par la CNSS pour les services listés d'autre part.

Le prix réel payé par les familles pour les consultations est détaillé dans le tableau 7.15 et celui pour les services utilisés autres que consultations dans le tableau 7.16. Ensuite nous avons calculé le coût laissé au détriment des familles concernant les services utilisés hors consultations et par la suite consultations incluses.

Le prix des consultations est limité en comparaison avec celui des autres services utilisés notamment tout ce qui est lié aux soins du cancer et de la dialyse malgré le taux de remboursement situé jusqu'à 90% pour ces catégories-là.

Pour évaluer l'impact du coût des soins sur les budgets des familles, le salaire déclaré à la caisse correspond généralement au salaire minimum pour une grande partie des adhérents enquêtés. Ce salaire minimum est de 600 000 L.L. l'équivalent de 400$.

### 7.6.1. Coûts réels payés par les familles

Il s'agit des prix réels payés par les familles pour les consultations de généralistes et de spécialistes et les prix réels payés par les familles pour les services utilisés autres que Consultations.

**Tableau 7.16. Prix réel payé par consultation par famille par an**

| Année | Nombre de familles par an | Minimum | Maximum | Moyenne | Total |
|---|---|---|---|---|---|
| 2012 | 89 | 20 000 | 1 355 000 | 284 542 | 20 771 600 |
| 2013 | 95 | 30 000 | 1 516 000 | 430 755 | 36 183 460 |
| 2014 | 99 | 30 000 | 1 350 000 | 430 333 | 37 439 000 |
| 2015 | 96 | 30 000 | 780 000 | 177 558 | 13 672 000 |
| **Grand Total** | **379** | **20 000** | **1 516 000** | **336 654** | **108 066 060** |

NB: Les données 2015 couvrent jusqu'à fin juin 2015.
**Source** : Réponses aux questions 5.1, 5.2, 5.11.

Cette question montre le coût minimum payé par consultation médicale effectuée. Un minimum de 20 000 L.L. est payé ; prix de consultation pouvant correspondre à celui d'une consultation d'un généraliste en général. C'était le prix adopté par la CNSS en 2012. Par la suite le prix s'est aligné sur la revalorisation du prix de la consultation généraliste par la Caisse.

Le salaire minimum par an est donc de 12 x 600 000 = 7 200 000 L.L. La moyenne pourrait atteindre 430 333 L.L. ce qui correspond à peu près à 16,8% du salaire.

Les dépassements des tarifications des consultations ses constatent dans les maxima décrits surtout en ce qui concerne les spécialistes. Certains oncologues peuvent avoir des prix de 120 000 L.L. à 175 000 L.L. par consultation.

Alors que pour les généralistes ce sont des prix qui peuvent être de 30 000 à 50 000 L.L. en général.

Il faudra signaler que les 102 familles de l'enquête peuvent ne pas figurer sur l'ensemble des années ou changer ou avoir des arrêts de prise en charge d'où le nombre des familles qui n'est pas toujours 102.

**Tableau 7.17. Coût total réel payé par famille pour services autres que consultations par an**

| Année | Nombre de familles par an | Minimum | Maximum | Moyenne | Total |
|---|---|---|---|---|---|
| 2012 | 89 | 146 390 | 13 531 656 | 2 510 849 | 223 465 601 |
| 2013 | 95 | 22 908 | 18 882 019 | 2 742 390 | 260 527 092 |
| 2014 | 99 | 84 281 | 15 128 986 | 2 973 587 | 294 385 145 |
| 2015 | 96 | 15 750 | 8 551 253 | 1 209 298 | 116 092 569 |
| **Grand Total** | **379** | **15 750** | **18 882 019** | **2 360 080** | **894 470 407** |

NB: Les données 2015 couvrent jusqu'à fin juin 2015.
**Source :** Réponses aux questions 5.1, 5.2, 5.13.

Le coût relatif aux autres services utilisés que les consultations constitue l'essentiel des dépenses en santé étudiées.

Le minimum payé est le plus élevé en 2014, mais les montants maximums par an peuvent dépasser le total des salaires déclarés et perçus par les adhérents. Les retards des remboursements pourront affecter les budgets des familles et contribuer à des difficultés socio-économiques majeures.

### 7.6.2. Coût restant à la charge des familles

Le coût réel restant à la charge des familles et qui peut constituer un poids socio-économique lié aux soins de santé est calculé dans les tableaux qui suivent. Etant donné les prix

limités des consultations, fut privilégié le coût laissé au détriment des familles pour les services utilisés autres que les consultations pour les inclure par la suite dans le calcul total des coûts laissés à la charge des familles.

**Tableau 7.18. Coût laissé à la charge de la famille/an pour les services utilisés autres que consultations**

| **Coût laissé au détriment du patient autre que consultation par famille par an** | | | | | |
|---|---|---|---|---|---|
| **Année** | **Nombre de familles par an** | **Minimum** | **Maximum** | **Moyenne** | **Total** |
| 2012 | 89 | 33 844 | 3 248 696 | 636 834 | 56 678 194 |
| 2013 | 95 | 4 582 | 3 838 252 | 635 881 | 60 408 725 |
| 2014 | 99 | 16 856 | 4 838 576 | 760 106 | 75 250 491 |
| 2015 | 96 | 3 150 | 1 710 171 | 293 892 | 28 213 647 |
| **Grand Total** | **379** | **3 150** | **4 838 576** | **581 929** | **220 551 057** |

NB: Les données 2015 couvrent jusqu'à fin juin 2015.

**Source** : Résultats de calcul basé sur les réponses aux questions 5.13 et 5.15 selon les taux de remboursement fixés par la CNSS.

Les coûts laissés à la charge des familles constituent un poids handicapant pour les budgets des familles. La moyenne revient à un salaire minimum ou un peu plus par an.

**Tableau 7.19. Coût laissé à la charge de la famille/an pour consultations et autres services utilisés.**

| Coût laissé au détriment du patient par famille par an | | | | | |
|---|---|---|---|---|---|
| **Année** | **Nombre de familles par an** | **Minimum** | **Maximum** | **Moyenne** | **Total** |
| 2012 | 72 | 26 714 | 2 764 910 | 412 500 | 29 699 968 |
| 2013 | 84 | 19 742 | 2 165 034 | 484 046 | 40 659 903 |
| 2014 | 87 | 23 132 | 2 404 614 | 491 019 | 42 718 650 |
| 2015 | 77 | 12 246 | 1 710 575 | 234 268 | 18 038 616 |
| **Grand Total** | **320** | **12 246** | **2 764 910** | **409 741** | **131 117 137** |

**NB : Les données 2015 couvrent jusqu'à fin juin 2015.**

Source : Réponses basées sur les questions 5.11, 5.13 et 5.15.

En incluant tous les services utilisés, les remboursements de la CNSS présentent une moyenne régulière du coût moyen restant à la charge des familles. Il peut arriver à l'équivalent de 15% d'un salaire minimum mensuel.

## 7.7. Résultats et hypothèses

Les hypothèses numéros 1, 2 et 3 sont validées dans cette enquête à partir de la fréquence de consultations constatées par famille par an auprès des généralistes et des spécialistes qui se situeront dans une motivation à mieux contrôler la santé de ses membres. Le nombre de recours aux différents services utilisés révèle également la réduction des barrières de soins. Toutes les familles choisies accidentellement ont bénéficié des services étudiés et ont bénéficié des remboursements de la CNSS. Une fréquence d'une moyenne de visite par an et par famille d'une et demie à un généraliste et de deux visites à un spécialiste ressort des résultats, ce qui présente un lien continu avec les professionnels de santé et un accès régulier aux

pharmaciens et aux centres de santé des services prescrits et suivis.

Une baisse de l'automédication pourrait être également constatée par le nombre d'achat de médicaments sur ordonnance de médecins généralistes soient-ils ou spécialistes. C'est une moyenne qui tourne autour de deux ordonnances par mois et par famille.

Le contrôle sur la santé est également constaté dans les résultats par la régularité de recours aux consultations de généralistes et de spécialistes. Cette régularité s'observe dans un maintien d'une moyenne de fréquence stable sur les années étudiées. Ce contrôle est également favorisé par le recours à la consultation du généraliste en premier, considéré souvent comme le référent médical de la famille et dont la consultation est moins onéreuse pour le budget familial.

L'hypothèse 4 est également validée : le taux élevé de consultations des pédiatres et des gynécologues ainsi que celles de médecine interne pour les parents sont révélateurs de la priorité du recours en fonction de l'âge. Les consultations régulières par catégorie d'assurés tableau 7.12. sont révélatrices de la priorité donnée par type de maladie notamment pour le cancer, la dialyse et les maladies cardiaques.

Le lourd fardeau laissé à la charge des familles est constaté dans les résultats et répond à l'hypothèse 5. Le coût des soins restant après remboursement dépasse les revenus moyens des familles enquêtées déclarés à la CNSS.

La contribution de la CNSS au remboursement des consultations allège la moyenne laissée à la charge des familles et participerait à une meilleure régularité dans l'accès aux soins. Cependant, le mystère demeure concernant ces dépassements des coûts en comparaison avec les revenus des familles au Liban.

Le nombre d'emplois non déclarés comme les petits emplois, les dépannages, le travail de l'agriculture et le commerce, etc. d'une part et la contribution des Libanais de l'émigration au soutien de leurs familles au Liban pourront être une explication à ce phénomène économiquement inégal et impossible. En effet, l'étude de Kasparian (2014) a démontré que 55% des émigrés libanais dans le monde font des virements réguliers à leurs familles pour essentiellement : 64,4% pour de la nourriture ; 58,9% pour des frais de logement et 53,9% pour améliorer la vie quotidienne.

Ces résultats et ces hypothèses seront discutés conceptuellement dans le chapitre 8 conjointement avec les résultats de l'étude qualitative dans le cadre conceptuel adopté de Kreuter and Green qui comprend les composantes de Aday et Anderson ainsi que les déterminants du comportement planifié de Azjen et Fishbein.

# Chapitre 8
# Discussion des résultats de cette recherche

La discussion des résultats obtenus dans cette recherche se fera sur la base du modèle conceptuel de Green et Kreuter. Une évaluation des déterminants sociaux et psychosociaux des comportements en santé adoptés par la population cible sera discutée à la lumière de la littérature internationale.

Les facteurs influençant le comportement étudié sont classés en trois catégories : prédisposants, facilitants et de renforcement. Ils sont présents dans le modèle d'Anderson et Aday décrit dans la littérature, mais seront abordés dans l'approche encore plus globale de Green et Kreuter pour favoriser une proposition d'une stratégie adaptée en promotion de la santé. Le modèle du comportement planifié sera également une référence pour la discussion des facteurs prédisposants au comportement de recours aux soins pour la pertinence de nos résultats.

## 8.1. Facteurs prédisposants

Les facteurs prédisposants comportent des caractéristiques sociodémographiques et culturelles du malade ou de son entourage immédiat. Ils abordent des opinions sur le système de soins, des croyances et valeurs concernant la santé et la maladie et des connaissances au sujet de la maladie. Ceux-ci incitent à concevoir une attitude envers un certain comportement, le recours ou non

en cas de besoin, à un service de santé (Beaudry, Hamelin, 2006). Les facteurs prédisposants retenus pour cette recherche sont les facteurs sociodémographiques et culturels, les composantes de la perception de la santé, les croyances et les connaissances thérapeutiques, les émotions de peur et de crainte ainsi que les attitudes envers les établissements.

### 8.1.1. Facteurs sociodémographiques et culturels

#### *Âge*

Parmi les variables sociodémographiques, l'**âge** du malade, est sans doute une composante essentielle ayant un impact sur la décision de consulter ou non un service de santé et sur le choix du type de recours. Il semble se dégager une tendance à l'utilisation préférentielle des soins modernes pour les enfants, surtout les plus jeunes. Par contre, les adultes dans un contexte de ressources financières limitées, recourent davantage aux thérapies traditionnelles.

Cette enquête CNSS a montré une prévalence dans des consultations des pédiatres pour les enfants et celles de cardiologie pour les hommes et de gynécologie obstétrie pour les femmes.

Le Liban a plus d'unités de chirurgie cardiaque par habitant que l'Allemagne, mais souffre d'une insuffisance de programmes de prévention et de sensibilisation autour des maladies cardiovasculaires dans la communauté libanaise (Ammar, 2003). En effet, en 2010 plus de 4 000 procédures d'intervention cardiaque étaient financées par Le ministère de Santé publique ce qui a monopolisé une grande partie des dépenses publiques en santé (Statistical Bulletin 2010, 2013).

Les enfants et les soins à la maternité pour les femmes en âge de procréer sont des priorités et cela se révèle dans la prévalence élevée des consultations des pédiatres et des

gynécologues. Une étude plus poussée sur le contenu des ordonnances des pédiatres pourra renseigner sur les pics d'infections, sur les vaccinations et déterminer plus clairement des périodes ou des situations d'enfants à risque pour contribuer à la réduction de la mortalité infantile (9/1 000) et la mortalité maternelle (18/100 000) qui restent élevées au Liban (MOPH, 2016).

### *Entre hommes et femmes*

Dans cette recherche, il était identifié et approuvé que les hommes interviewés aient plus tendance que les femmes à être passifs en cas de maladie et à avoir moins recours aux services de santé, un fait qui rejoint des résultats internationaux comme ceux de Shields et Shooshtari (2001).

Généralement, les hommes rencontrés durant les entretiens semi-directifs préfèrent économiser les frais dispensés en santé pour financer d'autres besoins plus élémentaires de leurs familles. Leurs repères de l'**image masculine** leur imposent de se montrer forts, capables de supporter la douleur. Ceci se révèle notamment dans le discours des hommes interviewés qui habitent la montagne.

### *Religion, culture et genre*

Concernant la **religion**, la recherche n'a pas montré des différences remarquables dans l'accès aux soins. Ceci est dû à la représentativité limitée de la religion islamique (11/53) dans notre population. Pourtant quelques particularités ont été relevées concernant la perception de la santé et la présence élevée de médecins traditionnels dans les zones habitées par une majorité musulmane.

Le déterminant du genre se conjugue à celui de la religion pour favoriser un recours culturel chez une professionnelle de santé du même sexe, notamment le choix des femmes notamment « voilées » et « de quartiers

populaires défavorisés du Liban » d'une sage-femme pour leur suivi gynécologique et de grossesse au sein des dispensaires.

*Niveau d'éducation*

Le **niveau d'éducation** des adultes est observé en lien direct avec la décision du recours. Les personnes rencontrées, ayant suivi des études universitaires ont tendance à utiliser en premier les services médicaux, élément retrouvé également chez Guyon (1988), Fassin et Aäch (2004). Les personnes qui ont un niveau éducatif supérieur ont tendance à mener un mode de vie sain et à adopter des mesures préventives face aux maladies, mais l'intention est parfois bloquée par des obstacles financiers. Cette dimension rentre dans les déterminants sociaux de santé et peut refléter une disparité structurelle des inégalités sociales en santé (Fassin et Aïach, 2004).

### 8.1.2. Perception de la santé

La définition de la santé dans cette étude a ouvert le volet des **croyances**, des **connaissances** et des **valeurs personnelles** qui composent la **perception de la santé**. Toutes les définitions données à la santé ne la limitent pas à une conception biomédicale, mais l'étendent aux différentes **représentations sociales et culturelles** selon les individus et les groupes sociaux.

La santé, définie sous diverses formes, reste pour la majorité des interviewés la grande richesse de la personne. Qu'elle soit un don de Dieu, une absence de maladie, un équilibre psychologique, physique et spirituel, elle est notamment reliée à la capacité de mener une vie productive, sans douleur et sans souffrance. C'est l'appréciation globale selon Levasseur (1995) que l'individu fait de son propre état de santé en y intégrant ses

connaissances et son expérience de la santé ou de la maladie.

Dans ce cadre-là, l'équilibre physique et psychique mène à une vie saine, surtout que les personnes soulignent l'importance de conserver leur santé afin de pouvoir assurer leurs obligations de vie quotidienne et professionnelles et de produire des profits financiers qui seront par la suite utilisés comme un capital dans la couverture médicale.

La présence de maladies chroniques et l'âge avancé servent à expliquer selon les chercheurs **la perception négative de la santé** (Henchoz et al. 2008).

**La valeur de la santé** et la gravité de la maladie se sont démontré d'importants déterminants du choix du recours ou du non-recours aux soins. En effet, une **gravité perçue** élevée, tend à pousser à la consultation de spécialistes de santé plutôt qu'à se contenter de l'automédication. La gravité peut évoluer au cours du temps parallèlement à l'évolution de la maladie.

Ainsi, une maladie considérée au début comme légère sera traitée à domicile par l'automédication ou les soins de type traditionnel qui peuvent prendre pour certains le sens d'un **évitement du système de soins** et pour d'autres la valorisation d'une **norme d'autonomie** à l'égard de la santé (Bergot-Le Floch et al., 2015). Finalement la maladie sera perçue comme plus grave si les soins procurés à domicile débouchent à un échec. L'itinéraire thérapeutique suivi et les comportements en santé sont donc la conséquence de **l'évaluation continue de l'état de santé** faite par le malade et son entourage ainsi la perception de l'état de santé se relierait aux mesures d'incapacité fonctionnelle et de limitation des activités (Levasseur, 1995). Il en va de même de **l'urgence perçue** d'une intervention ; pour les cas urgents, la rapidité d'intervention domine souvent la recherche de l'efficacité

maximale, quitte à, dans un deuxième temps s'adresser à un service plus qualifié si nécessaire. En contrepartie, le recours aux médecins traditionnels peut être adopté par le malade après échec de la médecine conventionnelle.

Face à la gravité perçue de la maladie, **le diagnostic établi** par le médecin se révèle un facteur influençant le choix thérapeutique. En effet, les maladies chroniques graves diagnostiquées comme le diabète, le cancer... provoquent la peur chez le malade et l'incitent à consulter régulièrement les spécialistes. En contrepartie, d'autres facteurs surtout économiques apparaissent comme obstacle et obligent le malade à renoncer aux soins.

Les résultats quantitatifs confirment ce facteur de gravité perçue de la maladie. Les bénéficiaires de la CNSS, les coûts les plus élevés des médicaments et des services utilisés sont ceux du cancer, de la dialyse, du diabète, du cœur... malgré la couverture arrivant à 95% du seuil fixé par la CNSS pour certains médicaments. Le problème du seuil de tarification et du poids financier laissé au détriment des familles en cas de maladies graves se dresserait comme une entrave à un meilleur recours aux soins.

En ce qui concerne les maladies chroniques, un accès primaire et secondaire sont observés à travers une régularité du recours vers les généralistes (une consultation et demie/mois/famille). Ce recours au généraliste comme référent médical de la famille **réduit une probabilité de renoncement aux soins selon l'étude de Valmy** et al. (2016).

Le recours au spécialiste à une moyenne de deux visites par mois par famille est également révélateur de la prise de conscience de la gravité de la pathologie et de la nécessité de consulter malgré le retard de remboursement qui pourrait faire renoncer certains à effectuer ce recours.

### 8.1.3. Croyances et connaissances thérapeutiques

Le recours aux soins dépend significativement **des représentations** ou **des croyances** des individus. L'analyse des données a montré que la majorité des interviewés étaient en contact permanent avec des pratiques curatives par des procédés traditionnels basés sur l'utilisation ou la consommation de produits thérapeutiques végétaux ou alimentaires. Ces consommations s'appuient en général sur des **savoirs hérités** de la famille ou sur des recettes retirées des livres traditionnels. Le rapport à ces produits apparaît alors en lien avec la façon dont les malades s'inscrivent dans la prise en charge de leur maladie. C'est en lien avec l'acceptabilité des soins selon Perchansky et Thomas (1981) dans son aspect culturel et social. Certains individus trouvent ces produits comme **des ressources disponibles** dans l'environnement et accessibles à tous afin de gérer par soi-même la maladie (Bergot-Le Floch et al., 2015). Pour d'autres, ces produits révèlent une rupture de dépendance à l'égard de la médecine moderne surtout en évitant la prise de médicaments perçus comme dangereux ou qui peuvent engendrer une addiction. Selon eux, ces produits pris quotidiennement permettent un entretien du corps et répondent aux besoins de différents cycles de la vie. En revanche, cet usage libre, renvoie à une **démarche plus autonome** dans la gestion individuelle des soins. Enfin, la consommation de ces produits répond à une multiplicité de besoins des malades qui cherchent le soulagement ou la guérison.

### 8.1.4. Peur, crainte et choix du recours

Ces deux émotions, évoquées fréquemment dans le discours des interviewés, sont aussi à la base de la notion du recours ou du non-recours aux soins médicaux. Elles jouent un double rôle, l'un positif et l'autre négatif. Le

côté positif touche la dimension du recours aux soins et de la persévérance dans la prise des médicaments par peur de tomber malade ou par crainte d'aggraver la situation ; émotion basée sur l'expérience vécue de la maladie au cours du parcours de vie. Le côté négatif est essentiellement relié à l'élaboration d'un diagnostic que le patient ne désire pas entendre ou à une anxiété envers la prise de médicaments ou leurs effets secondaires. Cette crainte compose une barrière au recours aux soins qui pourrait être rompue par la communication où une transmission d'informations entre les professionnels de soins et les patients se fera dans un échange équilibré. C'est la prise en considération de la place de la vie psychique et sociale dans la santé et la maladie (Straet et Picard, 2007).

### 8.1.5. Attitudes envers les établissements

Les résultats de cette recherche révèlent **l'importance de la perception** que les individus ont des établissements sanitaires. Qu'elle soit négative ou positive, cette perception influence le recours. En effet, si les patients avaient le choix, rares sont ceux qui fréquentent un hôpital public ou un dispensaire. La préférence pour l'hôpital et les cliniques privés est globalement forte. Mais ces institutions sont généralement considérées par les patients admis en secteur public comme un luxe qui ne leur est pas accordé.

Concernant le secteur public certains le trouvent comme une structure spécifique destinée « aux pauvres ». D'autres le voient comme une solution, l'important pour eux c'est d'avoir un recours. Par contre, des personnes qui ont choisi de consulter les établissements publics ont été rencontrées et elles ont exprimé leur satisfaction.

Concernant les hôpitaux privés, les personnes bénéficiant d'une couverture médicale, trouvent comme

meilleure institution sanitaire les hôpitaux localisés dans la capitale « Beyrouth », ceci est expliqué par les différentes **représentations sociales** autour des services de meilleure qualité à la capitale.

La perception est généralement bâtie suite à des **expériences vécues**. Ces dernières sont rattachées à l'accueil, à la durée d'attente, à l'attention donnée, à la qualité des services et à l'assiduité du suivi.

Ce qui a été exposé rejoint en effet la définition du **contrôle comportemental perçu** défini comme la facilité ou la difficulté perçue à effectuer un comportement et il est censé refléter l'expérience passée aussi bien que les empêchements et les obstacles anticipés (Ajzen, 1987). Dans la théorie du comportement planifié, la réalisation ou non du comportement dépend donc non seulement de **l'intention,** mais aussi de **facteurs non motivationnels** tels que **l'opportunité** ou **les ressources à disposition**, soient les aptitudes individuelles ou l'environnement physique qui se traduisent en trois facteurs facilitants dans cette étude.

## 8.2. Facteurs facilitants

### 8.2.1. Accessibilité financière

Elle renferme deux volets, le niveau économique et la couverture médicale des ménages.

**Le niveau économique** des ménages influence directement l'accès aux soins de santé, qu'il soit un soin de santé primaire ou secondaire. Au Liban, toute consultation d'un spécialiste même effectuée dans un dispensaire doit être payée. Très rares sont les privilégiés bénéficiant de soins payés à l'avance ou remboursés directement. Durant les entretiens, des personnes à revenu limité sont rencontrés. Face à ce constat, l'hypothèse d'un

lien entre le niveau économique des ménages et les comportements du recours aux soins s'impose.

En effet, les problèmes financiers n'influencent pas seulement la question du recours, mais aussi celle du renoncement. Le renoncement, comme décrit dans la littérature, se produit après la phase du recours aux soins jusqu'à la délivrance du soin nécessaire. Chez les interviewés de cette étude, il prend différentes formes : ne pas consulter de nouveau un médecin, ne pas acheter le traitement prescrit, ne pas faire les examens demandés. C'est ce qui est également observé en ce qui concerne la couverture complémentaire dans les pays développés où sans couverture complémentaire c'est le reflet de l'effet prix qui délimite par exemple l'acquisition du médicament moins bien ou plus du tout remboursable (Dourgnon et Sermet, 2002). Le renoncement peut être soit temporaire soit définitif. Le budget des ménages qui renoncent aux soins est en quelque sorte en tension et ne peut être chargé de dépenses excédentaires sur le plan de la santé (Lombrail, Pascal, 2005).

S'orienter vers un établissement offrant des services semi-gratuits ou renoncer aux soins pour des motifs financiers, sont vécus par certains de nos interviewés comme une épreuve de privatisation, de frustration liée souvent au décalage entre le souhait d'un soin et la réalisation de ce dernier.

Les résultats de cette étude rejoignent la littérature et montrent clairement qu'un niveau économique bas ou moyen limite l'accès aux soins, notamment aux soins désirés. Par contre, les ménages à revenu élevé, ont toutes les **opportunités de recours**, ce qui crée une inégalité dans l'accès aux soins au Liban (Levasseur, 1995).

Cependant, la **faiblesse des ressources** constatée et le manque de couvertures médicales provoquent un sentiment d'insécurité et d'angoisse continu chez les

individus. Jusot (2010) a mis d'ailleurs en évidence le lien entre pauvreté et mauvais état de santé. Ce sont également des éléments essentiels déterminant l'orientation vers l'établissement sanitaire. En effet, **l'absence de couverture médicale** intervient fortement dans le recours vers l'institution sanitaire qui offre une accessibilité financière facile telle que les dispensaires au Liban.

Pourtant, malgré la situation économique précaire, il faut relever la capacité d'une part des ménages à mobiliser les ressources nécessaires devant un besoin indispensable. Diverses stratégies en premier, internes au ménage, sont mises en place : vente d'un terrain, utilisation de fonds cachés, dettes... Si ces pratiques sont insuffisantes ou absentes, il est souvent possible de mobiliser d'autres **ressources familiales (**de l'émigration et autres**) ou environnementales** reliées aux associations caritatives ou religieuses. D'autre part, trouver un traitement alternatif, moins cher, sera une option adoptée au besoin.

Dans l'étude qualitative, deux types de **couvertures médicales sont étudiées :** la CNSS et l'assurance privée.

### *CNSS*

La CNSS, couvrant plusieurs catégories de professions exposées dans la littérature, est la garantie d'une sécurité psychologique interne pour certains des interviewés. Ses bénéfices, pour les interviewés de l'étude, sont multiples allant de la couverture de 80% du coût des traitements et des examens médicaux jusqu'à la couverture de 90% des frais de l'hospitalisation (Chamseddine, 2012). Pour eux, elle donne au patient **la liberté de choisir** l'établissement sanitaire désiré et favorise **l'accès géographique** vers l'institution de proximité.

En contrepartie, certains la considèrent comme la couverture la plus injuste à cause de son arrêt à 64 ans, âge de la retraite (Chamseddine, 2012).De nombreux inconvénients ont été aussi relevés : payer les frais de

consultations et de traitements puis attendre plusieurs mois pour être remboursé, payer le montant restant de la facture médicale, faire face à des problèmes d'admission à l'hôpital et à des procédures administratives difficiles. Ceux-ci forment des **obstacles** entravant le recours aux soins et poussant les individus à renoncer au suivi.

Cette enquête sur les dossiers des adhérents de la CNSS révèle effectivement les délais des remboursements qui restent longs et les formalités administratives diverses et compliquées : accord préalable, le nombre de papiers administratifs et civils à fournir pour le remboursement… (Éléments et propos notés lors de la présence du chercheur au remplissage des questionnaires et l'observation du déroulement du travail de remboursement. Ceci peut contribuer selon Moatti et Ventelou (2009) à un renoncement aux soins du fait d'une préférence adaptative prenant en compte les priorités des besoins des ménages par rapport à l'amélioration de leur état de santé.

Le coût des soins laissé au détriment des familles adhérentes à la CNSS contrastent avec la moyenne des revenus et selon l'OMS les paiements directs des frais de santé dans les pays en développement peuvent aller jusqu'à mobiliser 40% des revenus nets des ménages (Moatti et Ventelou, 2009).

### *Assurance Privée*

Quant à l'assurance privée, et selon cette étude, elle est majoritairement attribuée aux ménages ayant des revenus supérieurs à 2 250 000 LL, vu que la cotisation de cette couverture constitue un fardeau lourd pour les ménages à revenu limité. Pourtant, elle se présente comme la seule alternative de couverture aux personnes ne bénéficiant d'aucune protection sociale. Les membres adhérents rencontrés mentionnent qu'ils profitent d'une hospitalisation payée à 100% sans problème administratif quant à l'admission. Pour certains d'eux, l'équipe

soignante offre aux admis en première classe une meilleure qualité de prise en charge. Malgré tous ces avantages, le grand problème de l'assurance reste le risque d'arrêt de la prise en charge en cas de déclenchement d'une maladie chronique.

### 8.2.2. Offre de soins

La présence des ressources ne suffit pas pour accéder aux soins. Il est intéressant de savoir qu'une **sous offre de soins** à l'égard des besoins des patients peut contribuer à l'explication des formes du non-recours aux soins. En effet, les difficultés rencontrées se concentrent essentiellement autour de l'absence de régulation de médecins spécialistes aux dispensaires et de la qualité de soins offerts. De plus, dans les hôpitaux publics, le nombre de lits fonctionnels est très restreint et la majorité des services sont fermés. A titre indicatif, le Ministère de Santé publique a financé en 2013 : 57 257 lits en hôpital public et 163 779 en hôpital privé (Statistical Bulletin, 2013).

Ces statistiques montrent une nette préférence pour les hôpitaux privés en ne comptant pas le refus de plusieurs hôpitaux privés d'admettre des patients sur des lits du ministère selon Ammar (2012).

Quelques remarques ont été relevées par les interviewés portant sur l'insuffisance de choix. Ils ont évoqué par exemple, le manque d'alternative de dispensaires autour de leur lieu de résidence et le nombre limité d'hôpitaux publics retrouvés dans les régions étudiées, ainsi que **l'absence d'un hôpital privé** dans la montagne du Kesrouan.

D'autres entretiens retracent les problèmes induits par les horaires d'ouverture des dispensaires et la durée d'attente dans les urgences hospitalières du secteur public. Les propos des interviewés ont aussi montré une forte

plainte envers la présence des syriens qui, selon eux, a influencé l'accès aux soins des Libanais et a augmenté le prix des services rendus par quelques centres.

Il s'agit donc d'un manque de disponibilité des services dans la production des services surtout après les conséquences de la crise syrienne et la présence massive de réfugiés syriens en quête de soins et assimilés aux classes défavorisées. La stigmatisation interculturelle d'une part, et l'insuffisance d'une offre de soins adéquate aux besoins de la population libanaise et syrienne présente sur le territoire d'autre part, sont des barrières effectives au recours aux soins et constituent un véritable enjeu de santé publique au Liban.

### 8.2.3 Accessibilité géographique et proximité des services

**L'accès géographique** est un des facteurs déterminant le recours aux soins, prenant en compte la mobilité des patients, la durée, la distance et le coût du trajet, c'est une mesure de proximité (Barlet et al., 2012).

Plusieurs interviewés se dirigent vers le centre sanitaire le plus proche de leur milieu de résidence. Néanmoins, il est bien clair que parfois en cas d'urgence les services de proximité sont délaissés au profit de services plus lointains soit pour rechercher un niveau supérieur de prise en charge, soit pour rechercher des services semi-gratuits.

Les habitants des régions rurales présentent également des **difficultés dans l'accès géographique** aux hôpitaux privés et publics. Ceci influence le choix du recours des habitants à l'automédication et à la médecine traditionnelle.

Concernant les adhérents de la CNSS, ils ont le choix de consulter les professionnels et les institutions de soins de leur choix. Privilégier la proximité se montrait surtout dans le choix des généralistes (élément constaté lors du

remplissage des questionnaires et au cours des interactions avec les employés du centre CNSS).

## 8.3. Facteurs de renforcement

Les facteurs de renforcement valorisent le comportement et contribuent à son maintien. Ce sont des facteurs qui ont des influences positives ou négatives provenant de l'entourage (Baril-Gingras, 2007). Dans l'analyse des données recueillies, trois types de facteurs de renforcement sont identifiés : le milieu social et environnemental, l'influence des pairs, et la relation avec l'institution sanitaire et l'équipe soignante.

### 8.3.1. Milieu social et environnemental

Le milieu social et environnemental exerce une influence sur le patient qui le pousse vers le recours ou le non-recours aux soins. Durant les entretiens, **l'influence du soutien familial** est constatée dans le recours ou non aux soins ou dans l'adoption ou l'abandon d'un comportement en santé. En effet, **l'entourage familial** représente une ressource sur laquelle la personne malade peut compter. Cette ressource apparaît chez les interviewés de l'étude sous deux formes principales. La première est reliée à la présence de quelqu'un à côté du malade. Cette personne peut assurer au malade le support nécessaire, l'encourager à continuer la prise en charge, lui préparer le traitement, l'accompagner au centre sanitaire et lui effectuer les procédures administratives.

La deuxième forme renvoie au support financier. Ce dernier est assuré soit en payant au membre les frais d'une couverture médicale, les frais d'hospitalisation ou même en lui procurant le médicament.

En opposition à cette présence familiale, il fallait faire face à des personnes souffrant de solitude et d'absence

d'un entourage soutenant engendrant un non-recours aux soins. Le sentiment d'être délaissé aboutit en fait au rejet du soin. Ceci rejoint les résultats de la recherche de Roy et al. (2006) qui montrent que l'absence de support familial influence négativement le bien-être de l'individu et le pousse à négliger sa santé.

Devant toute urgence incontrôlable, ces individus cherchent à trouver un support du voisinage ou des associations caritatives, mais ce support reste insuffisant et temporaire.

### 8.3.2. Influence des pairs

L'entourage pousse les patients à adopter différents comportements. Ainsi **l'influence des expériences vécues par le milieu familial ou environnemental** renforce souvent le comportement des patients du recours ou du non-recours vers un service de santé. En effet, cette étude a fortement montré le lien entre l'apparition d'une maladie grave ou le décès d'un parent, d'un proche ou d'un ami suite à une négligence et une inattention attribuée à la santé et entre le recours aux soins. L'impact de ce vécu favorise en fait l'appel aux soins devant toute symptomatologie même la plus banale.

Toutefois, le milieu social et environnemental exerce une influence opposée sur l'individu en le poussant vers le recours aux soins à domicile à travers différentes recommandations d'un savoir empirique qui permet de conseiller (Bergot-Le Floch et al. 2015). Ces derniers peuvent cependant être à l'origine d'une utilisation irrationnelle de l'automédication et des soins traditionnels.

### 8.3.3. Relation avec l'institution sanitaire et l'équipe soignante

La relation avec l'institution et l'équipe soignante est aussi à prendre en considération dans le comportement du recours ou du non-recours aux services de santé du patient. En effet, les résultats de cette étude soulignent trois niveaux relationnels encourageant ou freinant les interviewés à maintenir un comportement en santé.

Tout d'abord, **la relation médecin-malade** s'avère importante dans la conservation d'un comportement en santé. Cette relation contient un double paradoxe. D'un côté, le patient se remet au médecin en lui confiant sa santé et en suivant ses directives. De l'autre côté, il abandonne le suivi suite à un sentiment de déception ou par manque de confiance. D'ailleurs, la relation médecin-malade découle d'un acte de communication (Scheen et al, 2006) ; la qualité de cette relation pourrait influer positivement ou négativement sur le vécu du patient vis-à-vis de sa maladie, mais aussi de son traitement, car le médecin perçoit le soin à travers une consultation et une prescription, mais le patient y perçoit en plus du soin, sa maladie, sa souffrance et ses craintes (Sheen et al. 2006 ; Straet et Picard, 2007).

Ensuite, l'attitude des soignants a été notée comme capitale pour les patients en quête de soins. Le simple fait que la **relation équipe soignante-malade** se personnalise, suffit parfois à pousser le malade à adopter un comportement en santé. Le patient cherche dans la **structure sanitaire** un contexte sécurisant, un accueil chaleureux, une approche humble et des services de qualité, ce qui le pousse à visiter davantage le centre à chaque malaise. De même, la connaissance ultime de son histoire médicale et de ses antécédents par les professionnels de santé de cet établissement l'incite à y adhérer. C'est le lien institutionnel bienveillant et soutenant face à la maladie et à la souffrance (Saliba Sfeir, 2013). Cependant les recherches ont montré

que certains patients surtout des milieux défavorisés sont intimidés par le tas de démarches administratives à effectuer et que se voir refuser ou être déçus par un soin médical seraient des facteurs prédictibles d'un renoncement aux soins (Valmy et al., 2016).

# Conclusion et recommandations

Cette étude a cherché à comprendre le recours aux soins au Liban et a fait ressortir les déterminants sociaux et environnementaux de l'adoption ou du renoncement à ce recours chez la population libanaise.

L'approche empirique adoptée au niveau qualitatif et quantitatif a permis de définir dans quel contexte l'individu adopte ou n'adopte pas un comportement de recours aux soins. Les barrières aux soins se sont révélées multiples et rejoignent celles constatées dans les pays en cours de développement ou ce que nomment Chevalier et son équipe (2002) les pays en situation de précarité définis comme ceux où il y a une absence de sécurité ou de stabilité économique sociale ou politique.

Les obstacles se sont avérés multiples touchant à des caractéristiques du système de soins et de la population libanaise. Certains de type socio-économique aboutissent à un renoncement aux soins surtout chez les personnes ne bénéficiant d'aucune couverture médicale ou bien même chez celles bénéficiant de la couverture CNSS faute de remboursement ou de remboursement tardif. Le coût laissé à la charge des familles reste très important en comparaison avec la moyenne des seuils minimums de ressources, de l'accessibilité financière et en économie de santé à bénéficier des services de santé.

D'autres obstacles au recours aux soins sont liés à la priorité et la valeur accordées à la santé ainsi qu'à l'évaluation souvent personnelle de la gravité de la maladie. Cette évaluation conjuguée à un niveau économique bas et à une offre de soins onéreuse peuvent

faire jouer des préférences adaptatives d'une survie immédiate aux dépens d'une aspiration à une meilleure santé. Le regard que l'individu porte sur l'établissement sanitaire et la confiance qu'il a envers le médecin et l'équipe soignante ont une influence majeure sur le comportement de recours.

L'environnement psycho-social joue un rôle dans l'orientation du choix du recours ou du non-recours à travers la densité du réseau de soutien moral et matériel au niveau familial et social.

La présence d'une couverture médicale telle celle prodiguée par la CNSS réduit déjà ces obstacles pour les populations les plus fragiles (enfants, malades chroniques et graves, femmes enceintes) et favorisent un recours aux soins réguliers.

La couverture des soins reste insuffisante ou inexistante à plusieurs niveaux (dentaire, ophtalmologie, physiothérapie...) et certains seuils de remboursement sont tellement inférieurs par rapport au coût réel payé que les adhérents n'y ont recours que quand leur vie devient en danger.

Le cadre conceptuel de Kreuter et Green de cette recherche permet de formuler des recommandations en promotion de la santé qui tiennent compte à la fois des aspects individuels et des réalités environnementales. Il s'agit de permettre aux individus de gagner un plus grand contrôle sur les déterminants de leur propre santé ; en considérant la santé comme une ressource de la vie quotidienne.

L'amélioration de l'état de santé des populations contribue au développement économique (Moatti et Ventelou, 2009) et à une meilleure justice sociale. La réduction des inégalités sociales se fait par une offre aux soins accessible à l'ensemble de la population comme un droit au bien-être et un droit de citoyenneté.

Sur ce, une proposition d'une stratégie de promotion santé sera basée sur les axes de la charte d'Ottawa en ce qui concerne le recours aux soins chez les Libanais favorisant davantage l'équité sociale.

***Elaboration de politiques pour la santé***

-Inscrire la santé à l'ordre du jour des responsables politiques libanais de tous les secteurs et à tous les niveaux. Des mesures législatives et financières doivent favoriser le recours aux soins en augmentant la contribution de l'état au financement du Ministère de la Santé Publique qui est à ce jour de 3% du budget national d'une part et au renforcement de l'ouverture des possibilités de couverture médicale à l'instar de celle de l'hospitalisation sur le compte du ministère pour les soins primaires pour éviter des refus de soins vitaux faute de moyens de paiement.

-Plaidoyer auprès du parlement libanais de la nécessité d'une loi pour élargir la gamme de couverture des soins de la CNSS, du MSP et des autres mutuelles ainsi que l'amélioration du remboursement à temps des frais de soins aux hôpitaux et aux structures de santé pour éviter une stigmatisation des patients et un renoncement ultérieur des soins.

-Sensibiliser autour de la nécessité d'instaurer une assurance vieillesse et une assurance retraite pour toute la population à l'instar des organismes de l'état : 54,9% des personnes âgées de 65 ans et plus n'avaient aucune assurance maladie en 2007 selon Osta et al. (2012). Le ministre de la Santé au Liban annonce la couverture des soins hospitaliers à 100% par le ministère de Santé publique pour les personnes de plus de 64 ans à partir de novembre 2016, mais les modalités ne sont pas encore fixées (MOPH, 2016).

-Considérer les mesures en santé comme un input pour la réduction de la pauvreté, la croissance économique et le

développement à long terme. En effet, un traitement médical efficace permet de restaurer la productivité affectée par la maladie selon l'OMS.

***Création de milieux favorables***

- Développer la qualité des services rendus dans les centres de santé et les dispensaires pour compenser la difficulté financière du recours aux soins.
- Créer un partenariat stratégique entre les ministères (MSP, MAS…) pour diffuser une sensibilisation au droit à la santé primaire et augmenter le nombre des professionnels en santé pour améliorer les services rendus malgré la surcharge représentée par le nombre important des réfugiés syriens.
- Assurer les moyens pour des horaires flexibles de ces centres couvrant la totalité de la journée en mettant les moyens qu'il faut : multiplier le nombre des professionnels, assurer les moyens logistiques nécessaires…
- Créer des hôpitaux publics dans les hautes montagnes et les zones rurales.

***Acquisition des aptitudes individuelles***

- Sensibiliser la population libanaise sur l'importance de la santé comme ressource de vie et de justice sociale.
- Développer et appuyer des stratégies des campagnes en santé autour de la nécessité du recours à la santé et de la prévention des maladies en lien avec l'augmentation de l'espérance de vie.
- Diffuser les différents moyens de contrôler au mieux sa santé en assurant l'information nécessaire autour des services existants et des bénéfices d'une couverture médicale à mettre en place pour faire face au risque de maladie et assurer une sorte de sécurité face à ce risque qui peut chambouler des vies et appauvrir des familles.
- Mobiliser l'Ordre des médecins et les représentants des professionnels de santé pour une meilleure stratégie

des services dispensés dans les centres de santé et favoriser les services de santé dans les milieux ruraux, dans les quartiers défavorisés pour réduire les disparités en santé.

- Sensibiliser les professionnels de santé sur l'importance des rôles des équipes soignantes sur le recours ou le renoncement dû à la perception de la relation soignant/soigné.

- Agir sur les croyances erronées et favoriser la valeur de la santé en insistant sur la qualité des services de soins à revendiquer et au droit du recours aux soins dans la dignité en modifiant les perceptions de la population vis-à-vis des services de santé des dispensaires et des hôpitaux publics.

***Réorientation des services de santé et renforcer l'action communautaire***

- Renforcer le travail interministériel autour de la question du non-recours aux soins de la population libanaise pour contribuer à réduire la précarité existante et favoriser un sentiment de sécurité malgré l'instabilité politique et régionale.

- Elargir les missions des services de santé existants en développant un partenariat et un travail en réseau décentralisé pour évaluer les besoins en santé dans chaque région et élaborer les propositions adéquates aux décisionnaires.

- Impliquer les Municipalités, écoles, universités, ministères et population dans des actions ciblées en santé où portes ouvertes, conférences, films seront organisés conjointement avec les instances locales concernées par les secteurs des centres et des structures de la santé.

- Déléguer des comités formés par les employés, des représentants associatifs et municipaux des dispensaires et des centres de santé pour transmettre régulièrement les

besoins en santé au MSP et au MAF et assurer les moyens pour la continuité des services offerts.

***Développer des recherches universitaires et créer des bases de données***

- Contribuer à la mise en place d'enquêtes épidémiologiques pour développer une base de données par observation systématique des inégalités en santé.
- Développer le secteur de la recherche multidisciplinaire en santé spécialement en champ de santé notamment en sociologie et psychosociologie, épidémiologie, psychologie et en économie de santé pour développer des connaissances spécifiques au contexte libanais concernant les déterminants sociaux et environnementaux de la santé au niveau du pays en respectant les spécificités du système culturel et politique existant.
- Créer un réseau interuniversitaire de recherches et favoriser un partenariat université/ministère autour des thématiques de santé de la population.

Finalement, cette recherche exploratoire n'a fait qu'éclairer certains déterminants sociaux et environnementaux des inégalités sociales en santé au Liban sur un secteur représentatif limité. Ses résultats pourront être un leitmotiv pour un élargissement du spectre vers une étude au niveau national des dimensions du recours et de l'accès aux soins dans l'expérience des Libanais et autour du système de santé pour favoriser une réforme du système de santé libanais, une évolution des perceptions positives en santé de la population et pour contribuer au développement d'un droit citoyen à la santé pour tous au Liban.

# Références bibliographiques

1.Aday L-A., Andersen R-M. (1974). « A framework for the study of access to medical care », *Health Services Research*, vol.9, n°3, p.208-220, disponible sur http://www.ncbi.nlm.nih.gov/pmc/articles/PMC1071804/, consulté le 13/04/2014.

2.Alexopoulos E. C. et Geitona M. (2009). « Self-Rated Health: Inequalities and Potential Determinants », *International Journal of Environmental Research and Public Health,* 6, 2456-2469, disponible sur https://www.ncbi.nlm.nih.gov/pubmed/19826556?dopt, consulté le 28 novembre 2015.

3.Ammar W. (2012). التوجهات الاستراتيجية للنظام الصحي في لبنان, Ministère de la Santé publique, Liban, disponible sur : http// www.moph.gov.lb, consulté le 14 octobre 2013.

4.Azar S. (2000). « La politique de santé au Liban depuis 1945 », United Nations Development Programm [UNDP], Conference on Linking Economics Growth and Social Development, Beyrouth, p.143-163, disponible sur http://www.undp.org.lb/communication/publications/linking/Session6.pdf, consulté le 10/04/2014.

5.Azar S. (2015). « La politique familiale I, Enjeux, typologies et modèles », *Les Sciences Sociales*, CRSS, 18 mars, p. 28-48.

6.Azar S. (2016). « La politique familiale II, Evolution, enjeux et impact redistributive au Liban », *Les Sciences Sociales*, CRSS, 22 pages, en cours de publication.

7.Baril-Gingras G. (2007). « Conditions et processus menant à des changements à la suite d'interventions en

santé et en sécurité du travail : l'exemple d'activités de formation ». *PISTES : perspectives interdisciplinaires sur le travail et la santé,* n°9, disponible sur http://pistes.revues.org/2998?=en, consulté le 23/11/2014.

8.Barlet M., Coldefy M., Collin C et al. (2012). *« L'accessibilité potentielle localisée (APL) : Une nouvelle mesure de l'accessibilité aux médecins généralistes libéraux »*, Etudes et résultats, Direction de la recherche, des études, de l'évaluation et des statistiques [DREES], 8p., disponible sur http://www.drees.sante.gouv.fr/IMG/pdf/er795.pdf, consulté le 10/11/2014.

9.Bazin F., Parizot I., Chauvin P. (2006). « Déterminants psychosociaux du renoncement aux soins pour raisons financières dans cinq zones urbaines sensibles de la Région parisienne en 2001 », *Sciences sociales et santé*, Volume 24, n°3, p. 11-31

10.Beaudry M. et Hamelin A-M. (2006). « Introduction à la partie « PRECEDE » du modèle « PRECEDE-PROCEED » pour planifier et évaluer des programmes de promotion de la santé – son application en nutrition publique », *Cahier de nutrition publique*. Université Laval, n°3, disponible sur http://poledfn.org/wpcontent/uploads/2013/05/introduction PRECEDE.pdf, consulté le 5/12/2014.

11.Benattar F. (2010). « Regards aigus sur les inégalités sociales de santé », *Santé Autrement Magazine*, disponible sur http://www.santeautrementmagazine.fr/2010/regards-aigussur-les-inegalites-sociales-de-sante/, consulté le 05/05/2014.

12.Benattar F. (2012). « Des inégalités en santé à l'équité en santé », *Santé Autrement Magazine*, disponible sur http://www.santeautrementmagazine.fr/2012/des-inegalites-en-sante-alequite-en-sante/, consulté le 05/05/2014.

13.Bergot-Le Floch A-L. Moulin P. Haxaire C. (2015). « L'autonomie en matière d'automédicamentation et ses limites telles que perçues dans les comptes rendus de « pharmacies familiales » en pays messin », in *Actes des Rencontres Nord/Sud de l'automédication et de ses déterminants*, Cotonou, mars, disponible sur https://f.hypotheses.org/wp-content/blogs.dir/2003/files/2015/12/ACTES_5_Bergot-Le-Floch_Moulin_Haxaire.pdf, consulté le 30 septembre 2016.

14.Blanchet A. et Gotman A. (1992). *L'enquête et ses méthodes* : l'entretien, Paris, Nathan.

15.Bonnet P. (2002). *Le concept d'acceptabilité et d'accès aux soins,* dossier de DEA GEOS Université Paul Valéry, Montpellier 3.

16.Bourdieu P. (1993). « Comprendre », in Bourdieu P. (dir.), *La Misère du Monde*, Paris, Le Seuil, p. 903-939.

17.Bourgueil Y., Marek A., Mousques J. (2009). « Trois modèles types d'organisation des soins primaires en Europe, au Canada, en Australie et en Nouvelle-Zélande », *Questions d'économie de la santé,* n°141, p 1-6, disponible sur http://www.irdes.fr/Publications/Qes/Qes141.pdf, consulté le 13/05/2014.

18.Braveman P., Gruskin S. (2003). « Defining equity in health », *Journal of epidemiology & Community Health*, n°57, p. 254-258, disponible sur http://www.ncbi.nlm.nih.gov/pubmed/12646539, consulté le 10/05/2014.

19.Cantoreggi N. (2010). *Pondération des déterminants de la santé en Suisse*, Université de Genève, GRES (Groupe de recherche en environnement et santé).

20.Chamseddine H (dir.). (2012)., « Code de la sécurité sociale », in قوانين العمل والضمان الاجتماعي , éditions des publications juridiques, p. 33-60.

21.Chen B., Cammett M. (2012). « Informal politics and inequity of access to healthcare in Lebanon », *International Journal for Equity in health*, vol.11, n°23, p.1-8, disponible sur http://www.equityhealthj.com/content/pdf/1475-9276-11-23.pdf, consulté le 14/04/2014.

22.Chevalier A., Beauquesne I., Gagnayre R. (2002). « Analyse des conditions préalables à la mise en œuvre de formations en santé dans le cadre de l'aide humanitaire », *Santé Publique*, n°1, vol. 14, p. 37-46.

23.Clark R., Coffee N. (2011). « Why measuring accessibility is important for public health: a review from the Cardiac ARIA project », in Dermott R. (dir.), *Public Health Bulletin SA Rural health in the 21st century: challenges and opportunities*, Government of South Australia, vol.8, n°1, p.3-8, disponible sur http://www.health.sa.gov.au/pehs/publications/Public%20Health%20Bulletin%20Vol8%20No1-phcc-March2011.pdf, consulté le 15/04/2014.

24.CNSS. (2010). *Book Madmoun,* دليل المضمون disponible sur https://www.cnss.gov.lb/index.php/book-madmoun consulté le 31 janvier 2016.

25.CNSS. (2014). Nombre des contractuels CNSS. المؤسسات والهيئات الصحية المتعاقدة مع الصندوق, disponible sur https://www.cnss.gov.lb/index.php/statisctics/cnssmc, consulté le 31 janvier 2016.

26.CNSS. (2014).احصائيات المضمونين والمستفيدين disponible sur https://www.cnss.gov.lb/index.php/statisctics/cnssstatprod, consulté le 31 janvier 2016.

27.Dourgnon P., Sermet C. (2002), *La consommation de médicaments varie-t-elle selon l'assurance complémentaire?*, CREDES (Centre de recherche et d'études documentaire en économie de la santé), France.

28.El Osta N.et al. (2012). Vieillissement de la population libanaise : démographie, évaluation sanitaire et impact en santé bucco-dentaire. IAJD Revue arabe internationale de dentisterie, disponible sur http : //www.ojs.usj.edu.lb/ojs/index.php/iajd/article/view/23/15, consulté le 18/10/2015.

29.Fassin D. et Aïach P. (2004). « L'origine et les fondements des inégalités sociales de santé », *la Revue du Praticien* ; 54 : 2221-7.

30.Ghiglione R. et Matalon B. (1995). *Les enquêtes sociologiques, Théories et pratique*, Paris, Armand Colin.

31.Godin G. (1991). « L'éducation pour la santé : les fondements psycho-sociaux de la définition des messages éducatifs », *Sciences Sociales et Santé*, vol.9, n°1, p.67-94, disponible sur http://www.persee.fr/web/revues/home/prescript/article/sosan_02940337_1991_num_9_1_1185, consulté le 23/09/2014.

32.Green L.W. and Kreuter M.W. (2005). *Health Program Planning: An Educational and Ecological Approach.* 4th edition. NY: McGraw-Hill Higher Education, 2005.

33.Green L.W. et Kreuter M. W. (1991). *Health Promotion Planning: An Educational and Environmental Approch.* (Second Edition ed.). Mountain View: Mayfield PublishingCompany.

34.Grignon M., Naudin F. (2002). *Etude de faisabilité d'une évaluation des dispositifs à la prévention*, Centre de Recherche D'étude et De Documentation En Economie De La Santé [CREDES], disponible sur http://www.evaluation.gouv.fr/cgp/fichiers/ei/faisabilite.pdf, consulté le 14/12/2014.

35.Grigoriev P., Grigorieva O. (2011). « Self-perceived Health in Belarus : Evidence from the income and

expenditures of households survey », *Demographic research,* vol.24, n°23, p.551-578, disponible sur

36.Guyon L. (1988). « La perception de la santé à travers l'enquête Santé Québec », *Cahiers québécois de démographie*, vol.17, n°2, p.193-212, disponible sur http://www.erudit.org/revue/cqd/1988/v17/n2/600639ar.pdf, consulté le 23/09/2014.

37.Henchoz K., Cavalli S., Girardin M. (2008). « Perception de la santé et comparaison sociale dans le grand âge », *Sciences sociales et santé*, vol.26, p.47-72, disponible sur http://www.carin.info/revue_sciences_sociales_et_santte_2008_3_page_47.htm, consulté le 13/9/2014. http://www.demographic-research.org/volumes/vol24/23/, consulté le 25/09/2014.

38.INED (Institut National d'Etudes Démographiques), (2004) et (2009), disponible sur http://www.ined.fr/fr/france/mortalite_causes_deces/mortalite_infantile/, consulté le 29 janvier 2016.

39.Inserm, (2013). *Les morts maternelles en France, mieux comprendre pour mieux prévenir*, Rapport du Comité National d'experts sur la Mortalité Maternelle 2007-2009, octobre, disponible sur http://www.inserm.fr/espace-journalistes/mortalite-maternelle-diminution-de-la-mortalite-par-hemorragies, consulté le 28 février 2016.

40.Institut de recherche et documentation en économie de la santé [IRDES]. (2013). *La géographie de la santé*, 139p., disponible sur http://www.irdes.fr/documentation/syntheses/la-geographie-de-la-sante.pdf, consulté le 14/04/2014.

41.Institut national de prévention et d'éducation pour la santé [inpes]. (2014). *Planifier pour mieux agir,* traduction francophone de Precede/Proceed, disponible sur

http://www.inpes.sante.fr/ressources-methodologiques/outils/precede.asp, consulté le 25/09/2014.

42.InVS (Institut National de Veille Sanitaire), (2010). *La mortalité infantile en France, Bilan 2001-2006*, Rapport du Comité national d'experts sur la mortalité maternelle (CNEMM) 2001-2006. Unité Inserm 953, Institut de veille sanitaire. Janvier 2010.

43.Jusot F. (2010). *Inégalités sociales de santé : Quels constats ? Quels leviers d'action ?* , LEDA-LEGOS, Université Paris-Dauphine, IRDES.

44.Kasparian Ch. (2014). *L'apport financier des émigrés et son impact sur les conditions de vie de Libanais*, Observatoire universitaire de la réalité socio-économique (OURSE) de l'Université Saint-Joseph de Beyrouth.

45.Kronfol N. (2003). « Case Study: Lebanon », in Abeykoon P., Brodsky J., et al., *Long-term care in developing countries: ten case studies*. The world health organization, Geneva, Edition World Health Organization, coll. « On long term care ». p. 171-216, disponible sur http://www.who.int/chp/knowledge/publications/case_study_Lebanon.pdf, consulté le 05/05/2014.

46.Lambert D.-C. (1985).« Le mythe de l'équidistribution des états de santé », *Revue d'Economie Régionale et Urbaine,* numéro spécial,p. 389-419.

47.Legal Agenda (2015), السلطة الأبوية والحضانة في قوانين الأحوال الشخصية اللبنانية, 31mars, disponible sur http://www.legal-agenda.com/newsarticle.php?id=919&lang=ar, consulté le 20 janvier 2016.

48.Levasseur M. (1995). « Perception de l'état de santé », in Bellerose C., Lavallee C., Chenard L. et Levasseur M., *Santé Québec et la santé, ça va en 1992-1993*, Rapport de l'enquête sociale et de santé 1992-1993, vol.1,

Montréal, Ministère de la Santé et des services sociaux, gouvernement du Québec, p. 199-209, disponible sur http://classiques.uqac.ca/contemporains/quebec_sante_quebec/rapport_enquete_92_93_t1/t1_chap_11_perceptions_etat_de_sante/sante_qc_perception_etat_sante.rtf, consulté le 20/09/2014.

49.Loiselle C. et Profetto-McGrath. (2007). *Méthodes de recherche en sciences infirmières, approches quantitatives et qualitatives*, Québec, Editions ERPI.

50.Lombrail P., Pascal J. (2005). « Inégalités sociales de santé et accès aux soins », *Revue les tribunes de la santé*, n°8, p.31-39, disponible sur http://www.cairn.info/revue-lestribunes-de-la-sante-2005-3.htm, consulté le 23/05/2014.

51.Mayer R., Ouellet F., St-Jacques M.C., Turcotte D. (2000). *Méthodes de recherche en intervention sociale*, Québec, Gaetan Morin.

52.Melki R. (2000). « La protection sociale au Liban, entre reflexe d'assistance et stratégie d'assurance », UNDP, conference on Linking Economic Growth and Social Development, Beyrouth, p. 187-210, disponible sur http://www.undp.org.lb/communication/publications/linking/Session8.pdf, consulté le 05/05/2014

53.Moatti J-P., Ventelou B. (2009). « Economie de santé dans les pays en développement, des paradigmes en mutation », *Revue économique*, 2, Vol. 60, p. 241-256, disponible sur http://www.cairn.info/revue-economique-2009-2-page-241.htm, consulté le 25 février 2016.

54.MOPH. (2016) إعلان عن بدء التغطية الإستشفائية الكاملة للمسنين الشهر المقبلdisponible sur http://www.moph.gov.lb/ar/Pages/17/9151/announcement-of-the-start-of-full-hospitalization-coverage-for-the-elderly-next-month, consulté le 2 octobre 2016.

55.OMS. (1978). « Déclaration d'Alma Ata sur les soins de santé primaire », disponible sur

http://www.who.int/topics/primary-health-care/alma-ata-declaration/fr, consulté le 11/05/2014.

56.OMS. (1986). « Charte d'Ottawa pour la promotion de la santé », Première conférence internationale pour la promotion de la santé, Ottawa.

57.Penchancky R., Thomas J-W. (1981). « The concept of access: definition and relationship to consumer satisfaction », *Medcare*, vol.19, p.127-140, disponible sur http://www.ncbi.nlm.nih.gov/pubmed/7206846, consulté le 10/04/2014.

58.Picheral H. (2001). *Dictionnaire raisonné de la géographie en Santé*, Cahiers GEOS (Géographie de la Santé), Université de Montpellier.

59.Potvin L., Moquet M-J., Jones C. (2010). *Réduire les inégalités sociales en santé*, Saint-Denis : Institut National de prévention et d'éducation pour la santé [inpes], Editions Yves Géry, coll. « santé en action », disponible sur http://www.inpes.sante.fr/CFESBases/catalogue/pdf/1333.pdf, consulté le 14/04/2014.

60.Pouëzat J. (2002). *Santé Publique bucco-dentaire et société*, Bull. Acad. Natle Chir.dentaire.

61.Quivy R. et Campenhoudt L.V. (2006). *Manuel de recherche en sciences sociales*, Paris, Dunod.

62.Renaud L. et Gomez Zarnudio M.(1998). *Planifier pour mieux agir*, Québec, REFIPS.

63.Rochaix L., Tubeuf S. (2009). « Mesures de l'équité en santé. Fondements éthiques et implications », *Revue économique*, vol.60, p.325-344, disponible sur http://www.cairn.info/revue-economique-2009-2-page-325.htm, consulté le 20/05/2014.

64.Roy Sh., et al. (2006), *Itinérance et accès aux services : problèmes et enjeux*, Collectif de recherche sur l'itinérance, la pauvreté et l'exclusion sociale, CRI-UQÀM, Québec-Canada, disponible sur

www.er.uqam.ca/nobel/cri/spip/IMG/pdf/rapport_Itinerance_Acces, consulté le 3-10-2015.

65.Salameh P.et Barbour B. (2011). "Pattern of obesity and associated diabetes in Lebanese adolescents: a pilot study", *Eastern Mediterranean Health Journal* (EMHJ), vol. 17, n° 3, p. 226 – 30.

66.Saliba Sfeir C. (2013). *Parentalité, addiction et travail social.* Paris, Editions L'Harmattan, coll. Logiques sociales.

67.Scheen A.J., Parada A., Giet D. (2006). « Conseils pour une meilleure prescription médicamenteuse », *Revue Med Liège* ; 61 : 5-6, p. 493 – 488, disponible sur http://orbi.ulg.ac.be/bitstream/2268/7877/1/20060506_31.pdf, consulté le 25 janvier 2016.

68.Shields M. et Shooshtari S. (2001). « Determinants of self-perceived health », *Health reports*, vol.13, n°1 (décembre), p.35-52, disponible sur http://www.ncbi.nlm.nih.gov/pubmed/15069807, consulté le 25/09/2014.

69.Statistical Bulletin 2013 (50 pages), disponible surhttp://www.moph.gov.lb/Statistics/Documents/StatisticalBulletin2013.pdf, consulté le 28 février 2016.

70.STRAET A. & PICARD C. (2007). « Le patient et sa maladie : tout un vécu à prendre en compte », *La Revue de la Médecine Générale*, n° 248, 12/2007, p. 430-432.

71.Université Saint-Joseph [USJ], OMS, MSP. (2012). « Recueil national des statistiques sanitaires au Liban », p.29-33, disponible sur http://www.igspd.usj.edu.lb/docs/recherche/recueil/2fr.pdf consulté le 20/9/2014.

72.Valmy et al. (2016). Prevalence and predictive factors for renouncing medical care in poor populations of Cayenne, French Guiana. *BMC Health Services Research* 2016, 15 p.1-11, disponible sur

http://www.biomedcentral.com/1472-6963/15/1 /, consulté le 25 février 2016.

73.Valmy L. et al.: Prevalence and predictive factors for renouncing medical care in poor populations of Cayenne, French Guiana. BMC Health Services Research 2016 15:

74.Vie Publique. (2014). « Systèmes bismarckien et bévéridgien : quelles caractéristiques ? », disponible sur http://www.vie-publique.fr/decouverte-institutions/financespubliques/protection-sociale/definition/systemes-bismarckien-beveridgienprotection, consulté le 25/04/2014.

75.World Bank. (2013). « Lebanon: Economic and Social Impact Assessment of the Syrian Conflict» 8p., disponible sur http://www.worldbank.org/content/dam/Worldbank/document/MNA/LBNESIA%20of%20Syrian%20Conflict-%20EX%20SUMMARY%20ENGLISH.pdf, consulté le 14/12/2014.

76.Zakia T. (2008). « Réforme de la protection sociale au Liban. Atelier n°47- les reformes de la protection sociale », 33eme conférence mondiale du CIAS, France, disponible sur http://www.icsw.org/doc/0047_8f_Zakia_Fr_Abstract.doc, consulté le 05/04/2014.

77.Zitouni S et Ezzina R.(2007). *Mesure de l'effet des variables individuelles sur l'intensité d'adoption de l'EAD par les étudiants tunisiens : approche par la théorie du comportement planifié,* TICE Méditerranée.

# Annexes

# Annexe 1

**المؤسسات والهيئات الصحية المتعاقدة مع الصندوق**

| عدد المؤسسات والهيئات الصحية المتعاقدة مع الصندوق **بتاريخ ٣٠-٠٩-٢٠١٤** | |
|---|---|
| الأطباء | ١١٣٤٥ |
| الصيدليات | ٣٠٢٠ |
| المعالجين الفيزيائيين | ١٥٤٩ |
| المختبرات | ٤٦١ |
| مراكز الأشعة | ٢٤٨ |
| مراكز المعالجين الفيزيائيين | ١٧٦ |
| المستشفيات | ١٤٨ |
| القابلات القانونية | ٨٤ |
| مجازين تقويم السمع | ٣٢ |
| اخصائي أطراف إصطناعية | ٣٢ |
| اخصائي صناعة أحذية طبية | ٦ |
| المجموع | ١٧١٤٦ |

# Annexe 2
## Guide d'entretien effectué auprès des patients

**<u>Guide d'entrevue</u>** <u>N°</u>: …….

**Nom de l'établissement :** ………………………………

**Secteur de l'établissement :** ☐ Public ☐ Privé

**1- Informations générales concernant les membres du ménage**

<u>Religion</u> : ☐ Chrétien ☐ Musulman ☐ Druze ☐ Autre : ………………

<u>Milieu de résidence</u> : ………………………

| Membre de la famille / Caractéristiques sociodémographiques | Chef du ménage | Epouse | Enfant 1 | Enfant 2 | Enfant 3 | Enfant 4 | Enfant 5 | Autre |
|---|---|---|---|---|---|---|---|---|
| Age | | | | | | | | |
| Sexe | | | | | | | | |
| État Marital | | | | | | | | |
| Niveau d'éducation | | | | | | | | |
| Occupation | | | | | | | | |
| Couverture sociale | | | | | | | | |

<u>Revenu du ménage</u> : ☐ < à 675.000 L.L ☐ 675.000 L.L – 1. 250.000 L.L ☐ 1.250.000 L.L – 1.750.000 L.L ☐ 1.750.000 L.L – 2.250.000 L.L ☐ > à 2.250.000 L.L

| N° | Questions | Relances | Objectifs |
|---|---|---|---|
| **1** | Quels sont les centres sanitaires dans votre région ? | | Connaissances sur les structures sanitaires, accessibilité géographique. |
| **2** | Comment définissez-vous la santé ? | | Perception de la santé, connaissances. |
| **3** | Que signifie pour vous votre consultation de ce centre ? Qu'attendez –vous ? | A quand remonte votre dernière consultation chez un médecin?<br>Quand envisagez-vous la prochaine consultation?<br>Y a-t-il eu un rendez-vous chez un médecin cette année auquel vous ne seriez pas allé? Pour quelles raisons? | Priorité des soins, perception du centre. |
| **4** | Quels comportements adoptez-vous lorsque vous vous sentez malade ? | Quelles sont les structures sanitaires que vous fréquentez ? | En pratique, les attitudes et les comportements face à la maladie. |
| **5** | D'habitude quand l'un des membres de votre famille tombe malade à qui vous vous adressez en premier ?<br>Qu'est-ce qui vous pousse à faire ce choix ? | Quelqu'un des membres de votre famille souffre de maladies? Pouvez-vous en parler ?<br>Quelle est la cause de la maladie ?<br>Quels sont les moyens de soins adoptés ? | Priorité de sa santé et comportements vis-à-vis des membres de sa famille. |
| **6** | Etes-vous soigné(e) par la médecine non conventionnelle ? racontez- nous. | | Perception, croyances, valeur de la santé, pratique face à la maladie. |

| N° | Questions | Relances | Objectifs |
|---|---|---|---|
| 7 | Lorsqu'un médecin vous prescrit des médicaments, prenez-vous l'ensemble de ce qu'il a marqué sur l'ordonnance ?<br>De manière générale, prenez-vous les traitements prescrits jusqu'au bout ? Pour quelles raisons? | | Comportements, valeurs, perception du traitement.<br>Influence économique. |
| 8 | Comment vous payez les frais de soins de votre famille ? Depuis quand êtes-vous dans cette situation ? | Pensez- vous que votre état économique influence votre santé ? Racontez-nous. | Influence économique sur la santé de la personne et de sa famille et sur le choix du traitement. |
| 9 | Avez-vous déjà renoncé à des soins pour des raisons financières ?<br>Quels types de soins ? Quand ? Depuis quand ?<br>Y avez-vous renoncé définitivement ou les avez-vous reportés? | | Influence économique sur la santé de la personne et de sa famille et sur le choix du traitement. |
| 10 | Comment pour vous la couverture sociale influence le choix du traitement ? | A votre avis, la couverture sociale influence- t- elle la qualité de la prise en charge ? Comment ?<br>Selon vous, quelle est la couverture sociale la plus efficace dans le cas de maladies au Liban ? | Perception de la couverture. |
| 11 | Durant ces deux années, parler nous d'une maladie qui vous a touché (e) ou a touché un membre de votre famille ? (Nature de la maladie, durée avant la prise en charge, type de remèdes, coût des soins, résultat du traitement, raisons du choix du traitement) | | Description du parcours de soins. |

# Annexe 3
# Guide d'entretien effectué auprès des patients
## (traduit en arabe)

| رقم | السؤال | |
|---|---|---|
| ١ | ما هي مراكز الخدمات الصحية في مكان إقامتكم؟ | |
| ٢ | كيف تعرّفون الصحة؟ | |
| ٣ | ماذا يعني لكم اللجوء إلى هذا المركز الصحي؟ ماذا تنتظرون منه؟ | متى قمتم بآخر معاينة طبية؟ متى تنوون زيارة طبيب؟ هل تأخرتم أو عدلتم عن زيارة طبيب خلال السنة الحالية؟ ما هي الأسباب؟ |
| ٤ | عندما تشعرون بتوعك، ما هي أولى الخطوات التي تقومون بها؟ | ما هي المراكز التي تقصدونها؟ |
| ٥ | عندما يتوعك أحد أفراد الأسرة، إلى من تلجأون؟ ما الذي يدفعكم للإقدام على هذا الخيار؟ ما هو نوع العلاج الذي تستخدمونه؟ | هل يعاني أحد أفراد أسرتكم من مرض؟ ما هو؟ ما سبب المرض برأيكم؟ ما هي سبل علاجه المعتمدة؟ حدّثونا. |
| ٦ | هل سبق و تعالجتم بالطب البديل؟ حدّثونا. | |
| ٧ | هل تأخذون الدواء المسجّل على الوصفة الطبية بانتظام؟ لماذا؟ | |
| ٨ | كيف تأمّنون كلفة العلاج؟ منذ متى أنتم على هذه الحالة ؟ | |
| ٩ | هل سبق وأرجأتم أو عدلتم عن العلاج بسبب الأوضاع المالية؟ ما هو نوع العلاج؟ منذ متى؟ | هل تظنّون أنّ وضعكم الاقتصادي ينعكس على صحتكم؟ كيف؟ |
| ١٠ | كيف تؤثر التغطية الصحية على اختيار نوع العلاج؟ | هل تظنّون أن التغطية الصحية تؤثر على نوعيّة الخدمات الصحية وجودتها؟ كيف؟ برأيكم ما هي التغطية الصحية الأكثر فعاليّة في لبنان؟ |
| ١١ | خلال السنتين المنصرمتين، هل عانيت أو عانى أحد أفراد أسرتك من أي مرض؟ ( نوع المرض، نوع العلاج، أسباب اختياره، فترة العلاج، ثمنه، نتيجته) | |

# Annexe 4

## Tableau n°2 : présentation des caractéristiques sociodémographiques des interviewés dans les dispensaires

| Identité | Sexe | Religion | Age | Niveau d'éducation | Milieu de résidence | Taille du ménage | Couverture sociale | Revenu par 1000L.L./ Mois |
|---|---|---|---|---|---|---|---|---|
| E1 | Femme | Chrétien | 67 | P | Bourj Hamoud | 1 | S.C | SR |
| E2 | Femme | Chrétien | 29 | P | Bourj Hamoud | 5 | CNSS | 675-1250 |
| E3 | Femme | Musulman | 21 | P | Jdeideh | 3 | S.C | 675-1250 |
| E4 | Femme | Chrétien | 60 | P | Bourj Hamoud | 4 | CNSS | 1750-2250 |
| E5 | Femme | Chrétien | 37 | S | Byakout | 4 | Ass | 1250-1750 |
| E6 | Femme | Chrétien | 47 | C | Bourj Hamoud | 3 | S.C | <675 |
| E7 | Femme | Chrétien | 70 | C | Bourj Hamoud | 1 | S.C | SR |
| E8 | Femme | Chrétien | 39 | U | Hrajel | 4 | Ass | >2250 |
| E9 | Homme | Chrétien | 50 | P | Fakra | 6 | CNSS+Ass | 1750-2250 |
| E10 | Femme | Chrétien | 30 | U | Hrajel | 4 | CNSS | >2250 |
| E11 | Homme | Chrétien | 28 | S | Hrajel | 4 | S.C | 1750-2250 |
| E12 | Femme | Chrétien | 48 | U | Ain El Rihani | 4 | Ass | >2250 |
| E13 | Femme | Chrétien | 39 | S | Shayle | 4 | CNSS | >2250 |
| E14 | Femme | Chrétien | 41 | C | Kfardebian | 5 | Ass | 1750-2250 |
| E15 | Femme | Chrétien | 55 | U | Ain El Rihani | 3 | S.C | 1750-2250 |
| E16 | Femme | Chrétien | 41 | U | Ain El Rihani | 6 | Ass | >2250 |
| E17 | Femme | Chrétien | 55 | P | Ain El Rihani | 3 | Ass | 675-1250 |
| E18 | Homme | Chrétien | 65 | P | Achkout | 5 | CNSS | 1750-2250 |
| E19 | Femme | Chrétien | 29 | U | Jeita | 4 | Ass | 1750-2250 |
| E20 | Homme | Chrétien | 55 | S | Adonis | 2 | S.C | 675-1250 |
| E21 | Femme | Musulman | 34 | C | Tayouneh | 6 | S.C | >2250 |
| E22 | Femme | Musulman | 42 | C | Tehwita | 6 | CNSS | 1750-2250 |
| E23 | Femme | Musulman | 33 | S | Tayouneh | 4 | S.C | 675-1250 |
| E24 | Femme | Musulman | 25 | U | Bourj Al Barjaneh | 2 | CNSS | 1250-1750 |
| E25 | Femme | Musulman | 42 | C | Bourj Al Barjaneh | 5 | S.C | 1250-1750 |
| E26 | Femme | Musulman | 28 | S | Chweifat | 4 | S.C | 675-1250 |
| E27 | Femme | Musulman | 25 | S | Chweifat | 5 | CNSS | 1250-1750 |
| N total = 27 | | | | | | | | |

P : Primaire
C : Complémentaire
S : Secondaire
U : Universitaire
S.C : Sans couverture
Ass : Assurance
SR : Sans revenu fixe

# Annexe 5

## Tableau n°2 : présentation des caractéristiques sociodémographiques des interviewés dans les hôpitaux privés

| Identité | Sexe | Religion | Age | Niveau d'éducation | Milieu de résidence | Taille du ménage | Couverture sociale | Revenu par 1000L.L/ Mois |
|---|---|---|---|---|---|---|---|---|
| E42 | Femme | Chrétien | 50 | C | Reyfoun | 1 | Ass | 1250-1750 |
| E43 | Homme | Chrétien | 49 | S | Reyfoun | 4 | CNSS | 1250-1750 |
| E44 | Homme | Chrétien | 38 | U | Feytroun | 2 | Ass | >2250 |
| E45 | Femme | Chrétien | 42 | U | Bouar | 4 | CNSS | 1750-2250 |
| E46 | Homme | Chrétien | 33 | U | Jeita | 2 | CNSS | >2250 |
| E47 | Homme | Chrétien | 22 | U | Ghazir | 4 | CNSS | 1750-2250 |
| E48 | Homme | Chrétien | 51 | U | Dhour chweir | 3 | Ass | >2250 |
| E49 | Homme | Chrétien | 63 | U | Dbayeh | 3 | Ass | >2250 |
| E50 | Homme | Chrétien | 68 | P | Zouk Mikael | 2 | CNSS | 675-1250 |
| E51 | Homme | Chrétien | 59 | U | Beit mery | 4 | Ass | >2250 |
| E52 | Homme | Chrétien | 36 | U | Bikfaya | 3 | CNSS+Ass | >2250 |
| E53 | Femme | Chrétien | 48 | U | Baouchrieh | 2 | Ass | >2250 |
| N total = 12 | | | | | | | | |

P : Primaire
C : Complémentaire
S : Secondaire
U : Universitaire
S.C : Sans couverture
Ass : Assurance
SR : Sans revenu fixe

# Annexe 5

## Tableau n°2 : présentation des caractéristiques sociodémographiques des interviewés dans les hôpitaux publics

| Identité | Sexe | Religion | Age | Niveau d'éducation | Milieu de résidence | Taille du ménage | Couverture sociale | Revenu par 1000L.L./ Mois |
|---|---|---|---|---|---|---|---|---|
| E28 | Homme | Musulman | 44 | P | Bourj Hamoud | 1 | S.C | 675-1250 |
| E29 | Femme | Musulman | 53 | P | Ain El Remaneh | 3 | S.C | <675 |
| E30 | Femme | Chrétien | 22 | U | Bourj Hamoud | 4 | CNSS | 1250-1750 |
| E31 | Homme | Chrétien | 55 | P | Hsarat- Jbeil | 2 | S.C | <675 |
| E32 | Femme | Chrétien | 62 | C | Okeibeh | 2 | S.C | <675 |
| E33 | Homme | Chrétien | 81 | P | Haddath | 2 | S.C | 675-1250 |
| E34 | Femme | Chrétien | 86 | P | Bejje | 1 | CNSS | 675-1250 |
| E35 | Homme | Chrétien | 77 | C | Mayrouba | 3 | S.C | 1250-1750 |
| E36 | Femme | Chrétien | 87 | P | Nahr Ibrahim | 1 | S.C | <675 |
| E37 | Homme | Chrétien | 66 | C | Yahchouch | 5 | S.C | 1750-2250 |
| E38 | Femme | Chrétien | 60 | C | Sarba | 1 | S.C | SR |
| E39 | Homme | Musulman | 74 | U | Kfour | 1 | S.C | SR |
| E40 | Homme | Chrétien | 60 | P | Sarba | 1 | S.C | 675-1250 |
| E41 | Homme | Chrétien | 62 | C | Batroun | 1 | S.C | 675-1250 |
| N total = 14 | | | | | | | | |

P : Primaire
C : Complémentaire
S : Secondaire
U : Universitaire
S.C : Sans couverture
Ass : Assurance
SR : Sans revenu fixe

# Annexe 7
# Lettre et accord de la CNSS

**FSP**
UNIVERSITE LIBANAISE
FACULTE DE SANTE PUBLIQUE
Section II

١٢٥٦
٥ ايار ٢٠١٥

الى جانب مدير صندوق الضمان الاجتماعي في جونيه

الدكتور جان بيار بطرس الجزيل الاحترام،

المستدعية : د. كريستيان صليبا ، استاذة في الجامعة اللبنانية

تحية وبعد،

في اطار مشروع بحث اكاديمي اقوم به في الجامعة اللبنانية بعنوان Recours aux soins et couverture médicale ندرس من خلاله الشروط و الحالات التي تحيط طلب المعالجة والعناية الطبية من قبل المواطنين، نتقدم من ادارتكم ومن خلال هذا الكتاب بطلب لدرس ملفات العناية الصحية في الضمان الاجتماعي لمتطلبات هذه الدراسة.

ونود بالتذكير بان غاية هذا التحليل هي اكاديمية فقط، والدراسة تلتزم بالسرية اللازمة وعدم التسمية و تضمن احترام الشروط المرعية في اطار العمل في الصندوق

نرجو من ادارتكم الموافقة على دراسة 70 الى 100 ملف بحسب متطلبات البحث و المستلزمات العلمية له.

ولكم مني فائق الاحترام

حرر في 22 نيسان 2015

# Annexe 8
# Questionnaire CNSS

Date :

N° Bénéficiaire : Code :

1 - Type de travail :

2 - Période totale de couverture à la CNSS :

3 - Caractéristiques sociodémographiques et couverture

| 3.1. Ménage | 3.2. Sexe | 3.3. Date de naissance | 3.4. couverture | 3.5. Raison | 3.6. Durée de couverture des parents à charge | |
|---|---|---|---|---|---|---|
| Ayant Droit (B) | | | | | | |
| Epoux/se B (EB) | | | | | | |
| Enfant 1 (E1) | | | | | | |
| Enfant 2 (E2) | | | | | | |
| Enfant 3(E3) | | | | | | |
| Enfant 4 (E4) | | | | | | |
| Enfant 5(E5) | | | | | | |
| Parent 1 | | | | | | |
| Parent 2 | | | | | | |
| | | | | | | |
| | | | | | | |

**4 - Nombre total de demandes cumulées de remboursement de recours aux soins entre 2012 et 2015 :**

**5 - Détails des recours par demande de remboursement déposée (DRD) :**

| 5.1. Bénéficiaire des soins | **5.2. Date des soins** | 5.3 C | 5.4 $C^2$ | 5.5 CS | 5.6 $CS^2$ | 5.7 Médocs **F4** | 5.8 Labo **F3** | 5.9 Rayons **F2** | 5.10 IRM Scan et préalable F1 | 5.11 Prix réel C payé | 5.12 Tarif CNSS pour Consults | 5.13 Total factures médocs et autre que Consults | 5.14 Total payé tarif CNSS **autre que Consultations** | 5.15 Remb CNSS 80% | 5.16 Spécialisation médecin |
|---|---|---|---|---|---|---|---|---|---|---|---|---|---|---|---|
| | | | | | | | | | | | | | | | |
| | | | | | | | | | | | | | | | |
| | | | | | | | | | | | | | | | |
| | | | | | | | | | | | | | | | |
| | | | | | | | | | | | | | | | |
| | | | | | | | | | | | | | | | |
| | | | | | | | | | | | | | | | |
| | | | | | | | | | | | | | | | |
| | | | | | | | | | | | | | | | |
| | | | | | | | | | | | | | | | |
| | | | | | | | | | | | | | | | |
| | | | | | | | | | | | | | | | |
| | | | | | | | | | | | | | | | |
| | | | | | | | | | | | | | | | |
| | | | | | | | | | | | | | | | |
| | | | | | | | | | | | | | | | |
| | | | | | | | | | | | | | | | |
| | | | | | | | | | | | | | | | |
| | | | | | | | | | | | | | | | |

**6 - Accord Hospitalisation : oui non Indications :**

# Table des matières